THE PATIENT AS
VICTIM AND VECTOR

THE PATIENT AS VICTIM AND VECTOR

Ethics and Infectious Disease

With a new Preface

Margaret P. Battin
Leslie P. Francis
Jay A. Jacobson
Charles B. Smith

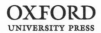

OXFORD
UNIVERSITY PRESS

OXFORD
UNIVERSITY PRESS

Oxford University Press, Inc., publishes works that further
Oxford University's objective of excellence
in research, scholarship, and education.

Oxford   New York
Auckland   Cape Town   Dar es Salaam   Hong Kong   Karachi
Kuala Lumpur   Madrid   Melbourne   Mexico City   Nairobi
New Delhi   Shanghai   Taipei   Toronto

With offices in
Argentina   Austria   Brazil   Chile   Czech Republic   France   Greece
Guatemala   Hungary   Italy   Japan Poland   Portugal   Singapore
South Korea   Switzerland   Thailand   Turkey   Ukraine   Vietnam

Published by Oxford University Press, Inc.
198 Madison Avenue, New York, New York 10016

www.oup.com

Oxford is a registered trademark of Oxford University Press

Library of Congress Control Number: 2020949057

ISBN 978-0-19-756454-7(pbk.)

Printed by Marquis, Canada

CONTENTS

PREFACE TO THE 2021 EDITION: VICTIMS, VECTORS, AND THE COVID-19 PANDEMIC

COVID-19, the disease caused by the novel coronavirus SARS-CoV-2, is new, but the ethical issues it raises aren't novel at all. This book, *The Patient as Victim and Vector*, explores questions that arise in all of the many, often ineffective ways human beings have tried to protect themselves from contagious infectious disease. Throughout the past, we've used quarantine, isolation, cordon sanitaire, forced treatment, social distancing, crude and more sophisticated forms of testing, surveillance, and contact tracing. These practices raise hard ethical issues: self-protection and privacy, individual choice and harms to others, the risks and potential gains of untested forms of treatment, the role of government and the scope of individual rights, justice in the allocation of scarce medical resources, obligations of providers to treat even when there are risks to themselves, and our responses to the dying. And they show us tragedies of too many patients facing inadequate resources, reveal living and working situations where too many are inadequately protected from disease spread, and lay bare structural injustice and deep fissures in the social fabric.

This book's novel theoretical perspective—that we are all victims *and* vectors to one another—was developed over a decade ago. With this perspective, we sought to analyze how bioethics had emerged without real attention to the challenges of infectious disease, but our more important goal was to develop a new way of seeing ethics in healthcare through the lens of infectious disease. This lens, which we call the *patient-as-victim-and-vector* perspective—PVV for short—is all too relevant today.

Ethics and Infectious Disease at the Outset of the Twenty-First Century

The original Preface to this volume opens with a class of undergraduates, taught by three of the four authors—a bioethicist and two infectious disease physicians—hearing distant reports early in 2003 about a mysterious respiratory illness, originating in Hong Kong, spreading in China, and leaping to Toronto, where it killed 44 people. Uncertainty and fear were in the air. That disease was SARS, for "severe acute respiratory syndrome," a coronavirus illness of high lethality but apparently less contagious than its newer cousin, COVID-19. SARS terrorized the world for several months while it infected some 8,000 people and killed 774, but it was contained relatively quickly.

By contrast, COVID-19 has become a global pandemic, and as of this writing, is still spreading rapidly around the world. We do not know whether it will ever be fully contained, continue in secondary waves, or subside into an endemic disease like influenza, always with us in virtually every corner of the globe. The fear of a lethal SARS pandemic gripped the world only briefly, as the transmission of that earlier coronavirus was interrupted and controlled. Yet after a spate of planning in response to SARS and then fears of avian influenza, many societies let preparedness lapse. Funding for public health has steadily eroded, too. What COVID-19 shows us is that those fears of SARS nearly 20 years ago were not unrealistic after all—it's just that the disease more to be feared hadn't yet come along. We are facing it now.

COVID-19 confronts us directly with some of the characteristics of person-to-person contagious infectious disease that raise special ethical issues. We give communicable diseases to each other, sometimes without ever knowing whom we have infected, when, or how. Infectious disease can strike slowly, like leprosy or tuberculosis, or strike quickly like bubonic plague. Formerly healthy people can become deathly ill or die in a matter of hours. Communicable infectious diseases, including those that have nonhuman intermediate vectors, seem to strike from outside, like invading enemies. Rates of recovery, incomplete recovery, and death vary widely among infectious diseases. Some kill only a few of those they infect; others, like the Spanish flu of 1918–1919, kill vast numbers. We may try to depend on herd immunity—the percentage of the population needed to be immune to a disease, either through prior infection or through vaccination—in order to prevent disease spread. However, with a novel infection there is no herd immunity at the start; that's part of why a disease like COVID-19 spreads so inexorably. When mortality is high, the disease is unfamiliar, or the disease strikes both the well and the already-frail with impunity, fear may become overwhelming.

Pandemics that spread quickly and extensively are especially frightening. If large numbers of the population are naïve to the infection, virtually everyone is at risk. We have seen the effects of contagious infectious disease on naïve populations in the past: bubonic plague killed an estimated 60% of the population of Europe in the 14th century, and smallpox, brought by Europeans as early as the 16th century and continuing through the 19th, wiped out much of the entire indigenous population of the New World. With a novel agent like SARS-CoV-2, the virus that causes COVID-19, the entire globe lacks prior immunity. We may not know how the infection is spread, how deadly it is, or whether or how it can be treated. We may not know how the infection is spread, how deadly it is, or whether or how it can be treated.

When an infection is novel, we may also not know for many years what the consequences are of having been infected. How long does it take to recover? Do some people never recover fully? Will some experience lifelong consequences, like the increasing muscle weakness from polio, or recurrences in a different form, like shingles in older age from chicken pox infection as a child? Will initially disturbing findings about persistent difficulty in breathing or cardiac inflammation persist? We don't know now, but we will eventually find out, to our relief—or to our sorrow.

Published in 2009, this book has been recognized as the first authored book on the general topic of ethical issues associated with infectious disease. There's a reason for its appearance then. As a collaboration between a bioethicist, a bioethicist/lawyer, and two infectious disease specialist physicians, we recognized in reflecting on that 2003 outbreak of SARS how little attention the bioethics literature paid to the ethical issues raised by transmissible infectious disease. Indeed, as Part I of this volume argues, issues of infectious disease had been largely "left out" of concern in bioethics. The U.S. Surgeon General is famously reported—apparently incorrectly—to have said, sometime between 1969 and 1972, that it was "time to close the book on infectious disease." This time period was just when bioethics was coalescing as a field, and just before HIV/AIDS took epidemic form. The supposed remark seemed realistic at the time. The belief was widespread that infectious disease was a thing of the past, controlled by public sanitation, effective treatment, and vaccines.

Moderate or even severe outbreaks threatened this complacency, however. Almost immediately there was HIV/AIDS. There were outbreaks of avian flu, H1N1 swine flu, Middle Eastern respiratory syndrome or MERS, Ebola, Zika, and others, many involving viruses that had jumped from animals to humans as a consequence of cultural practices and human impact on the environment. Nonetheless, through most of these outbreaks it had been easy to assume that effective treatment would eventually be found and/or a vaccine developed. To us, on the other hand, still aware of HIV and in the wake of SARS, it seemed important to resist this complacency by developing a general account of how best to think about contagious disease overall—not only about past outbreaks, but also about current and especially future ones.

Now, as the COVID-19 pandemic spreads around the globe, bioethics and all areas of healthcare and political and social policy are consumed with attention to it. We must reflect on how efforts to control disease transmission can place enormous social and economic burdens on traditionally vulnerable and underserved populations. At the same time, as we attend to these issues posed by COVID-19, what is sometimes missing is the resonance of the long history of human affliction by varied forms of infectious disease and the ethically trenchant lessons that responses to earlier outbreaks can have for us today.

The PVV Perspective

In this volume, we develop a picture of the human being as a "way-station self," both a "breeding ground" for infectious agents and a "launching pad" to other people. As human beings, we are caught in a "web of disease," whether to a lesser or greater extent. Our way-station selves are mutually at risk from one another. Each of us is potentially *both* victim *and* vector, at one and the same time. A morally acceptable policy, program, or practice must take both these aspects of human existence into account.

As victims, we become ill, suffer, and possibly die. We need treatment, comfort, symptom management, and end–of-life care. We lose jobs, income, security, and loved ones. We may become "long haulers" slow to recover or permanently disabled: one of the most frightening aspects of COVID-19 is that we do not know the extent to which people will fully recover or experience damage that may be lifelong.

As vectors, we are the source of disease to others. With COVID-19's very high rate of asymptomatic infection, we may be vectors without ever knowing that we have harbored the virus. We are under surveillance for our potential contacts, tested for disease when testing is available, and examined for symptoms. If we are suspected of having been exposed, we may be quarantined, sometimes where we cannot protect ourselves from increased risks of infection. If we stay home from work, we lose pay or possibly even our jobs. When we get sick, we are likely to be isolated and alone. Even if we have tried to stay safe, we may feel guilty or be blamed or shamed for passing disease on to family, friends, or unknown others. Supposed "superspreaders" or hosts of "superspreading" events may be blamed or shamed, even if they lacked full awareness of the risks of spread.

But there is more. As victims and vectors, we are mutually vulnerable. In the phrase that has become ubiquitous in the COVID-19 pandemic, "We're all in this together." No one of us can be sure that we won't become victims, and no one of us can be sure that we won't be vectors, either. We live in uncertainty about whom disease will strike next and who will be the source of disease. COVID-19 is especially sneaky since people can be vectors without ever having been symptomatic, and whole communities can become victims practically overnight. The Italian town Bergamo's joy at its soccer team Atalanta's victory over Valencia in the European Champions League, February 19, 2020, when some 40,000 fans traveled the 35 miles to Milan, turned into what a respected doctor called a "biological bomb," spreading the pandemic in northern Italy. The month-long Mardi Gras street party celebrations in late February 2020 brought death to New Orleans. And countless funerals and weddings have introduced disease into unprepared and unsuspecting communities.

At the same time, we are not equal in our susceptibility, our knowledge about our risks, or our ability to protect ourselves. For COVID-19, we do know that if we are elderly, immune compromised, or have other underlying illnesses, we are disproportionately likely to become sick or die of COVID-19. We know that if we have jobs that allow us to telecommute, live in areas with plenty of outdoor space, or can pay for delivery of food and supplies, we can self-protect. We know that some jobs place us at far greater risk, such as working in a meatpacking plant, driving a bus, or working in a nursing home. We know that if we are confined to congregate settings such as nursing homes, prisons, immigrant detention centers, or refugee camps, we are at high risk of becoming ill once infection is introduced into that environment. And COVID-19 is taking a disproportionate toll on communities of color, although we don't fully know whether the explanation lies in social determinants of health, inadequate access to healthcare, biological differences, overt or covert racism, or some combination of all of these.

This is the ethical framework of PVV, the *patient-as-victim-and-vector* view, from which we must approach pandemic contagious disease. We are waystations of disease, all potential victims and vectors to one another. We're in a state of uncertainty about our actual situation as victim and vector at any given time—that is our common lot. But we're also in a state of partial knowledge and privilege that can pull us apart unless we remember that each of us may become both victim and vector, too.

Infectious Disease Now: PVV and COVID-19

Many of the ethical issues that we discuss in this volume remain in full force today. But much has changed, too, in the intervening decade since this book was first published. Science has advanced, particularly our capacities to test people, track contacts, and model the spread of disease. Research in the development of vaccines and effective treatments is far more sophisticated than a decade ago. Social media and smartphones are widely used across the globe, allowing rapid sharing of not only information but also misinformation. Conflict has increasingly arisen between political agendas and scientific and public health concerns. And, at least in some countries, especially the United States, political polarization and inequality have continued to widen as the pandemic has spread.

Issues familiar in past outbreaks arise again with new visibility in the COVID-19 pandemic, thanks partly to media exposure. When diseases are highly contagious, isolating the ill seems imperative, but this means some people will die alone, without the comfort of family, the support of friends and coworkers, the solace of a religious advisor, or even the chance to say good-bye. In Chapter 9, for example, we argue that isolation of the gravely ill must ethically be accompanied by recognition of the reality of their victimhood, using imaginative methods of comfort, like bringing a dying man's dog to his bedside; today, forms of video contact may partly substitute for this loss.

Fast-moving illnesses may overwhelm available resources for treatment. Ethical triage, as we discuss in Chapter 19, must take into account each individual as a victim. To avoid discrimination on the basis of disability or age, patients must be assessed individually rather than as members of a category in order to assess their need for and likelihood of benefitting from treatment. Pandemic plans must be developed through processes that are transparent and fair. Ethics also must also not ignore other forms of victimhood—including people who need treatment for diseases other than COVID-19, like heart disease or cancer or other conditions that can prove fatal.

As another example, we owe healthcare workers and other essential workers adequate protective equipment so they will not become victims—or vectors—themselves. If essential workers do become victims, reciprocity may require ensuring them access to treatment or compensation for harm. Reciprocity also requires considering who is essential and how we can reduce risks. Chapter 18 considers some of these issues, including compensation when harm has occurred.

Testing, contact tracing, and vaccination may place individual rights to choose at apparent odds with the public good. Testing and the confidentiality of test results were issues at the forefront of the HIV/AIDS pandemic; they are issues for COVID-19 too, although its mechanisms of transmission are not associated with behaviors that have otherwise been stigmatized. Anti-vaccination movements have grown over the last decade; suspicion about COVID-19 vaccines are already beginning to emerge, especially concerns about the safety of a vaccines that have been rapidly developed. As we confront these apparent tensions, we must remember that we are at once victims and vectors, all in this together, and that vaccines affect us in both those roles.

In attempts to control the spread of COVID-19, quarantine, isolation, cordon sanitaire, shelter in place, home-based lockdown, contact tracing, mandatory masking, and social distancing are all being used. Isolation must be draconian to be effective; if so, it will predictably exacerbate loneliness and psychological distress. Quarantine may be unjust if it herds the well but exposed together with the sick. Cordon sanitaire must cut everything off from the geographical area being encircled and only works if the disease has not already escaped or spread widely within a larger geographical area. Shelter in place, contact tracing that results in quarantine recommendations for possible contacts, and social distancing are potentially economically devastating to those who cannot work; to children who lose out on adequate instruction, nutrition provided by school lunches, and socialization; and to businesses that must close. Questions of justice that we discuss in this volume come to the fore: What costs are we willing to bear to stop pandemic spread? How should these costs be distributed? And what should be our response if, as we are increasingly becoming aware, these costs are not at all borne equally?

Much has changed also since we began this book. Central to our interest in re-releasing this book is to stimulate thinking about how technical and other advances affect the ethical issues. We can act more quickly: It took 5 months to sequence the SARS virus in 2003; for the novel coronavirus emerging in Wuhan, it took less than a month. Our capacities to rapid test for current and prior infection have greatly increased. Dizzying amounts of further research are underway, with pharmacology groups sifting through a huge range of possibly effective drugs and at one point well over 100 labs around the globe vying for the prize of developing a safe and effective vaccine. People are eagerly signing up as subjects in research to test possible vaccines for safety and efficacy, despite the possible risks.

But there is cause for concern as well. There is still so much we don't know and so much we are trying out. Publication practices have changed, with electronic methods bringing much that has been written into wide circulation before full peer review, raising questions about trade-offs between accuracy and speed. In the United States, potentially promising treatments for COVID-19 are given quick authorization for emergency use despite unknown risks. Only recently have we come to understand, based on real-time and retrospective studies in Wuhan, how community spread took place even before the novel virus was recognized. If we don't yet know how to test for the earliest phase of asymptomatic or presymptomatic infection when there is not yet enough viral replication to be detectable and hence cannot tell whether someone who has been exposed is indeed infected, we have to recommend quarantine even for exposed, test-negative individuals. And, of course, our models of disease spread, with peaks and recurrences, are based on still-limited information, both about other pandemics and about this one.

Social media and smartphones are another major technological change since we wrote this book. The first tweets were sent in 2006, and the first iPhone was marketed in 2007; the term *Web 2.0* for the interactive web was introduced in 2004, and Google searches were first personalized in 2005. These technologies allow information—and misinformation—to travel instantly, exponentially, and globally. They also allow for new forms of surveillance. Artificial intelligence identifying unexpected patterns in immense data sets enables syndromic surveillance for outbreak detection. Smartphones can be used to track movements and contacts; methods for encrypting data and relying on data storage on individual devices rather than central repositories can protect privacy but with potentially less efficacy for contact tracing. Social media not only can be used to educate people about disease risks and prevention, but also can directly target them as victims. Some countries, notably South Korea and Taiwan, made initially effective use of these technologies: There, the pandemic was virtually contained and almost averted where protective equipment had been stockpiled and well-known infection control measures had been augmented by new technologies, including contact tracing and proximity detection by smartphone. Nevertheless, after relaxation and reopening, new spikes occurred.

However, perhaps most disturbingly, especially in the United States, political polarization and inequality have continued to grow since we began this book. Both make pandemics more difficult to address. Political polarization has undercut support for public health and magnified mistrust in government; ordinary citizens from mask-wearers to public health officials have become the targets of protests and threats. Tensions between the demands of careful science and feelings of loss of freedom, exacerbated by directives to stay at home, wear masks, keep schools and churches closed, prohibit large public gatherings, and not assemble in groups of more than a handful of people, have escalated. A small but significant percentage of the US population reportedly believes that COVID-19 is a hoax. Many others believe that it is a problem for urban areas but not for where they live. Early signs of social solidarity in controlling the pandemic have rapidly disintegrated, at least in the United States, and data are mounting about the unequal effects of the pandemic, especially on people of color, people who have lost jobs or livelihoods, and people who must work in settings where they are put at disproportionate risk.

Infectious disease and public health communities have traditionally warned vigorously about the risks of new respiratory viral infections and specifically about avian influenza or another animal-to-human spread, and the Centers for Disease Control and Prevention and the infectious disease community have been concerned about emerging pathogens for decades. Nevertheless, to the dismay of many experts, the US Global Health Security and Biodefense unit, responsible for pandemic preparedness, has been merged into other offices; China has been blamed for the pandemic although it may turn out to have been more successful in controlling the disease within its own borders than many Western countries have, and the prospect of U.S. withdrawal from the World Health Organization became highly controversial, potentially undermining that organization's ability to gather global information about outbreaks, encourage international cooperation, help with research and treatment, and enforce the World Health Regulations.

Yet there is reason for optimism. Perhaps most importantly, new testing methods could allow us to avoid many of the inequities and injustices of the traditional methods of pandemic control if we can get them deployed quickly enough. For example, what was sheer science fiction at the time of the original edition of this book, posed as a thought experiment about rapid testing in airports and other places of public contact in Chapter 15, may be coming closer to reality. In an airlines industry first, April 15, 2020, Emirates pioneered on-site rapid testing of passengers for its Dubai-to-Tunisia flight; testing was conducted by the Dubai Health Authority in the group check-in waiting area for the flight, using a quick blood test that yielded results within 10 minutes. Some months later, in September 2020, Helsinki airport was reported to be testing sniffer dogs trained to detect COVID-19 in passengers on arrival, using a sweat sample obtained by wiping their necks—the dogs can detect an infected person in 10 seconds, even if asymptomatic, and earlier than a polymerase chain reaction test, known as PCR. Sniffer dogs trained in Germany were reported to detect COVID-infected people using saliva samples with 94% accuracy, it was claimed. Were such testing, high tech or low tech, fully effective and universally used—it is neither one today, but is certainly much improved—it could prevent disease transmission as people fly from one location to another, -even, we can imagine, the intercontinental transmission of COVID-19 from Asia to the New World or the other way around.

That may be still partly fantasy, but even in the real world of today, if we could rapid test for infection, including asymptomatic and presymptomatic infection, with adequate sensitivity and specificity, we wouldn't need to isolate people unless it were clear that they actually have the virus. We could reduce the need for social distancing, especially global social distancing that shuts down entire industries and wreaks economic havoc. A contemporary cordon sanitaire could be permeable, allowing people who test negative on the most sensitive and specific tests to come and go through the barrier. Quarantine that confines people who are not ill with those who are, thus incubating further spread, would be obsolete; only true positives, whether on a cruise ship or in a nursing home, would be required to isolate. And sheltering in place wouldn't be necessary either, unless, as in the current COVID-19 pandemic, the disease had already moved far beyond our capacity to contain it. That's part of the irony involved in reissuing this volume: We've already seen that many of these traditional tactics pose ethical challenges, and we now have the scientific and technological potential to decrease our reliance on them. Unfortunately, we've done far less than we could have done and are suffering as a result.

As we reflect on early days of the COVID-19 pandemic, we hope that our PVV tool, insisting that we always see the patient as *victim AND vector*, can shed light on some of the ethical questions we are now facing. PVV, we think, gives us a way to see what's "half-right" in the way we are dealing with the current coronavirus pandemic and what skews the balance too far to one side or the other. It can help us to recognize that we are at risk from one another and that even as we try to protect ourselves from these risks we must also respond to one another as victims of the diseases we transmit to them. Fairness requires no less—as does our success in ultimately addressing the pandemic together. The PVV perspective is just as useful in this outbreak as in the previous ones, and, we believe, it will also be useful for the virus next time. After all, COVID-19 is neither the last nor the worst pandemic we can expect.

It is much too soon to know the long-term outlook for the current pandemic: Is this another pestilence we can control or one that will become endemic, a permanent part of our environment, one with ongoing infection and always risking substantial rates of death? As of this writing—almost a year after the initial cases of a novel coronavirus were recognized—there still was no fully effective treatment, but with multiple candidates from labs around the world, we are seeing some promise of safe and effective vaccines. Yet attention to the ethical issues in COVID-19 isn't just a matter of the next several months, but perhaps of the next 5 years—or 10, or 20. If COVID-19 finally comes under control, attention to the ethical issues it raises is still immensely important in order to brace ourselves for the next outbreak to come along—and the one after that, and the one after that. The metaphor of COVID-19 as an "enemy" with which we're at war is sometimes used, but the problem with contagious disease is far greater: It's an enemy with a boundless supply of fresh troops and remarkably clever new tactics for invasion.

Thus this is, ironically, the perfect moment to reissue this volume, while the threat of a new pandemic disease remains real and feared and before any full solution has been found—that is, before COVID-19 has been eclipsed, if this is ever to be the case, by effective treatment and vaccines and thus fades into past history. We can so easily forget. But COVID-19 is neither the last nor the worst outbreak the future may bring. This volume's basic lessons can perhaps help equip us to think carefully about the ethics of the policies we construct and the choices we make, not only for the virus this time but for the virus next time as well. This volume looks in detail at tuberculosis, HIV/AIDS, human papilloma virus or HPV, and many other communicable infectious diseases. We bring it forward again in the conviction that its analysis of ethical issues prior to COVID-19 will illuminate how to think about the current pandemic as well. COVID-19 is, after all, just another in the very long human history of vulnerability to infectious disease. What we have learned in facing epidemics of the past can help us now.

In the spring semester 2003, not long after we began to write this book, three of us taught an undergraduate honors seminar designed to explore ethics issues in infectious disease. It was January when the course began, and we found a group of eager, well-prepared, advanced honors students, many of whom expected to enter medical school. We covered the basics of ethical theory and the microbiology of infectious disease. We read famous cases in the annals of public health. We discussed dilemmas of medical management and the obligations of the physician, especially in times of plague. But we also found ourselves mentioning a few reports coming from the Centers for Disease Control and Prevention—this was in early January 2003—of a couple of cases of a previously unrecognized syndrome, trickling in from China.

We did not pay much attention to it in the first week or two of class, while we were learning the basic science of infectious disease, how various viruses function, and by what mechanisms human-to-human and animal-to-human transmission occurs. We had read about classic problems like the plague in Greece at the time of Thucydides and in medieval Europe, but those were problems of the past whose only contemporary analogue was AIDS. But those new cases kept trickling in—there were a handful of cases when the class met one week, and a few dozens of cases when it met a week later, and cases in the hundreds when it met the week after that. At the beginning, although the new condition had been given a name, Severe Acute Respiratory Syndrome or SARS, nobody knew how to stop it or treat it. It was spreading, and often with fatal outcome.

Many of the members of the class were pre-med students. As the number of SARS cases grew, it was becoming clear that this devastating disease affected health-care workers with unusual frequency. Now the class was becoming more than academic, and much more serious: "do physicians have an obligation to treat patients with potentially lethal infectious diseases?" we wondered. Some argued yes, appealing to codes of ethics from the AMA and elsewhere; some argued no, reminding us that the risk to themselves might also be a risk to their spouses and their children.

Meanwhile, the strength of the SARS epidemic was increasing, with new cases reported not just in China but next door, in Toronto, on this continent, just a short plane ride away. We still did not know how far it would go or how to stop it. What precautions ought a society take against a disease whose causes and mechanism are still poorly understood? Now the class debated the ethics of universal involuntary quarantine for anyone exposed, state-required immunization if a vaccine were ever to be developed, and issues of distributive justice about who should get first access to treatment and how health-care resources should be prioritized. We were all scared, students and teachers alike, because we understood all too fully what could be at stake and how deeply troubling the moral issues it raised were.

As the seminar continued, we all felt the sense of vulnerability that we would later come to associate with what we call "embeddedness" in a "web" of infectious disease —that sense of threat, an unknown peril, a potential disaster, from a new and not-yet-understood disease breaking out among humankind. And we began to think more seriously about the ethical issues in infectious disease, not merely as an academic exercise in an honors class but as a deeply disturbing human issue.

Fortunately, SARS was contained shortly afterward, at least as far as we currently know. Just the same, none of us, we think, will forget this class: this was physicians and prospective physicians and ethicists working together in real life, in real time, to try to address issues of compelling personal and social concern. This book is in part the fruit of these reflections.

The Plan of the Volume

The book is divided into five parts. Part I, Chapters 1–5, sets the background: what are (some of) the ethical problems associated with infectious disease, what needs to be understood about the microorganisms that cause infectious disease, and what is distinctive about infectious disease—its characteristic acuity, treatability, potential lethality, and association with social circumstances like disruption and poverty. This section also explores—and documents—the fact that infectious disease got "left out" of early bioethics, reflected both in the kinds of cases it discussed and in its institutional separation from public health. Public health, for its own part, also missed some of the central ethical issues in infectious disease, concerned as it became with other matters—asbestos exposure, tobacco use, and obesity, for example—that are not biologically communicable in the way that infectious disease is. Thus this first section both sets the stage and shows why the stage is furnished the way it is—or, rather, barely furnished at all. It shows why there is little if any adequate reflection about ethical issues in infectious disease: these questions were virtually never addressed by those who might have been able to do so.

In Part II, Chapters 6 and 7, we develop the theoretical position we call the *patient as victim and vector* view, or *PVV* for short, that is central to this book.

We begin this section with an account of the patient—the person—as physically embedded in a web of disease, a "way-station self" who is breeding-ground and launching-pad for some trillions of microorganisms, many of which are benign or crucial to human functioning but some of which are dangerous or lethal, the germs that cause disease. The central ethical issues, as we develop them in the further chapters of the book, have to do with our efforts to respond to its damage and to try to extricate ourselves from this web of disease. The seven chapters of Part III, 8–14, explore attempts to deal with or control infectious disease in a variety of real-world contexts: isolation of those exposed and of those who are dying, human experimentation, mandatory testing and reporting, blocking of maternal/fetal transmission, conflicts of interest in the development of antimicrobial resistance, and required immunization. These are all real-world situations that look different under the lens of the PVV view.

Part IV, Chapters 15–19, focuses more directly on constraints. Chapter 15 proposes a thought-experiment about universal surveillance (beginning with airports!) in order to explore the limits of acceptable constraints. Chapter 16 examines general considerations in the justification of constraints, developing a set of procedural and substantive guidelines for their use, and Chapter 17 employs these guidelines to examine certain proposed constraints for the control of a possible avian influenza pandemic. Chapter 18 develops an argument that compensation is required for some cases of harm due to pandemic constraints. Chapter 19 explores justice within pandemic planning, bringing our PVV perspective to bear on decisions about prioritization of pandemic influenza prevention and treatment. But the issues of justice raised by pandemic planning are not only about prioritization *within* plans; they are also about the justice *of* pandemic planning itself. Pandemic planning, we contend, is but one example of how our PVV perspective can be used to develop an important line of argument for global concern with health security worldwide.

To conclude the book, Chapters 20 and 21 in Part V both examine the present and push into the future. Chapter 20 "thinks big," observing the importance of infectious disease in the current momentum for improving global health (the most visible global effort at the moment is to reduce the enormous burden of disease from HIV/AIDS, tuberculosis, and malaria, but attempts to eliminate or control many other infectious diseases are under way as well), and asking what might be involved in a global effort to eradicate, eliminate, or control infectious disease. As we point out, this is not just a practical or scientific question, but a moral one. Viewing it from our PVV perspective, we see the effort to extricate human beings in general from the web of infectious disease as a continuing part of a *Comprehensive Global Effort* begun with Jenner, who vaccinated a boy against smallpox in 1796; the question is whether we can not only realistically but ethically pursue this effort further. In our optimistic moments we think the answer is yes; in our pessimistic ones, we are aware of the threats of newly emerging diseases, overwhelmed infrastructure, and the risks of biowarfare.

In the final Chapter 21, the many threads of the volume are brought together in two ways as we utilize our PVV view as a "tool." We first use the PVV view as a challenge to several forms of philosophical thought: our examples are principlist bioethics, the capabilities approach in social justice theory, and the underlying liberal theory that has informed western thinking since John Stuart Mill. Second, we use PVV as a tool for examining past, present, and projected public policy, observing whether a given policy overemphasizes vectorhood and underemphasizes victimhood or the other way around. Thus, the PVV view can display what is "lopsided" about disease-control policies in the historical past—for example, the isolation of lepers and suspected lepers on Molokai in the Hawaii of the late 1800s or the quarantine of Chinese for plague in San Francisco in 1900—but also important, what is half-right about them, even when their violations of basic ethics are so extreme.

Even in the most egregious of cases, we argue, there is something half-right as well as wrong; our PVV perspective lets us see what is otherwise often obscured from view. This does not excuse what was wrong, but allows us to understand the complexities of disease-control policies, as we have been seeing in many contexts in this volume. The PVV view can also show what makes policies ethically controversial, like Cuba's HIV-positive containment policy, and what makes it possible to say that policies are ethically as close to satisfactory as possible, like Canada's current exit policy for people with active, communicable tuberculosis who want to travel abroad. Thus PVV is a theoretical view, but it is also a practical, usable tool for continuing policy analysis.

On Joint Authorship

As always, with a jointly authored publication, it is very difficult to sort out independent contributions of the authors. This book is no exception, especially as it has grown over a considerable period of time. The original idea for a book about bioethics and infectious disease was hatched by Peggy Battin; she, Jay Jacobson, and Charles Smith developed the course on ethics and infectious disease, mentioned above, first taught in the honors program at the University of Utah in 2003—the year that SARS erupted. The philosophical theory that is the basis of the book was developed together by Leslie Francis and Peggy Battin, and the medical expertise and wisdom, as well as public-health experience, has been the contribution of Jacobson and Smith.

Together with Michael Selgelid, one of the earliest writers to insist that "the topic of infectious disease should be recognized as one of *the* most important topics for the discipline of bioethics,"[1] Battin and Smith co-edited a journal issue and a subsequent volume of papers, *Ethics and Infectious Disease*;[2] Francis and Jacobson were among the reviewers for these works, and we have all profited from the many excellent papers submitted to each of them. We have variously participated in many discussions, workshops, panels, and meetings, and been extensively influenced by others there. Among them have been the meetings of the American Philosophical Association (a panel on the global threat of infectious disease that included John Harris, David Fidler, Andrew Jameton, and Richard Miller); the American Society for Bioethics and Humanities; the Uehiro Center at Oxford University (thanks to Julian Savulescu and Matthew Liao, as well as many participants listed in chapter 20); a conference on law and bioethics at the University of London (organized by Michael Freeman); and the various meetings of the International Association of Bioethics in Australia, Brasilia, and in Beijing, including satellite meetings of InterPHEN—the International Public Health Ethics Network, organized by Angus Dawson and Marcel Verweij; the meetings of the European Society for Philosophy of Medicine and Health Care in Barcelona and in Cardiff, and a Florida pandemic planning project that included Robert Hood, Heidi Malm, Tom May, Saad Omer, and Daniel Salmon. Our project has thus been influenced by many colleagues interested in ethics issues related to infectious disease around the world, and we are grateful to them. We have presented various parts of this work in these and other venues, and we are grateful to many for the extensive discussion we have received.

For those who want to know who wrote which chapters of this book, we insist that we have all been involved in all of them. With respect to individual chapters, however, it is possible to identify distinctive emphases. Jacobson is lead author on Chapters 2 and 11. Smith is lead author on Chapters 3, 9, 12, and 14. Battin and Francis were lead authors on Chapters 1, 6, and 7. Battin is lead author on Chapters 15, 20, and 21. Francis is lead author on Chapters 4, 5, 8, 10, 13, and the series on constraints and pandemic planning, Chapters 16–19. Jacobson and Smith, both physicians who are infectious disease specialists, are the sources of the materials on biology, medicine, and public health, and they both draw on their extensive clinical experience both in the United States and at hospitals and AIDS clinics in Kenya. Battin, a bioethicist also trained as a fiction writer, is particularly responsible for the thought-experiment components of the volume, evident especially in Chapters 15 and 20.

---

1. Michael J. Selgelid, "Ethics and Infectious Disease," *Bioethics* 19, no. 3 (June, 2005): 272–289, p. 273.
2. Michael J. Selgelid, Margaret P. Battin, and Charles B. Smith, *Ethics and Infectious Disease*. Special issue of *Bioethics* 19, no. 4 (August 2005); expanded as a book (Oxford: Blackwell Publishing, 2006).

Francis, a professor of health law as well as philosophy, took the lead in the documentation of how infectious disease got left out of bioethics as well as the analyses of pandemic planning and other public policy issues. As is also inevitable with co-authored works, the authors do not always agree about everything—we think that will be reflected in many of our discussions, though we hope it results in a fruitful complexity. We have all worked jointly, however, on every chapter in the book—reading each line by line together, sometimes many times, and what we do agree about most earnestly is the importance of these issues of infectious disease and the need for ongoing dialogue.

Acknowledgments

We want to thank a number of people who have worked with us briefly or extensively on some or all of this book. Some are co-authors for earlier versions of parts of it (identified in the first footnote of the relevant chapter): Jeffrey Botkin, M.D., James O. Mason, M.D., Larry Reimer, M.D.; others are colleagues and associates: Jim Tabery, Donald Granger, M.D., Warren Pettey (working together with Amanda Pettey), and Linda Carr-Lee; others have reviewed specific chapters: Jaqueline Colby, Ph.D., Robert Rolfs, M.D., M.P.H., and Jennifer Van Horn, M.D.; still others are former students, including Emily Asplund, Gretchen Domek, and Alexandra Weill; and some are our research assistants or research contributors over the years, Sara Taub, Beverly Hawkins, Constance Orzechowski, Charity Williams, Ashley Chadwick, and Daniel Jarvis.

Support for this project has come from a variety of sources. Early work on the book was supported by a College of Humanities interdisciplinary seed grant at the University of Utah to Battin and Francis. Some of the public policy work was supported by a grant from the Florida Department of Health and the University of Florida to Francis. All along, research for the volume has been supported by the Division of Medical Ethics and Humanities at the University of Utah and LDS Hospital, of which Jacobson is chief and Francis and Battin are members. Finally, work on the volume has also been supported by our home departments and programs, through the Excellence in Research and Teaching fund at the University of Utah S.J. Quinney College of Law, the Honors College, and the Department of Philosophy. We are grateful to all who have been with us over time.

PART I: SEEING INFECTIOUS DISEASE AS CENTRAL

1

SEEING INFECTIOUS DISEASE AS CENTRAL

Only decades ago, infectious disease was thought to be on the verge of being vanquished. Developments in sanitation, immunization, and antibiotics, together with other public health and scientific milestones, were heralded as announcing the imminent end of infectious disease. Smallpox had been eliminated; polio was nearly conquered; and the U.S. Center for Disease Control, as it was then called,[1] had a plan for eliminating tuberculosis in the United States by 2010.[2] Diphtheria, tetanus, typhoid, yellow fever, and syphilis were largely controlled by immunization or treatment, and other once-feared infectious diseases were the subjects of promising research. The U.S. Surgeon General is famously reported to have said in a burst of optimism sometime between 1969 and 1972 that it was time to "close the book" on infectious diseases.[3] That this story is quite likely apocryphal, and that in any case he was probably primarily thinking of the developed country whose Surgeon General he was at the time, is barely relevant; the legend remains alive.

The Birth of Bioethics amid the Seeming Decline of Infectious Disease

The new field of bioethics, born in the 1950s and 1960s, was maturing in the 1970s and 1980s. Bioethics began with observations about the dilemmas physicians faced, such as whether to tell dying patients the truth, reveal confidential

---

1. The Center for Disease Control became the Centers for Disease Control in 1980, and became the Centers for Disease Control and Prevention in 1992. It is universally referred to as the CDC.
2. Ronald Bayer and Laurence Dupuis, "Tuberculosis, Public Health, and Civil Liberties," in *Ethics and Infectious Disease,* ed. Michael J. Selgelid, Margaret P. Battin, and Charles B. Smith. (Oxford: Blackwell, 2005), 120, citing the Centers for Disease Control and Prevention, "A Strategic Plan for the Elimination of Tuberculosis in the United States," *Morbidity and Mortality Weekly Report* 38, suppl. S-3 (1989): 1–23.
3. See, e.g., Roxanne Nelson, "Tougher Bugs, Few New Drugs: Dearth of New Antibiotics Threatens Public Health," *Washington Post,* March 31, 2004, http://www.washingtonpost.com/wp-dyn/articles/A34467-2004Mar29.html (accessed December 29, 2007). While this phrase is quoted in many places and the quotation is typically attributed to testimony before Congress, we have not been able to corroborate it with an original source. See further discussion in Chapter 4.

information, or limit patients' liberties for their own good. The early salient issues in bioethics ranged from those surrounding life-extending technologies in coma and terminal illness; to organ transplantation and dialysis; to reproductive failure, abnormal pregnancy and neonatal deficit; to experimentation with human subjects. The issues most discussed involved patients with congenital anomalies, brain injuries, disseminated cancers, renal failure, and heart disease. These conditions largely involve malformation, deterioration, or destruction of organ function or physical structures of individual patients. These early core issues and the clinical cases associated with them presented the challenges of newly developed life-extending technologies in already compromised persons. Problems of social justice also eventually received attention: access to health care, and discrimination based on race, age, or disability. However, during the formative period of bioethics, infectious disease played virtually no role. As concern with infectious disease seemed to be waning, interest in bioethics was growing apace; the two never really met, to the disadvantage of bioethics—or so we contend.

Bioethics began as case-based, but only a few of the cases that generated extensive discussion during the initial decades of the field involved infectious disease. These included the notorious Tuskegee study of deliberately untreated syphilis in black men, the Willowbrook research on institutionalized children infected with hepatitis, and occasional reference in end-of-life controversies to letting terminally ill patients succumb to pneumonia—"the old man's friend."[4] However, in each of these controversial cases that did involve communicable infectious disease, the discussions that consumed bioethics pointed largely away from the fact that the diseases involved could be transmitted from one person to another. Instead, matters of concern were the vulnerability of the study populations, coercion in institutional settings, civil rights, and racial discrimination and exploitation—not infectiousness per se. Perhaps the most notorious example is the outcry about the Tuskegee syphilis study, which largely ignored the syphilis study's potential impact on the sexual partners and children of the men in the study, at least until President Bill Clinton's apology in 1997.

Canonical accounts of principles in bioethics—such as Beauchamp and Childress's autonomy, nonmaleficence, beneficence, and justice[5]—were also not tested by infectious disease examples. Even Jonsen, Siegler, and Winslade's four-cell framework for clinical decision making—patient preference, quality

---

4. The original of this phrase was "friend of the aged." William Osler, *The Principles and Practice of Medicine: Designed for the Use of Practitioners and Students of Medicine,* 7th ed. (New York: Appleton, 1909), 165.

5. Tom L. Beauchamp and James F. Childress, *Principles of Biomedical Ethics,* all editions, 1978 to present (Oxford: Oxford University Press).

of life, medical indications, and other considerations[6]—focused attention less on transmissibility than on the situation of the individual patient, although it did include infectious disease case examples along with legal requirements under "other considerations."

Left aside in bioethics were problems that are particularly characteristic of infectious conditions: the importance of rapid diagnosis; the significance of acute onset; the risk of transmissibility to family, friends, caregivers, and even strangers; the function of surveillance; the role of screening, prevention, and immunization; the constraints of quarantine and isolation; and the effects of treatment of a given patient on the health of others. To be sure, these issues of infectiousness have been the traditional bastions of public health. Public health's areas of focus, however, were the causes of epidemics and the control measures invoked to try to protect populations, rather than the individual bedside dilemmas that were the early concern of bioethics. Public health, in the words of Dan Brock and Dan Wikler, took a "bird's eye" view of population health—a view they urged bioethics to take as well.[7] Moreover, during the formative period of bioethics, public health, too, was largely engaged by topics such as asbestos exposure, insecticide use, smoking, and pollution that pointed away from the ethical issues raised by infectious disease; and these fashionable new issues of focus in public health were by and large matters that did not involve *communicability*.

Scholars trained in bioethics after the emergence of AIDS may find our picture of the development of the field of bioethics particularly surprising— if not outright wrong. When AIDS was recognized in the early 1980s and the cause had been identified as a virus, ethical issues were widely raised in bioethics about illness where the disease could be transmitted from one person to another. By the time the AIDS epidemic had emerged in full force, however, the field of bioethics had already been largely defined, with areas of inquiry laid out and a core set of normative principles enshrined as the prevailing philosophical approach. Moreover, rights-based political activism shaped responses to the AIDS epidemic, making AIDS in important ways an exceptional case of infectious disease. Abigail Zuger identified AIDS as the "first disease on record to spawn a huge, vocal, visible, angry grass-roots patients' rights movement that changed the course of history."[8] And AIDS, given its mode of transmission, does not press some of the characteristics of infectious disease that

6. Albert R. Jonsen, Mark Siegler, and William J. Winslade, *Clinical Ethics: A Practical Approach to Ethical Decisions in Clinical Medicine* (New York: Macmillan, 1982).
7. Daniel Wikler and Dan W. Brock, "Ethical Issues in Population Health: Mapping a New Agenda," paper presented at the 7th World Congress of Bioethics, International Association of Bioethics, University of New South Wales, Sydney, Australia, 2004.
8. Abigail Zuger, "What Did We Learn from AIDS?" *New York Times*, sec. F, November 11, 2003.

are most challenging for traditional paradigms of bioethics, such as rapid lethality or widespread transmission among persons who have had no direct contact with each other. In short, during the development of bioethics, concern with infectious disease was never central—and indeed, with the later exception of AIDS—barely evident at all.

It is this remarkably unfortunate lapse, given the intensified threats of infectious disease both in the developed world and especially globally, that we hope to rectify. Our initial concern in much of this volume will be to explore the kinds of issues that bioethics addresses, issues like truth-telling, privacy and confidentiality, patient autonomy, human experimentation, reproductive dilemmas, dilemmas about dying, surveillance, required testing, mandated immunization, and the imposition of constraints, in the light of infectious disease. But while we focus primarily on bioethics issues, we also hint that the account we give of human reality in the context of infectious disease—that of a "way-station" self "embedded" in a "web of disease"—has broader implications, not just for bioethics but for social ethics and indeed philosophical ethics far more generally. We thus seek not only to repair what we see as a gap in bioethics, but to pursue an augmented, and we think more nuanced, conception of human reality in many other contexts.

In a sense, looking at the human being in his or her *physical* interrelatedness as giver and receiver of disease is to see something of the human condition that thinkers in the liberal tradition, and indeed in much of philosophy in general, have largely failed to see. Paul Ramsey's groundbreaking *The Patient as Person*,[9] whose title we deliberately echo in our own, saw (as did Joseph Fletcher,[10] Samuel Gorovitz,[11] and other progenitors of bioethics in their varying ways) that what is central to ethics in medicine is that the individual who is ill—the patient—be recognized as a *person*, a being worthy of respect. However, when disease is communicable, as we will explain, the patient—the person—cannot be seen solely as an "individual." The patient, this person, is in relationship to others: the sources of infection, others who might become infected from the patient, and those who will be affected by how the patient is treated. The infectious disease patient is at least potentially both *victim* and *vector*. Both the individualistic perspective that prevailed in early bioethics and the characteristic population view of public health must

9. Paul Ramsey. 1970. *The Patient as Person. Explorations in Medical Ethics.* New Haven: Yale University Press.

10. Joseph F. Fletcher, 1954. *Morals and medicine: The moral problems of the patient's right to know the truth, contraception, artificial insemination, sterilization, euthanasia.* Princeton, N.J.: Princeton University Press.

11. Samuel Gorovitz, Ruth Macklin, Andrew L. Jameton, John M. O'Connor, and Susan Sherwin, eds. 1976. *Moral problems in medicine.* Englewood Cliffs, N.J.: Prentice–Hall.

be incorporated within a new, broader way of viewing bioethics in light of infectious disease. While we do not reject the importance of autonomy and rights, we do contend in this volume that the ethical understanding and implications of these concepts need to be rethought in the light of disease that is communicable, including disease that is serious and often fatal. The infectious disease patient is a *patient-in-disease-relationships*, not just a *patient with a disease*, and philosophical approaches to bioethics and to ethics in general must come to terms with this fact.

The PVV View

We call the view we develop in this volume the *"patient as victim and vector"*— or *PVV* view. We see it as an augmentation of existing bioethics theory and ethics generally, not a replacement for them. The PVV view is not intended as a comprehensive theory and it is not hostile to existing accounts of ethics, social, and political theory, or metaphysics; rather, it views them as incomplete in taking account of human reality. Human beings are capable of comparative independence—that free, autonomous, tall-standing individual that is the paradigm of liberal theory—but only when they have succeeded in extricating themselves from what we call the "web of disease," that pattern of ongoing transmission either from human to human or through intermediate vectors that characterizes infectious disease. To a considerable degree this extrication has occurred in developed countries, where the eradication, elimination, and control of infectious disease has been extensive. To a dismaying degree, in the poorest, least developed nations, infectious disease still kills so many, whether because immunization or treatment is not available for financial or social reasons, or because the diseases are ones we do not know how to prevent or treat.

The PVV view we develop is complex, involving as we will see three intertwined perspectives through which to view issues of infectious disease. It can be stated simply:

> *Ethical problems in infectious disease should be analyzed, and clinical practices, research agendas, and public policies developed, that always take into account the possibility that a person with communicable infectious disease is both victim and vector.*

But its full formulation requires more detailed analysis. Developing this principle, exploring applications of it in practice, and examining its philosophic and policy consequences are the extended tasks of this book.

Developing and Using the PVV View

The starting-point of our project will be to examine what is interestingly different about infectious disease. These characteristics include communicability and acuity, as well as facts about treatment of many infectious conditions. It may be apparent quite quickly whether treatment is working; individuals may recover fully or die; and treatment may vary widely in price, from pennies to thousands of dollars. Infectious disease also presents collective issues, such as the possibility of "herd" immunity or the impact that failure to treat some people has on the health of others who might be infected. All human beings are vulnerable to infectious disease; in this sense, everyone is (potentially) both victim and vector. All human beings are potentially (and often actually) both *persons-in-need* and *persons-as-threat*. As victims, people are in need of care. They may also be in need of protection, because those who are vulnerable or perceived as threats are at risk of victimization. Moreover, when disease is contagious the victim-perspective—the perspective that sees people as in need—cannot be detached from the vector-perspective—the perspective that views people as posing risks of harm to others. This characterization of individual agents facing the possibility of infectious disease, we contend, requires rethinking the ethical significance of many traditional concepts in bioethics. Included here are what respect for autonomy requires, how to understand duties to prevent harm, and what to conclude about people as responsible agents in the roles of both patients and health-care providers.

Our PVV perspective, the theoretical account of human beings as victims and vectors, is the bedrock of this volume, and we are concerned to explore the implications of this view. Central to our project is modifying and enhancing the understanding of what autonomy means for people who are interrelated as victims and vectors. Some of the recent contributions to the theory of autonomy are relevant; for example, feminist and narrative conceptions of autonomy as relational. We will also try to show how some of the particular characteristics of some infectious diseases undercut familiar assumptions about autonomy; for example, how the acuity of infectious disease militates against reflective decision making and how the capacity for permanent prevention may reshape assessments of risk and benefit.

But more than relationality is involved here. Human beings are embodied—that is, they are physical beings with attendant limitations. Human physical limits are also often recognized in the theory of autonomy: people cannot fly, even if they wish to, people cannot see in the dark or hear sounds above their hearing range. It is human to invent machinery to help in doing these things; though invention is often brilliantly successful, human beings remain finite, physical beings. Similarly, people invent preventatives and treatments and after-the-fact restoratives to try to cope with disease, and while many innovations—like immunization against smallpox—are wonderfully successful, human beings remain organisms at risk. As we shall see, in proximity and physical as well as emotional closeness to each other people must recognize that they are all vulnerable to acquiring disease from each other. This fundamental fact about human agency is part of what an enhanced bioethics, informed by our PVV perspective, must capture, both for infectious disease and beyond.

In one sense, everyone is an individual; bioethics has focused on protecting this individuality. But in another, the one we focus on here, people are also "way-stations" for disease; it is public health that has recognized this latter fact. Our view, explored here, is that these concerns are interrelated. An adequate understanding of these concerns suggests both recognition of the complexity of risks people pose to each other and respect they have for each other as persons.

To view human beings in this "biologicized" way also necessitates development of a positive theory of what people owe each other as they confront a world of transmissible infectious disease. As autonomous agents, people must understand their interconnectedness—that they are not only victims but also vectors. As members of a public, they must understand their individuality—that they are not only vectors but also victims. Infectious disease challenges bioethics to develop new ways of understanding autonomy and the related concepts of harm and responsibility in light of biological reality. Infectious disease also raises the very real possibility that constraints may be necessary, and that compensation may be morally, if not legally, required if those constraints are imposed.

Another way to put these facts of our basic biology is to remind ourselves that human beings are animals, members of a distinctive species but animals just the same. Not only are humans like animals in communicating diseases to each other, within the herd, but humans contract diseases from animals—including dangerous zoonoses like Ebola, SARS, rabies, and, potentially, human-to-human avian flu. People do not always adequately recognize that they have much in common with other species beyond certain morphological similarities, genetic commonalities, and behavior patterns: for example, disease runs through the human species, from one member of the pack to another and so on; like many animal species, we shun sick members of a group However, we humans have better defenses. We know how to keep our water clean, to wash our hands, to develop immunizations and antibiotics. We can understand epidemiology, pandemic modeling, and the germ theory of disease. We have foresight, at least to some degree, and we have some understanding of when to take future predictions seriously and how to distinguish fear from risk. We can recognize progress in the past, and we can construct hopes for the future. We know how to think about the utility and ethical characteristics of such measures as quarantine and isolation, as well as the least-limiting ways of decreasing the risk of transmission. Just the same, however, we share with other animals our vulnerability to endemic, epidemic, and pandemic disease, passed along directly or through intermediate vectors from one of us to another.

Our PVV perspective is intended as a practical as well as a theoretical tool. It has real uses in analyzing both traditional and contemporary ethical issues involving infectious disease, including among others many of the familiar ethical issues in medicine such as confidentiality and informed consent. It addresses medical practice and health policy questions like the imposition of serious constraints, as in the example we explore—the poignant and clinically troubling case of a patient dying of drug-resistant tuberculosis. Regulations governing research with human subjects, especially the issue of secondary subjects who might be put at risk by research, are a challenge too, as are the apparent inconsistencies in policies governing testing for vertically transmitted infectious disease and vertically transmitted genetic disease. New technologies also make a difference, raising issues about, for example, rapid testing for HIV/AIDS during pregnancy or during delivery, especially where, as in many places in the developing world, a pregnant woman first presents for medical treatment when she is already in labor.

Such issues reveal yet another concern as we explore ethical problems in infectious disease: to recognize the grave differences in infectious-disease issues in the wealthy, developed world, where public sanitation, immunization, and treatment are almost universally available, and the poor, less developed parts of the world, where poverty, warfare, ethnic cleansing, and inadequate infrastructure compound the risks of infection. These differences are dismayingly real, and in this book we seek to be alert to both of these situations, and all the intermediate positions in between.

A global focus, seen in a number of chapters of this book, is complementary to a focus on individual clinical situations. For example, there are difficult *ethical* issues raised by antibiotic resistance: should care for *this* patient take into account whether practices of antibiotic overuse may in the long run result in less effective care for everyone? What about the treatment of a patient dying of a resistant, highly transmissible, and dangerous form of disease that, even in his final days, he could transmit to others? Is a kind of paternalism appropriate in mandating immunizations, and what is the appropriate role of parental consent or objection? Thus we also address problems that have become the focus of intense controversy; for example, proposals for infectious-disease surveillance, travel restrictions, prioritization for access to care in the event of a pandemic, and in the United States a proposal to require vaccination against the principal strains of human papilloma virus responsible for cervical cancer—a proposal that would mandate immunization for school attendance for 11–12-year-old girls.

There has been as far as we know no attempt to develop a comprehensive account of the ethical issues raised by infectious disease that faces directly the challenge infectious disease presents both to the traditional paradigms of bioethics and to public health. This task is enormous; a single volume cannot hope to treat all of the issues raised by infectious disease. But it can do something we regard as crucial to the project of this volume: not only to see infectious disease as central among the issues in bioethics and indeed in public health, but to provide a systematic mechanism, a kind of tool, as we call it in its simplified form at the end, for exploring and evaluating these issues. It is this that we call the *patient-as-victim and vector* approach, or the PVV view.

It should go without saying that this project is urgent. Far from being a closed book, as the Surgeon General perhaps predicted decades ago, infectious disease is again on the public agenda, in sometimes deeply frightening ways. There is a pessimistic face to our concerns: threats of bioterrorism have led to controversial proposals for surveillance and other major new public health measures, such as the Model Emergency Health Powers Act[12] and the Turning Point Model State Public Health Act.[13] Emergent infectious diseases, such as West Nile, SARS, or the prospect of person-to-person avian flu, apparently know no borders. Hospitals are seen as incubators of infection, including the deadly methicillin-resistant Staphylococcus aureus (MRSA), passed easily not only from infected patients to others but from health-care personnel to patients, sometimes with a mere brush of the sleeve of a white lab coat.[14]

12. Lawrence O. Gostin, "The Model State Emergency Health Powers Act: Public Health and Civil Liberties in a Time of Terrorism," *Health Matrix* 13 (2003): 3–32. As of July 2007, 38 states had adopted at least some provisions drawn from the Model Act. Center for Law & the Public's Health, "Model State Public Health Laws," http://www.publichealthlaw.net/Resources/Modellaws.htm#MSEHPA(accessed August 2007).
13. As of August 2007, 17 states had adopted the quarantine and isolation provisions of the Turning Point Act. Center for Law & the Public's Health, "The Turning Point Model State Public Health Act State Legislative Matrix Table," http://www.publichealthlaw.net/Resources/Resources PDFs/MSPHA%20Matrix%20Table.pdf (accessed August 2007). The Act would authorize quarantine, under stringent conditions including that it be the least restrictive alternative, that patients who have been identified as ill be isolated from those in quarantine, and that all those in quarantine or isolation are provided with the means to meet their basic needs.
14. R. Monina Klevens et al., "Invasive Methicillin-Resistant *Staphylococcus aureus* Infections in the United States," *Journal of the American Medical Association* 298, no. 15 (2007): 1763–1771.

Environmental degradation, population growth, and poverty feed reservoirs of infection that are transnational and international matters of concern.[15] Both national and international law are striving to come to grips with the specter of pandemic infection and with a wide range of questions about the significance of infections in one part of the globe for people in other far-distant parts.

But there is also an optimistic face to our concerns. Infectious disease has come back into worldwide attention not as a closed book but as a reopened volume of grand proportions, stimulated by new attention to global health. It raises ambitious questions of what might be required by wide scale efforts—already clearly in progress—to eradicate, eliminate, or bring infectious disease under control by means of prevention, immunization, and effective treatment. These efforts, like those in the pessimistic aspects of our inquiry here, also require ethical reflection and analysis based on a thoroughgoing understanding of the significance of *communicable* disease. We seek to provide this analysis.

Within philosophical thinking there have been many other theories of individuality, relationality, communitarianism, and so on. However, they have not generally seen the *biological* point we make here. That is why we have to start with a chapter about bugs—the many kinds of microorganisms that inhabit both the internal and external parts of human beings—as a way of understanding the degree to which our account here is not just a flight of metaphysical fancy, but about what human life is like in the real world.

We are obviously concerned here to work out the implications of our PVV view for the way in which we attempt to prevent and treat infectious disease. But we also think the view may be far more powerful. To be sure, something analogous to transmissibility characterizes many social issues. For example, child abuse is said to be frequently vertically transmitted, passed along from parents to children, though presumably as a learned rather than a biologically wired-in behavioral model. The treatment of a patient with mental illness may have substantial consequences for others, much as does the treatment of a patient with infectious disease. Yet these causal connections are far less tight than those in infectious disease, where it is the microorganisms that inhabit us and are part of our very being that take advantage of our susceptibilities to cause disease.

We treat this human embeddedness as central, something ineluctably part of the human condition. In the end, it will remain a question for us whether

---

15. See, e.g., Paul Farmer, *Pathologies of Power: Health, Human Rights, and the New War on the Poor* (Berkeley: University of California Press, 2003); Paul Farmer, *Infections and Inequalities: The Modern Plagues* (Berkeley: University of California Press, 2001); David P. Fidler, *International Law and Infectious Diseases* (Oxford: Clarendon Press, 1999).

this is a necessary feature of human existence or whether it could ever cease to be true. This is one reason we do not develop our PVV view as a *replacement* for previous theories in bioethics, social justice theory, or liberal theory in general. Rather, we leave open whether the PVV view could ever become irrelevant—should a *Comprehensive Global Effort for the Eradication, Elimination, or Control of Infectious Disease* of the sort imagined in Chapter 20 to become fully realized. And we leave for further speculation how differently we might think of human reality were we all no longer mutually embedded in a web of disease.

2

THE BIOLOGICAL BASICS OF INFECTIOUS DISEASE

By one recent estimate, there are over 1,400 pathogens—viruses, bacteria, parasites, protozoa, fungi, and prions—that can infect human beings.[1] These pathogens reflect variations on a number of important themes for bioethics. Although fortuitous discoveries and assiduous investigations have made some of them among the best understood of human diseases, pathogen-caused diseases are still among the most disturbing disorders because of their acuity and severity, among other distinctive characteristics. Some are utterly nondiscriminatory and will attack any human, while others prey selectively on particular groups. Some infectious diseases affect primarily children or are most virulent in children, while others affect people of any age; indeed, we never outgrow our risk of infectious diseases. Many infectious diseases prey on the ill, malnourished, or weak, but some disproportionately affect the healthy and strong: for example, the flu of 1918 had its highest lethality rates in young adults ages 18–24.[2]

Many infectious diseases are quite easy to treat; they are are among the few diseases that are absolutely curable. Many are easily preventable or limited to a one-time occurrence. Paradoxically, however, some are extraordinarily difficult to manage and some remain untreatable. Others can be recurrent over a lifetime, such as the cold sores caused by the herpes virus. Still others, like chicken pox, can appear in one form—an itchy, generalized rash in childhood that resolves spontaneously—only to reappear six to seven decades later in another form, the sharply localized and painful rash called "shingles" that slowly recedes but can cause weeks or months of excruciating pain.

Consider some of these features that are characteristic of many infectious diseases:

— Onset of the disease is often acute and sudden. The patient typically has no prior experience with it.

---

1. John von Radowitz, "Animals Spreading Many More Diseases to Humans," *Press Association Newsfile,* February 20, 2006 (quoting Mark Woolhouse speaking at meetings of the AAAS).
2. John M. Berry, *The Great Influenza* (New York: Penguin Books, 2004).

— The disease, if untreated, changes rapidly and often worsens, but most infectious diseases then resolve by themselves.
— The patient is usually symptomatic.
— Diagnosis is usually relatively simple, swift, and certain.
— Symptoms can be managed specifically, but treatment of the infection may resolve all the symptoms.
— For most infectious diseases, treatment is relatively easy and safe to administer.
— Treatment is often, but by no means always, comparatively inexpensive and limited to a short course.
— Treatment often means this disease will not recur.
— The effectiveness of treatment is usually apparent quickly.
— The treatment of these diseases is usually associated with a high benefit to burden ratio.
— The outcome of successful treatment is often complete cure. Where effective treatment is available, permanent disability or chronic disease is uncommon.
— Most infectious diseases are not fatal.
— A cured patient is generally restored to his or her previous state of health.
— Survival of an infectious disease often means that this disease will not recur.
— The disease is often constructed as an attack by an enemy, not as a "natural" failure of an organ or the host. The patient or family that chooses to fight this battle has a good chance of winning—unlike the battle against most other medical diseases.
— People are often familiar with the types of treatment for acute infectious diseases and often expect successful treatment.
— Except where there are fiscal constraints, treatment of these diseases does not deprive others of a scarce resource like an organ.
— The incidence and types of infectious disease caused by these organisms are strongly influenced by geography, climate, environment, the condition of the host, and access to sanitation.
— Many but not all infectious diseases are either directly or indirectly transmissible.
— Because infectious diseases may be acute, may affect otherwise healthy individuals, may occur in epidemics, and may produce high mortality rates, they often provoke fear and intense emotional and often irrational responses.

Some of these features, such as acuity, are biological facts about particular infectious diseases. Others, such as the use of military language in speaking about infection—"attack," "fighting the battle," "surrendering" or "succumbing"—are social responses. Still others, such as the relatively low costs of treating many infectious diseases, are a combination of both biological facts and social responses to them. As we shall see, some, but not all, of these features are ethically important. Some are shared with non-infectious physical conditions;

others largely are not. Moreover, some infectious diseases exhibit few or virtually none of these characteristics. Our strategy in this volume is not to separate infectious disease as exceptional, but to identify the cluster of features of infectious disease that, taken together, present underappreciated challenges for bioethics and require rethinking standard paradigms of understanding issues in the field in light of the patient as victim and vector.

This chapter introduces, first the organisms that cause disease, and then central aspects of the pathogenic mechanics of infectious disease that will be critical to the issues to be examined in this volume. The audience for this particular chapter is the non-specialist who, we assume, is relatively unfamiliar with the biology of infectious disease. The next chapter continues for a broader audience by presenting a number of the distinctive features of infectious disease, together with our responses to it, that make up the core of the challenge of infectious disease for bioethics.

One important way that infectious diseases are distinguished from other diseases is the fact that they involve our interaction with another life form: that is, interaction between humans and another living organism or organisms. Humans not only can be affected by or acquire infectious diseases in conjunction with these other living organisms, but they also can carry and transmit them to other organisms, both human and nonhuman.

In an infectious disease, a pathogen invades a susceptible host. Most life forms that cause infection are or have stages that are too small to see without the aid of a light or electron microscope. These tiny microorganisms, collectively called *microbes*, are known as *human pathogens* if they can cause diseases in people. They are known as *opportunistic pathogens* if they only produce disease in people whose immune defenses are compromised. Not all interactions between microorganisms are pathogenic; some microorganisms are beneficial and even indispensable for human health. Nor are all infectious diseases communicable. However, the varieties of organisms and of modes of transmission of both mild and serious pathogens are legion. Because patterns of infection and transmission are so complex and variable, it is useful to define a number of terms in order to understand how infectious diseases occur and what strategies work to prevent or treat them.

Types of Infectious Organisms

Many types of tiny or microscopic organisms can cause disease. The classification system in common use includes five major types: parasites, fungi, bacteria, viruses, and prions, described here in descending order of size and complexity. The account in this and in the next sections includes at least one organism from each major category, an explanation of how it produces an infectious disease, and considerations about what can be done to control its exposure, transmission, and disease.

Parasites

Some of the largest parasites are the arthropods, generally visible to the naked eye, or at least with the help of a magnifying glass. A familiar example might be lice or "crabs." These tiny creatures are quite mobile on their jointed legs and they can crawl about on the skin or burrow into it. They lay their eggs on skin or on hair follicles. As they grow and move about, they can produce intense itching, scratching, and a characteristic skin lesion or rash. A clinical encounter with arthropods can be better termed an *infestation* than an infection. The medical response to arthropods is mechanical—physically removing them, as with a fine-tooth comb, and making their environment uninhabitable with strong soaps, shampoos, or lotions. Humans are the reservoir for *Sarcoptes scabei*, a mite that causes scabies—an itching condition of the skin identified by the red lines resulting from tracks under the skin made by the burrowing mite. Transmission can be by direct physical or sexual contact or by indirect means such as clothing and bedding. The incubation period is two to six weeks, and patients and fomites can transmit their infection until mites and eggs are destroyed.

Flat and round worms are other types of large parasites. Well-known examples of the former are tapeworms, and of the latter are pinworms (and *Ascaris lumbricoides*). The parasitic roundworms resemble their free-living close relatives, but they depend on a host or hosts for their survival. They typically spend part of their often-complex life cycle in the human gut, where they can produce no symptoms or disturbances in digestion, absorption, or elimination. Many are barely visible, but ascaris can be up to thirty-five centimeters long and the fish tapeworm up to twenty-five feet. The reservoirs for ascaris are humans and soil contaminated by feces. Transmission is by ingestion of contaminated soil, the incubation period is four to eight weeks, and the period of communicability is as long as the fertilized female worm lives in the gut, which may be up to twenty-four months. The female worm produces over 200,000 eggs per day. Control measures include sanitation and personal and food hygiene. The reservoir for the fish tapeworm, *Diphylobothrium latum*, is human beings with fish being the second intermediate host. Transmission is by eating raw or inadequately cooked fish. The incubation period is three to six weeks, and people can shed eggs for many years.

Protozoa, a smaller type of parasite, are unicellular organisms that are easily visible with a microscope. The term protozoan means "first animal." The ways that protozoa move, reproduce, consume, digest, and excrete are similar to what is associated with animals. Giardia—that bane of hikers who drink water from lakes or streams—may be a familiar example. The mobile trophozoite is about fifteen microns long and moves through a liquid medium by using its multiple whiplike flagella. The trophozoite lives and reproduces in the intestines of humans and other mammals. The cysts are excreted in stool and can survive in water and thus infect animals or humans that drink it. Exposure to giardia cysts often results in asymptomatic carriage, but can cause clinical infection in about one week. Carriers or symptomatic persons with diarrhea can excrete the cysts for months. Giardia can produce more serious and prolonged infection in persons with AIDS and thus could be an opportunistic pathogen in those hosts. Control measures focus on personal hygiene and treatment of water. Other protozoa like amoebas can also be acquired by drinking contaminated water. However, the plasmodia—the protozoans that cause malaria—require a vector, the mosquito, for their transmission to humans. This obviously leads to very different approaches and strategies for control, from insecticide-impregnated bednets that kill mosquitoes that have been attracted to a person sleeping inside, to swamp drainage and other forms of mosquito eradication.

Fungi

Fungi have distinctive cell wall characteristics and multicellular growth. All fungi are eucaryotes—cells with a distinct nucleus, containing DNA surrounded by a nuclear membrane. Fungi range greatly in size, from microscopic molds to large and visible mushrooms. Microscopic molds can produce a visible mass when they grow and multiply. They also include unicellular yeasts, some of which are familiar to bakers and brewers, while others are human pathogens such as candida species that cause thrush in babies and immune-compromised hosts, and vaginitis in women. Candida is an example of a yeast that can be a part of our normal intestinal flora, but also can, in particular situations, cause a skin or mucus membrane infection or an even more serious bloodstream or vital organ infection.

Aspergillus species are molds that live in decaying vegetation, soil, and dust. They can even be found in hospital buildings, especially during construction, when dust may be aerosolized and distributed through ventilation systems. The aspergillus fungus can grow in human tissue, especially in compromised hosts, but it also produces spores or conidia that circulate in the air. Aspergillus is a ubiquitous fungus, but an opportunistic pathogen. It is not communicated from person to person. Control measures focus on the environment and on air.

Bacteria

Bacteria (procaryotes) are very small, simple single-cell organisms. The DNA of bacteria is not within a nuclear membrane. Bacteria are most often rod-like (bacilli) or spherical (cocci). *Bacillus anthracis,* for example, is the cause of anthrax in animals, including humans. Its reservoir is soil. Transmission is by contact with infected soil or animal tissues, ingestion of contaminated material, or inhalation of spores in the air. The environment or contaminated materials may remain infectious for years. Person to person transmission is rare. The incubation period varies by type of exposure.

Measures for controlling anthrax bacteria are directed at preventing disease in animals and transmission to humans through vaccination and special occupational precautions. The stability of this organism and its potential for aerosol dispersion make this organism attractive for bioterrorists, as in the "anthrax letters" sent through the mail to public officials in the Senate Office Building, resulting in several deaths of postal and newspaper workers in October 2001.[3]

Viruses

Viruses are even smaller than bacteria. They can only be seen with the aid of an electron microscope. They are much simpler than bacteria, actually acellular, consisting of a core made of either DNA or RNA surrounded by a protein coat. They may have an additional lipid membrane called an envelope. Viruses lack self-sufficiency, for they are unable to reproduce without the cellular machinery of other organisms.

Human herpes virus 3, also known as varicella zoster virus (VZV) is the cause of chicken pox (varicella) and shingles (herpes zoster). The reservoir for this virus is humans. The virus is transmitted directly by contact with droplets and indirectly by airborne spread of blister fluid or respiratory secretions, or by articles soiled with infected material. The incubation period is two to three weeks, but exposed persons can transmit infection for up to five days before the typical rash appears and for about five days afterward or until the lesions are crusted. Everyone who has not had chicken pox and has not been immunized is susceptible to infection with VZV. Most infected children recover and are immune to a second infection. The virus, however, can remain latent in cells of the nervous system where it can reactivate years later and produce a localized rash or shingles. Immune-compromised patients are both more likely to experience severe chicken pox if they are exposed to the virus and to experience a reactivation of it if they have latent infection. Control measures include isolation or exclusion of exposed susceptible and infected persons, special protection for high-risk individuals, and routine population-based immunization.

Many viruses—but not all—have extraordinary ability to mutate. Although, for example, the varicella virus has a single strand of DNA and is quite stable,

---

3. See, e.g., Eric Lipton and Kirk Johnson, "A Nation Challenged: The Anthrax Trail," *New York Times*, sec. A, December 26, 2001.

influenza viruses have multiple strands of RNA and mutate rapidly. HIV also mutates rapidly; this instability explains in part why it has been possible to develop effective vaccines for chickenpox but very difficult for HIV. It also explains why influenza vaccines are modified annually to respond to the steady mutation of existing strains of the virus, and why it may be difficult to plan ahead to immunize people against new strains of flu virus.

Prions

A prion (proteinaceous infectious particle) is the smallest infectious particle known. A prion is a protein with no genetic material of its own, so simple that it hardly qualifies for the title "microbe." But prions can be extremely damaging. Because a prion is not really a living organism, it cannot be "killed" in the usual sense, but it can be rendered non-infectious by agents called proteases that destroy proteins. One of the best-known examples of a prion "infection" is bovine spongiform encephalopathy (BSE) or "mad cow disease." The reservoirs for BSE are cattle and humans, with transmission thought to be via consumption of infected or contaminated beef or direct contact with infected human tissue. Theoretically, transmission via blood from an infected donor is also possible. The incubation period may vary from 15 months to 30 years. The illness produced by the prion responsible for BSE is a progressive dementia and neurological disease. Tissues of the nervous system are infectious throughout symptomatic illness and may remain infectious long after they are removed from the host. Control measures have included testing and slaughter of infected cattle herds,[4] export and import restrictions, burial precautions when handling potentially infected human tissues, and exclusion of blood and tissue donation from infected or exposed individuals.

Transmission Mechanisms in Infectious Disease

All pathogens have a place where they normally reside, their *reservoir*. Reservoirs can be inanimate or living. Examples range from the soil in which anthrax spores reside, to water contaminated with cholera bacteria, to nonhuman mammals such as bats and raccoons that harbor rabies. Humans themselves can also be reservoirs, as they in fact are for tuberculosis and HIV.

For some pathogens, as already described, getting from the reservoir to humans requires a mechanism for transmission called a *vector*. These vectors can be alive, such as the mosquitoes that transmit malaria, snails that transmit

---

4. See, e.g., John Taglibue, "Mad Cow Disease (and Anxiety)," *New York Times*, sect. C, February 1, 2001.

schistosomiasis, or humans who transmit tuberculosis or HIV. Inanimate objects or materials can also be the means of transmission for pathogens. Examples include hospital equipment or solutions contaminated with pseudomonas bacteria, or undercooked meat that contains viable pathogenic *E. coli*. When inanimate objects found in the home or workplace serve as vectors, they are called *fomites*. Examples include a stethoscope used on more than one patient, a telephone in an office, or a dining room table surface in a home. One reason it is difficult to get rid of Norwalk virus on a cruise ship, it is said, is that passengers are always hanging onto the ship railing: one infected person may make a hundred disease-transmitting handprints. Although often impugned, however, toilet seats rarely have been implicated as a vector.

Transmission of an infectious disease can be direct or indirect. Direct transmission, also known as *case-to-case transmission,* occurs when disease passes directly from one affected person to another through some form of physical contact. Well-known examples are sexually transmitted diseases, including HIV/AIDS, syphilis, gonorrhea, Herpes simplex and chlamydia infections. Direct transmission also passes via hand-to-hand contact in the case of the common cold—where virally infected secretions find their way from mucous membranes to a patient's hands, thence to a second person's hands and to her mucous membranes. Shaking hands, a culturally accepted courtesy in some cultures, is a frequent route of direct transmission.

Indirect transmission can occur when infectious material enters the air or water. Examples include airborne tuberculosis transmission and waterborne cholera transmission. Indirect transmission can also occur via vectors and fomites. Indirect transmission also occurs when an infectious disease is acquired not from an infected and symptomatic person, but from a *carrier,* someone who is not ill or affected by the organism, but who harbors it.

Carriage can occur after a symptomatic infection or it can begin and continue without the patient experiencing any complaints attributable to the infection. Thus "infection" is not always synonymous with "disease." An example of this kind of indirect transmission is the development of typhoid fever following consumption of food prepared and contaminated by the hands of a person who is a gastrointestinal carrier of Salmonella typhi. Typhoid Mary, a cook who catered to the wealthy in New York around the turn of the twentieth century, has entered our language as a notorious example of a source of an outbreak attributed to this kind of transmission. Sexual relations with a partner who is an asymptomatic carrier of hepatitis B can also result in carrier-to-case transmission. For some diseases, it may be difficult to distinguish people who are asymptomatic and will remain that way from people who are asymptomatic but who may progress to clinical disease—a particularly clear example is hepatitis B. Early in the HIV epidemic, when the disease was less well understood, and to some extent even today, it was also unclear who would progress to active AIDS.

To further complicate matters, the mode of transmission does not necessarily predict or correlate with clinical consequences. Someone whose infection is acquired from a case may become a carrier or a case. Similarly, a person who acquires infection from a carrier may become either a carrier or a case. What transpires in the person who acquires the infection depends on their response to the infection, not on the mode of transmission. Bacterial meningitis is an interesting and perhaps surprising example. Many people are alarmed when exposed to a case of "spinal meningitis"—a redundant but scary name for a bacterial infection of the tissues that envelop the spinal cord due to the meningococcus bacterium. Most cases do not originate from exposure to a symptomatic patient, but from exposure to an asymptomatic carrier. Furthermore, most exposures to cases and to carriers do not result in disease. The far more likely result is no infection at all or asymptomatic carriage. Thus, isolation of a person with bacterial meningitis, while it may allay the fears of family members, acquaintances, and even health providers, does very little to curtail transmission of infection.

One factor that affects whether exposure to an infectious agent results in disease, carriage, or no infection at all is the prior experience of the persons exposed. *Antibodies* are specific proteins that target and/or neutralize an infectious agent. If persons have been previously infected with an agent, whether or not they experienced symptoms, and have antibodies, they may be *immune* or invulnerable to that agent. Familiar examples are the adults who have had or have been exposed to measles, mumps, chicken pox, or the meningococcus bacterium in their childhood who are later exposed, but rarely become ill, when their own children manifest those infections.

Prevention and Treatment

From the time of Jenner's development of the vaccine in 1798 and earlier in Arabic and Chinese cultures, variolation or immunization has been a mainstay of smallpox prevention. A *vaccine* is a modified form of an infectious agent or its toxin that stimulates the vaccinated person to develop antibodies but not symptoms of disease. Capitalizing on natural immunity, vaccines are derived from infectious agents. Some are derived from microbial components and toxins. Persons who are vaccinated successfully are artificially, but effectively, immune to a variety of pathogens. Vaccines have now been developed for many diseases, including measles, mumps, rubella, polio, influenza, diphtheria, tetanus, human papilloma virus (HPV), and several bacteria that produce meningitis and pneumonia. Most of the serious infections of childhood are now preventable with vaccines. However, vaccines are not available for many serious diseases, including some of the most significant causes of death from infectious disease worldwide: HIV/AIDS, malaria, most forms of infantile diarrhea, and, except for seasonal influenza, acute viral respiratory disease.

To prevent clinical or symptomatic infections, immunizations must generally be given prior to exposure. That is because the antibodies we require for protection generally take about two weeks to develop. In some cases, protection requires several immunizations administered months apart to produce the requisite level of antibodies. Therefore, vaccination is not always a rapidly effective strategy to counter an epidemic that is already under way. Fortunately, there are other ways and strategies to prevent infectious diseases that take advantage of modes of transmission and human and pathogen biology.

Before exposure, many approaches are effective. One strategy is to reduce or eliminate exposure itself, as when a patient with pulmonary tuberculosis is isolated and the patient and visitors are required to wear masks that exclude small aerosol particles. Another strategy is to sterilize surgical tools and syringes and wash or glove hands to prevent indirect transmission of pathogens from health-care providers to patients. Still another is to treat water and cook meat to minimize or eliminate exposure to infectious agents.

Once exposure has occurred, intervention can still prevent clinical infection during the *incubation period*—the time before the pathogen replicates sufficiently to produce disease and before the host or patient responds with signs and symptoms. For some disorders, like staphylococcal "food poisoning," the time to symptomatic response can be as short as 8 to 12 hours, because peoples' intestines respond violently to toxins that staphylococci produced in the food even before it was eaten. The incubation period varies from two weeks in the case of chicken pox up to decades for tuberculosis and HIV. These facts about timing afford more opportunities for prevention of disease. In the case of chicken pox, people can be injected with *immunoglobulin* (serum from immune persons) that contains antibodies that will provide short-term protection. Alternatively, an antiviral drug—acyclovir—can be administered to destroy the virus and thus prevent or ameliorate the infectious illness. In the case of asymptomatic tuberculosis, an antimycobacterial drug—isoniazid—is used to destroy the tubercle bacillus and prevent subsequent disease in a process called *chemoprophylaxis*.

Epidemiology and Epidemics

Epidemiology, the scientific discipline that addresses questions of when and where diseases occur and how they are transmitted within populations, can be descriptive, analytical, or experimental, and can focus on any disease or condition. Infectious diseases are a major focus of epidemiologic study because reasonably well-developed tools are available for diagnosis, treatment, surveillance, prevention, and control for this group of medical problems.

An epidemic of an infectious disease is of special concern both to the public and to epidemiologists. An *epidemic* is defined as a significant increase in the incidence of a disease above a baseline or normal rate. *Incidence* refers to the number of new cases that occur within a specified population in a fixed time period. For example, if we normally encounter 0 to 10 cases of influenza per 100,000 persons in a given region per month and the incidence increases to 1,000 per 100,000 in February, this would certainly constitute an epidemic. *Prevalence* refers to the number of people in a population with a given diagnosis at a given point in time. Epidemiologists describe the impact of diseases on populations by their *morbidity* rate (the incidence of the disease), their *mortality* rate (the incidence of deaths due to the disease), and the *case fatality* rate (the proportion of cases that result in death). Infectious agents' degrees of contagiousness are highly variable, depending on the type, severity, and location of the infection among other factors. For example, TB patients who have laryngeal involvement are much more contagious than patients with involvement of a joint. Similarly, the degree of infectiousness is highly dependent on the type of exposure: some infectious diseases such as HIV require direct contact with mucosal fluids or blood; some require exposure at sufficiently close range to breathe in aerosolized particles; and others involve a wide variety of exposure types. The efficiency of transmission can also be quantified, and may vary in different circumstances; for example, measles is more communicable than TB, even though both are aerosolized. Transmission efficacy factors are used in modeling the anticipated severity of possible epidemics.

Faced with an epidemic with serious morbidity and/or mortality, epidemiologists and public health officials consider a variety of prevention and response strategies, ranging from immunization, to screening, to isolation and quarantine, any of which may be mandatory or voluntary. These strategies can be very effective in controlling epidemics, but can also be expensive, potentially harmful to some individuals, and disruptive of personal privacy or liberty. Because infectious diseases involve not only human interaction with microbes but also interactions with loved ones and strangers, and because prevention, control, and treatment for one person has implications and impact on many people or perhaps on all people, infectious diseases compel us to examine personal ethical choices and public policy responses to individual cases and to potential and actual epidemics.

Conclusion

Further questions about how infectious diseases are caused, transmitted, treated, and prevented will be considered more fully in later chapters. It would be impossible (in less than the several thousand pages of the principal infectious-disease texts[5]) to provide full detail for the hundreds of types of infectious diseases. But with any specific ethical issue in infectious disease, it is crucial to understand the details of the particular type of infection(s) involved. Thus, later chapters will discuss, among others, the mechanisms of transmission of tuberculosis (Chapter 9), HIV/AIDS (Chapter 12), HPV (Chapter 14), and pandemic influenza (Chapters 17–19). These mechanisms for the organisms that cause these diseases are dramatically different, thus affecting what we say about cautions and constraints that may or may not be imposed on the human-to-human contacts involved. In Chapter 7, we will develop the notion of the "way-station" self as we explore our theoretical account of ethical issues, but trust that this background chapter serves as a reminder that infectious organisms, their modes of transmission, and their mechanisms of disease causation are astonishingly varied.

5. Gerald L. Mandell, John E. Bennett, and Raphael Dolin, eds., *Principles and Practice of Infectious Diseases*, 2 vols., 6th ed. (Philadelphia: Elsevier, 2005).

3

CHARACTERISTICS OF INFECTIOUS DISEASE
THAT RAISE DISTINCTIVE CHALLENGES
FOR BIOETHICS

Historically, infectious diseases such as leprosy, plague, smallpox, typhoid, cholera, tuberculosis have caused enormous fear and social distress. Early on, most of these deeply frightening diseases were recognized as contagious, even though the mechanisms of contagion were not understood. They often occurred in dramatic epidemics, wiping out entire villages or threatening populations on a large scale. Some of the ethical issues that are raised by infectious diseases are related to these diseases' powerful ability to engender fear in individuals and panic in populations. Such fear and panic may lead to rapid, emotionally driven decision making about the care of individual patients and about public health policies, even when these decisions challenge generally accepted principles of medical ethics such as patient autonomy.

However, the challenges to medical ethics posed by infectious disease are not simply the result of human responses based on irrational fear or misunderstanding. Instead, it is important to understand the specific characteristics of different infectious diseases that raise a wide range of ethical issues. Some infectious diseases may develop rapidly, leaving little time for reflective decision making between physician and patient. Communicable infectious diseases, especially if the transmission is swift and extensive, may have widespread social as well as individual effects.

Before we examine some of the features of infectious diseases that present distinctive ethical challenges for bioethics, an initial cautionary note is in order. Some infectious diseases do not share these characteristics. Some noninfectious diseases do. There is much to be learned from exploring the similarities and the differences between infectious and other diseases. Nonetheless, many of these features cluster with diseases that are both infectious and contagious; we believe that their significance has been underappreciated, and that consideration of them will be instructive for bioethics more generally.

An earlier version of this chapter appeared as Charles B. Smith, Margaret P. Battin, Jay A. Jacobson, Leslie P. Francis, Jeffrey R. Botkin, Emily P. Asplund, Gretchen J. Domek, and Beverly Hawkins, "Are There Characteristics of Infectious Diseases That Raise Special Ethical Issues?" *Developing World Bioethics* 4, no. 1 (May 2004): 1–16.

High Morbidity and Mortality

The high morbidity and mortality rates for many infectious diseases mean that there is a lot at stake when diagnosing, treating, and preventing them. Pressing ethical concerns are bound to emerge whenever large numbers of human lives are in the balance. While the same could be said for other non-infectious diseases with high morbidity and mortality rates, such as cancer and heart disease, infectious diseases have this quality to a greater degree and with greater rapidity than most other types of diseases. In the twenty-first century, infectious diseases continue to be among the leading worldwide causes of death and disability,[1] despite dramatic twentieth-century advances in the eradication, control, and treatment of infectious diseases such as smallpox, polio, and bacterial infections.

Generally, what sparks ethical debate because of the high morbidity and mortality rates of infectious diseases are fearful reactions to outbreaks, with government organizations, health professionals, and individuals altering their own behavior or requiring altered behavior in ways that are ethically questionable. When fear of these diseases becomes a principal force in clinical and public health decision making, serious ethical issues concerning human rights and the just distribution of resources are likely to arise[2].

For example, government support for programs of high social value such as education, nutrition, and economic development may be subordinated to the need for public health and medical funding to control and treat infections. The highly fatal and contagious Ebola virus, although only rarely transported out of Africa, has been a cause of worldwide fears that have influenced local economic, travel, and immigration policies.[3] In 2003, an outbreak of the frequently fatal albeit less contagious viral disease severe acute respiratory syndrome (SARS), both in and outside China, threatened economic havoc to entire cities as resources were diverted to meet needs for intensive hospital care and commerce was brought to a halt by quarantine and travel restrictions. Relative ignorance about the reservoir and source of SARS, as well as its mode of transmission, generated fear of the unknown and possible over-reaction by public health officials in the use of isolation and quarantine. In attempts to control the SARS epidemic in Taiwan, more than 130,000 individuals were placed in quarantine for 10 or more days with threat of fines and jail time for violators. Less than 0.3% of quarantined persons were subsequently diagnosed

---

1. World Health Organization, *The World Health Report* (Geneva: World Health Organization, 2001), 144–155.
2. R Barrett and PJ Brown Stigma in the Time of Influenza: Social and Institutional Responses to Pandemic Influenza. *Journal of Infectious Diseases* 197 (Suppl. 1) 2008: S34-37.
3. Laurie Garrett, *The Coming Plague: Newly Emerging Diseases in a World Out of Balance* (New York: Penguin Books, 1994), 192–221.

as suspect or probable SARS cases, and the net effectiveness of the quarantine program is still under evaluation.[4]

Human rights such as privacy and autonomy may come into conflict with the perceived needs of the community to utilize quarantine and forced therapies to control potentially fatal infectious diseases such as AIDS and tuberculosis.[5] In the early 1990s, the decision of New York City public health officials to move from an approach to therapy of tuberculosis that allowed free choice by patients to mandatory directly observed therapy, was in large part motivated by the recognition that new strains of tuberculosis were highly resistant to antibiotics—so-called multidrug-resistant tuberculosis (MDR-TB) and extensively drug-resistant tuberculosis (XDR-TB). Many patients, including health-care workers, were dying from this normally treatable infection. The management of the antibiotic-resistant tuberculosis outbreak in New York has been a rare example of good ethical policy arising from extensive dialogue between the public health officials, infectious disease specialists, and patient advocacy groups, as we shall discuss in Chapter 9.[6] Unfortunately, the more recent emergence of XDR-TB in South Africa and elsewhere presents a less hopeful picture; the World Health Organization (WHO) has categorized it a global health risk as serious as HIV/AIDS or avian flu.[7]

Although the WHO declared worldwide eradication of smallpox in 1980, the 30% mortality rate from smallpox and the potential for its reintroduction as a bioterrorism agent has introduced fear-driven discussions about public policies for quarantine and the public versus individual risks and benefits of widespread immunization.[8] Physicians, nurses, and other hospital clinical employees have been particularly conflicted about their public duty to take a vaccine to protect themselves and subsequently their patients and the public from the spread of smallpox. The conflict has arisen because of the well-defined potential risks of this live-virus vaccine causing serious and even fatal illness in the recipients of the vaccine or of spreading the vaccine to immune deficient patients at high risk of developing serious complications.

---

4. Centers for Disease Control and Prevention, "Use of Quarantine to Prevent Transmission of Severe Acute Respiratory Syndrome–Taiwan, 2003," *Mortality and Morbidity Weekly Report* 52, no. 29 (July 23, 2003): 680–683.
5. M.R. Gasner, K.L. Maw, G.E. Feldman et al., "The Use of Legal Action in New York City to Ensure Treatment of Tuberculosis," *New England Journal of Medicine* 340, no. 5 (February 4, 1999): 359–366.
6. N.N. Dubler, R. Bayer, S. Landesman, and A. White, *The Tuberculosis Revival: Individual Rights and Societal Obligations in a Time of AIDS* (New York: United Hospital Fund, 1992), 1–39.
7. World Health Organization, "New Plan to Contain Drug-resistant TB," http://www.who.int/mediacentre/news/releases/2007/pr32/en/index.html (accessed June 2007).
8. J.M. Neff, J.M. Lane, V.A. Fulginiti, and D.A. Henderson, "Contact Vaccinia—Transmission of Vaccinia from Smallpox Vaccination," *Journal of the American Medical Association* 288 (2002): 1901–1905.

Recent European outbreaks in cattle of the fatal neurological disease, bovine spongiform encephalopathy, have been associated with over 130 cases in humans of variant Creutzfeldt-Jakob Disease (vCJD), a similar fatal neurological disease.[9] The resulting attempts to control these diseases have led to widespread slaughter of cattle and embargoes on the import of beef from infected herds and countries. Although the number of human cases has been very small, the universal mortality of humans with vCJD has been a powerful force for drastic methods of control.

The continued high prevalence of potentially fatal infectious diseases can in part be attributed to the ability of microorganisms to mutate rapidly to become resistant to anti-microbials and vaccines.[10] In addition, the steady increase in the prevalence of these resistant pathogens has been attributed to increasing and often inappropriate use of antimicrobials in patient care and by the agriculture industry. This association, as we shall see in Chapter 13, has stimulated discussions of the ethical conflicts between the desires of individual patients for maximum antibiotic therapy and the interests of the community in reducing inappropriate antimicrobial use. Similarly, public policy debates are stimulated by the desires of the meat and poultry industries to speed animal weight gain by using antibiotics in animal feed—a practice that has been severely restricted or eliminated in Europe and Canada—and the public health needs for controlling the development of resistant microbial pathogens.

Invasiveness

Whereas many diseases arise from within the individual's own genetic makeup in interaction with some aspects of their lifestyle or environment, infectious diseases are caused by invasion or attack on humans by foreign micro-organisms. The common use of war-related words to describe infectious diseases (killer-viruses, flesh-eating strep, invasiveness, attack, and black death) reflects the fear that is associated with these diseases. This notion of enemy attack raises ethical questions similar to those faced in discussions of actual warfare. Consider, for example, these questions. What rights do individuals and communities have in defending themselves against such attacks? To what extent are different defensive measures justified? May individuals refuse to defend themselves if this refusal endangers others? Is a paternalistic response ever justified to force people to defend themselves? The rights of the individual and of the community to protection from attack are at stake when an outbreak occurs, as we can see in many examples.

---

9. Centers for Disease Control and Prevention, "Probable Variant Creutzfeldt-Jakob Disease in a US resident—Florida, 2002," *Mortality and Morbidity Weekly Report* 51, no. 41 (October 18, 2002): 927–929.
10. M. Lappe, *Breakout: The Evolving Threat of Drug-Resistant Disease* (San Francisco: Sierra Club Books, 1995), 69–92.

For millennia, militarists have attempted to utilize microbial pathogens or their toxins to kill or to immobilize their enemies either through the direct effects of these agents or by engendering fear and disruption of social and public health programs. The 2001 experience with the "anthrax letters" and the possibility of bioterrorism in the United States raised policy and ethics questions such as the justice of decisions about who should be screened for infection, who should receive the limited supply of prophylactic antibiotics, who should receive a vaccine of uncertain effectiveness and safety profile, and what services—for example postal—should be shut down to protect the public.[11] Although some have welcomed this bioterrorism-fear-induced infusion of public funds to support public health laboratories and programs,[12] others have expressed concern that the lack of truth telling and possible exaggeration of the risks of bioterrorism by military, FBI, and other government officials may ultimately damage public confidence in public health agencies, a confidence that is necessary for these agencies to be effective.[13]

The idea of enemy attack may also suggest innocence on the part of the victim. In the case of diseases such as HIV/AIDS, however, public opinion may see the infected individual who transmits as the attacker, a victim not of some foreign aggressor but of their own behavior, and the person to whom it is transmitted as the true victim—though often also a victim of his or her own behavior. Throughout this volume, we will question this view as simplistic. The notion of patient as *victim* as well as *vector* will prove to be a complex one, as we shall see as we develop our full PVV perspective.

Acuity

Infectious diseases can be the most quickly progressing of any diseases. Many infectious diseases, such as meningitis, pneumonia, bacterial septicemia, and hemorrhagic viral infections can develop and progress to a rapidly fatal outcome in less than a 24-hour period. This acuity leads to fear and the need for rapid decision making before a definitive diagnosis is available. Fear may in turn lead to hasty decisions that are poor public health policy or that deprive infected individuals of their rights.

The meningococcus is among the most rapidly invasive of bacterial pathogens; the time between the appearance of the first symptoms and death may

---

11. See, e.g., David E. Rosenbaum and Sheryl Gay Stolberg, "A Nation Challenged: The Vaccine," *New York Times*, sec. B, December 20, 2001.
12. M.R. Fraser and D.L. Brown, "Bioterrorism Preparedness and Local Public Health Agencies: Building Response Capacity," *Public Health Reports* 115 (2000): 326–330.
13. V.W. Sidel, R.M. Gould, and H.W. Cohen, "Bioterrorism Preparedness: Cooptation of Public Health," *Medicine and Global Survival* 7 (2002): 82–89.

be less than 24 hours. In outbreaks of meningococcal meningitis and septi-cemia, fear of this rapidly fatal infection has sometimes led school leaders and parents to close schools and leave the community, making it difficult for public health officials to conduct needed prophylaxis and immunization programs.

In circumstances of acute infectious disease, the rights of individuals un-derstood as autonomous agents to choose maximum therapy may conflict with the rights of the community to discourage prescription practices that in-crease the prevalence of resistant pathogens. For example, a patient with acute and rapidly progressive pneumonia of unclear etiology may initially be treated with multiple antibiotics, a practice that has potential therapeutic efficacy but one that has been shown to increase the prevalence of multiple drug resistant pathogens in the community.[14] Physicians and patient advocacy groups have collaborated to educate physicians about the need to change antibiotic therapy to a single effective drug based on subsequent laboratory reports. Significant efforts have also been directed to educate patients, and physicians, about the lack of effectiveness of antibiotics in treating common viral infections.[15] This collaboration is a good example of effective integrative ethics where public health officials, individual practitioners, and patients communicate to arrive at policies that meet the needs of individuals and communities.

Communicability

Many infectious diseases are directly communicable from person to person. Others are transmitted indirectly from one person to another. Communicabil-ity thus implicates people as vectors, and may raise questions of responsibility, at least in some sense. Different patterns of communicability may raise different ethical issues. At least three patterns will compel our attention here: first, when the patient is a risk to the community in general; second, when the patient is a risk to health-care providers; and third, when health-care providers pose a risk to their patients. In each of these scenarios we must identify who poses risks of communicability, who can best avoid communication, who should take pre-ventive measures, and who should bear the costs of these preventive efforts.

Communicability essentially involves the ways human beings interact—the various levels of intimacy they have with one another. When intimacy becomes a serious threat, it is necessary to change these interactions if the danger of in-fection reaches a certain threshold and the judgment is that it should be pre-vented. But what is this threshold? And which behaviors may society justifiably

---

14. M.R. Jacobs, "Emergence of Antibiotic Resistance in Upper and Lower Respiratory Tract In-fections," *American Journal of Managed Care* 5 (1999): S651-S661.
15. S.B. Levy, *The Antibiotic Paradox: How the Misuse of Antibiotics Destroys Their Curative Pow-ers*, 2nd ed. (Cambridge: Perseus, 2002), 304-308.

require to be altered? And what degree of force ought to be used to achieve this altered behavior? And who should bear the costs of the requirements? And how can society make it up to those who have borne costs, physical risks, or even death, to benefit everyone? Once again, difficult questions of moral principle, individual choice, and public health come to the fore at the threat of infection.

For example, the decisions of some communities to require patients with tuberculosis to accept therapy under strict observation, and in extreme cases to quarantine infectious patients who refuse, have engendered considerable debate among medical ethicists and political leaders.[16] Sometimes the public's fear of communicable infections far exceeds the actual risk. Sometimes it may not, as with the extensively resistant strains of tuberculosis that have become apparent in South Africa in Tugula Ferry, KwaZulu Natal Province.[17] Although leprosy is not very contagious, since Biblical times the public has tended to drive lepers from their communities and to exile them to remote islands and villages. Only recently, since antimicrobial therapy has been shown to control leprosy, has the practice of isolation and exile of these patients ceased in the United States. In Parts IV and V, we shall explore how such fright-induced and overly restrictive practices have failed to appreciate the victimhood of those they affected and thus violated basic principles about what we owe each other in the context of infectious disease.

Some social behaviors, including unprotected sex with multiple partners and intravenous drug use, are highly linked to the risk of acquiring infectious diseases such as hepatitis and AIDS. These behavioral associations with infectious diseases have led to considerable discussion about potential conflicts between autonomy, community moral values, and effective but controversial public health practices. For example, the regular use of condoms has been shown to be effective in reducing the spread of many venereal diseases such as syphilis, gonorrhea, and HIV infections. However, the effective public health practice of distributing condoms may conflict with community religious and moral values, and the spread of these diseases may not be adequately controlled because of the conflict. Similarly, the public health practice of providing clean needles and syringes to drug addicts that has been shown to decrease the spread of HIV and hepatitis virus infections has been discouraged in many communities because of conflict with local cultural and moral values.[18]

---

16. E.W. Campion "Liberty and the Control of Tuberculosis," *New England Journal of Medicine* 1340 (1999): 385–386.

17. World Health Organization, "The Global MDR-TB and XDR-TB Response Plan 2007–2008," http://www.stoptb.org/resource_center/assets/documents/Global%20MDR-TB_and_%20XDR-TB_Response%20Plan_2007–08.pdf (accessed June 2007).

18. See, e.g., Jonathan M. Mann, "Medicine and Public Health, Ethics and Human Rights," *Hastings Center Report* 28, no. 1 (1998): 6–13 (9).

The current worldwide AIDS epidemic has appropriately sensitized the public to the risks of being exposed to contaminated blood and body secretions. However, the fear of communicability is scientifically inappropriate and ethically an injustice to infected individuals when HIV-infected children like Ryan White are barred from schools, and when some physicians and other health care workers refuse to care for AIDS patients. These patients are victims, as much as they are vectors, and, as we shall argue, are deserving of our respect.

The concept that the patient may also be the vector of a potentially lethal infectious disease becomes particularly complicated when the patient is a physician, nurse, or other caregiver. Physicians, dentists, and nurses are at an increased risk of becoming infected with hepatitis viruses, and the HIV viruses that cause AIDS because of their exposure to blood and body fluids from infected patients, especially where universal precautions are not observed.[19] The ethics of professionalism are challenged when these caregivers refuse to treat infected patients because of this risk, and when caregivers infected with these viruses continue to practice their profession in ways that increase the risk of transmission of their infections to patients.[20]

A smallpox scare in a major U.S. city, Seattle, illustrates that institutions as well as individuals may react inappropriately due to fear of communicable diseases.[21] An airline passenger was detained at the airport upon landing because he had developed a generalized rash that resembled smallpox. The patient and the possibly exposed passengers were appropriately temporarily detained on the aircraft while expert clinical opinion was obtained. In the process of evaluating the patient, public health officials contacted the major hospitals in the city to determine which hospital would accept the patient for care if the diagnosis were confirmed. Every hospital refused to accept the patient. Although the diagnosis fortunately was not confirmed, this episode illustrated the need to identify and equip hospitals in each community to care for suspected smallpox patients as part of bioterrorism planning. It also illustrated the conflict between hospitals' missions to care for the sick, and possibly their fear that accepting such a patient would expose other patients to smallpox. It is possible that they were also concerned that accepting this patient would be costly and would hurt their business by discouraging patients from coming to their hospital.

19. G. Ippolito, V. Puro, J. Heptonstal et al., "Occupational Human Immunodeficiency Virus Infection in Health Care Workers: Worldwide Cases Through September 1997," *Clinical Infectious Disease.* 28 (1999): 365–383.
20. K.A. DeVille, "Nothing to Fear but Fear Itself: HIV-Infected Physicians and the Law of Informed Consent," *Journal of Law, Medicine, and Ethics* 22 (1994): 163–175.
21. Charles B. Smith, personal communication.

Communicable Diseases Typically Have No Respect for Political Boundaries

The need for international cooperation to control the spread of these diseases has been a powerful force in the development of international public health programs, such as the World Health Organization, and in the evolution of international quarantine laws. Epidemic communicable diseases, such as cholera, tuberculosis, and AIDS, have required negotiating common public health policies, rules, and regulations between communities that may have quite different values and ethical principles. Infectious diseases, it is often said, know no borders. For example, within a few months after religious leaders in the Nigerian state of Kano ordered the cessation of polio vaccination efforts, the disease had spread to 7 neighboring countries,[22] and eventually on to 19 countries overall.[23] SARS spread from Hong Kong to Toronto via a single index patient's intercontinental flight.[24] Avian flu, moving throughout Southeast Asia and beyond, is at the top of the current most feared list. Writers such as Larry Gostin[25] and David Fidler[26] have and continue to deal in systematic ways with questions of national and international law raised by the transmission of disease within and across borders. Meanwhile, enteric pathogens like salmonella, *Escherichia coli* 0157, cyclospora, and listeria travel easily across local and national boundaries in an increasingly international and consolidated food supply.[27] Other global problems, including environmental degradation, population growth, refugee migration, and widespread poverty, feed reservoirs of infection that are transnational and international matters of concern.

Preventability and Treatability

Most infectious diseases, as already noted, are preventable or treatable. While there currently are no therapies or effective methods for preventing some infectious diseases such as Ebola and SARS, there are effective preventive measures

---

22. Stephen Pincock, "Poliovirus Spreads Beyond Nigeria After Vaccine Uptake Drops," *British Medical Journal* 328 (2004): 310.
23. World Health Organization, *World Health Report 2007—A Safer Future: Global Health Security in the 21st Century*, http://www.who.int/whr/2007/en/index.html (accessed February 9, 2008), 21.
24. Tomislav Svoboda et al., "Public Health Measures to Control the Spread of the Severe Acute Respiratory Syndrome During the Outbreak in Toronto," *New England Journal of Medicine* 350 (2004): 2352–2361.
25. See, e.g., Lawrence O. Gostin, *Public Health Law: Power, Duty, Restraint* (Berkeley: University of California Press, 2000).
26. See, e.g., David P. Fidler, *International Law and Infectious Diseases* (Oxford: Oxford University Press, 1999).
27. Ann Marie Kimball, *Risky Trade: Infectious Disease in the Era of Global Trade* (Aldershot, UK: Ashgate, 2006).

or therapies, though not always vaccines, for most of those infectious diseases that are the greatest causes of mortality worldwide. This poses a dilemma that is at the root of many of the most heated discussions over ethical and social resource issues related to infectious diseases: if effective therapies and preventive measures are available, why are these diseases still major causes of mortality? Although effective preventive measures and therapies exist, individuals and communities may choose not to employ them for various reasons. Religious convictions are sometimes cited as reasons for refusing immunization; individuals may value their religious practices more than they value the decreased risk of infection that inoculation provides. Personal fears about side effects or concerns about the actual effectiveness of immunizations can also be reasons for refusal. Populations that would benefit from preventive measures against infectious diseases are not always ready or willing to employ such measures, and the extent to which more developed nations ought to impose these measures is a compelling question. Improvements in sanitation, availability of clean water, and relief of poverty and overcrowding conditions have all been major factors in the control of infectious diseases in developed countries. In developing countries, the need for resources to achieve these environmental improvements is often in competition with the need for resources for education, industrial development, military actions and, unfortunately, in some cases, the support of unethical rulers. Although improving, financial support from developed countries to those in need in the developing world still lags far behind what the WHO and other agencies perceive as reasonable contributions to improve world health.

The relative high cost of antimicrobials is a continuing reason why many patients in developed nations do not receive appropriate therapy for their infections. The recent heated dialogue over availability of much less expensive generic (non-patented) anti-HIV medications in developing countries such as Brazil, India, Kenya, and South Africa, is rooted in the ethical dilemma over the conflicting needs of patients in poor countries for these medicines and the desires of drug manufacturers to protect their patents and related profits. The issues raised by intellectual property rights related to antibiotics have also been a major cause of ethical argument in the United States. A major drug company stopped manufacturing oral Cefixime, an antimicrobial that had a valuable unique application in treatment of venereal diseases, because its patent had expired and profits were no longer attractive,[28] leaving practitioners with less satisfactory alternatives. .[29] Despite its clear advantages in the treatment of

---

28. Centers for Disease Control and Prevention, "Discontinuation of Cefixime Tablets—United States," *Mortality and Morbidity Weekly Report* 51, no. 46 (November 22, 2002): 1052.

29. Centers for Disease Control and Prevention, "Oral Alternatives to Cefixime for the Treatment of Uncomplicated Neisseria Gonorrhoeae Urogenital Infections," http://www.cdc.gov/std/treatment/cefixime.htm (accessed December 29, 2007).

gonorrhea, Cefixime remained off the market for six years until April 2008, when it was released by another manufacturer.[30]

As noted before, excessive and inappropriate use of antimicrobials by patients and clinicians—as well as in animal husbandry[31]—has been a major cause of development of resistance to antimicrobials. One cause of this excessive use has been an increasingly aggressive commercial advertising campaign by many drug companies to promote the use of the newest, most expensive, and most profitable patented antimicrobials. In Chapter 13, we take up this issue of antibiotic resistance in greater detail.

Vaccines for infectious diseases such as polio, measles, chickenpox, and smallpox have been effective in nearly eradicating these diseases from the developed world. These vaccines are effective not only for the individual recipients, but also to create "herd immunity"—that is, to reduce the incidence of these infections in whole communities. This dual effect has raised ethical issues when selected individuals, families, or religious groups assert rights to refuse vaccination and as a result increase the risks of the remaining population to infection.[32]

Host Susceptibility

The general health of the host determines susceptibility to many infectious diseases. While some infectious diseases such as Ebola virus and smallpox are so virulent that they will attack all humans regardless of their general health status, susceptibility to most infectious diseases is highly linked to the general health of the host. Susceptibility to infection and the resulting morbidity and mortality from such common infectious diseases as tuberculosis, enteric pathogens, and acute respiratory tract diseases is highly correlated with nutrition and general health status. The relatively high mortality rates for the common infant diarrheas and childhood respiratory tract infections seen in malnourished children in poor African nations and in wartime refugee camps dramatically illustrate this association. This realization leads to frequent debate about the just distribution of community resources. It has been argued that available but limited resources should primarily go toward providing adequate nutrition before resources are spent on more expensive and possibly less effective medical services.

---

30. Centers for Disease Control and Prevention. 2008. Availability of Cefixime 400 mg. Tablets. United States, April 2008. *Morbidity and Mortality Weekly Report* 57, no. 16 (April 25): 435
31. M.J. Gilcrist et al., "The Potential Role of Concentrated Animal Feeding Operations in Infectious Disease Epidemics and Antibiotic Resistance," *Environmental Health. Perspectives.* 115, no. 2 (2007): 313–316.
32. L.F. Ross and T. Aspinwell, "Religious Exemptions to the Immunization Statutes: Balancing Public Health and Religious Freedom.," *Journal of Law, Medicine & Ethics* 25 (1997): 202–209.

Ethical discussions about treatment of infectious diseases may also be involved in end of life cases. With many non-infectious conditions, the effectiveness of giving treatment to individuals whose health is already poor may be seen as not outweighing the costs of such treatment. In these instances, the cost and burdens may be very high, while the health benefit is low. Patients dying of cancer and other debilitating diseases are often more susceptible to infectious diseases such as pneumonia. With a patient who is near the end of life, and who then develops a treatable infectious disease, the cost and burdens of treatment may be quite low, but the benefit is also said to remain low. With treatment of the infection, the result may be simply a prolongation of the status quo, already a deteriorating condition. Just as they sometimes refuse respirators, chemotherapy, and other components of life-prolonging therapy, some patients choose to refuse antibiotics in episodes of pneumonia, thus letting themselves die. These issues are highly controversial in current medical ethics and will be discussed in Chapter 8.

Community and Global Susceptibility

The general health of the community environment determines susceptibility to many infectious diseases. The social and environmental health status of communities includes the provision of sanitation, hygiene, availability of clean air, water, and food, adequate nutrition, control of mosquitoes, and other vectors of infectious diseases. This social infrastructure has significant effects on the susceptibility of community members to infectious diseases.[33] The strong association of poverty and poor environmental health with infectious diseases raises ethical issues of justice and human rights.

The WHO estimates that at least two-thirds of the world's population lacks safe sanitation and one-quarter lacks access to safe water.[34] It is not surprising then that in these undeveloped communities infantile diarrhea continues to be a major cause of death worldwide. The poverty-associated crowding and lack of hygiene in central Africa has for more than 100 years been associated with a very high rate of meningococcal meningitis. In a 1996 outbreak, more than 15,000 Africans died of this acute and often fatal infection, and mortality remains high in the "meningitis belt" in Africa.[35]

Poverty-related lack of hygiene and associated increased susceptibility to infectious diseases continue to be problems even in highly developed countries

---

33. Jim Whitman, ed., *The Politics of Emerging and Resurgent Infectious Diseases* (New York: St. Martin's Press, 2000), 6.
34. Ibid., 2.
35. N.E. Rosenstein, B.A. Perkins, D.S. Stephens et al., "Meningococcal Disease," *New England Journal of Medicine* 344 (2001): 1378–1388.

such as France and the United States. Outbreaks of tuberculosis, diphtheria, and louse-borne trench fever have recently been observed in the homeless population in several cities in the United States.[36]

In most wars, morbidity and mortality from infectious diseases has exceeded that of military actions. War-associated refugee camps continue to suffer from high attack rates and mortalities from measles, cholera, infantile diarrheas, acute respiratory tract diseases, and malaria.[37] This phenomenon illustrates the effect of war-related disruptions of community socio-economic conditions on infectious diseases. The public realization that this link exists can generate considerable fear and influence decisions to abandon communities during wartimes and create refugee crises. Although not a direct form of biowarfare, the military strategy of disrupting social, economic, and public health systems and encouraging refugee migrations has the same effect of precipitating outbreaks of infectious diseases and killing large numbers of civilians.

It is a truism that infectious diseases know no borders. Try as one nation-state to close immigration to people who may bring diseases with them, these efforts will prove futile for at least some modes of disease transmission. Rats hop ships and spread the plague, mosquitoes stow away on airplanes or infest new regions as the climate warms, and birds migrate around the globe. Infections that emerge in one corner of the earth may cause deaths far away. Poor systems of public health or medical treatment and attendant injustices that foster disease may, quite literally, put everyone at risk. Infectious disease thus presents issues of international justice in starkest form.

High Socio-Economic Impact

Infectious diseases may lead to deterioration in community socio-economic status. In this regard, there is a tremendous amount at stake. The link between low community economic status and susceptibility to infectious diseases goes both ways. For centuries the devastating effects of worldwide epidemics, such as the plague and influenza, on local and even world economies have been well known. The outbreak of bubonic plague in Europe in the mid fourteenth century killed at least one-third of Europe's population, and the effects on local and regional commerce were extraordinary.[38] The 1918 worldwide influenza

36. P. Brouqui, B. Lascola, V. Roux, and D. Raoult, "Chronic Bartonella Quintana Bacteremia in Homeless Patients," *New England Journal of Medicine* 340 (1999): 184–189.

37. Jim Whitman, ed., "Refugee Infections," in *The Politics of Emerging and Resurgent Infectious Diseases* (New York: St. Martin's Press, 2000), ch. 6.

38. M. Drexler, *Secret Agents: The Menace of Emerging Infections* (Washington, DC: Joseph Henry Press, 2002), 4.

epidemic killed an estimated 21 million people, an effect on mortality and economic development that rivaled that of World War I.[39] This raises issues of the economic responsibility of societies to maintain conditions that discourage infections and to treat outbreaks. This is not to say that the primary reason to treat infectious disease is to improve economic outlook—the primary reason is relief of human suffering—but it is to point out that infectious disease is both contributor to and result of global poverty.

Most recently, awareness has grown of the destructive effects of the AIDS epidemic on the economies of countries where as many as 25% of the working age population can be taken out of the work force by this infection. The fear of continued spread of the HIV infection and resulting AIDS mortality has been compounded by the realization and fear that the decline in socio-economic and public health services is associated with epidemics of tuberculosis and other infectious diseases. These fears have led some community leaders to deny publicly the incidence of some infectious diseases, such as AIDS and SARS, a violation of the truth-telling ethic that has seriously delayed and obstructed needed community public health control measures.[40]

The 2002 Macroeconomics and Health Report to the World Health Organization recognized the synergy between economic development and infectious diseases by emphasizing that economic growth is not possible without a healthy population.[41] This realization speaks for a more just distribution of resources between the rich and poor nations. In the 2002 meeting of the World Health Assembly, the Commission on Macroeconomics and Health reported that the world now has the capability of ending poverty and poverty-associated diseases for the first time in history: the cost to the rich developed countries would only be one penny out of every $10 of gross national product (GNP).[42] By 2005, the UN had increased the suggested level of support to five pennies (0.5%) out of every $10 of GNP, and five countries (Norway, Denmark, Luxembourg, Sweden, and the Netherlands had each achieved a higher level

39. Jared Diamond, *Guns, Germs and Steel* (New York: W.W. Norton, 1999), 202.
40. Michael J. Selgelid discusses the failure of South Africa to tell the truth about their AIDS epidemic in *Ethics and Infectious Disease*, Michael J. Selgelid, Margaret P. Battin, and Charles B. Smith eds. (Oxford: Blackwell, 2006), ch. 1. For a discussion of the failures of Chinese leaders to acknowledge the presence of SARS, see L.O. Gostin, R. Bayer, and A.L. Fairchild, "Ethical and Legal Challenges Posed by SARS: Implications for the Control of Serious Infectious Disease Threats, " *Journal of the American Medical Association* 290 (2003): 3229–3237. See also P. Fritsch, M. Pottinger, and L. Chang, "Divergent Asian Responses Show Difficulties in Dealing with SARS," *Wall Street Journal*, sec. A, April 7, 2003.
41. D. Banta, "Economic Development: Key to Healthier World," *Journal of the American Medical Association* 287 (2002): 3195–3197.
42. Ibid.

by giving 0.7% of GNP.[43] Countries of the European Union had agreed to meet the 0.7% funding level by 2015.[44]

In Sum

The distinctive characteristics of infectious diseases that we have identified—high morbidity and mortality, invasiveness, acuity, communicability, spreading across borders, preventability and treatability, host susceptibility, community and global susceptibility, and high socio-economic impact—are not shared among all infectious diseases. In addition, although many of the characteristics of infectious diseases mentioned in this chapter may be present in non-infectious diseases, taken together they comprise a group of traits that raise far-reaching and distinctive ethical concerns. The distinctive characteristics of infectious disease all contribute to the difficulty of ethical issues in diagnosis, treatment, and prevention. Yet they have been underappreciated in bioethics, as we shall now explore.

43. Celia W. Dugger, "U.N. Proposes Doubling of Aid to Cut Poverty," *New York Times*, sec. A, January 18, 2005.
44. *US Fed News*, "World Summit Examines Progress in Meeting Development Financing Commitments Made Five Years Ago in Monterrey," September 14, 2005. For a follow up report, see World Health Organization, *Tough Choices: Investing in Health for Development* (Geneva: World Health Organization, 2006), http://www.who.int/macrohealth/documents/report_and_cover.pdf (accessed August 2007), 27.

4

HOW INFECTIOUS DISEASE GOT LEFT OUT
OF BIOETHICS

Bioethics emerged as a field between the late 1950s and the 1970s. This was the period of civil rights activism and legal responses, from *Brown v. Board of Education* in 1954[1] to the Civil Rights Act of 1964 and the Age Discrimination in Employment Act of 1967. It was also a period of growing environmental concern, fueled by the publication of Rachel Carson's *Silent Spring* in 1962[2] and implemented by the National Environmental Policy Act of 1964, the Clean Air Act of 1970, and the Clean Water Act of 1972. Medicare came on the scene in 1965, in the midst of other programs designed to end poverty.

The period of the late 1950s through the early 1970s, before the recognition of HIV/AIDS, was also a period when infectious disease was increasingly regarded as a receding problem, a health threat largely conquered. As we have seen in Chapter 1, the pronouncement attributed to the U.S. Surgeon General, purportedly closing the book on infectious disease, reflected this optimism. As we shall see in this chapter, this optimism—in retrospect so obviously unwarranted—was simply assumed as the field of bioethics developed. Perhaps even more surprising, similar optimism was to be found to a certain extent in the field of public health, with attention increasingly devoted to environmental hazards and to patterns of behavior identified as problematic such as smoking or weight gain. Only with HIV/AIDS—and then in the main limited to HIV/AIDS—did characteristic features of infectious diseases come to the fore for discussion in bioethics. Here, what were regarded as "exceptional" features of HIV/AIDS truncated appreciation of the more general theoretical challenges infectious diseases posed for bioethics.

An earlier version of this chapter appeared as Leslie P. Francis, Margaret P. Battin, Jay A. Jacobson, Charles B. Smith, and Jeffrey Botkin, "How Infectious Disease Got Left Out—and What This Omission Might Have Meant for Bioethics," *Bioethics*, special issue on ethics and infectious disease, ed. Michael J. Selgelid and Margaret P. Battin, also in Michael J. Selgelid, Margaret P. Battin, and Charles B. Smith, eds., *Ethics and Infectious Disease* (Oxford: Blackwell, 2006).

1. Brown v. Board of Education of Topeka, 347 U.S. 483 (1954).
2. Rachel Carson, *Silent Spring* (Boston: Houghton-Mifflin, 1962).

The discipline of public health continued to consider the spread of disease and the overall health of populations. But in public health discussions during the period of the early development of bioethics, attention had shifted away from infectious disease to problems such as the health effects of cigarettes or DDT and other environmental toxins.[3] Writers in public health, like writers in bioethics, viewed infectious disease as largely conquered; ethical problems like the protection of confidentiality were set aside as largely moot. Although the fields of public health and public health law featured discussions that recognized the differences between aggregative, population-based approaches and the individualism of clinical medicine, scholars in the field of bioethics and in the field of public health rarely engaged with each other in ways that brought their paradigms of analysis into fruitful dialogue. This has begun to change to some extent, as the American Public Health Association has published a code of ethics (in 2002) and a number of special issues of journals in bioethics have been devoted to the ethics of public health or to ethical issues that are highly salient to the field of public health, such as international human rights and health.[4] Nonetheless, until recently, as we demonstrate in this chapter and the next, the public health discussions and the field of bioethics developed separately, and the two never really met.

These formative developments—the absence of attention to infectious disease in early bioethics, and the failure of extensive dialogue between public health and the new field of bioethics—were not benign. Virtual omission of issues concerning infectious disease and lack of awareness of the characteristic features of infectious disease affected the choice, framing, and discussion of problems in bioethics. Bioethics issues were framed not only in the context of the individual physician/patient encounter, but also in terms of encounters that did not typically raise immediate issues of serious physical risks to others. This myopia reached the deepest theoretical levels, where basic normative commitments such as autonomy, and indeed the relationship between clinical medicine and public health, were understood without examination of the moral significance of communicable infectious disease.

We begin the discussion about how infectious disease got left out of bioethics and public health with a survey of the field of bioethics in its early years. In the next chapter, we continue with an account of the dialogue in public health

---

3. See, e.g., Carson, *Silent Spring*. The term "bioethics" actually originated in discussions of ethics and the biosphere, but quickly came to be applied to ethical issues in health care. It is interesting to speculate whether links between bioethics and public health might have been forged much earlier had "bioethics" continued to encompass not only human but also environmental health. See, e.g., Peter J. Whitehouse, "The Rebirth of Bioethics: Extending the Original Formulations of Van Rensselaer Potter," *American Journal of Bioethics* 3, no. 4 (2003): W21-W26.

4. See Public Health Leadership Society, *Principles of the Ethical Practice of Public Health*, Version 2.2, Public Health Leadership Society (2002), http://www.apha.org/NR/rdonlyres/1CED3CEA-287E-4185-9CBD-BD405FC60856/0/ethicsbrochure.pdf (accessed December 29, 2007).

during roughly the same period. Although it requires the meticulous documentation we present here, the survey in this chapter is a needed corrective to pictures of the field of bioethics that have been formed in the wake of HIV/AIDS. The absence of infectious disease in the discussions of the early period of bioethics was virtually complete, and may be particularly surprising to younger scholars whose entire conversance with bioethics and public health postdates the emergence of AIDS. Moreover, although HIV/AIDS reintroduced problems of contagion and therefore might have become a serious connecting point to public health, it did not press bioethics in the way a full consideration of the range of infectious diseases might have done. The discussion in these two chapters concludes with the significance of what has been regarded as the dual "exceptionalism" of HIV/AIDS, both in its characteristics as an infectious disease and in its highly politicized nature, and a response to the question of whether bioethics could have been different: indeed, it could have been, as it approached HIV/AIDS and other challenges.

Leaving Out Infectious Disease: The Early Texts in Bioethics

A review of the texts in a field can be remarkably informative about how the field understands itself. We have comprehensively inspected the early texts in bioethics, including the monographs, anthologies, and published case studies that constituted the literature of the emerging field, in order to see what issues and cases were seen as canonical. We cannot be certain we have uncovered everything, of course, but we can show that in the formal discussions of bioethics that actually made it to the printed page, infectious disease was indeed—with an apparent single exception—virtually left out.

The earliest texts in bioethics, as the field is currently understood, date from the 1950s. They were written and published primarily in the United States; active discussions and publication programs in bioethics in Europe, Asia, and elsewhere began to flourish a decade or more after the emergence of the field in the United States. We have reviewed 19 texts published before 1984 (and thus before the advent of HIV/AIDS) to determine the extent and manner of these texts' consideration of infectious disease. These include the texts most widely used in bioethics courses, such as Gorovitz, Macklin, Jameton, O'Connor, and Sherwin's famous *Moral Problems in Medicine*, the first of the bioethics anthologies.[5] They also include Beauchamp and Childress's now-canonical *Principles of Biomedical Ethics*, first published in 1979, also often revised and now in a

---

5. Samuel Gorovitz, Ruth Macklin, Andrew L. Jameton, John M. O'Connor, and Susan Sherwin, eds., *Moral Problems in Medicine*, 2nd ed. (Englewood Cliffs, NJ: Prentice-Hall, 1983) (originally published 1976).

fifth edition.[6] We also examined the text in most widespread clinical use, Jonsen, Siegler, and Winslade's influential *Clinical Ethics*—the compact medical-ethics reference published in 1982 that would fit into the pocket of a physician's white coat.[7]

Our finding is that systematic discussion of ethical problems raised by communicable infectious disease is manifestly absent from these early texts. Even cases and examples involving infectious conditions are rare at best. The only significant exception to this claim is the Jonsen, Siegler, and Winslade volume, which includes acute infectious disease as one model of clinical care and addresses this model at points in the ethical discussion. What follows is a comprehensive account of the appearance of infectious disease in the early texts. We have cited the entire reference where it occurs; the infectious disease examples that do appear typically are given very short discussion or perhaps only passing mention, not the kind of sustained treatment afforded other examples such as the withdrawal of life sustaining treatment in a patient in a persistent vegetative state.

In general, early texts in the field of bioethics mention infectious disease only sporadically, if at all. Several texts mention infectious disease only to dismiss it as a problem that has largely been resolved; for example, Beauchamp and Walters' *Contemporary Issues in Bioethics* (1978)[8] and Davis, Hoffmaster, and Shorten's *Contemporary Issues in Biomedical Ethics*, also 1978.[9] Only the Jonsen, Siegler, and Winslade text presents a systematic account of the characteristics of infectious disease that might be ethically relevant, such as its acuity and unexpected nature, but even this text does not recognize the full range of characteristics of many infectious diseases that we have presented in Chapter 3.[10]

Where infectious disease was discussed and examples drawn from infectious disease were used, patient confidentiality was typically regarded as the primary issue of concern for bioethics. Four of the early texts consider the conflict between patient confidentiality and protection of others in brief discussions of infectious disease examples such as tuberculosis or sexually transmitted diseases.[11] Notably, neither of the two widely used early texts—Gorovitz et al.'s

6. Tom L. Beauchamp and James F. Childress, *Principles of Biomedical Ethics* (New York: Oxford University Press, 1979).

7. Albert R. Jonsen, Mark Siegler, and William J. Winslade, *Clinical Ethics* (New York: Macmillan, 1982).

8. Tom L. Beauchamp and LeRoy Walters, eds., *Contemporary Issues in Bioethics* (Encino, CA: Dickenson, 1978), 58.

9. John W. Davis, Barry Hoffmaster, and Sarah Shorten, eds., *Contemporary Issues in Biomedical Ethics* (Clifton, NJ: Humana Press, 1978), vi.

10. Jonsen, Siegler, and Winslade, *Clinical Ethics*, 18–20.

11. These four are Joseph Fletcher's seminal *Morals and Medicine* (Princeton: Princeton University Press, 1959 and 1979), 56–57; Jonsen, Siegler, and Winslade's *Clinical Ethics*, 154; Thomas A. Mappes

1976 *Moral Problems in Medicine*[12] and Robert Veatch's 1977 *Case Studies in Medical Ethics*[13]—considers a single infectious disease example in the context of whether it is appropriate for a physician to violate patient confidentiality. Jonsen, Siegler, and Winslade's pocket reference is a counterexample; it uses an acute infectious disease—meningitis—initially as a dilemma posed for the physician in clinical care when the patient refuses treatment and then as an example of whether there is a duty to warn others who may be put at risk by the patient's refusal.[14] Their handbook also analyzes the relatively standard example of a husband refusing to inform his spouse about a venereal disease, as well as the remarkably contemporary example of whether a physician is obligated to report a health care worker who is hepatitis B positive to the director of a dialysis unit.[15]

Infectious disease examples also sometimes appear in discussions of the need to protect health-care workers or the public. Healy's 1956 *Medical Ethics* mentions the duty of a physician to alert a nurse to the presence of infection in order to allow her to protect herself.[16] A few texts mention quarantine in the face of an epidemic.[17] Just one text, Reiser, Dyck, and Curran's *Ethics in Medicine: Historical Perspectives and Contemporary Concerns*,[18] presents materials that consider ethical problems in public health in a sustained manner, including mention of the socio-economic impact of infectious conditions such as yellow fever. Only Hunt and Arras portray control of an infectious condition (viral hepatitis) as a "foremost" problem in preventive medicine; this discussion occurs in the context of their treatment of the problems of research ethics raised by the Willowbrook experiments on transmission of infectious hepatitis among institutionalized children.[19]

Several of the most notorious scandal cases in research ethics involved infectious diseases. In the Willowbrook experiment, children in a facility for people with intellectual impairments were deliberately exposed to hepatitis A as part of a study of transmission of the disease in institutional settings. The researchers

and Jane S. Zembaty, *Biomedical Ethics* (New York: McGraw-Hill, 1981), 117; and the very early text by Charles J. McFadden, *Medical Ethics*, 4th ed. (Philadelphia: F.A. Davis, 1956), 435.

12. For the discussion of confidentiality, see Gorovitz et al., *Moral Problems in Medicine*, 157.

13. For the discussion of confidentiality, see Robert M. Veatch, *Case Studies in Medical Ethics* (Cambridge: Harvard University Press, 1977), 127.

14. Jonsen, Siegler, and Winslade, *Clinical Ethics*, 18–20, 172.

15. Ibid., 154, 174.

16. Edwin F. Healy, *Medical Ethics* (Chicago: Loyola University Press, 1956), 26.

17. Robert Hunt and John Arras, *Ethical Issues in Modern Medicine* (Palo Alto, CA: Mayfield, 1977), 334; Jonsen, Siegler, and Winslade, *Clinical Ethics*, 171; McFadden, *Medical Ethics*, 433; and Wade Robison and Michael Pritchard, *Medical Responsibility* (Clifton, NJ: Humana Press, 1979), 30.

18. Stanley Joel Reiser, Arthur J. Dyck, and William J. Curran, eds., *Ethics in Medicine: Historical Perspectives and Contemporary Concerns* (Cambridge: MIT Press, 1977), 554.

19. Hunt and Arras, *Ethical Issues in Modern Medicine*, 291.

argued that because virtually all children in this hospital would eventually get hepatitis A, it was permissible to infect them deliberately in the interests of better understanding the epidemiology of the disease. A number of the early bioethics texts mention the ethical dilemma posed by Willowbrook—but largely as a problem about coercion and vulnerable subjects.[20] Several other texts refer to vaccine testing on children as examples of problems in the ethics of research.[21]

In the Tuskegee syphilis study, perhaps the most infamous example of the abuse of research subjects in the United States, the U.S. Public Health Service continued to observe the natural history of syphilis in untreated African-American males long after effective therapy had become available. The researchers did not tell these "subjects" that effective treatment was available, and deliberately concealed this option from them, yet monitored their condition under the guise of offering care. The Tuskegee study was stopped in 1972 after several high-profile newspaper reports, but there is virtually no mention of the study or the moral issues it raised in the early bioethics texts. Even when the study was finally discussed, the consequences of not treating this transmissible disease for others in addition to the men themselves are still not a focus of concern, as we shall show in Chapter 10. As Chapter 10 details more fully, the treatments of Willowbrook, Tuskegee, and other cases of problematic research involving infectious disease were notable for the absence of attention to the possible contagiousness of the conditions under research, concentrating instead on the vulnerability of the study populations, coercion in institutional settings, and racial discrimination and exploitation. These cases were discussed as examples of research malfeasance, but without raising concerns specific to the contagiousness of the conditions under study. No attention was given in the early bioethics literature to whether latent syphilis, the condition under primary study in the Tuskegee experiment, was transmissible or not. Although the 1979 edition of Beauchamp and Childress, for instance, uses the Willowbrook example, it does not discuss Tuskegee at all.

In addition, the early texts contain a limited number of references to how infectious disease may affect patient decision making or the role of the physician in the physician–patient relationship. The possibility that contagion might justify compulsory lifesaving treatment is mentioned in Beauchamp and Walters's 1978 *Contemporary Issues in Bioethics*[22] and in Jonsen, Siegler, and Winslade.[23] Gorovitz et al. discuss the case of pneumococcal meningitis as an

20. Gorovitz et al., *Moral Problems in Medicine*, 603; Paul Ramsey, *The Patient as Person*, 3rd ed. (New Haven: Yale University Press, 1973), 47; Veatch, *Case Studies in Medical Ethics*, 275.

21. Ramsey, *The Patient as Person*, 15–17; Reiser, Dyck, and Curran, *Ethics in Medicine*, 456.

22. Beauchamp and Walters, *Contemporary Issues in Bioethics*, 58.

23. Jonsen, Siegler, and Winslade, *Clinical Ethics*, 62, 78 (meningitis).

example of how delay in treatment might be related to severity of outcome—
thus recognizing the acuity of some infectious conditions—but do not give
the case more systematic discussion.[24] In his 1982 *Doctors' Dilemmas: Moral
Conflict and Medical Care*, Gorovitz mentions the risk of reactions to smallpox
vaccination in the course of discussing the importance of characteristics of
the individual patient to decision making.[25] This discussion, however, focuses
on the risks to the individual patient rather than on the implications for others of the failure to immunize or the potential infectiousness of the person
vaccinated; it is presented as part of a discussion of risks to patients rather
than of the implications of contagiousness. Finally, Edmunds and Scorer's
Ethical Responsibility in Medicine: A Christian Approach gives the example of
maternal rubella in discussing the morality of abortion.[26] Here again, the emphasis is on the significance of the potential damage to the fetus, not the fact
that the damage was acquired by vertical transmission from the mother. In
Chapter 11, we discuss whether there are special features of vertical infectious
transmission in comparison to vertical transmission of genetic traits. Vigorous
discussions of issues about transmissibility appeared in venues outside the
bioethics literature; for example, the medical journals published multiple discussions of the risks and benefits of using live in comparison to killed polio
vaccine, recognizing that immunization of one child with a vaccine that sheds
live virus in a household where there was another, immune-compromised
child might pose risks to that sibling. But as we shall detail in Chapter 10,
these discussions historically were not framed as "ethics" issues and they were
not scrutinized within the field of bioethics.

Things change somewhat by the early 1980s, when HIV/AIDS was recognized. But the changes were less than might have been expected, at least in the
standard textbooks. Although HIV/AIDS is discussed, infectious disease more
generally is not. To assess the extent of the changes brought by HIV/AIDS, we
have compared the fifth and latest edition of the primary theoretical text in
the field, Beauchamp and Childress's *Principles of Biomedical Ethics*, published
in 2001, to its first edition, which appeared in 1979, before the entry of HIV/
AIDS onto the bioethics scene. Infectious disease is slightly more prominent
in the later edition, but the difference is due almost entirely to HIV/AIDS, not
to greater attention to the overall significance of infectious disease. The 1979
edition had mentioned infectious disease only twice. Once, in discussing the
physician–patient relationship, it had considered the example of a physician

24. Gorovitz et al., *Moral Problems in Medicine*.
25. Samuel Gorovitz, *Doctors' Dilemmas: Moral Conflict and Medical Care* (New York: Oxford
University Press, 1982), 27.
26. Vincent Edmunds and C. Gordon Scorer, eds., *Ethical Responsibility in Medicine: A Christian
Approach* (London: E. & S. Livingstone, 1967), 64.

performing an employment physical who might not think of the person being examined as his/her patient. If the physician discovers the person has tuberculosis, Beauchamp and Childress had concluded, the physician has a moral (but not a legal) duty to disclose the information to the patient and to withdraw from the relationship if inappropriate disclosures to the employer are required.[27] Each edition of the Beauchamp and Childress text contained a series of cases for discussion in an appendix. The second appearance of infectious disease in the 1979 volume was in the case appendix, where Willowbrook was the twenty-sixth case presented.[28] But it is the only infectious disease example among the nearly 30 cases, and is presented as raising concerns about experimentation on vulnerable populations rather than as exemplifying issues raised by communicability.

The 2001 edition of Beauchamp and Childress features HIV/AIDS more prominently. HIV/AIDS is viewed as posing a conflict between the autonomy (of the patient) and beneficence (to others)[29] and a potential conflict between the health-care provider's obligation to treat the patient and the risks of transmission to the provider.[30] It is also treated as an example of the need for express consent to certain forms of testing[31] and as an example of the role of uncertainty in treatment.[32] The implications of HIV/AIDS for patient privacy are emphasized: it is discussed as an example of how various proposals for screening threaten patient privacy; of balancing patient privacy against public policy reasons that support mandatory screening or treatment; and of justified infringement of rules of confidentiality.[33] These references to HIV/AIDS are the only additional references to infectious diseases in the 2001 edition, beyond the references in the 1979 edition. Notably, the discussion of conflicts of fidelity and divided loyalties does not reference infectious disease examples—even in 2001.[34] Willowbrook remains the only infectious disease case presented in the appendix.[35] Outside of HIV/AIDS, drug-resistant tuberculosis, and hepatitis at Willowbrook, no other infectious conditions draw mention in the 2001 edition. At late as 2001, in this text at least, the attention to HIV/AIDS had not been translated into more general attention to the challenges infectious disease might pose for bioethics.

We are not alone in the observation that infectious disease has been virtually left out of bioethics. Perhaps prodded by similar reflections, Michael Selgelid

---

27. Beauchamp and Childress, *Principles of Biomedical Ethics* (1979 ed.), 219–220.
28. Ibid., 276–277.
29. Beauchamp and Childress, *Principles of Biomedical Ethics* (2001 ed.), 20.
30. Ibid., 43.
31. Ibid., 67.
32. Ibid., 201.
33. Ibid., 293, 297–300, 309–310.
34. Ibid., 312–319.
35. Ibid., 428–430.

reports that "'Infectious disease' is hardly found even in indexes of standard bioethics texts."[36] Bioethics' neglect of infectious disease is easily demonstrated via searches on the Internet, Selgelid reports. In March 2005, for example, a Google search of the phrase "ethics and infectious disease" yielded only 35 entries, while "ethics and genetics" yielded 5,100.[37] In April, 2008, the gap had narrowed to merely ten-fold, due in large part to citations of works by Selgelid and earlier versions of chapters of this volume: 623 (infectious disease) and 6610 (genetics). PubMed searches (conducted by Selgelid in May 2004)—in titles and abstracts— for the terms "ethics" and "infectious disease" yielded a total of 195 citations. "Ethics" and "abortion," in the meantime, yielded 4,000; "ethics" and "genetics" yielded 8,400; "ethics" and "euthanasia" yielded 8,288.[38] Selgelid viewed these results as an "embarrassment" for the discipline of bioethics, which appears to be guilty of a misdistribution of research resources analogous to the divide in medical research, in which less than 10% of the dollars go to conditions that account for more than 90% of the global burden of disease—largely infectious diseases.[39] A different PubMed search conducted by the authors in April 2008 was even more discouraging: 5249 entries for "ethics and abortion," 10140 for "ethics and euthanasia," and a paltry 87 for "ethics and infectious disease."

Leaving Out Infectious Disease: The Dilemma-Cases of Bioethics

Much of the work of early bioethics consisted in the discussion of dilemma-cases. Bioethics began as a case-based field, and re-examining bioethics' early dilemma-cases is crucial in an account of the characteristic concerns of bioethics.

---

36. M. Selgelid, "Ethics and Infectious Disease," *Bioethics* 19, no. 3 (2005): 272–290 (283).

37. A similar search in 2002 yielded only 11 entries, 6 of which were to our own work. Selgelid's discussion was originally presented at the meetings of the International Association of Bioethics in 2002. In response to discussion challenging the claims about the virtual absence of infectious disease, Selgelid writes: "There have of course been books and anthology sections on ethical issues associated with AIDS in particular. And Internet searches of 'Ethics and AIDS,' as was pointed out by Peter Singer in discussion, will yield more results—i.e. 408 results on 1 March 2004. The fact remains, however, that discussion of infectious diseases in general (which would likely inform discussion of particular diseases such as AIDS) is lacking. In my opinion even AIDS—with the exception of doctor-patient relationship issues (especially the "duty to treat") and AIDS related international research ethics (especially the debate over "standards of care")—has not received adequate attention in mainstream bioethics literature, given the magnitude of the problem. On 1 March 2005, in any case, a Google search of 'ethics and tuberculosis' yielded only 42 results (though tuberculosis kills two or three million persons per year) and 'ethics and malaria' yielded zero (though malaria kills one million per year). On the same date, 'ethics and stem cells' yielded 440 results—despite the newness of stem cell research (in comparison with AIDS)" (Selgelid, "Ethics and Infectious Disease," 283, n. 41).

38. PUBMED numbers were provided by Kathleen Montgomery in collaboration with M. Selgelid.

39. Selgelid, "Ethics and Infectious Disease," 273.

Whether to tell a patient a fatal diagnosis, how to handle the distribution of a scarce resource such as dialysis, and whether to countenance highly risky experimentation with human subjects, such as that involving the artificial heart, were the daily fodder of bioethics discussions. It is, of course, difficult to know what actually went on as these issues were raised in bedside discussions of difficult treatment decisions, in fledgling hospital ethics committees, in hospital or university corridors, in medical school classes, or in the many college and university bioethics courses springing up all over the United States. Bioethics cases did make it into print, however, and became the paradigm cases for consideration in the field. Here too, in the dilemma-cases that were discussed and rediscussed in print, infectious disease was virtually absent. We have already indicated that the case appendix to the Beauchamp and Childress volume featured only one infectious example—Willowbrook—and not for its communicability. A similar absence of infectious disease can be documented in other standard compendia of bioethics cases.

The most longstanding series of case discussions in bioethics is a feature of the *Hastings Center Report*. These involve a case presentation followed by discussion by experts in the field. Two (overlapping) compendia of cases from early days of the *Report* have been published, first in 1982 and the second in 1989.[40] In the 1982 compendium, there were dilemmas of reproduction, such as using a fetus for organ donation or sterilizing a "retarded" child; dilemmas of the physician–patient relationship, such as proxy consent or choosing a therapy when physicians disagree; dilemmas in mental health treatment, such as the questionably competent patient or the treatment of convicts; dilemmas in death and dying, such as demands to die or the role of nurses in DNR orders; dilemmas in human subjects research, such as parental consent when the subjects are pregnant teenagers; dilemmas in allocation, such as the famous "last bed in the ICU"; and dilemmas in public policy.

The cases in this last group, public policy dilemmas, are particularly revealing. It is here that one might expect to find cases involving risks to others besides the index patient himself or herself. Yet the complete list of dilemmas discussed is this: laetrile, interns and residents on strike, baby making and the public interest, regulating anti-aging drugs, drinking on the job, mentally retarded hepatitis B carriers in public schools, health risks and equal opportunity, state mandates of infant car seats, and police informants in the hospital. Only one of these public policy dilemmas—the most likely home of discussions of public health concerns or concerns raised by infectiousness—featured an infectious condition, hepatitis B. The case, published in the 1982 compendium

40. Carol Levine and Robert M. Veatch, eds., *Cases in Bioethics from The Hastings Center Report* (New York: Hastings Center, 1982); Carol Levine, ed., *Cases in Bioethics: Selections from The Hastings Center Report* (New York: St. Martin's Press, 1989).

(before the emergence of issues about HIV), concerned mainstreaming of children with intellectual impairments into public schools when those children were hepatitis B positive. In the presentation and discussion of the case, the issues raised by infectiousness were mingled with the issues raised by intellectual impairment and inclusion in the community in general, despite the fact that hepatitis B as an infectious condition in the public school population is not limited to children with intellectual impairments.

Of the 42 cases in the 1982 collection, only one other case, "The Homosexual Husband and Physician Confidentiality," involved an infectious disease.[41] The details of this case are truly stunning. As this case was presented, the patient, "David," was a young man of marriageable age, pressured by his father to meet ideals of "male" success. But he had refused to go to college, refused to participate in athletics, gained a draft exemption for homosexuality, and been "treated for gonorrhea, asthma, and infectious hepatitis." When David contemplates marriage—predictably and conveniently to "Joan," another patient of his physician—the physician has to decide whether to tell Joan about David's homosexuality. After the marriage—so the case narrative continues—Joan learns of David's homosexuality when the marriage is not consummated. She is devastated and angry with the physician for his failure to reveal her husband's homosexuality to her. The case is thus framed as one about homosexuality and confidentiality, not as one about infectiousness and confidentiality—although presumably the possibility that David might be infected with communicable diseases posed a very real risk to Joan.

The commentaries reflect this framing, with none of the commentators focusing on the infectious character and transmissibility of David's illnesses. Daniel Callahan's discussion does note that the rule of confidentiality admits of exceptions in the case of legal reporting requirements, for "e.g., dangerous communicable diseases and gunshot wounds."[42] But there is no comparable, known public rule about breaking confidentiality in the case of homosexuality so, Callahan concludes, it would have been a violation of David's trust for his physician to have revealed his sexual orientation to Joan. Eric Cassell, in his comment, notes that David had gonorrhea and infectious hepatitis, "both diseases of increased prevalence among male homosexuals," but does not return to these features of the case.[43] Instead, he treats the case as involving conflicting obligations between patients and concludes that patient trust requires keeping confidences. In his commentary, Robert Veatch does not mention the risk of transmission of infectious conditions to Joan or for that matter to

41. Harvey Kuschner, "The Homosexual Husband and Physician Confidentiality," in *Cases in Bioethics*, ed. Levine and Veatch, 20.
42. Daniel Callahan, "Commentary," in *Cases in Bioethics*, ed. Levine and Veatch, 21.
43. Eric J. Cassell, "Commentary," in *Cases in Bioethics*, ed. Levine and Veatch, 21–22.

David's male sexual partners; his focus, too, is entirely on the revelation of David's homosexuality. Veatch recommends that professional organizations should adopt rules about confidentiality and that providers should discuss their practices with patients before the issue arises. Absent prior ground rules, Veatch concludes that the best course of action in such difficult conflicts between patients is for the physician to arrange an alternative source of care for Joan.[44]

The 1989 compendium of cases from the *Hastings Center Report*—some 60 cases—omits the case of the homosexual husband. It retains the case involving "mentally retarded hepatitis B carriers in public schools." Alongside cases such as "Using a Cadaver to Practice and Teach," "When Baby's Mother Is also Grandma—and Sister," "When the Doctor Gives a Deadly Dose," and "Two Cardiac Arrests, One Medical Team," appear two new cases devoted to HIV/AIDS: "AIDS and a Duty to Protect" and "If I Have AIDS, Then Let Me Die Now!" The first case replaces the case of the "homosexual husband," and features a bisexual, HIV-positive patient who refuses to tell his fiancée of his infection.[45] One commentator, Morton Winston, concludes that the physician can best mediate his conflict between a duty of confidentiality to his patient and a duty to warn by trying to persuade the patient to reveal his condition to his fiancée. If the patient refuses, Winston recommends, the physician "must seriously consider revealing the information himself," after consulting appropriate authorities, if the risk to the fiancée is "significant and if all other means of persuading the patient to accept his moral responsibility have failed."[46] The other commentator, Sheldon Landesman, worries that breaching confidentiality about HIV test results will discourage possibly infected persons from seeking counseling and treatment. Landesman concludes that in the absence of a legal mandate, although the "difficult ethical dilemma is one of balancing long-term societal benefits against short-term benefit to an individual," maintaining confidentiality should be paramount.[47] As this case is framed and discussed, the autonomy and interests of the individual patient are pitted against the potential concerns of the public—a flat, conflictual analysis that fails to grasp the deeper problems raised by contagious infectious disease. In Chapter 7, we reconsider confidentiality and other classic bioethics issues in light of our PVV perspective, which gives thoroughgoing attention to infectious disease.

The discussions of the second HIV case in the 1989 Hastings Center compendium, "If I Have AIDS, Then Let Me Die Now!"[48] raise many problems

---

44. Robert M. Veatch, "Commentary," in *Cases in Bioethics*, ed. Levine and Veatch, 22–23.
45. "AIDS and a Duty to Protect," in *Cases in Bioethics*, ed. Levine and Veatch, 39–42.
46. Ibid., p. 40.
47. Ibid., p. 42.
48. "If I Have AIDS, Then Let Me Die Now!" in *Cases in Bioethics: Selections*, ed. Levine, 127–132.

about end-of-life decision making—autonomy, competence, burdens of care on others, the rationality of choosing death, potential feelings of depression or guilt about homosexuality, possibilities of survival, and the availability of a supportive network. Transmissibility appears, but only obliquely; one commentator, A-J Rock Levinson, notes that family caregivers might try to dissuade the patient from refusing treatment if they knew the facts about transmission and the availability of support systems to help with care.[49] This marks something of a turning point in bioethics: with AIDS, attention is given to transmissibility, but it is hardly generalized beyond this disease.

Such myopia was not confined to the United States. An early collection of British cases that emerged from the Radcliffe Circle of bioethics seminars at Oxford University begun in 1983, also left issues of infectious disease completely out.[50] The cases discussed (and their authors) are when life begins (Michael Lockwood), whether to prescribe contraception to a 15-year-old (Ian Kennedy), non-therapeutic research on children (R.M. Hare), compulsory removal of the elderly from their homes (J.A. Muir Gray), patient autonomy and the refusal of consent to needed medical care (Raanon Gillon), slippery slopes (Bernard Williams), in vitro fertilization (Mary Warnock), experimentation with embryos and the Warnock Report (Michael Lockwood), and telling patients the truth about dire diagnoses (Roger Higgs).

A compendium of bioethics cases that looks back historically on the development of cases in this new and maturing field is Gregory Pence's *Classic Cases in Medical Ethics*, produced first in 1990 and updated to a fifth edition by 2008.[51] Here, too, infectious disease is not at center stage in the unfolding bioethics scene. The Tuskegee syphilis study is one of two cases in which a communicable infectious disease appears.[52] The case is viewed as an example of research ethics gone wrong—a judgment with which we heartily agree as we explore further in Chapter 10 and again in 21—but not as primarily an example of transmissible infectiousness. Pence's discussion outlines many critical ethical issues in the case: deception, racism, study design, media coverage, justice, and harm to subjects. Nearly all of the discussion among various critics takes place without reference to the transmissibility of syphilis, however.

49. Ibid., p. 129.
50. Michael Lockwood, ed. *Moral Dilemmas in Modern Medicine* (Oxford: Oxford University Press, 1985).
51. Gregory Pence, *Classic Cases in Medical Ethics* (Boston: McGraw-Hill, 1990, 1995, 2000, 2004, 2008).
52. Pence, *Classic Cases in Medical Ethics* (1990 ed.), 184–205. There was ample opportunity for infectiousness to appear in other cases, but it does not. The discussion of the transplant of a baboon heart into Baby Fae ignores concerns about zoonoses; the discussion of preventing undesirable teenage pregnancies ignores sexually transmitted diseases.

There is one very important exception: Pence's observation that "an especially troubling fact to critics was that no effort was made to survey syphilis in wives and children of subjects," and that the researchers thus took a chance on the possibility that wives of subjects might be infected or reinfected or children might be born with congenital syphilis.[53] Pence's observation is virtually unique among critics of the Tuskegee study.

Pence's 1990 compendium also includes a case on mandatory testing for HIV/AIDS in the section titled "classic cases about individual rights and the public good." Here, mandatory testing is presented as pitting utilitarian benefits against protection of privacy and protection against stigmatization. The other cases in this section on rights and the public good deal with homelessness and involuntary psychiatric commitment (Joyce Brown), preventing undesirable teenage pregnancy, and genetic testing for Huntington's Disease (Nancy Wexler). The 1995 updated and revised edition of Pence's compendium highlights the "effects on subjects' families" as a subhead of the ethical wrongs apparent in the Tuskegee study. It adds a case on Medicare policy to the section on individual rights and the public good. But other than Tuskegee, mandatory HIV/AIDS testing remains the sole representative of infectious disease among the 18 cases given full treatment in the volume. The 2004 edition replaces the case on HIV/AIDS testing with a case titled "Preventing the Global Spread of AIDS." Its focus is on the conflicts between sexual moralism and protecting public health. Although the case is highly critical of the "exceptionalism" of HIV, attention to infectiousness has not pervaded the remainder of the volume.[54] Nor is Pence's approach unique; other contemporary casebooks in bioethics continue to ignore infectious disease entirely or to limit discussion to HIV/AIDS.[55]

Leaving Out Infectious Disease: Histories of the Field of Bioethics

In the more sweeping histories of the field of bioethics infectious disease is virtually absent, even in the background. Al Jonsen's "chronicle of ethical events" from the 1940s to the 1980s goes like this:[56]

> 1947: the doctors' trial at Nuremberg
> 1953: DNA—the secret of life

---

53. Pence, *Classic Cases in Medical Ethics* (1990 ed.), 203.
54. Pence, *Classic Cases in Medical Ethics* (2004 ed.).
55. See, e.g., Peter Horn, *Clinical Ethics Casebook* (Belmont, CA: Wadsworth, 2003). In this casebook, not a single one of the nine cases on "communication and confidentiality" involves whether information about risks of disease spread should be shared.
56. Albert R. Jonsen, *A Short History of Medical Ethics* (Oxford: Oxford University Press, 2000), 99–114.

1954: renal transplantation
1960: oral contraceptives
1960: renal dialysis and the Seattle selection committee
1967: heart transplantation
1968: Harvard definition of brain death
1972: the Tuskegee revelations
1973: *Roe v. Wade*
1975: the *Quinlan* case
1978: baby Louise Brown (IVF)
1982: Baby Doe
1982: the artificial heart
1983: the AIDS epidemic

On this list, the revelations concerning the syphilis experiment at Tuskegee are the only example of case involving infectious disease before HIV/AIDS; notably absent, just to take a few other infectious disease possibilities during the same time period, are the patent for mass manufacture of penicillin (1948) and ethical issues about use of and just distribution of life-saving antimicrobials; the development of the Salk (1955) and Sabin (1957) vaccines and issues about the respective risks of live and killed vaccines; the reported premature pronouncement of the closure of the book on infectious disease (sometime around 1969) and its consequences; the eradication of smallpox (announced by WHO in 1967; last reported case in 1977); and the long history of expected and required immunization that led to this and other public health triumphs.

Jonsen's *Birth of Bioethics*, perhaps the best-known history of bioethics, begins with the theological, philosophical, and political origins of the field. It then takes up the core initial areas of concern: experimentation with human subjects, genetics, organ transplantation and artificial organs, the ethics of death and dying, and reproductive ethics. Nine scattered references to infectious disease occur along the way in this 400-page volume, largely in discussions of experimentation with human subjects, such as the development of penicillin, the announced conquest of infectious disease, the eradication of polio, early experimentation with smallpox vaccination and yellow fever immunization, Nazi experimentation with infection and immunization, Tuskegee, and research on infectious disease involving prisoners.[57] HIV/AIDS is treated in an epilogue: HIV/AIDS came on the scene largely but, it should be noted, not entirely after the formative period of bioethics and Jonsen's announced end-date to his historical account, 1987.[58] Nowhere in the discussions

---

57. Albert R. Jonsen, *The Birth of Bioethics* (Oxford: Oxford University Press, 1998), 12, 13, 16, 126, 128–29 (yellow fever), 135 (Nazi experimentation), 146–148 (Tuskegee), 156, and 395.
58. Jonsen, *The Birth of Bioethics*, 406–410.

of genetics, organ transplantation, the ethics of death and dying, or reproductive medicine, does infectiousness enter the stage. In the epilogue, in light of HIV/AIDS, there is a promissory note:

> As AIDS came into the ken of bioethics, it evoked the need for better ways to think about the individual's relation to the community. Not only did the carefully crafted ethics of research and the ethics of care for the dying have to be revisited, but community—as carrier of distinct cultures, source of power, and repositories of strength for individuals—had to be introduced into bioethical reflections as a balance to individualism.[59]

Although we agree with Jonsen about the challenges posed by infectious disease, we will argue in this book that these challenges are usually put in a deeply misleading way, as a matter of the individual in conflict with the community. We will argue that autonomy and the nature of individual agency itself might have been viewed differently, had infectious disease been as present in the formation of bioethics as chronic disease, coma, and reproductive anomalies. In order to address our status as victims and vectors adequately, we will contend, bioethics needs to reconsider some of its fundamental conceptual building blocks, most basically autonomy but also responsibility, harm, and other related notions.

Another, far less sympathetic, treatment of the development of the field of bioethics is David Rothman's *Strangers at the Bedside*.[60] A historian, Rothman explores how external actors—bioethicists, lawyers, and regulators—have increasingly constrained medical practice. He locates the development of the field in the context of the development of civil rights more generally, but concludes that this development has come at a price: the protection of rights against a more "contractual, prescribed, and uniform" medical practice, which patients experience as "powerful and impersonal, a more or less efficient interaction between strangers."[61] In Rothman's account, infectious disease examples were on the scene early on: the public health concerns to conquer yellow fever, to avert influenza epidemics, to immunize against diphtheria or dysentery, or to protect soldiers against venereal disease pressed researchers into many of the examples of unethical research highlighted by Henry Beecher in his stirring critique in the *New England Journal of Medicine*.[62] Here is Rothman's description of the effects of infectious disease on research: "the medical

---

59. Ibid., 410.

60. David J. Rothman, *Strangers at the Bedside: A History of How Law and Bioethics Transformed Medical Decision Making* (New York: Basic Books, 1991), 261–262.

61. Ibid.

62. Henry K. Beecher, "Ethics and Clinical Research," *New England Journal of Medicine* 274 (1966): 1354–1360.

researchers learned in their first extensive use of human subjects . . . that ends certainly did justify means; that in wartime the effort to conquer disease entitled them to choose the martyrs to scientific progress. They learned, too, that the public would accept such decisions, and that so long as the researchers were attentive to potential areas of dispute, the support for research was considerable."[63] Other than setting the stage in this way for the development of concern for human rights in bioethics, however, infectious disease never reappears in Rothman's book, either in his account of the development of regulatory structures or in his understanding of the role played by patient autonomy and civil rights. "Public health" is not an entry in Rothman's index, despite the pressures of public health concerns that were apparent in his characterization of the early experiments.

Rothman's history of clinical medicine in the time of the development of bioethics stands in sharp contrast to Robert Veatch's recent historical portrait of clinical medicine before the nineteenth century. Up to and including the Enlightenment period, Veatch contends, medicine and humanistic philosophy were deeply intertwined. Only with the advent of separatist professionalism did medicine become detached from the larger ethical and political dialogues of the day, including concerns for public health. In Veatch's view, the separation between the ethics of clinical medicine and broader social concerns is an unusual feature of the nineteenth and twentieth centuries, remedied only by the reintroduction of humanist concerns into the clinic with the development of bioethics in the 1970s.[64] Yet in Veatch's account of the dynamically reconnected conversations of the 1970s and beyond, the syphilis studies at Tuskegee are the lone example of a communicable infectious disease, characterized once again as an example of research abuse. Veatch's list of all the "key topics" covered in the resurgent medical ethics courses tells it all: "death and dying, fertility control, human subjects research, and health insurance."[65]

From this survey—first of principal texts in the field, and then of the traditional dilemma-cases and histories of the field—it seems fair to conclude that infectious disease was not at the forefront and perhaps not even on the back burner of the earliest discussions in bioethics. HIV/AIDS has changed this picture somewhat, but apparently not in systematic or thoroughgoing ways, if the canonical texts like Beauchamp and Childress in their latest editions are to be taken as an example. In the most recent journals, texts, monographs, and other publications, work on infectious disease is beginning to appear— for example, the leading journal *Bioethics* devoted a special issue to the topic

---

63. Rothman, *Strangers at the Bedside*, 50.
64. Robert Veatch, *Disrupted Dialogue: Medical Ethics and the Collapse of Physician-Humanist Communication, 1770–1980* (Oxford: Oxford University Press, 2005).
65. Ibid., 213.

in 2005.[66] Listservs such as INTERPHEN (the International Public Health Ethics Network, an affiliated group of the International Association of Bioethics) also are springing up, but this is a very recent development in the life of bioethics. Even so, despite some of this recent attention, prognoses about the most pressing contemporary issues in the field continue to focus on matters like the human genome project, or on access to care[67]—but only at best indirectly on the kinds of concerns we raise in this volume. Case compendia continue to be published with limited attention to infectious disease examples, and examinations of the problems these cases pose simply as conflicts between the individual's privacy and the rights of others or the public rather than as more sweeping challenges to the field of bioethics.[68] For almost all of bioethics' young history, both throughout its formative period and continuing until today, infectious disease has simply been left out. One might ask whether attention to HIV/AIDS has sufficiently provoked attention to issues raised by communicable infectious disease—attention to confidentiality, duty to warn, risks to providers, or the just distribution of resources when people pose risks of harm to each other. We will return to this question at the end of the next chapter, in a fuller discussion of how the significance of HIV/AIDS has been shaped by a kind of exceptionalism that has restricted its impact on the field of bioethics as a whole.

Could Bioethics Have Been Different?

How, we might ask, would things have been different if infectious disease had been more fully present at the "birth of bioethics"?[69] Bioethics began in the context of physician–patient encounters; this focus no doubt encouraged the kind of individualism we have detailed but would not by itself direct attention

---

66. *Bioethics, Special Issue: Ethics in Infectious Disease Control*, ed. Michael J. Selgelid and Margaret P. Battin, vol. 19, no. 4 (2005).

67. See, e.g., Stephen Wear, James J. Bono, Gerald Logue and Adrianne McEvoy, *Ethical Issues in Health Care on the Frontiers of the Twenty-First Century* (Dordrecht, the Netherlands: Kluwer Academic, 2000).

68. See, e.g., Judith C. Ahronheim, Jonathan D. Moreno, and Connie Zuckerman, *Ethics in Clinical Practice*, 2nd ed. (Gaithersburg, MD: Aspen, 2000). This volume contains three infectious disease cases, among 31 cases presented. A married man with syphilis is treated as a conflict between his confidentiality, risks to his wife, and public reporting requirements. A case of a health-care worker's refusal to be tested for possible TB is explored in terms of public health concerns about drug-resistant infections and the permissibility of directly observed therapy. Whether mandatory testing violates the health-care worker's autonomy is viewed in terms of the worker's implied consent to testing in virtue of her job—not in virtue of what her autonomy in such cases might really mean. The case of surgical delay in an HIV-positive patient is treated in terms of whether health-care workers have an obligation to take risks in treating patients and when there might be exceptions to the duty to treat.

69. The phrase is Albert R. Jonsen's, *The Birth of Bioethics* (Oxford: Oxford University Press, 1998).

away from the issues raised by infectious diseases. With the exception of Jonsen, Siegler, and Winslade's volume, however, even the clinical encounter was not portrayed in the context of infectiousness and theoretical developments in the field were not tested in terms of features that are typical of infectious disease.

Communicable infectious disease forces us to recognize that individuals are socially situated in a distinctive way—not just as individuals who are located in a social nexus, but as foci of victimhood and vectorhood in relation to others. Some philosophers and bioethicists have criticized the individualism that was characteristic of early bioethics as inadequate to describe human reality: Thomas May, for example, rejected the "impoverished, atomistic" view of the individual that characterizes earlier accounts in bioethics in favor of a view of individuals as "socially located."[70] Al Jonsen, in a passage quoted in this chapter, urged that bioethics should take into account conflicts between the individual and the community. But these observations about social location—together with the more communitarian concerns of public health—are incomplete as well, we shall contend. Moreover, they encourage a picture in which the community is seen as in conflict with the individual. A contention we shall ultimately develop in our PVV view is that if infectiousness were more central to bioethics, individual autonomy and its requirements and constraints would be seen differently. Had infectiousness been more central earlier on, the theoretical paradigms would not simply have been the extremes of individualism—the patient against the community, or communitarianism— the patient as identified with the community. The patient would be seen as, among other things, both victim and vector, embodied, vulnerable, and in relationships of contagion and transmission to others in many different ways. How we should understand the concept of autonomy against such a background is a primary task of this volume.

Before turning to a thoroughgoing exploration of what the presence of infectious disease might have meant for bioethics and its theoretical bases, however, we will look briefly in the next chapter at the parallel developments within the field of public health—where the more general concerns about population health were voiced largely without dialogue with the developing field of bioethics.

---

70. Thomas May, "The Concept of Autonomy in Bioethics: An Unwarranted Fall from Grace," in *Personal Autonomy: New Essays on Personal Autonomy and Its Role in Contemporary Moral Philosophy*, ed. James Stacey Taylor (Cambridge: Cambridge University Press, 2005), 299–309.

5

CLOSING THE BOOK ON INFECTIOUS DISEASE: THE MISCHIEVOUS CONSEQUENCES FOR PUBLIC HEALTH

Unlike bioethics, public health is a field of longstanding origins. From the construction of aqueducts and sewers in ancient Rome, to efforts to combat plague in medieval Europe, to the origins of the U.S. Public Health Service in the care of injured merchant seamen in 1798,[1] to Dr. John Snow's famous attribution of cholera to London's Broad Street pump in 1854, efforts to improve population health have been a matter of public concern. Bioethics, by contrast, as we have seen, is a relative latecomer as a field, emerging during the period of the late 1950s through the 1970s. Given the respective backgrounds of the fields, the relative optimism in bioethics about infectious disease may seem less startling than the concomitant optimism found in public health during the same time period. The discipline of public health never quite forgot its origins in preventing the spread of disease and promoting the overall health of populations. However, in public health discussions during the early development of bioethics, attention had, to a considerable degree, shifted away from infectious disease to other kinds of problems in the health of populations.

Infectious disease might have brought the fields of bioethics and public health together in an area of common concern, with bioethics scholars emphasizing the situation of the individual patient and public health concerned to protect populations from disease spread. Had this interplay occurred, the victim-paradigm of bioethics might have been tested against the vector-paradigm of public health. As it happened, however, the developments in the field of public health we document in this chapter, as much as the origins of bioethics, contributed to the failures of either field to challenge the other.

A previous version of this chapter appeared as Leslie P. Francis, Margaret P. Battin, Jay A. Jacobson, Charles B. Smith, "Closing the Book on Infectious Disease: The Mischievous Consequences for Bioethics and for Public Health," in Angus Dawson, ed., *The Philosophy of Public Health* (Aldershot: Ashgate, 2008).

1. U.S. Department of Health and Human Services, "About the Commissioned Corps: History," http://commcorps.shs.net/aboutus/history.aspx (accessed December 29, 2007).

Public Health and Bioethics: Differing Paradigms

Ethical issues raised by infectious disease and transmissibility might seem properly to be the core domain of public health rather than part of the problems of clinical medicine that were the focus of bioethics. If so, it may seem unsurprising that bioethics ignored issues of infectiousness, perhaps working on the assumption that these issues were the provinces of a different field. Historically, infectious disease was the staple issue of public health and continued to garner attention during the formative period of bioethics. Nonetheless, the discussions in public health at the time also were marked by optimism about infectious disease.

Long before the mechanisms of infectious disease transmission were understood, public health originated in societal attempts to try to control the spread of disease by isolating lepers, attaching bells to plague victims, imposing quarantines on ships entering a harbor and similar measures. With increasing understanding of the microbial basis of infectious disease toward the end of the nineteenth century, practical public health measures became more effective, reflected in improved public sanitation, immunization, the application of the germ theory of disease in encouraging doctors to wash their hands between seeing patients, and many other public health measures aimed at reducing transmission. Indeed, at least until the mid-twentieth century, the containment of communicable infectious disease was the central concern of public health.

For the most part, public health has been population-focused rather than individual-focused, involving societal, governmental, or institutional measures aimed at protecting or improving the health of populations by containing or preventing transmission of disease rather than treating disease in individual patients. The generally accepted short definition of the field was formulated by the Institute of Medicine: "what we, as a society, do collectively to assure the conditions for people to be healthy."[2] In a classic statement regarding the "protean field of public health," Charles Winslow wrote:

> Public Health is the science and art of preventing disease, prolonging life, and promoting physical health and efficiency through organized community effort for the sanitation of the environment, the control of communicable infections, the education of the individual in personal hygiene, the organization of medical and nursing services for the early diagnosis and preventive treatment of disease, and the development of the social machinery to insure everyone a standard of

2. Institute of Medicine, *The Future of Public Health* (Washington, DC: National Academy Press, 1988), 19; also in Public Health Leadership Society, *Principles of the Ethical Practice of Public Health, Version 2.2*, Public Health Leadership Society (2002), http://www.apha.org/NR/rdonlyres/1CED3CEA-287E-4185-9CBD-BD405FC60856/0/ethicsbrochure.pdf (accessed December 29, 2007), preamble.

living adequate for the maintenance of health, so organizing these benefits as to enable every citizen to realize his birthright of health and longevity.[3]

Concomitantly, ethical paradigms in the field have been largely utilitarian in character, emphasizing protection of the community as a whole.[4] To be sure, public health has not ignored questions of distributive justice or even the treatment of disease in individual patients,[5] but its motivations for supporting health-improvement measures and for encouraging treatment have paralleled its motives for employing containment measures such as immunization and quarantine—to promote overall population health and to prevent the spread of the disease to other persons in the population as a whole. Public health is primarily concerned with securing the greater overall good, even if that might involve unhappy tradeoffs for those comparatively few individuals who would be quarantined, forcibly immunized, isolated, or otherwise constrained.[6] To take just one example of the utilitarian theme in public health analyses, consider this quotation, from a widely used public health text of the 1970s:

> A large part of public health law in the United States is concerned with the control of communicable diseases. The most important basis on which rests the enactment and enforcement of public health law is the police power . . . It will suffice here to remind the reader of the folly, even in a democracy, of allowing individuals complete freedom of action. In fact individual freedom, in order truly to exist, must be limited to the right to engage in all activities except those that may be detrimental to the common welfare. An individual infected with a disease transmissible to others must necessarily forfeit some of his personal freedom for the common good.[7]

More recently, the Principles of the Ethical Practice of Public Health of the American Public Health Association, adopted in 2002, contrast the individual, provider–patient focus of clinical medicine with the population-based, prevention-emphasizing purview of public health.[8]

3. Charles E.A. Winslow, "The Untilled Fields of Public Health," *Science* 51 (1920): 23–33 (23, 30); quoted in Wendy K. Mariner, "Law and Public Health: Beyond Emergency Preparedness," *Journal of Health Law* 38 (2005): 247–285 (251–252).

4. Dan E. Beauchamp, "Public Health: Alien Ethic in a Strange Land," *American Journal of Public Health* 65 (1975): 1338–1339.

5. Winslow, for example, wrote in 1920, that "the public health worker needs the physician," and that "such organized medical care must be made available not merely for the very poor and very right but for the entire community." (*Untilled Fields*, 28).

6. See, e.g., Daniel Markovits, "Quarantines and Distributive Justice," *Journal of Law, Medicine, & Ethics* 33 (2005): 323–338; Mariner, "Law and Public Health"; Daniel Callahan and Bruce Jennings, "Ethics and Public Health: Forging a Strong Relationship," *American Journal of Public Health* 92 (2002): 169–176.

7. John J. Hanlon, *Public Health Administration and Practice*, 6th ed. (St. Louis: C.V. Mosby, 1974), 401.

8. Public Health Leadership Society, *Principles of the Ethical Practice of Public Health*.

Bioethics, in contrast, as we saw in the previous chapter, was born at the bedside of the individual patient who has been ill; it has been the illness of this patient and the way it affects him or her that has been the field's primary focus. Autonomy was the first of the four canonical principles in the field of bioethics, followed by nonmaleficence, beneficence, and justice; although this order was not meant to represent a prioritization, it nonetheless appears on the printed page almost uniformly in this order and has often been taken as a genuine priority-ranking in practice: autonomy has pride of place. Most forms of illness that concerned bioethics in its early days were not infectious, and, if infectious, were not addressed primarily with their potential for transmission in mind. The focus of bioethics has been the plight of *this* patient suffering *this* illness, and how this patient's interactions with physicians and others involved in decision making about his or her care should proceed. To put the contrast in a nutshell, bioethics has been primarily interested in the patient as *victim*, public health in the patient as *vector*.

Perhaps contributing to this difference in focus, the field of bioethics developed in a manner that was for the most part institutionally independent of the field of public health. Bioethics grew up in schools of philosophy, theology, and in medical schools; schools of public health were institutionally distinct, often located at a distance, with comparatively little crossover in courses of study or faculty. Robert Veatch's history of the disrupted dialogue between humanists and physicians—as well as its reconnection in the 1970s—contains only a single mention of bioethics appointments in schools of public health—the appointment at the Harvard School of Public Health of two scholars associated with the Harvard Divinity School, Arthur Dyck and Ralph Potter—notably, to work on moral issues of policies related to fertility and migration.[9] A handful of well-known contemporary bioethicists like Ruth Faden and Jeffrey Botkin and health lawyers such as George Annas and Wendy Mariner have degrees in public health, but this has not been the norm. Perhaps the most longstanding relationships between bioethics and public health ethics have been located at the Department of Health Law, Bioethics, and Human Rights at Boston University, founded in the 1980s,[10] and at Columbia University's Mailman School of Public Health, where Ronald Bayer is a longstanding member of the faculty. The Bloomberg School of Public Health at Johns Hopkins University is a relatively later development in the field, and the Phoebe R. Berman Bioethics Institute, affiliated with the School and now a leading

9. Veatch, *Disrupted Dialogue*, 185–186.
10. The Department's website describes it as having been active for "more than two decades," http://sph.bu.edu/index.php?option=com_content&task=view&id=66&Itemid=94 (accessed December 29, 2007).

supporter of work in bioethics, was not founded until 1995.[11] The migration of well-known bioethics scholars Dan Brock, Norman Daniels,[12] and Dan Wikler to the Harvard School of Public Health is a twenty-first century development.

The Shifting Concerns of Public Health

Public health measures have been astonishingly successful in transforming morbidity and mortality, especially for the developed world: up through the middle of the nineteenth century most people in most parts of the world died of infectious diseases. By 1984, just before the outbreak of AIDS, infectious diseases—with the exception of pneumonia and septicemia—were no longer the leading causes of death in the developed world. They had been displaced by heart and circulatory disease, cancer, and various forms of degenerative organ system failure.

As the threat of infection seemed to have receded, public health increasingly turned its attention to other factors affecting the health of populations—matters like asbestos exposure, cigarette smoking, toxic waste, and obesity. While human behavior plays a major role in these conditions, none of them involves biologically transmissible disease. Indeed, we can document for public health some of the same optimism that infectious disease had been conquered that we have already shown to pervade the development of the field of bioethics. During the formative period of bioethics—from the late 1950s to the advent of HIV/AIDS, attention in public health was to some extent pointed away from infectious disease. This affected discussions in public health ethics, just as it did in bioethics.

This change in focus within public health is displayed, for example, in the classic public health text, *Maxcy-Rosenau*, now in its 14th edition. The volume, reissued approximately every eight years, is a compendium of articles on topics in public health written by authorities in the field. The 8th edition, dating from 1956, devotes nearly 600 pages to the prevention of communicable diseases, without discernable attention to ethical issues such as confidentiality in the investigation and control of disease spread.[13] By 1978, the 10th edition, featuring

---

11. See Johns Hopkins Berman Institute of Bioethics, "About the Institute," http://www.bioethic-sinstitute.org/web/page/387/sectionid/387/pagelevel/1/interior.asp (accessed December 29, 2007).

12. The appearance of Daniels' new book, *Just Health* (New York: Cambridge University Press, 2008), as this book was going to press, illustrates the fruitful possibilities of better connections between philosophy and public health. *Just Health*, in comparison to Daniels' earlier *Just Health Care* (Cambridge: Cambridge University Press, 1985), is centrally embedded in an understanding of the social determinants of health. Even in this new volume, however, infectious disease is not at the center of the analysis; issues such as aging and workplace safety draw extended attention and the primary infectious disease example is HIV/AIDS in the developing world.

13. Kenneth Maxcy, ed. *Rosenau Preventive Medicine and Public Health*, 8th ed. (New York: Appleton Century Crofts, 1956).

a new section on population dynamics, devoted fewer pages to communicable diseases, again with no attention to the ethical issues they raise.[14]

The first entry in *Maxcy-Rosenau* specifically devoted to ethics and public health law appears in the 11th edition, dated 1980. This entry is nothing short of remarkable. It attributes the importance of attending to a legal framework for public health activities to the movement in public health from disease prevention to health promotion and access to health services.[15] It treats the use of traditional methods of infection control such as quarantine and surveillance with breathtaking brevity. Ironically, this optimistic observation was published in 1980, scarcely a year before the initial reports of puzzling cases of immune-deficiency were published:

> Except for [tuberculosis and venereal diseases], measures to control reservoirs of infection tend not to be utilized. With most of the infectious diseases having been brought under control and with increased effectiveness of treatment resulting from the advent of antibiotics, the right to the individual to be free to move about at will took precedence over the needs to restrict him in the interest of protecting the public as a whole.[16]

Instead, the bulk of the discussion attends to the issues of paternalism and restrictions on liberty attendant on such public health interventions as cigarette smoking or exposure to toxic substances.

By the 13th edition of *Maxcy-Rosenau* in 1992, communicable diseases had shrunk to just over 300 pages in the volume. Environmental health occupied almost 400 pages; behavioral health, chronic illness and disability another almost 400 pages. The final essay—a mere 10 pages in the nearly 1,200-page volume, is devoted to "ethics and public health policy." It reviews the canonical principles of bioethics—autonomy, beneficence, nonmaleficence, and justice—as helpful in public health dilemmas. The overall perspective of the analysis is that the rights of individuals must be balanced against the needs of communities, both where diseases are communicable and where they are not. More specifically, the author of this essay, John Last, suggests that "a useful guideline is to consider the ethical principles of beneficent truth telling, distributive justice, and nonmaleficence: what is the truth about the situation and which of the competing priorities will harm the fewest people over the longest period?"[17]

14. Philip E. Sartwell, ed., *Maxcy-Rosenau Preventive Medicine and Public Health*, 10th ed. (New York: Appleton Century Crofts, 1973).

15. Sidney Shindell, "Legal and Ethical Aspects of Public Health," in *Maxcy-Rosenau Preventive Medicine and Public Health*, 11th ed., ed. Jerald A. Last and Philip E. Sartwell (New York: Appleton Century Crofts, 1980), 1834–1845.

16. Shindell, "Aspects of Public Health," 1837.

17. John Last, "Ethics and Public Health Policy," in *Maxcy-Rosenau-Last Public Health and Preventive Medicine*, 13th ed., ed. John M. Last and Robert B. Wallace (Norwalk, CT: Appleton and Lange, 1992), 1187–1196.

This relative oversimplification of ethical issues in public health was not the full story. Appreciation of the tension between the contrasting paradigms of utilitarianism and respect for individuals appeared in the literature, both in discussions of behavioral interventions[18] and in discussions of research ethics.[19] Regular columns in the *American Journal of Public Health*, by William Curran, George Annas, Leonard Glantz, Ronald Bayer, and others, treated issues of law, ethics, and public health, such as workplace hazards, abortion rights, and patient dumping. In the decades since the appearance of HIV/AIDS, these discussions have become far more robust.

At least three trends are increasingly apparent in the most recent public health literature. One is the continuing debate about whether public health should confine itself to problems that are in some sense "collective": problems of infection, sanitation, environmental hazards, and the like. Issues of "population health"—conditions that affect many in the population, such as obesity and diabetes, lack of exercise, and smoking—encompass far more than these collective problems, and have garnered as much attention in the public health literature as they have in the popular press. This approach has been picked up in bioethics too, with scholars such as Dan Brock and Dan Wikler urging bioethics to take a "bird's eye" view of ethics in health care.[20] The first of the anthologies to address ethics and public health directly, Dan Beauchamp and Bonnie Steinbock's *New Ethics for the Public's Health* (1999), devotes only four of its twenty-nine essays exclusively to infectious diseases, with human rights, access to health care, obesity, drug use, violent injury, gene therapy, infertility, tobacco, alcohol, and criminal justice occupying large sections of the volume.[21] Critics such as Richard Epstein have decried the implicit paternalism of these "new" public health efforts to improve population health through behavior change.[22]

A second trend in public health is the move beyond "international health," the effort to stop the spread of disease across national borders, to "global health," the effort to address the overall burden of disease worldwide. Linkages between health and international human rights, drawn by the late Jonathan Mann,[23]

---

18. See, e.g., Beauchamp, "Public Health: Alien Ethic."
19. See, e.g., Charles E. Lewis, Mary Ann Lewis, and Muriel Ifekwunigue, "Informed Consent by Children and Participation in an Influenza Vaccine Trial," *American Journal of Public Health* 68, no. 11 (1978): 1079–1083; Margaret E. Martin, "Statisticians, Confidentiality, and Privacy," *American Journal of Public Health* 67, no. 2 (1977): 165–167.
20. Dan Brock and Dan Wikler, paper presented at the International Association of Bioethics, Sydney, Australia, November 2004.
21. Dan E. Beauchamp and Bonnie Steinbock, eds., *New Ethics for the Public's Health* (Oxford: Oxford University Press, 1999).
22. Richard A. Epstein, "In Defense of the 'Old' Public Health: The Legal Framework for the Regulation of Public Health," *Brooklyn Law Review* 69 (2004): 1421–1470.
23. Jonathan M. Mann, "Medicine and Public Health, Ethics and Human Rights," *Hastings Center Report* 27, no. 3 (1997): 6–13.

by Paul Farmer,[24] and by others in the fight against HIV/AIDS, drug-resistant tuberculosis, and the myriad diseases of poverty have greatly enriched ethics discussions in public health at the beginning of the twenty-first century. The major impetus for this linkage between international human rights and global health has been renewed focus on the burdens of infectious disease in impoverished areas of the world,[25] including the efforts of Mann at UNAIDS and of Farmer in Haiti. Some theorists have gone so far as to argue that global disparities in health and human rights go hand in hand.[26] The journal *Health and Human Rights* (published since 1994), the creation of centers such as the François-Xavier Bagnoud Center for Health and Human Rights at Harvard in 1993 and the Center for Public Health and Human Rights at Johns Hopkins in 2004, and the devotion of a chapter in the *Oxford Textbook of Public Health*[27] to human rights all testify to the burgeoning role played by international human rights in the discipline of public health. In the United States, Larry Gostin has pressed the role of international human rights in protecting persons with HIV and the importance of civil rights in constructing a framework for domestic public health law.[28]

A third development in public health has been the field's self-conscious attention to its own ethical principles. Along with growth in public health education came attention to whether schools of public health taught ethics; in 1976, at least, the answer was largely "no,"[29] but by 1999 all but two of twenty-four schools responding offered courses in the field.[30] In 2002, the American Public Health Association adopted a code of ethics, the *Principles of the Ethical*

24. Paul Farmer, *Pathologies of Power: Health, Human Rights, and the New War on the Poor* (Berkeley: University of California Press, 2003).

25. Theodore M. Brown, Marcus Cueto, and Elizabeth Fee, "The World Health Organization and the Transition from 'International' to 'Global' Public Health," *American Journal of Public Health* 96 (2006): 62–72.

26. Solomon R. Benatar, "Global Disparities in Health and Human Rights: A Critical Commentary," *American Journal of Public Health* 88, no. 2 (1998): 295–300; Milton Roemer and Ruth Roemer, "Global Health, National Development, and the Role of Government," *American Journal of Public Health* 80, no. 10 (1990): 88–92.

27. Sofia Gruskin and Daniel Tarantola, "Health and Human Rights," in *Oxford Textbook of Public Health*, ed. Roger Detels, James McEwen, Robert Beaglehole, and Heizo Tanada, vol. 1, 4th ed. (Oxford: Oxford University Press, 2002), chap. 4.1.

28. Lawrence O. Gostin and Zita Lazzarini, *Human Rights and Public Health in the AIDS Pandemic* (New York: Oxford University Press, 1997); Lawrence O. Gostin, *Public Health Law: Power, Duty, Restraint* (Berkeley: University of California Press, 2000). See also James F. Childress and Ruth Gaare Bernheim, "Beyond the Liberal and Communitarian Impasse: A Framework and Vision for Public Health," *Florida Law Review* 55 (2003): 1191–1219.

29. Naomi R. Bluestone, "The Teaching of Ethics in Schools of Public Health," *American Journal of Public Health* 66, no. 5 (1976): 478–479 (10 out of 15 schools responding had no ethics course; only Harvard and Columbia indicated significant ethics offerings).

30. Steven S. Coughlin, Wendy H. Katz, and Donald R. Mattison, "Ethics Instruction at Schools of Public Health in the United States, "*American Journal of Public Health* 89, no. 5 (1999): 768–770.

Practice of Public Health.[31] A primary rationale for this code of ethics was that the field of public health had treated ethical principles as implicit but needed to make them explicit and public. The code begins with the affirmation that human beings have a right to the resources necessary for health; it continues by asserting that humans are inherently interdependent and social values of trust, community, and participation are core ethical concerns. Development of the code was the occasion for systematic reflection on the ethical structure of public health[32] as well as calls for increased cooperation between the fields of public health ethics and bioethics.[33] Public health scholars have increasingly been exploring the foundations of the field: in equity,[34] in the harm principle of liberal theory,[35] and in a balance between liberalism and communitarianism.[36]

To sum up, throughout the formative period of bioethics and through the end of the twentieth century, public health ethics has not only been institutionally separate but has occupied a separate sphere of discussion from bioethics. This separateness may be a function of deeper incompatibilities between the conceptual and theoretical paradigms in use in the fields. Clinical ethics—the original core of bioethics—has to a large degree assumed a respect-for-persons view, in which principles like autonomy, truth-telling, confidentiality, informed consent, and other individual-centered, individual-respecting principles are central, while public health is rooted in a far more utilitarian, population-based, "good-of-the-whole" ethical view.[37]

Closing the Gap: Convergence Between the Ethics of Public Health and Bioethics

Since approximately the beginning of the twenty-first century, the gap between bioethics and public health ethics has been closing. To some extent, this convergence has been stimulated by the self-conscious attention to ethics by scholars in public health.[38] Moreover, work in bioethics has begun to address

31. Public Health Leadership Society, *Principles of the Ethical Practice of Public Health.*
32. Nancy E. Kass, "An Ethics Framework for Public Health," *American Journal of Public Health* 91, no. 11 (2001): 1776–1782.
33. Betty Wolder Levin and Alan R. Fleishman, "Public Health and Bioethics: The Benefits of Collaboration," *American Journal of Public Health* 92 (2002): 165–167; Callahan and Jennings, "Ethics and Public Health."
34. Sudhir Anand, Fabienne Peter, and Amartya Sen, eds., *Public Health, Ethics, and Equity* (Oxford: Oxford University Press, 2004).
35. Stephen Holland, *Public Health Ethics* (Cambridge, UK: Polity Press, 2007).
36. Ronald Bayer, Lawrence O. Gostin, Bruce Jennings, and Bonnie Steinbock, eds., *Public Health Ethics: Theory, Policy, and Practice* (New York: Oxford University Press, 2007).
37. This is the picture presented by Kass, "An Ethics Framework."
38. Examples include Beauchamp and Steinbock, *New Ethics for the Public's Health;* Coughlin, Soskolne, and Goodman, *Case Studies in Public Health Ethics;* Gostin, *Public Health Law and Ethics;*

points of contact between the fields, both in terms of particular issues and possibilities for theoretical convergence. There has been significant interest among the bioethics journals, as exhibited for example in the special issues of the *Journal of Law, Medicine & Ethics* (winter 2003 and its Special Supplement) devoted to population health and to public health and law, the issue of *Bioethics* devoted to public health in 2004,[39] and the issue of *Bioethics* devoted to infectious disease in 2005.[40]

These are but beginnings. To date, no fully systematic account has attempted to see whether the insights of one field warrant extensive reassessment of the other, in either direction. Instead, the picture remains one of the need to mediate the tensions between the individualism of bioethics and its privileging of autonomy on the one hand and the concern of public health for the good of all on the other. Ron Bayer and Amy Fairchild put it bluntly: "As we commence the process of shaping an ethics of public health, it is clear that bioethics is the wrong place to start when thinking about the balances required in defense of the public's health."[41] This apparent gap between bioethics and public health, we believe, is exacerbated and reflected in the somewhat different ethical paradigms these fields employ, and it is part of our project in this volume to see whether the gap can be closed. We think that bridging this gap will require rethinking paradigms of analysis along the lines of the PVV perspective we develop here for bioethics.

HIV "Exceptionalism"

Although HIV/AIDS impelled dialogue between bioethics and public health, it unfortunately did not sufficiently press the paradigms of either field. The link between bioethics and public health ethics first began to be forged when HIV/AIDS was emerging in the early 1980s. HIV was in some respects a wake-up call for bioethics, bringing a reinvigoration of traditional public health concerns about communicable disease.[42] In other respects, however, HIV may have been doubly "exceptional," to use Ron Bayer's term, and thus not have

---

and Michael Boylan, ed., *Public Health Policy and Ethics* (Dordrecht, the Netherlands: Kluwer Academic, 2004).

39. Wendy Rogers and Dan Brock, eds., "Ethics and Public Health," special issue, *Bioethics* 18, no. 6 (November 2004).

40. Michael J. Selgelid and Margaret P. Battin, eds., "Ethics and Infectious Disease," special issue, *Bioethics* 19, no. 4 (August 2005); also expanded as Michael J. Selgelid, Margaret P. Battin, and Charles B. Smith, eds., *Ethics and Infectious Disease* (Oxford: Blackwell, 2006).

41. Ronald Bayer & Amy L. Fairchild, "The Genesis of Public Health Ethics," *Bioethics* 18(6): 474-492, p. 474 (2004).

42. An excellent discussion of the ethical issues raised by HIV is Ronald Bayer, *Private Acts, Social Consequences* (New York: Free Press, 1989).

been seen to pose the more thoroughgoing theoretical challenges to bioethics (and perhaps also to public health) that we explore in this volume. This is for several reasons, both biological and political. For one thing, the transmission routes of HIV infection—through the exchange of bodily fluids—are more likely than transmission routes such as sneezing to be the subjects of both awareness and control. For another, the politics of HIV have been shaped by rights-based analyses. In neither of these ways does HIV reflect the fuller range of infectious diseases.

HIV is transmissible only by routes that today can largely be controlled by the agent or identified others such as health-care providers: primarily sexual intercourse, sharing of syringes in IV drug administration, and exposure to contaminated blood products or other bodily fluids. While HIV is like many other infectious diseases in that it can be (and very often is) transmitted unknowingly or unintentionally, the mechanisms of transmission are nevertheless open in principle to the agent's control, both for the transmitter and the transmittee, especially with adequate education. There are even reported incidents of deliberately conducted transmission of HIV, including a website for "bugchasers" who wish to receive or transmit HIV.[43] This is quite a different picture from diseases that are aerosolized or transmitted through intermediate vectors like mosquitoes; here, the human agents—both transmitter and transmittee, even with the conscientious use of such measures as insecticide or bed nets—have very much less control over whether the disease is passed along. HIV is also quite different from diseases that have common reservoirs—water or soil—because these reservoirs are far more difficult for ordinary people to avoid. Both vector-limitation and victim-protection are thus easier to construct for HIV than for infectious diseases such as influenza. Moreover, these mechanisms of HIV transmission and prevention became known within a few years of identification of the syndrome.

To say that HIV is in many ways exceptional is certainly not to say that there is a sharp distinction between HIV and other infectious diseases—they share many features—nor that HIV is unique. But the fact that the HIV virus is not transmitted casually or by diffuse routes such as aerosolization or intermediate vectors, but only by the limited routes of exchanges of bodily fluids normally subject to agent control is a very significant difference. It may be especially telling that the first extensive efforts of modern bioethics to deal with an infectious disease were focused on HIV, one of the least instructive and least challenging cases for understanding the *theoretical* implications of infectious disease for bioethics more generally, despite its enormous and devastating global impact.

---

43. See Gregory A. Freeman, "Bugchasers: The Men Who Long to Be HIV+," *Rolling Stone* (February 6, 2003), http://www.solargeneral.com/library/BugChasers.pdf (accessed December 29, 2007).

That HIV is transmitted by well-identified and potentially manageable routes has been an attractive draw for public health interventions in at least some countries. Cuba, for example, quarantined HIV-positive persons and has comparatively successfully contained the spread of the infection in that country.[44] Brazil has also been successful in controlling its epidemic, by using largely education and access to treatment rather than forcible constraint.[45] Constraints such as Cuba's are controversial, as we shall see in Chapters 16 and 21—but it is the mode of transmissibility of HIV that makes it seem more tractable to relatively straightforward public health interventions—testing, reporting, and restraining—than many other infectious diseases. Claims that changing transmission behavior is easier for HIV than for other infectious diseases may be culturally relative, but it is at a minimum true that HIV is not contracted—as some infectious diseases are, like flu—just by walking around.

The pressures on confidentiality and on liberty presented by the possibility of effective public health interventions against HIV resulted in demands for the protection of civil liberties in countries such as the United States that have strong rights-protective legal regimes. These demands for rights-protections were greatly intensified by the overall climate of concern for civil rights generally and rights for sexual liberty particularly that obtained during the late 1970s and early 1980s, the initial era of HIV.[46] Zita Lazzarini gives this account of the exceptionalism argument about HIV:

> Supposedly, the argument goes, public fear was so great, the political power of gay men so substantial, and concern over stigmatization and discrimination so real, that public health authorities abandoned 'traditional' and effective approaches to communicable disease control in favor of a civil liberties-focused approach. This resulted in policies that emphasized pre- and post-test counseling, anonymous testing, and stringent protections of confidentiality as opposed to named reporting, targeted screening, and partner notification.[47]

Abigail Zuger, as we noted in Chapter 1, identifies AIDS as the "first disease on record to spawn a huge, vocal, visible, angry grass-roots patients' rights movement that changed the course of history."[48] AIDS activists have been very effective in forcing public health officials and legislators to consider the rights of patients to privacy, autonomous decision making regarding their care, and

---

44. For a sympathetic account of Cuban HIV policy, see Farmer, *Pathologies of Power*, especially ch. 2.

45. See, e.g., P.R. Teixeira, M.A. Vitoria, and J. Barcarolo, "Antiretroviral Treatment in Resource-Poor Settings: The Brazilian Experience," *AIDS* 18, suppl. 3 (2004): S5-S7.

46. The U.S. Centers for Disease Control and Prevention (CDC) identified the syndrome in 1981; the virus was identified in 1984.

47. Zita Lazzarini, "What Lessons Can We Learn from the Exceptionalism Debate (Finally)?" *Journal of Law, Medicine & Ethics* 29 (2001): 149–151.

48. Abigail Zuger, "What Did We Learn from AIDS?" *New York Times*, sec. F, November 11, 2003.

the rights of infected patients to justice in the distribution of health-care resources. Conversely, the relation of AIDS communicability to specific human
behaviors has forced individual practitioners to be more open about questioning patients' private behaviors, to be more concerned with educating patients and the public about high-risk behaviors, and to consider classical public health methods for reducing communicability. In multiple ways, AIDS and
many other infectious diseases require us to consider the patient as both a *victim*
with individual needs and rights and as a potential *vector* of disease that is of
concern to the community.[49] But the way in which a person contracting AIDS
is a victim and that same person transmitting AIDS is a vector is different from
many other forms of communicable infectious disease.

At the time HIV came on the scene, there was increased legal emphasis on
liberty in intimate sexual relationships. The initial primary mode of transmission that introduced HIV into the United States—sexual activity among gay
men—made it seem particularly difficult to regulate. Ron Bayer pointed out
quite early in the discussions of HIV that it was being treated differently from
other infectious diseases, with an emphasis on individual rights, for example
on counseling before testing. Bayer describes in extensive and regretful detail
how gay activism made it difficult even to regulate the bathhouses in San
Francisco and New York that were a major locus of HIV transmission.[50] Bayer
is very sensitive to the ironies of the interventions that would be required for
survival, just when gay men were achieving freedom, as well as to the disastrous risks of stigmatization given ongoing attitudes about gay sexuality. At
the same time, Bayer relates, the public health law of disease control remained
mired at the turn of the twentieth century in yellow fever and quarantine
cases where state power had been left relatively unfettered regardless of the rationale for the intervention. Even with modern due process law, however,
Bayer believes that there are important conflicts between civil rights (including individual choices about intimate behavior) and the fact that efforts to
stop the spread of this deadly disease would have required decisions to change
intimate behavior. A full account of ethics in infectious disease must explore
whether this conflictual view—sexual liberty over against the protection of
the community—is too limited; we believe that it is.

As AIDS has come to be thought of as a chronic disease in areas of the
world where effective anti-retroviral therapy is available, there have been calls
for its "normalization."[51] Examples of such normalization include routine

---

49. Mann, "Medicine and Public Health."
50. Bayer, *Private Acts, Social Consequences,* esp. ch. 2.
51. See, e.g., Ronald Bayer, "Public Health Policy and the AIDS Epidemic: An End to HIV Exceptionalism?" *New England Journal of Medicine* 324 (1991): 1500–1504; Ronald Bayer, "Clinical Progress and the Future of HIV Exceptionalism," *Archives of Internal Medicine* 159 (1999): 1042–1048;

reporting, contact tracing, routine prenatal testing, over-the-counter test kits, and the use of rapid tests not requiring long waiting periods for results. There have, however, been calls for the reintroduction of the fully utilitarian paradigms of public health, such as mandatory testing and contact tracing, as HIV infection rates have begun to increase.[52]

To be sure, bioethics developed tremendously in response to the crisis of HIV/AIDS. Discussions of issues like obligations to treat, personal responsibility for disease, confidentiality, public surveillance, justice in international research, and the stigmatization of gay men and intravenous drug users have assumed great importance in bioethics. The growth in bioethics has been extraordinary; but these concerns have still been largely discussed within the traditional framework of bioethics, based in liberal theory and its standard constructions of autonomy and the harm principle. What these discussions have not taken fully into account has been characterized as the dual exceptionalism of AIDS: its mode of transmission and the rights-activism that accompanied it. HIV/AIDS has not presented the full range of challenges other infectious diseases might to standard liberal paradigms in bioethics. Thus the conclusions reached in bioethics about HIV/AIDS have not been—and could not easily have been—extended to infectious disease as a whole, as we discussed earlier in this chapter. Calls for the normalization of responses to HIV and for the application of public health ethics to the case of HIV may prove useful, but are, we think, also incomplete. They, too, require development of the more robust structures for bioethical analysis that we explore in the following two chapters.

Looking Ahead

In understanding the ethical implications of communicable infectious disease, we believe, something is needed over and above the familiar postures of bioethics and of public health. The patient is a current victim of infectious disease; the patient is also an actual or potential vector of infectious disease. Seeing any individual person in both ways at once requires a revised theoretical paradigm, one that can make possible a genuine union or at least a real connection between the sort of traditional clinical medicine that has been the concern of bioethics and the population-wide view that has been the concern

Lainie Friedman Ross, "Genetic Exceptionalism vs. Paradigm Shift: Lessons from HIV," *Journal of Law, Medicine & Ethics* 29 (2001): 141–146.

52. See, e.g., Jay F. Dobkin, "HIV Management: Time for a Public Health Approach?" *Infections in Medicine* 23 (2006): 48–49; Thomas R. Frieden, Moupali Das-Douglas, Scott E. Kellerman, and Kelly J. Henning, "Applying Public Health Principles to the HIV Epidemic," *New England Journal of Medicine* 353, no. 22 (2005): 2397–2402.

of public health. A revised theoretical paradigm, as we develop in this volume, must be capable of seeing the patient in *both ways at once*—not just flipping back and forth from one view to the other. Both public health ethics and bioethics will gain, not so much by replacing the basic paradigm of bioethics with that of public health, or the other way around, but by modifying and enhancing what each has developed so far. Both fields require rethinking of basic theoretical notions—autonomy, the individual patient, the harm principle, the public—in light of the idea that human beings are all, always, in some sense both victims and vectors at one and the same time. To be sure, some attempted fusions of moral concerns are best described, as Mark Sagoff puts it, as "bad marriage, quick divorce,"[53] but other deep-level fusions are fruitful indeed, and we think that this is possible—and urgent—between bioethics and public health.

---

53. Sagoff's reference is to environmental ethics and animal rights. See Mark Sagoff, "Animal Liberation and Environmental Ethics: Bad Marriage, Quick Divorce," *Osgoode Hall Law Journal* 22 (1984): 297–307.

PART II: THEORETICAL CONSIDERATIONS

6

EMBEDDED AUTONOMY AND THE "WAY-STATION SELF"

In Chapter 4, we documented the virtual absence in early bioethics of attention to infectious disease; in Chapter 5, we probed the gap between bioethics and public health that has been associated with bioethics' failure to examine the issues raised not just by disease, but by communicable infectious disease. In this chapter and the next, we begin the ethically urgent task of rethinking fundamental areas of theory in bioethics in light of the challenges of the distinctive features of contagious infectious disease. Our basic contention is that because bioethics' fundamental concepts—among them, autonomy, the harm principle, and responsibility—were rooted in an individualistic picture of actors drawn from liberal theory, bioethics has overlooked or misunderstood our vulnerability to each other as both victims and vectors, a vulnerability characteristic of communicable disease. As a result, it has relied on paradigms of analysis that are too impoverished to deal with the newly apparent challenges of infectious disease—paradigms that in retrospect we can now see were problematic from the beginning. In this and the following chapter, we supply a corrective, designed to augment this earlier and, we think, simplistic view. This corrective is not unique to infectious disease but, as we then argue in Chapter 8, can inform more traditional issues in bioethics as well.

This chapter begins the development of our new theoretical perspective. Understanding our vulnerability requires that we see ourselves in new ways, not only as the individuals we ordinarily think we are, but also biologically and indeed ecologically—as what we will call "way-station" selves. As way-station selves, we exercise autonomy that is embedded in a web of biological relationships. Such embedded autonomy requires us to rethink four theoretical aspects of traditional liberal bioethics: the accounts of the individual agent, of autonomy, of the harm principle, and of responsibility. In this chapter, we re-examine each of these fundamental notions in light of the biological and social facts of infectious disease. We argue that the traditional liberal picture is classically characterized by flat, conflictual analyses, in its treatment both of autonomy as respect for an individual's choices limited by the harm principle, and of responsibility as the obligations of some individuals toward others.

Reunderstanding the Individual Agent

Communicable infectious disease forces us to recognize that individuals are not only socially but also physically situated in a distinctive way. Individual people are foci of victimhood and vectorhood in physical relation to other humans and to the biological world. As bioethicists and especially feminist bioethicists have long understood, people stand in a nexus of social relationships among each other. We now also need to see that people stand in a broader nexus of biological relationships as well—not just the biological ties of family, ancestry, and reproduction, but the interrelationships of contagion and vulnerability to contagion—as well as the non-biological ties of society and culture.

In recent years, philosophers increasingly have recognized the inadequacy of individualistic metaphysical accounts of the agent. Thomas May's rejection of the "impoverished, atomistic" view of the individual in favor of a view of individuals as "socially located" was mentioned in Chapter 4.[1] Feminist writers have developed important accounts of relational autonomy.[2] These views emphasize familial and caring relationships: partners, parents, caregivers and the ones cared for.[3] An important observation for our discussion here is that such social relationships are also often physical ones, involving touching, holding, containment (as in pregnancy), penetration, and genetic continuity.

As this observation suggests, attention to social locatedness is not enough. "Physical locatedness," to adapt May's term, is critical as well. The theoretical paradigms of liberalism typically see the individual as a physically discrete entity, however tightly individuals may be socially related, and not as physically connected except in largely elective actions such as shaking hands, hugging, fist-fighting, undergoing surgery, and of course making love. But these paradigms are simplistic and misleading, as ecologists and bioethicists of an ecological bent have recognized.[4] Infectiousness is an especially direct reminder of how misleading the paradigms of individualism can be. The notion that a person is a discrete individual is not exactly wrong, but is seriously abbreviated. Indeed, discussions of an evolutionary basis for human biological interrelatedness with transmissible microorganisms have been appearing in the recent popular and scientific literature.[5]

---

1. Thomas May, "The Concept of Autonomy in Bioethics: An Unwarranted Fall from Grace," in *Personal Autonomy: New Essays on Personal Autonomy and Its Role in Contemporary Moral Philosophy*, ed. James Stacey Taylor (Cambridge: Cambridge University Press, 2005), 299–309.
2. Catriona MacKenzie and Natalie Stoljar, *Relational Autonomy: Feminist Perspectives on Autonomy, Agency, and the Social Self* (New York: Oxford University Press, 2000).
3. See, e.g., Sara Ruddick, *Maternal Thinking: Toward a Politics of Peace* (Boston: Beacon Press, 1989).
4. See, e.g., Bruce Jennings, "The Liberalism of Life: Bioethics in the Face of Biopower," *Raritan Review* 23, no. 4 (Spring 2003): 132–146.
5. See, e.g., Marlene Zuk, *Riddled with Life: Friendly Worms, Ladybug Sex, and the Parasites That Make Us Who We Are* (Orlando, FL: Harcourt Books, 2007).

Just as physical relationships among human beings may be personal and intimate or accidental and among strangers, victims and vectors may pass disease along either in intimate relationships or without any awareness of each other. The feminist emphasis on relationality, while it reminds people of their sociality, interconnectedness, and even physicality, does so in a more local and less universal way than does infectious disease. After all, contagion may occur despite whether the victim knows the vector, and despite whether the victim can even identify the vector or the time of contagion. Transmission can be reciprocal, chained in a sequence of transmissions, or exponentially widespread. Any person can be both victim and vector simultaneously, or victim of one disease but at the same time vector of another; this is particularly true where one disease affects susceptibility to or transmissibility of other infectious diseases, like HIV and tuberculosis or genital herpes and other sexually transmitted diseases. One individual can transmit the same disease over and over again. And people can transmit disease utterly anonymously, without any social connection at all: think of the hotel guest whose viruses or bacteria remain on the telephone handset or the light switch in the bathroom long after she has checked out, ready to infect the next guest.[6]

The only possibility of being a true non-vector may seem to be hermit-like isolation. But even isolation will not fully protect people from the nexus of infectious diseases. Many infectious diseases are not transmitted directly from person to person; there may be animal or inanimate reservoirs such as soil or water involved in transmission, as discussed in Chapter 2. If someone is bitten by a mosquito, even though she has no contact with other humans, she can still transmit malaria; if she defecates near the stream even in a remote forest, she still may pass disease along. For some diseases, the patient can largely control transmission—in HIV/AIDS, for example, by not donating blood, having sex, or sharing needles; this is one aspect of the exceptionalism of HIV we discussed in Chapter 5. Moreover, the efficacy of control mechanisms may vary widely with the mode of transmission. For example, the availability of effective vaccines often lags behind the appearance of new strains of influenza. For other diseases, immunization may prevent infection and isolation may reduce the likelihood of spread. But such control measures are not available or effective for many infectious diseases, such as malaria, schistosomiasis, or giardiasis. Cultural practices are also relevant in controlling transmissibility, such as bowing rather than shaking hands as a greeting or not eating meat as a factor in avoiding the transmission of variant Creutzfeldt-Jakob disease (vCJD, the human form of "mad cow" disease). In some contemporary Asian cultures,

---

6. J. Owen Hendley, "Hotel Rooms Have Unseen Guests," study presented at the Interscience Conference on Antimicrobial Agents and Chemotherapy, San Francisco, CA., September 26–27, 2006.

people wear masks to avoid spreading disease. But even with all of these measures people are never in full control of their status as either victim or vector.

As physically located bodies, human beings are always "embedded" in potential circumstances of exchange. One person's transmission of disease to others—to person x and x_1, and from x_1 to x_2, and from x_2 to x_3, and so on along a chain or chains, branching out to perhaps many others—may be easy to track. But it is also critical to understand that a given infectious condition, or something like it, may rebound back to that person—from x_3 to x_2 to x_1 to the original person, among many others—whether by the original or other transmission routes. Although reinfection with the same disease is not always possible because of developed immunities, some diseases can recur in the same individual multiple times: gonorrhea, for example. And already infected people may be reinfected with different types of the same microbe, as with the human papilloma virus (HPV) or the human immunodeficiency virus (HIV). People may be both agents and patients at the same time, at staggered times, at times with long intervals in between, or simultaneously. Even where one episode of disease may confer immunity to that disease (and sometimes to related conditions), individuals are still at risk for transmission of other or even related diseases.

Thus human beings all live together with each other in a web of potential and actual disease, all the time, even when they are not currently overtly ill and not aware of the possibility of transmission. While many infectious diseases are comparatively innocuous and mild, some are rapid-moving, fatal illnesses. With some infectious diseases, people are literally well one day, gravely ill the next, and either dead or fully recovered the next—infections such as meningitis can move exactly this fast. This vulnerability is not one people can always choose to avoid by taking precautions, for instance by gloving, masking, or becoming immunized. As long as there are unpreventable, uncontained infectious diseases in the human population, this agent/patient/agent relationship will remain an ineluctable feature of human moral life. No matter how people try, they cannot avoid the fact not just that they are at risk of infection from others but that they in turn pose risks to others and thus perhaps to others far distant from themselves.

Biologically speaking, the human "individual" must be seen for what he or she is: a large organism carrying and inhabited by a host of smaller ones that move easily from their habitat in one "person" to another. The human organism is a way-station, a breeding-ground, a launching-pad for enormous multitudes of smaller life. The "individual" human organism, after all, is colonized by tens of trillions of microorganisms, both internally and on its surfaces. One recent study catalogued 182 different species of bacteria, belonging to 91 genera, just on small patches of forearm skin from six healthy human subjects—and of these only four species were found on all six subjects, and species rapidly replaced each other in later testing.[7] The immense numbers of bacteria, viruses, and other microorganisms that inhabit the throat and nasal passages, the gut, and elsewhere in the body, are far more diverse.

That human individuals are colonized by microorganisms is familiar and not always threatening. Many of these microorganisms are beneficial and indeed indispensable for human survival—for example, the bacteria that are involved in the digestive tract. Others, such as the chickenpox virus that can recur many years later as shingles, inhabit the individual for the most part innocuously but can become dangerous when that individual is under stress or is immune-compromised. Still others invade from outside, opportunistically, like fungal infections in the environment of the immune-suppressed host, or even when the human host is in full health. Some microorganisms, like the staphylococcus bacterium, kill cells directly. In other cases, such as tuberculosis, it is the host's immune response to the invading organism that causes tissue damage. Many infectious disease organisms cause disease in the malnourished, the elderly, and infants. And some are most damaging to the vigorous—for instance, as we have seen earlier, the flu of 1918–1919 that killed an estimated 40-100 million people or more worldwide was most fatal in healthy young adults, those with the most active immune systems that literally overwhelmed them physically in fighting off disease.[8]

These biological vulnerabilities and capacities for physical threat and threatenedness evident in infectious disease must be part of a full normative account of human agency. This is why it is urgent to reassess the conventional liberal notion of the independent individual. Human beings are not the tall-standing, health-enjoying, competent, rational, individually discrete figures envisioned in many accounts in liberal normative theory, so central in bioethics. Instead, they are complex and vulnerable constellations of organisms always under threat and always capable of causing threats to others, yet also dependent on some of these organisms, without which they would die. To dichotomize the individual and the environment is misleading, in that people *are* their microbial environment. This is the physical picture of the human individual to keep in mind. This is not metaphysical nonsense; this is biological fact. But it *is* metaphysically significant for bioethics: patients—the field's "unit of analysis," as it were—are interconnected as victims and vectors and cannot be seen as individual "units" apart from this microbial environment.

---

7. Zhan Gao, Chi-hong Tseng, Zhiheng Pei, and Martin J. Blaser, "Molecular Analysis of Human Forearm Superficial Skin Bacterial Biota," *Proceedings of the National Academy of Sciences* 104 (February 2007): 2927–2932.

8. See John M. Barry, *The Great Influenza: The Epic Story of the Deadliest Epidemic in History* (London: Penguin Books, 2004).

To be sure, burdens of infectious disease are not equally shared, and perhaps cannot be equally shared. People have immune systems of differing capacities, and live in different social circumstances. Chances of exposure, response to exposure, and ultimate likelihood of succumbing to disease, are not the same. Some of this is a matter of biological differences that John Rawls described as "arbitrary from a moral point of view"[9] and that other philosophers have regarded as "brute luck."[10] But at least as much of it, if not a great deal more, is due to social circumstances (or physical conditions that have their roots in social circumstances) that are not only arbitrary from a moral point of view in Rawls's sense, but also profoundly unjust.[11] These observations press the recognition that our starting point must not be regarded as an idealization, a picture of the human condition that might seem more relevant to "ideal" theory than to the realm of "partial compliance theory,"[12] the theorizing under conditions of injustice that is the typical locus of problems in applied ethics. In the discussions to follow, we will need to attend to the challenges posed by the roles of brute luck and social injustice in generating differential susceptibilities. Whatever we say about such differences, however, they are exacerbations, not rejections, of our underlying point that in the end human beings, however well protected, are all in some sense susceptible to illness both from and to each other.

Finally, with respect to infectious disease, people are also historically situated individuals. All are embedded in a web of disease, the continuing transmission of pathogenic microorganisms from one person to another, with or without intermediate vectors in between. But this web itself can be historically mapped. Transmission chains stretch backwards to the emergence of a pathogen—as far back at least as the times of the pharaohs for smallpox, for example; or as recently as the spring of 1973, for an apparently novel transmission from deer mice to humans of a previously unidentified hantavirus;[13] and still more recently for other emerging infections. Transmission chains in general stretch forward into an indefinite future, even if occasionally fully stopped— smallpox in 1977, for example. Other transmission chains may also be fully stopped in the future: the hope once again is that the chain of polio transmission, including that emanating from the outbreak in northern Nigeria in 2003,

9. John Rawls, *A Theory of Justice* (Cambridge: Harvard University Press, 1971).

10. Thomas Nagel, "Moral Luck," in *Mortal Questions* (New York: Cambridge University Press, 1979), ch. 3.

11. See, e.g., Paul Farmer, *Pathologies of Power: Health, Human Rights, and the New War on the Poor,* (Berkeley: University of California Press, 2003).

12. The distinction between "ideal" and "partial compliance" theory is Rawls's, who drew it only to leave partial compliance theory aside; it will be discussed more fully in Chapter 19.

13. Ann Marie Kimball, *Risky Trade: Infectious Disease in the Era of Global Trade* (Williston, VT: Ashgate, 2006).

may be broken in the early decades of the twenty-first century. Human individuals each occupy a distinct historical point in that web of disease, though of course when they are coughing, sneezing, or enduring rashes or hemorrhagic bleeding, they rarely think of themselves as just one link in a perhaps short or possibly millennia-long, transmission chain.

Rethinking Autonomy

Thus the picture of the individual agent requires modification in the light of social and physical situatedness with respect to infectious disease. Such situatedness also forces modifications in the understanding of autonomy, as well as what might follow from it such as claims about liberty or rights.

Autonomy, although characterized by early and later writers in a wide variety of differing ways, has most centrally been viewed in terms of self-determination. Yet particular characteristics of some infectious diseases undercut familiar conditions for the exercise of autonomy. For example, the acuity of some infectious diseases militates against reflective decision making; the capacity for permanent prevention may reshape assessments of risk and benefit; and the complex infective mechanisms of communicable disease may work against some philosophical accounts of autonomy as informed by plans. Acuity can be regarded as an unusual, impaired circumstance, but prevention is an ongoing, ubiquitous issue. The prospect of communicable disease is ever-present and complex, even if a person is not at the moment ill. We do not deny the importance of autonomy, rights, plans, and related notions as appropriately central concepts in bioethics (and law). Our point is rather that the ideal of the thoughtful chooser, deciding in accord with his or her preferences and interests, is upset by our picture of the embedded agent. As a result, we must enhance our understanding of autonomy and its implications.[14]

It might seem that the absence of infectious disease in bioethics is an oversight that can be corrected relatively easily within standard bioethical analysis: just add infectiousness to the mix, as one more factor for the autonomous agent to consider. The agent in exercising autonomy then would be expected to attend in her choices to the risks of infectiousness that she experiences and constitutes. But are things so simple? Behind an easy grafting of infectiousness onto the consideration of these and other issues in bioethics lurk deeper tensions. For example, the agent who lacks time for reflection about whether to go to work while experiencing symptoms of flu is not just an ordinary decision maker in a hurry or under pressure who should be urged to consider choices

---

14. Centers for Disease Control and Prevention, "Progress Toward Interruption of Wild Poliovirus Transmission—Worldwide, January 2006-May 2007," *Mortality and Morbidity Weekly Report* 56, no. 27 (July 13, 2007): 682–685.

more carefully. She is a risk to others, and they in turn are risks to her. These are sometimes unrecognized threats of unknown urgency, gravity, or magnitude. Of course, someone who holds a hidden bomb may also be a risk of which others are unaware. But infectiousness is a reminder that all may pose risks to each other, all of the time, whether they know it or not, not just because of a weapon they carry, knowingly or perhaps unknowingly, but because of the very kind of organism they are. Sometimes these are direct risks of reciprocal transmission, where two parties mutually infect each other. But the far more general point holds as well, that people are always potential victims and potential vectors to each other and to the natural world.

Traditional accounts of autonomy fail to recall these possibilities of unknown and interlocking risks in transmissible infectious disease. We will explore a number of traditional dilemmas in bioethics in Chapter 8—dilemmas of truth-telling, informed consent, privacy and confidentiality, withholding and withdrawing care—and will see that in all of them, traditional accounts prove inadequate when the issue is raised in the context of transmissible infectious disease. Furthermore, as we shall see in later chapters, the prospect of transmissible infectious disease may also challenge the relationship between autonomy and justice.[15] What if there are conflicts between the choices of an autonomous, highly contagious agent to refuse treatment or to be treated in certain settings, and the achievement of justice for others? What of trade-offs with justice, such as between achieving a decent minimum of health care for everyone within a society, and the means needed to provide sufficient health care and vector management to reduce the risk of reservoirs of infectious disease? As victim, the patient may tend to see his plight as the responsibility of others, deserving care as a result; as vector, the patient may ignore his effects on others, thus creating otherwise avoidable needs for resources by his individual choices.

One conclusion to draw here might be that such tensions are inevitable, especially under circumstances of less than perfect justice. Individual patient choice just may be a complex matter, both as it affects the person herself and as it conflicts with the choices or needs of others. Traditional autonomy theory treats the former as self-regarding choices, for the individual alone to make, and the latter as the tension between competing actors, susceptible to analysis in terms of the individual's responsibility not to harm others. On this traditional view of autonomy, bioethics must simply live with these tensions, resolving them as best it can by providing patients with fuller information and other protection for the rationality of their choices, and by helping patients think through which values are most important in the solution of a given problem.

---

15. Rosamond Rhodes, "Justice in Medicine and Public Health," *Cambridge Quarterly of Health Care Ethics* 14, no. 1 (2005): 13–26.

We believe, however, that this may be giving up too soon. The roots of seeing decision making in this binary and conflictual way—the agent against others—lie initially in the limited way in which the autonomous agent has been understood in bioethics. Autonomy is not simply a matter of the choices of separate and separable agents who affect one another only contingently. It is a matter of the choices of embedded agents, way-station selves, who must take into account the ever-present possibility of their unavoidable biological connections with each other. The normative implications of these biological facts have been insufficiently developed, as discussion of the harm principle will show.

Rethinking the Harm Principle

Standard liberal theory has developed accounts of the permissible limits to patient autonomy and political liberty. Libertarians, who hold that people have rights to do whatever they want so long as they do not interfere with the rights of others, limit individuals' choices about how to move their fists by others' rights not to be punched. Liberals in the tradition of John Stuart Mill struggle with questions about the extent to which individuals are morally obligated to take into account the effects of their actions or omissions on others. Whether people are obligated to rescue someone who is drowning, calculate the effects of their energy use patterns on others, or refrain from taking jobs that are important to them despite the fact that they might sometimes perform them in a way that is risky to others, are sources of ongoing discussion in liberal theory and accommodation in the law. In addition, there are now some discussions of whether people have obligations not to go to work if they are contagious, not to travel if they have been exposed to certain infectious diseases, or not to reproduce if they might transmit infectious conditions to their offspring.

The "harm principle," famously set out (although not named) by Mill, holds that "the only purpose for which social power can be rightfully exercised over any member of a civilized community, against his will, is to prevent harm to others."[16] Like other harms, risks of contagion may legitimate social intervention under the harm principle. Quarantine, restricting a person's liberty to move about in the world, is one of the most extreme constraints that has been imposed to prevent people from risking harm to others. But other constraints have also been imposed in order to control infectious disease: for example, restrictions on sexual activity (e.g., closing bathhouses), on attending

---

16. John Stuart Mill, *On Liberty* (London: Oxford University Press, 1859), http://books.google.com/books?id=qCQCAAAAQAAJ&printsec=titlepage (accessed December 29, 2007), ch.1.

school (e.g., requiring immunization), on keeping matters secret (e.g., contact tracing), on refusing medical interventions (e.g., directly observed therapy), or on getting health-care treatment from one's chosen providers (e.g., requiring mainstream medical treatment rather than alternative health care).

Discussions in bioethics and the law have typically treated the solutions to these dilemmas as a matter of taking sides in a conflict between the liberty of the individual patient and the rights of others to be protected from harm. Our proposal, it may be thought, merely reflects an application of the familiar harm principle to infectious disease. To those who would press this objection, our reply is that the harm principle too requires a deeper understanding. The harm principle as it is sometimes presented treats the patient and those she might harm as in a situation of conflict. The liberty of the one must be curtailed if others are to be protected. Or protection must depend on voluntary self-restraint. Susan Okie also asks whether a person might be obligated to take an "altruistic" vaccine, such as a transmission-blocking vaccine against malaria that is designed to induce an immune response against the stage of the malaria parasite that develops inside the mosquito, a vaccine that would not protect the recipient of the vaccine but would prevent that person's blood from infecting a mosquito, which could transmit the parasite to someone else.[17]

On this "either liberty or coercion" view, cases of contagion are analogized to the standard "harm principle" cases in liberal theory, such as shooting another, stealing another's property, or shouting "fire!" in a crowded theater and causing a fatal stampede as people rush for the exits. In these cases, people are understood as actors, capable of refraining from shooting, stealing, or shouting false alarms. People "assault" each other by "delivering" their infectious microorganisms to each other, something they could avoid, albeit at perhaps significant costs to their own preferences. Society expects people who are infected with dangerous, transmissible diseases to sacrifice their interests for the overall social good, either altruistically or in response to coercion. Altruistic action involves the individual's sacrificing her own interests for the good of others. The constraints permitted by the harm principle are seen as arising externally from the agent who might want to shoot, steal, or shout "fire." They are not seen as connected to his agency in any deep sense; the harm principle permits limits on liberty that are imposed from outside.

On our view, however, this "harm principle" picture is simplistic. The contagious patient is not simply a known vector-threat to victim-others. She is also a victim-other to their vector-threats. When a patient is both victim and vector, the question of preventing harm arises not just from the outside, as a matter of preventing harm to separate others. A person who might harm

---

17. Susan Okie, "Betting on a Malaria Vaccine," *New England Journal of Medicine* 353, no. 18 (2005): 1877–1881 (1880).

others by transmitting disease is in a position to harm them, but by the same act might also be harmed by them. Moreover, these dimensions of interconnected risk may be unknown and difficult to know, at least in real life and time. People may be contagious before they are even aware that they are infected or before currently available forms of medical diagnosis could detect their infectiousness. In other cases, the sources of harm may be unknown to anyone.

The challenge the standard interpretation of the harm principle presents is not just the problem of extending the harm principle's legitimization of interference with liberty to cases in which the harm is merely probabilistic or speculative. Rather, we must move away from the model of one identifiable person posing risks to identifiable others, to the recognition that all live in a surrounding environment of microorganisms that regularly travel from one human "individual" to "another" as their mode of life. People are thus non-electively related in their vulnerability, in part because they are not biologically discrete beings whose physical interactions with each other are always under their own control. "Their" interests are not always so clearly distinct from "the interests of others," or from "our" interests, or from those of "society" as a whole. We must think through how to deal with these situations so that all are protected from infectious disease, and so that the burdens of our protection are fairly shared.

Constraints protect the actual and potential victim, just as they constrain the actual and potential vector. But it is not always certain who is who, and in any case everyone occupies all these roles. The traditional harm-principle separation between a realm of self-regarding and therefore socially free actions, and a realm of other-regarding and therefore socially subjected actions, breaks down in the context of these features of infectious disease.

Our point here is not that liberty should be overridden to protect everyone from risks of contagion. We are not arguing that autonomy should be abandoned, or that the rights it engenders should be thought of as a nuisance. Nor do we want to ignore the insights from the more population-based approach often found in the public health literature. Yet we need an account that can serve both the view of clinical medicine—in which the patient is characteristically seen primarily as victim—and the view of public health, in which the patient is seen as potential vector. What we want is an account in which the patient can be seen as both *victim* and *vector* at the same time, a person simultaneously occupying both morally relevant roles.

Consider how such an account might look. The earliest accounts of autonomy in bioethics are focused around reasonable preferences, including preferences that involve other parties, are altruistic, and so on. Individuals can have interests in the interests of others—in how their children, their partners, or their friends fare. Interests in global issues are seen in terms of effects on these individualized interests and may be more or less attenuated as a result. By contrast, individuals' interests start to look different when transmission is at issue.

Beyond individuals' own sets of interests and subsidiary concerns about how they affect others, and beyond any possible assumptions about whether people may be motivated by altruism, people have interests in not transmitting diseases because they are embedded among other people who, like them, are also at once victims and vectors. To put it most simply, as rational agents accepting a plausible view of moral responsibility, we do not want this to be the way we all live.

To be sure, individuals are most likely to transmit and acquire communicable diseases in more localized and relatively predictable ways: to and from people with whom they have close, physical contact, including family members, co-workers, sexual partners, in some cases sports partners (think of wrestlers and flesh-eating strep), and also nurses and physicians involved in treatment. Individuals are also likely to pass on disease within groups that they identify with—occupational, religious, recreational—primarily because these are the groups with which they have the most contact. Although they may not have contact with every member of those groups, those to whom they do transmit may pass infection on among the groups' internal web of contacts. Such "groups" are not necessarily residential, geographic, or interest-based; they may be stable over long periods or come together in a unique situation. A "group" may come together in a particular situation of stress but be otherwise unrelated, like passengers on an airliner with a recirculating air system or people interned in the same refugee camp. Examples also include religious groups, such as those that oppose immunization or share potato salad at a church picnic. Such groups may be affiliational or behavioral—for example, gay men and HIV, or adventure travelers and malaria, or dormitory roommates and meningitis. Or it may be a more-or-less accidental connection: Haitians quarantined on entering the United States, residents of a SARS-infected apartment building in Hong Kong, or poultry farmers in Asia. And, of course, groups intersect with other groups societywide.

Mutual disease transmission within families is a familiar phenomenon—one family member gets a cold and others in the family do too—as is the way in which disease may be transmitted throughout a group even when individual members have contact with only some of the individuals composing that group. How disease travels around the world is also familiar—ordinary flu does this every year. But the full moral implications for each and every person are rarely recognized. Human beings live in a world in which they transmit their diseases to others, whether they wanted to, intended to, or knew they were doing so—and in which others have already transmitted their diseases to them and to others, whether they wanted to, intended to, or knew they were doing so.

Clearly, people have an interest in not transmitting disease not only to people who are close to them and to people in groups they identify with, but also to the world more generally. To put the point more exactly, everyone has an interest in not being part of a mutually disease-transmitting family, group, or society—and, for that matter, globe. After all, as we shall see more clearly in our airport thought-experiment in Chapter 15, distant parts of the globe are just a plane ride away, and disease—whether mild, moderate, or lethal—can travel in a matter of hours on an airliner from one side of the earth to the other, from them to us, or from us to them. The moral implications of this picture do not rest simply on an enhanced or more sophisticated conception of self-interest. They rest on a modified and deepened picture of the self involved—a relational, embodied self who is unavoidably both threatened with harm and constitutes a threat of harm to others. This deepened picture of embedded agency also has implications for judgments not only about what we ought to do, but about ourselves as responsible agents.

Rethinking Responsibility

Judgments of responsibility include both whether people can be held responsible at all and what they can be held responsible for. Start with a fairly standard picture—flat and conflictual, as we have said—of the responsible agent, able to control whether she exceeds the appropriate limits of autonomy by violating her obligations not to harm others. This standard picture supposes that if she cannot exercise self-control, it is because of flaws in her—impairments, bad will, or lack of self-control. If she causes harm because of a mental disease or defect, she may be judged not to be responsible for what she has done, because there are flaws in her understanding or in her ability to conform her conduct to the requirements of law. If she is judged not to be responsible, it is because she falls short of full human agency—she is in some respects a deficient agent, thus not to be judged by the standards of ordinary agency.

Embeddedness as we understand it, however, is part of the structure of our agency, not merely a feature of defective agency. With some forms of contagiousness, control of whom and when individuals infect is not possible. With other forms, capacity for control may vary in many ways; it may be partial, or fluctuating, or time-dependent, as during periods of pre-symptomatic infectiousness. Compare judgments about the absence of responsibility in cases of mental illness with the partial or complete lack of control someone has when a sneeze dissipates droplets. She may not know ahead of time that she is about to sneeze; and sneezes cannot always be stifled successfully, even with effort. People can cover their mouths when they sneeze but that may not obviate contagion. People often act inadvertently or carelessly; for example, someone may think to cover his mouth when he sneezes but then put his hand on the stair railing right afterwards. But even with great care about infection-control measures, the only way to completely limit potential vectorhood would be simply to stay away from everyone else, to become a human isolate—to the extent possible a very costly and indeed inhumane solution over the long term. Even then, as we have seen, we may not be able to fully obviate either our vectorhood or our victimhood, for they extend beyond other human beings to the natural world.

Of course, many aspects of infectious disease are congruent with the picture of a person who can choose to avoid risks presented by others or to avoid imposing risks on them. That is, in many cases individuals have a measure of control over whether they become infected or infect others. Individuals do have choices about their actions in light of what they know about contagion, and they can be held responsible for those choices, at least when they knowingly infect others or put them at risk. Deliberately sneezing on one's competitor, having sex when one is aware of the possibility of transmitting disease, like chlamydia or syphilis—these are (ir)responsible acts. Similar notions of responsibility, praise, and blame apply to them, as to other reckless acts that put persons at risk: leaving toxic waste near a playground, having sex without protection against unwanted pregnancy, and so on. And they also apply to more sinister acts involving infectious agents, such as the plots of bioterrorists or the deliberate transmission of HIV as an act of revenge. But the point is that our ongoing presence in the web of infectious disease is part of our very nature in the context of which we make these choices and go about our daily lives without making choices about particular aspects of infectiousness at all.

Thus there is more to the context of infectious disease than whether control can be voluntary. People are often unaware that they are infectious or even ill or at risk of being ill, at the very point disease is most likely to be transmitted to others. Whether to transmit disease or not may not even be the subject of agency; with respect to some infectious diseases, spread to susceptible hosts may occur despite our very best efforts at prevention. Moreover, long transmission chains compound the issue; it may be difficult or impossible to trace these chains and thereby connect harm done to one person to the acts of another. Blameworthiness for transmission may be further affected by factors such as susceptibility in downstream parties, sometimes comparatively easily foreseen but often unpredictable. For example, with a simple sneeze someone might transmit an infectious agent that has no effect on herself but is utterly devastating to others, as a pneumonia might be simple to resolve in a healthy young adult but fatal in an elderly or immune-compromised person. Leaving a rainwater-filled old tire in the back yard during mosquito-breeding season in a West Nile virus-endemic area might be merely a nuisance if the neighbors are a college dormitory full of healthy young adults, but a lethal threat if a nursing home is next door.

Thus "source patient" imagery, the frequent picture in public health, can be misleading, especially when translated into moral-theoretical contexts for identifying agents responsible for given harms. Source patient imagery suggests a chain with a starting point, as disease moves on to others but does not further affect the originating party. Except for new mutations in emerging diseases and final eradication (like the last wild smallpox patient on Earth, in Somalia in 1977), there is no one "source" patient and no end-point terminus; the disease keeps traveling from one person to another. Source patient imagery tends to fail to see the web of interlocking and interplaying mutual, multiple transmissions, especially within groups of associated individuals. People may be appropriately held responsible for transmitting disease to others—that is, blamed—if they do so knowingly. But others are responsible, perhaps also blameworthy, for transmitting diseases along to still others. People are all implicated in a web of relationships that establish themselves without their knowing and that may be difficult to sort out in a linearly traceable way—even when it is possible to identify specific strains of a virus, for instance, that have been transmitted from one person to another along transmission chains that begin with the first emergence of a pathogen and continue on into the indefinite future, but which branch, overlap, mutate, and recombine along the way. This is because it is not just single occasions of disease transmission that each person is responsible for, but the whole web of disease relationships in which all participate.

It may be tempting to shrug these cases off as unpredictable, requiring too omniscient a capacity for foreseeing outcomes of individual choices and so not a violation of responsibilities to avoid harming others. After all, a person cannot be held responsible for what he or she cannot realistically predict. But we cannot grant this point. The more complex metaphysical status of human beings as individuals—their physical as well as social *locatedness*, their *embeddedness* among others who are also way-stations and launching-pads for dangerous as well as benign microorganisms—cuts against binary judgments that people are either responsible or not responsible, blameworthy or not blameworthy. Human beings are too immersed in infectious illness too much of the time to claim that they cannot know that all are parts of chains and webs of transmission all of the time.

If people are "embedded" in a physical as well as social nexus, judgments of responsibility are too simplistic if they merely point fingers at blameworthy originators of harm. Notions of blame must take into account that although someone may be blameworthy for transmitting a specific disease if he can avoid doing so, at the very same time he may be justified in blaming others, as are those who transmitted it to him if they could have avoided doing so. But such judgments must also take into account that he may put others in the same situation as himself, even though no one intends that this occur, and that all of this transmission may take place at one and the same time. Thus individual finger-pointing does not adequately take into account what it is to be caught in—and contributing to—a complex web of mutual transmission, ongoing all the time. Judgments of individual responsibility, appropriate in the cases of deliberate transmission or known risks, must be supplemented by judgments about how we together are responsible for reservoirs of infectiousness we both endure and perpetuate.

7

THE MULTIPLE PERSPECTIVES OF THE *PATIENT AS VICTIM AND VECTOR* VIEW

In the previous chapters we argued that traditional concepts in bioethics have failed to appreciate our dual status as both victims and vectors. Bioethics' normative analyses have been classically characterized by flat, conflictual ways of seeing issues that typically 1) assess autonomy as respect for an individual's choices but limited by the harm principle that attends to the effects of those choices on others, and 2) see responsibility as the obligations of some individuals toward others to whom they owe duties of fidelity, care, protection, and so on. The fuller *patient as victim and vector* view we explore here, which we nickname the *PVV view*, augments traditional ethical analyses within bioethics and public health by making positive use of the tensions in the different perspectives we do and should employ in thinking about communicable infectious disease. Our PVV view both incorporates these different perspectives and explains their significance in normative analysis. We think of this view as usable in various ways: identifying and analyzing problems, indicating where conflicts remain ineluctable, and deciding how clinical practices and public policies must address the reality of human interconnectedness in a web of infectious disease.

Tensions over issues in communicable infectious disease emerge within and among at least three distinguishable, but overlapping analytic perspectives. The first perspective is the vantage point of ordinary life, from which the individual characteristically views his or her own disease status—well or sick, safe or at risk. A second perspective is how groups and populations are doing overall, with individuals as data-point entities within a population-wide view, a view associated (not always accurately) with public health. A third is a hypothetical way of viewing the same matters suggested by our biologicized notion of the self, a kind of naturalized Rawlsian thought experiment perspective from which every human being's disease-relevant situation can be seen, but in which it is not possible to know which aspects of this situation are paramount at any given point in time. Each of these three perspectives yields insights that are centrally important in understanding communicable infectious disease. Each adds to and requires correction from the perspective of the others to yield an agenda for thinking about communicable infectious disease—a broader view intended to enrich the field of both bioethics and public health, and a view from which we will then develop a normatively defensible account of how to act and what kinds of policies to develop with regard to communicable infectious disease. Dealing with communicable infectious disease involves both seeing what is there and figuring out what to do. Neither is a simple task, and both are essential to our PVV project.

Understanding Multiple Perspectives

The role of different, initially descriptive perspectives in our PVV view can best be explained by analogy, though each of the analogies we offer here is imperfect in certain ways. Perceptual illusions are a well-known way of illustrating distinct and often incompatible views; here are a handful of examples from the history of philosophy and experimental psychology that approach the internal tensions over issues in infectious disease that we believe are important to see. Our concept of "internal tension" is not captured fully accurately by any of these analogies, but each of them approaches an aspect of what we have in mind.

Plato famously supported his view that everyday "reality" is illusory by pointing to what people see when they look at a stick in a glass of water. They *know* that the stick is straight. But they *see* a stick that is bent; and this, for Plato, confirms the fact that everyday perceptions are unreliable. In our account here, we are less interested in the reliability of perception than in the fact that there can be a gap, a tension, between what people (think they) know and what they (seem to) see.

The *Mona Lisa*, easily the most famous of Leonardo da Vinci paintings and perhaps the best-known painting in western art, portrays an enigmatically smiling woman. But her smile appears different if the painting is viewed from slightly off side to the left than if it is viewed from slightly off side to the right: either way, she seems to be smiling *toward* the onlooker. The perspectival illusion is found in many forms of art and architecture—witness staircase designs that appear to face the observer from any direction—but what is relevant here is that one entity, the portrait of a woman, can be seen in different ways even though nothing about the painted canvas itself has changed.

Again somewhat differently, consider the "duck-rabbit" figure that the twentieth-century philosopher Ludwig Wittgenstein adapted from an earlier Gestalt perception theorist:[1]

---

1. Ludwig Wittgenstein, *Philosophical Investigations*, 3rd ed., trans. G.E.M. Anscombe (Cornwall, UK: Blackwell, 2003 [2001]), 194 (figure reprinted by permission).

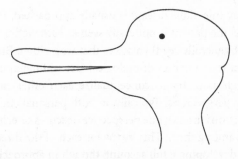

Look at the figure. Is it a duck? Or is it a rabbit? Can it be seen as both duck and rabbit at the same time? Or, if it is thought of as a duck, does any suggestion of rabbitness melt away, and vice versa? Although Wittgenstein himself was principally interested in the conceptual nature of perception rather than the phenomenon of mutual exclusiveness, what is instructive about the "duck-rabbit" figure for our purposes is that two aspects of seeing it—the "duck" way of seeing it and the "rabbit" way of seeing it—are impossible to entertain at the same time.

Or, consider the cube figure familiar to anyone learning perspective in drawing:

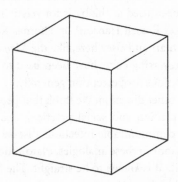

Here, there is no "reality" at all, even though the picture is a drawing of a geometrical solid, a cube; it is a line drawing that is normally perceived as a cube, but can reverse in perception—so that the cube is seen backwards from the initial view. This typically requires a deliberate act of re-perceiving the drawn cube: the viewer has to *try* to see it the other way around.

Our PVV view—the view of the "patient as victim and vector"—incorporates something of what each of these examples involves in permitting two different ways of seeing something at once, like but not exactly like the alternatives that characterize each of these examples. Put metaphorically, there is something akin to Plato's bent-looking stick in water, the *Mona Lisa's* shifting smile, Wittgenstein's duck-rabbit, and the reversing-perspective cube that

characterizes the way infectious disease is usually approached. In the context of infectious disease, the patient is not easily seen as *both* victim and vector at once. People do not generally see themselves that way, either. But everyone *is* both victim and vector as a matter of biological fact and metaphysical understanding; the struggle is to try to conceptualize each other simultaneously from these differing perspectives. Typically, in both personal and professional thinking about infectious disease, one perspective obscures or eclipses another, even as people shift among them. This is true for each of the three tensions we hold as essential in developing a full account, though in approaching any specific issue it is hard to hold the different perspectives in view at once. That is what contributes to the characteristic instability and inadequacy of ethical thinking about infectious disease.

The images from Plato, Leonardo da Vinci, Wittgenstein, and the drawing of a cube can be deployed to make various points not just about perception but about larger matters as well. Plato employed the example of the stick in water to expose not only the unreliability of perception but to support an entire metaphysical theory about reality. Wittgenstein used the duck-rabbit image to argue that perception is not merely a matter of what the eye sees, but is in some way conceptual—or, in the language of later writers, "theory-laden."[2] Plato's point has been used to support non-realist and idealist views of reality; Wittgenstein's view has been used as the basis for relativistic views in science such as those of Norwood Russell Hanson[3] or Thomas Kuhn.[4] Observations from perspectival shifts in art and elsewhere, like the *Mona Lisa*'s smile, directional staircases, or the reversing cube, have been used to make many points about the cognitive conditions for perception generally.

Our point goes in the other direction. We think that people experience their ordinary lives, conduct medical and social practices, and develop programs and policies concerning communicable infectious disease in ways that are to some degree like the tensions in these analogies. Plato's stick in water can only be *seen* as bent, even while it is *known* to be straight. The *Mona Lisa*'s smile is *necessarily* seen as one-directional by anyone standing to one side or the other (though now that the painting is protected by heavy bullet-proof glass, it is harder to achieve this effect, and it does not occur in the same way with poor-quality reproductions)—it is a smile *toward* the viewer, wherever positioned,

---

2. See, e.g., Chris Swoyer, "Relativism and the Constructive Aspects of Perception," *The Stanford Encyclopedia of Philosophy (Spring 2003 Edition)*, ed. Edward N. Zalta, http://plato.stanford.edu/entries/relativism/supplement1.html (accessed December 29, 2007).
3. Norwood Russell Hanson, *Patterns of Discovery: An Inquiry into the Conceptual Foundations of Science* (Cambridge: Cambridge University Press, 1958).
4. Thomas Kuhn, *The Structure of Scientific Revolutions* (Chicago: University of Chicago Press, 1970).

even though the paint on the canvas does not move. Wittgenstein's duck-rabbit *cannot* be seen in both ways at once—after all, the faces point in opposite directions; it is either a duck or a rabbit, or perhaps a flat line drawing in which it is neither. And the reversing-perspective cube can be easily drawn by anyone—in this sense, the tension is self-created—but cannot be drawn without incorporating the dual perspectives, unless of course it is drawn so clumsily that it is not a cube at all.

At the simplest level of our account, a person's and indeed a society's experience with infectious disease has something in common with these tensions: it is partly misleading, it is perspectivally shifting, it is conceptually influenced, and it is it partly self-created. But where our point heads in the other direction is this: whereas Plato and others have found such tensions deceptive, we see them as also partly informative. Understanding them and how they can shift back and forth from one to another is indispensable in the real world of infectious-disease practice and policy. Our PVV view seeks not to dismiss or efface these tensions (though it does believe they can be reduced), but to make positive use of them to analyze both practical and theoretical issues in bioethics.

PVV Perspectives

Our PVV account builds on multiple perspectives from which to view infectious disease. We have mentioned at least three earlier; there may be more, but at least these three are illuminating. No single one of these perspectives is sufficient or even fully accurate by itself, and each, we will show, will contribute to our complete PVV normative account of infectious disease.

First Perspective: The Experiences of Individual People with Infectious Disease in Real Life

The first of the three perspectives reflects an individual's actual, personal situation as victim or vector of infectious disease in the real world. This perspective reflects what people actually experience and presses the importance of these experiences for real people. Some are ill; some are not. Some are aware of the possibility that they might become ill; others are not. Some fear communicable disease; others do not even understand the etiology of disease, attributing it perhaps to evil spirits or to their own wrongdoing. Many people are not ill with major symptomatic transmissible diseases most of the time, at least not in the developed world outside the winter cold-and-flu season; nevertheless they recognize that they could become ill with a transmissible disease.

Except for hypochondriacs and people in the grip of fear during an epidemic, people do not normally experience the threat of becoming ill in a vivid way if they are not at the moment actually ill. Nor do they normally experience themselves as (potential) vectors if they are not at the moment actually ill. Especially with non-chronic illness, infectious disease in the developed world is typically experienced as transitory before return to a healthy state. So for those who feel relatively insulated from infection, it is difficult to bring into view what it is like to be a victim or, indeed, a vector.

But then there is the victim-side. Some people become victims, where the possibility of illness is all too real and they are sick: vomiting, coughing, aching, itching, fainting, hemorrhaging. The Heideggerian term "thrownness"— which describes how temporal beings experience the immediacy of their factual circumstances —eerily captures the immediacy of illness. For victims, too, it is difficult to imagine themselves outside of the immediacy of their circumstances, especially if illness is sudden and severe and they are in desperate need of care and treatment. An additional feature of the circumstances of victims is that victimhood may lead to victimization—to the fear, hatred, or worse, that may attend those perceived as threats to others. This is the insight we need to draw from the first perspective of our PVV view: the importance of considering what it is like for real people to be really ill or to be the source of illness to others. Yet even these experiences are typically temporary, at least for those who live in comfortable circumstances and feel themselves relatively insulated from disease: even when experiencing illness as victims, they remember and anticipate non-illness as their "normal" state. Illness is temporally located and limited: one may be well today, ill tomorrow, and well again not long after that. Someone may also be well today, a threat to others tomorrow, and cease to be a threat again not long after that. This is the lived experience of infectious disease in its acuity and rapidity, as we discussed in Chapter 3; and while it is not so true of chronic infectious conditions for which there is no effective treatment, it is true of many or even most communicable diseases.

Well or ill, these are the vantage points of individual patients in particular life contexts, from which much of the discussion in the field of bioethics has been initiated. These vantage points are in tension: victims want treatment, care and concern, as well as their confidentiality protected. Those who believe themselves to be safe nonetheless want protection from vectors: from someone sneezing on the subway or from foreign diseases now suddenly present in birds or mosquitoes. Of course, many people know what provides protection, both as victims and vectors—they get routine immunizations, drink pasteurized milk, wash their hands when visiting a friend in a hospital, practice safe sex with an intimate partner, and take only appropriate antibiotics when they are ill. But they are still at risk in many ways: some recognized, others unknown or unpredictable.

These vantage points of ordinary life make up many of the current dilemmas of bioethics, to which we will be returning in Part III: for example, should a patient's confidentiality be sacrificed to protect another person from disease? Should a person be forcibly immunized or isolated to protect others or to protect the population as a whole? The vantage points are, we will contend, crucially limited; seeing infectious disease from one point or the other alone is what gives rise to the analysis we have criticized as flat and conflictual. But this does not mean they should be ignored; any fully adequate normative account of infectious disease must respect the lives of real individuals as they are actually lived, and must have succeeded in seeing them as they are.

Second Perspective: The Population-wide View

In real life, individuals are members of groups and populations. There is insight to be drawn from this perspective, by considering how infectious diseases are distributed within and affect groups or populations. The distribution of illness within groups or populations matters to individuals directly as, for example, members of a religious sect, a refugee population, or a nation investing in health policy, or indirectly as members of all humankind. Knowledge about how the groups or populations of which they are members fare may be critical to bettering the circumstances of individuals as well as to assessing what might be going right or wrong for them. For example, without population-wide data, it may be difficult to tell whether certain groups are being disadvantaged, whether burdens of disease are rising or falling overall, or whether emerging threats are on the horizon.

This population-wide perspective starts with people seen not as individuals in specific, personal circumstances, but as members of populations that have distinctive characteristics and disease distributions. Persons are data points in the population under examination, rather than individuals; what is of interest is what they do or do not have in common with others in a population identified in the same way. For example, for what diseases are incidence rates rising or falling? Are some groups in the population affected more than others? Are prevalence levels of some conditions sufficiently high to warrant public health intervention?

The risk of a population-wide perspective is that individuals are seen solely as data-points to be taken into account in identifying disease threats or measuring progress in responding to disease spread. Any population-wide view invites the construction of policy objectives that focus on achieving given results in a population without reference to the identity of specific individuals. It is thus best reconstructed in classical utilitarian theory that judges actions or policies in terms of whether they further the overall good. Critics of this classical ("total") utilitarian view argue that it treats everyone's interests as though they were part of one giant decision function—as data points into the overall good—rather than as the individuals that they are.[5]

A population-wide perspective thus must be reminded of the importance of not losing focus on how what happens to the population overall has consequences for individual lives. For example, the World Health Organization's "3 by 5 initiative" against HIV/AIDS in Africa sought to provide treatment for 3 million HIV-positive patients by the year 2005. Even though the goal was not reached by 2005, the program has been praised for getting treatment to millions who otherwise might not have received it. Nonetheless, it has also been criticized as a somewhat misplaced initiative from the perspective of public health in that it focuses on treatment rather than on less expensive and potentially overall more effective measures to reduce disease spread.[6] Our take on that specific dispute is that there is something right about both contentions: the treatment goal focuses on the circumstances of those who are already victims, whereas the goal of reducing spread focuses on overall disease prevalence.

Our normative PVV view insists that we recognize the insights of these multiple viewpoints. Programs to stop the spread of AIDS are surely laudable in reducing the overall burden of disease—something that, as we will see, everyone has an interest in as victim and vector. We must not underestimate the at least partial success of a program like the 3 by 5 initiative in providing treatment to many of the 3 million that was its goal. Simultaneously, we also must not overlook the unmet need for treatment of the other 37 million out of the estimated 40 million HIV-positive individuals who would not have received therapy, even had the program been fully successful in meeting its goal. Prevalence-reduction programs in general fail to recognize that *each* of those who suffer from the disease in question is a victim, and that a program is not "successful" from the point of view of each victim if it does not treat them all—even if it is "successful" in the sense that it reduces or even halts the transmission of a disease to many others.

Similar reminders are in order in the way a solely population-oriented view characterizes individuals. To say of the population of, for example, Botswana that it has a 34% prevalence rate of HIV infection is to say of each individual that he or she has a 34% chance of being HIV positive as a member of the population considered in an undifferentiated manner, but nothing more—at

---

5. Total utilitarianism is identified with the model of the impartial spectator, deciding for all as for a single person. See, e.g., Roderick Firth, "Ethical Absolutism and the Ideal Observer," *Philosophy & Phenomenological Research* 12 (1952): 317–345. For the criticism that this view subsumes individuals, see, e.g., John Rawls, *A Theory of Justice* (Cambridge: Harvard University Press, 1971), 187.

6. See Jim Yong Kim and Arthur Ammann, "Is the '3 by 5' Initiative the Best Approach to Tackling the HIV Pandemic?" *PLoS Medicine* 1, no. 2 (November 30, 2004): e37.

least, nothing more is included in this claim alone, without other specifying features. But some claims may cloak others. To say of women in the United States who have had only one sex partner that they have an 11.5% chance of being HPV-infected[7] is to say of each such woman (again and importantly, without other differentiating factors) that she has a slightly more than 1 in 9 chance of being infected even if she is chaste in this way, but it is also to indicate something about the sexual lives of husbands or partners, though this is rarely made explicit in public discussions about HPV. Yet it does not say anything about the husband or partner of *this* monogamous woman or for that matter anything about *her*, even though it is sometimes interpreted in that way.

To put the point most bluntly, the population view if taken alone overlooks the immediate specificity and humanity of victims; this was the particular focus of our first perspective. And it forgets the specificity and humanity of vectors, too, if it regards them solely as points of disease-reduction. It does not capture the real uncertainties that will be part of our third perspective, even as it loses focus on the real individuals for whom disease matters. But this population-wide view does bring into focus the overall picture of whether burdens of disease are being reduced, as well as patterns of disease across populations. It may, for example, call attention to the fact that disease prevalence rates are much higher in some population subgroups than others, with all the consequences that might result: loss of cultures, social disorganization, or unrest and disintegration. It may also call attention to the roles played by economic injustice or discrimination in the distribution of diseases across populations. But it must also not lose focus on the real individuals for whom disease matters.

Third Perspective: Theoretical Uncertainty About Infectious Disease

Neither the perspective of the real-life individual—with pressing personal concerns—nor the perspective of an entire population, fully captures our picture of the way-station self, who may be victim or vector or both, and may not be able at any given time to know which. The third perspective is essential in capturing what is inadequate about the real person's real, lived experience as the perspective for understanding communicable infectious disease; it does not fully incorporate the degree of theoretical uncertainty that infectious disease involves and hence does not see the full power of the idea of the way-station self. As we have portrayed the embedded self, there is both an actual and a metaphysical sense in which all humans on the planet are both victims and vectors to each other. The shape this takes varies in real-world situations; and even in the actual

---

7. Dunne E.F., Unger E.R., Sternberg M. et al., "Prevalence of HPV Infection Among Females in the United States," *Journal of the American Medical Association* 297 (2007): 813–819.

world there is a very real sense in which the variance is difficult to predict: everyone is in a state of uncertainty about their given circumstances of victimhood and vectorhood, despite a (partly naive) sense of security when not currently ill. Embedded in a "web of transmission," anyone still could contract illness at nearly any time and could also pass it on to others. To be sure, in the real world people are vulnerable to infectious disease in largely specific ways, primarily as a function of where they live, what their society's infrastructure and sanitation arrangements are, whether they have been immunized, and what their personal health and sexual practices are. In real life, some people are vulnerable to some diseases, but some are not, and can know themselves to be exempt from such risks. However, there is a deeper theoretical understanding of uncertainty that captures our underlying metaphysical picture of the way-station self—a theoretical sense that presents something like a naturalized version of the familiar Rawlsian thought experiment known as the "veil of ignorance."

John Rawls, without doubt the best-known moral philosopher writing in English in the latter half of the twentieth century, developed a conjecture about the veil of ignorance as an analytic framework to use in justifying principles of justice.[8] Rawls's idea was that, in an "original position" in which people are imagined as selecting principles of justice to govern a society in which they will live their entire lives, they should imagine themselves to be stripped of any knowledge of personal circumstances from which they might tailor those principles to their own advantage: sex, race, age, natural talents, circumstances of birth, education, wealth, and so on. Thus deprived of information about themselves, Rawls contended, hypothetical choosers of principles of justice would be unable to use information that is arbitrary from a moral point of view. Their choice of principles of justice can then be defended as fair—to everyone affected by the principles. It is important that the veil-of-ignorance hypothetical justification speaks to each, Rawls emphasized. If it does, even those who end up worse off than some others do in the circumstances of their actual lives, can understand from the veil of ignorance experiment that the arrangements are fair for everyone. No one can choose principles biased in their own actual favor—because they are ignorant of what that favor would be.

In our adaptation, the possibility of communicable infectious disease poses what might be regarded as an expanded, naturalized version of the Rawlsian thought-experiment: understanding this is essential in seeing the deeper issues in infectious disease. Given each individual's physical embeddedness among other humans who, like everyone else, are all way-stations, launching-pads, and breeding-grounds for billions of microorganisms on the surface of and within their bodies, there is a real sense in which everyone is a potential vector

---

8. Rawls, *A Theory of Justice*.

and a potential victim of infectious disease all the time. However, no one fully knows—and perhaps cannot know—when the exact circumstances of being victim, vector, both or neither, will arise. This tension between what any given person actually knows about himself or herself as an individual—their real-life situation at the first level of analysis we have just discussed, where individuals have knowledge, for instance, about whether they have been immunized against a particular disease, whether they do or do not practice safe sex, or whether they do or do not live in a country where treatable diseases nevertheless remain endemic, and how they would think if they assumed they were all of the time both victim and vector but blinded from which at any given moment—is the linchpin for construction of just policies about infectious disease. It is what brings together the perspectives of actual victims and what in theory is the case—but could also actually be the case—into a coherent, more complex, view.

Importantly, our naturalized version is both broader and much stronger than the actual Rawlsian thought experiment. The infectious-disease version of the veil of ignorance blinds people not only to their own individual susceptibilities, immunities, and disease-courting or disease-preventing behaviors, but also to the susceptibilities and immunities of the specific population in which they find themselves—although it does not strip away the knowledge that they are, as biological beings, ever susceptible. In this, the infectious-disease version of the veil of ignorance goes well beyond Rawls. Rawls, at least the classical Rawls, thought principles of justice could be developed within societies rather than on a global scale, and while the Rawlsian veil stripped choosers of knowledge of their individual circumstances, it did not screen off knowledge of their society's capacities, economic and otherwise. With infectious disease, however, one society cannot be walled off from another; birds, boats, airplanes, and mosquitoes make infectious disease a global phenomenon, exacerbated both by social phenomena like refugee movement and natural phenomena like climate change.

Moreover, the Rawlsian veil treated the condition of ignorance of one's own characteristics and situation as something imagined in a hypothetical thought experiment. For Rawls the veil of ignorance does not create uncertainty about who people are in the real world; it is only (hypothetical, imaginary) people behind the Rawlsian veil who do not know their actual circumstances in life. The Rawlsian veil did not introduce uncertainty about these actual circumstances—they are whatever they turn out to be. Once out from behind the veil, as Rawls saw it, people are assumed to occupy whatever kinds of positions they have in real life. With infectious disease, however, the uncertainty also runs to the circumstances of real life.

This uncertainty is essential to comprehend. Much about infectious disease cannot be known in advance: new diseases emerge whose properties and forms of transmission are not initially understood; diseases may affect societies in unanticipated ways; and there is uncertainty about whether science—for instance in matters like developing antimicrobials that outrun resistance—will keep up with them. Thus the unknown plays a more pervasive role in the application of Rawls's thought experiment to infectious disease than it did with the traits he had in mind, like race, sex, or specific talents or disabilities. Our PVV infectious disease "veil" is a reminder not just of imaginary or hypothetical uncertainty, but of the *real* uncertainty with which we live. It is a reminder to think about susceptibility on a global level and under sometimes near-complete uncertainty, not just under uncertainty about any given person's actual circumstances.

Behind the veil of ignorance—the deepest theoretical perspective—there is a sense in which everyone faces risks of infectious disease. No one can be sure that they will continue to occupy the same position with respect to infectious disease, either in terms of their individual characteristics or those of their society, which they now actually occupy. This uncertainty holds for everyone adopting Rawls's "original position" in an effort to discover what sorts of policies about HIV would be just, to take only one example. Is someone a celibate man, say an observant monk in a religious order, or a young woman at risk, perhaps in a society in which sexual contact is often non-voluntary or is required in specific context, or whose way of survival in the world involves promiscuous or commercial sex? In theory, if their own characteristics are veiled from view, they must recognize that they could be either one, the monk or the prostitute, or one of many other sorts of people as well. They might be the person who eats the raspberries imported from Guatemala that were contaminated with *Cyclospora cayetanensis*, who contracts whooping cough in Salt Lake City, or who is one of the children paralyzed in the polio epidemic that emanated from northern Nigeria, or, for that matter, is a victim of some new disease yet to emerge.

This third, Rawls-like victim/vector perspective of course faces a ready challenge from actual individuals' apparent real-life experiences. A likely response to the Rawlsian victim/vector perspective is that in real life people are not all equally victims and vectors. Actual life circumstances—those of everyone's victim/vector duality in real life—do make it reasonable for people to think that they can predict at least some of their likely susceptibility to infectious conditions, and do make incorrect the alleged portrayal of everyone as at equal risk for HIV or any disease—at least at any given moment. In real life, someone may have been immunized against a specific disease—say, hepatitis B—or may not have been, whether or not she engages in the sexual behaviors that risk transmission. Or someone's health status may be less than robust, making him more susceptible to opportunistic infections than his more fortunate counterparts—for instance, he might be a cancer patient undergoing chemotherapy, suddenly at heightened risk of West Nile virus because of his compromised immune status. People who live in rural or urban areas of the world where infectious diseases are endemic may be at ever-present risk of exposure to diseases like malaria, especially if they are among the vast numbers of the globe's inhabitants who are malnourished and who live without adequate sanitation or basic health care. Even in such conditions, some may have developed natural immunities—but, of course, they may be unable to tell if they have these immunities or not. On the contrary, those who live in wealthy countries, and who are relatively well off, may be able to remain, at least most of the time, relatively oblivious to epidemics elsewhere. This is not to say that they *should* be oblivious, either prudentially or morally, just that they *are* likely to be so. With yellow fever, cholera, and polio epidemics a fear of the apparently distant past in most of the western half of the globe (though not yet in Africa, India, or the Middle or Far East), and emerging epidemics like SARS and person-to-person avian flu still not occurring (as of this writing) on a global scale, people in states of relative privilege may indeed think that the book on infectious disease can be closed—for them. But the exceptional force of the naturalized Rawlsian thought-experiment when applied in the context of infectious disease is that *everyone* is in some sense always genuinely (and not merely theoretically) uncertain about prospects for self-protection. Their picture of infectious disease as "over there" and far away is a matter of unwarranted and ultimately self-destructive complacency. That uncertainty is thus endemic to the way-station self helps in explaining why it would be mistaken to gamble on policies that seem to protect those in positions of relative safety without considering the circumstances of others; this will be essential in drawing normative implications from our initial exploratory, partly descriptive look at the multiple tensions in thinking about infectious disease. This is not to derive *ought* from *is*, as philosophical methodology cautions against, but rather to say that normative views must be informed by clear perceptions of what is—and could be—the case.

Rawls developed his thought-experiment as an alternative to utilitarianism, in its more modern economic formulation of maximizing the average welfare of population members.[9] In the 1950s, the economist John Harsanyi had originally

---

9. There are many different forms of utilitarianism as a moral theory and deep theoretical complexities attend the choice of the form of utilitarianism. One basic difference is between "average" and "total" utilitarianism. Average utilitarianism selects the action or policy that will produce the highest average utility within a population; total utilitarianism selects the one that will produce the greatest total utility. (Of course, the two reach the same conclusion in a constant population, but will recommend quite different population policies, for example, if the population size may change.) Total utilitarianism is identified with the model of the impartial spectator, deciding for all as for a single person. See, e.g., Firth, "Ethical Absolutism." Average utilitarianism is identified with the idea of decision making under risk: the highest average is the weighted sum of the probability of being in a certain position times the utility associated with that position. See, e.g., John Harsanyi, "Cardinal Welfare, Individualistic Ethics, and Interpersonal Comparisons of Utility," *Journal of Political Economy* 63 (1955): 309–321; John Harsanyi, "Cardinal Utility in Welfare Economics

proposed the idea of a veil of ignorance to model a decision problem: what decisions would people make if they assumed they had an equal probability that they might be any individual in society? Harsanyi argued that maximizing average utility was the solution to this decision problem.[10] In reasoning to this conclusion, Harsanyi treated the choice problem as one of what economists call "decision making under risk"—that is, decision making that selects among available choices by looking at the welfare associated with each outcome that might follow the choice, multiplying that welfare by the probability of the outcome's occurring, and summing the results for each choice.[11] What this represents is a gamble: trading off probabilities of better outcomes for probabilities of worse outcomes, so long as the overall average is not reduced. This may prove to be a very bad gamble for some, albeit a better one for others.

and in the Theory of Risk Taking," *Journal of Political Economy* 61 (1953): 434–435. In the history of public health, the predominant view has been average utilitarianism. However, there are strands of thinking that seem to approach more closely the total utilitarian idea of treating the social choice as the choice of an (albeit enlarged) individual. The eugenics movement, for example, might be viewed in this way: those individuals who are "defective" are viewed as "diseased" parts of the organism—the body politic, or the whole society—to be excised if needed for overall organism health. Justice Holmes, exploiting an analogy to control measures for infectious disease in *Buck v. Bell*, wrote: "We have seen more than once that the public welfare may call upon the best citizens for their lives. It would be strange if it could not call upon those who already sap the strength of the State for these lesser sacrifices, often not felt to be such by those concerned, in order to prevent our being swamped with incompetence. It is better for all the world, if instead of waiting to execute degenerate offspring for crime, or to let them starve for their imbecility, society can prevent those who are manifestly unfit from continuing their kind. The principle that sustains compulsory vaccination is broad enough to cover cutting the Fallopian tubes" (274 U.S. 200 [1927], 207).
10. Harsanyi, "Cardinal Welfare," and "Cardinal Utility."
11. To illustrate, consider a simplified example of a health policy problem with two choices: whether the United States should continue to rely on employer-provided insurance or implement a system of publicly funded health care for all. For each choice, there would be welfare outcomes for persons in different social positions: the employed, the unemployed, and the socially funded. Suppose that for the choice of employer-provided insurance, there is a .5 probability of being employed and hence having insurance and a welfare level of 200 associated with that position; a .3 probability of having socially funded insurance and a welfare level of 80 associated with that position; and a .2 probability of being unemployed with an insurance and a welfare level of -20 associated with that position. The weighted sum would then be: 100 + 24 − 4 = 120. Suppose that for the choice of socially funded insurance there is a 100% probability of having socially funded insurance and a welfare level of 80 associated with that position. The weighted sum for this choice would be 80. The first choice—employer-provided insurance—would have the higher average, despite the fact that it has some positions that are far worse than any positions under socially funded insurance.
    The probabilities and welfare levels assigned in this example are clearly artificial at best—despite the popularity of rhetoric opposing socially funded insurance, why would the welfare associated with being employed be that much higher than the welfare associated with socially provided insurance unless the benefits were very different?—but the assignments illustrate the crucial point about average utilitarianism.

With infectious disease, the trouble is uncertainty at a deep level about how well the gamble will pay off.

Indeed, Rawls thought, in response to Harsanyi, that average utilitarianism represented an irrational gamble. Despite an overall higher average, Rawls argued that people behind the veil of ignorance would refuse to gamble, given the importance of the sacrifices—essentially, sacrificing minimal conditions of a decent life. Moreover, Rawls contended that the veil of ignorance should not be thought of as a problem of risk (in which we know the probabilities that each social place will occur, but do not know which of the places we will occupy), but as a problem of uncertainty (in which the probabilities themselves cannot be estimated). So, Rawls concluded, choosers behind his veil of ignorance would opt for a "maximin" principle, tolerating inequalities only when they worked to the advantage of the least well off. That is because no rational person would choose policies under which he or she might get stuck with the worst outcome in a social-policy gamble where the stakes are high.

Our naturalized version of the infectious disease veil, we think, reveals the power of the Rawlsian point against Harsanyi. The worst outcome in contexts of epidemics is, after all, death, especially death preceded by unrelieved suffering and compounded by deaths of others one cares about. And the probabilities of being infected, being safe from infection—as well as overall levels of infection—are uncertain, and are particularly uncertain with emerging, potentially pandemic diseases, of which person-to-person avian flu is the current most pressing example, though others may well arise in the future. As dually victims and vectors, not knowing which or when, people would adopt a "we are all in this together" perspective, striving to do the best, as a matter of solidarity; that is, maximize the minimum for each and every one—rather than generating a better average—with respect both to our susceptibility to disease and what is needed to reduce the overall burden of disease.

The Perspectives Working Together

These perspectives—the individual in real life, the population view, and the naturalized Rawlsian uncertainty of the way-station self—shift and intertwine, and it is difficult to get a handle on all of them at once. Each is a crucial part of our full PVV picture. For example, although we as individuals do know some things about our potential for being infected based on our specific social circumstances and health status—that is from the first level—we do not know enough to be sure we can protect ourselves on our own. Uncertainties about some individual risks for specific diseases may be reduced as science improves—for example, whether meningococcus will cause multisystem collapse in a given individual is not currently understood, nor it is currently possible to tell who will contract HIV in a given exposure and who will not, but might become predictable and even preventable as a result of future research. Improved methods of disease understanding and control may also reduce identified risks for populations or even as diseases such as smallpox or polio are eradicated, for all humankind.

New uncertainties about personal risk may always be on the horizon as new diseases emerge in unpredictable fashion. Despite what is already known, the overall reality of infectious disease—both current and emerging—is that it is ultimately unpredictable who will get sick, from what, by what mode of transmission, from whom, and when. It is also largely unpredictable at least for many diseases which individuals an ill person will infect. Confronting infectiousness, people are more like Hobbesian man, never able to be sure they can protect themselves fully in the face of the power of others; there is always a possibility that infectious disease will unpredictably strike even the apparently healthiest. No one can know who or when that will be. So the perspective of the naturalized veil of ignorance is always a critical corrective. But it, too, should not obscure the insights from real individuals and from consideration about populations. It is the situations of real, flesh and blood victims and vectors—people in their ordinary lives—that serve as continual reminders that infectious disease policy must try to do the best for each. At the same time, the population view gives an overall picture of patterns and progress, albeit one that risks losing focus on the real individuals for whom the progress is meaningful.

Despite the challenges of holding all perspectives in view, our PVV view points in an ultimately constructive direction. We believe that it is theoretically possible—and consummately important—to see the patient to the fullest extent possible as victim *and* vector, but as the kind of being for whom uncertainty is endemic about which and when. The importance of this perspective, enriched by what we know about individuals and about populations, is the central message of this book. Our normative view takes elements from each, embracing some, rejecting others, to distill a view that can be phrased in a comparatively compact way. It rejects the flat, conflictual view of one individual limiting the rights of another that characterizes much of liberal theory and bioethics, which we consider inadequate. Our view insists on full awareness of personal human reality: what it is like to be ill, and what it is like to be aware that one may be a vector. It insists that although population-wide patterns are of relevance and that what happens both to population groups of which one is a member and to the human population as a whole matters, a morally adequate view cannot lose sight of the fact that persons must not be treated as mere data-points or that those not favorably affected by a policy do not matter. And it insists that a full awareness of both actual and theoretical uncertainty inform both our moral prescriptions and policies.

Our normative view—phrased as economically as possible, is this:

> *Ethical problems in infectious disease should be analyzed, and*
> *clinical practices, research agendas, and public policies developed,*
> *that always take into account the possibility that a person with*
> *communicable infectious disease is both victim and vector.*

Coming to understand the multiple perspectives essential to understanding the moral issues concerning infectious disease in all of their shifting ramifications is partly like looking at the *Mona Lisa*, becoming aware of the antecedent position in which we stand; partly like looking at Wittgenstein's duck-rabbit, recognizing that it is difficult to entertain both views at once; partly like looking at Plato's stick in water, recognizing that what we see may not be an accurate reflection of whatever reality might be; and a great deal like looking at the reversing cube: we must make a conscious, deliberate effort to see it the other way.

In the following chapters, we turn to the application and development of our normative view to both traditional issues in bioethics and to novel issues identified in some cases by the PVV perspective. In the final sections of this volume, we will return more explicitly to theory in our discussion of the issues of justice posed by efforts to control infectious disease, and the uses of the PVV view in critiquing both philosophical theory and public policy.

PART III: HEALTH CARE DILEMMAS THROUGH THE LENS OF INFECTIOUS DISEASE

8

OLD WINE IN NEW BOTTLES: TRADITIONAL ISSUES IN BIOETHICS FROM THE VICTIM/ VECTOR PERSPECTIVE

Bioethics, as we have already explored, began out of the effort to protect the choices and rights of individual patients. Traditional dilemmas in the field— truth-telling, informed consent, privacy and confidentiality, end-of-life decision making, and how to respond to the patient when the physician makes a mistake, among many others—were issues where individual autonomy took center stage. In this chapter, introducing Section III on both familiar and new health-care dilemmas seen through the lens of infectious disease, we employ the PVV perspective to enrich accounts of several of the most discussed traditional dilemmas in a way that goes beyond the standard binary picture of one patient's choices against the interests of others. Some of what we say consists in eliciting elements of the PVV perspective that have been implicit in bioethics discussions all along, but it is the overall, analytic framework of *the patient as victim* and *vector* that is new. Because any person, at any time, might be victim and vector, treatments of these problems as pitting the interests of one against another must be complemented by the understanding that the interests involved are also of one and the same person—that is, of anyone and everyone.

Telling the Truth About Infection

Consider truth-telling, a staple bioethics dilemma. Here, the standard way of posing the ethical dilemma concerned the patient's own condition: should the physician tell Susan that her cancer has recurred or Sam that his emphysema is likely to result in decline and death?[1] The past 40 years have seen remarkable shifts in physician behavior, from general concealment of dire diagnoses to continuing discussion of nuanced issues such as patients' abilities to comprehend complex information or the impact on patients of learning bad news.[2]

---

1. For the traditional view, see Mack Lipkin, "On Telling Patients the Truth," *Newsweek*, June 4, 1979, 13, reprinted in Ronald Munson, *Intervention and Reflection: Basic Issues in Medical Ethics*, 8th ed. (Belmont, CA.: Thomson/Wadsworth, 2008), 152–154.
2. See, e.g., N.A. Bostick, R. Sade, J.W. McMahon, R. Benjamin, "Report of the American Medical Association Council on Ethical and Judicial Affairs: Withholding Information from Patients,

The contemporary consensus, put roughly, is that patients should be told as much as they want to know and that information should be withheld only at the patient's request or if it is absolutely clear that more gradual sharing of information would be beneficial to the patient.[3] Respect for autonomy seems to require no less: tell the truth if the patient wants to know it, but remain silent or go slowly if the patient clearly refuses the information or would be disastrously harmed by it.

Against the background of this consensus, discussions of genetic information have questioned whether it is ethical for patients to refuse to acquire knowledge that might be beneficial to family members—that is, to refuse to be told the truth. Here, too, respect for autonomy has been paramount,[4] although some critics have contended that it is incoherent for a person both to favor autonomy and to choose to remain in ignorance.[5] Where information gleaned from genetic testing might seem important to the health of other family members, defenders of autonomy point out that, with the human genome project, such information is becoming less critical. In many cases it may be possible to provide family members with information while still respecting an individual's right to refuse to know.[6] James Watson, a founder of modern genetics, for example, has sequenced his own genome, but has announced that he does not want to know whether or not he has a susceptibility gene for Alzheimer's.[7] Conflicts between the choices of an autonomous patient and others who might benefit from genetic information have thus been deflected, though not fully resolved.

In comparison, should patients be able to refuse to learn the truth about their infectious state? Here, the conflicts cannot be so easily circumvented: a patient's own knowledge may be critical not only to her ability to protect herself, but to her ability to protect others. For example, a patient who refuses testing for tuberculosis, yet goes about his daily life, may put others at risk of

Rethinking the Propriety of 'Therapeutic Privilege,'" *Journal of Clinical Ethics* 17, no. 4 (2006): 302–306; Anthony G. Tuckett, "Truth Telling in Clinical Practice and the Arguments For and Against: A Review of the Literature," *Nursing Ethics* 11, no. 5 (2004): 500–513.

3. American Medical Association, "Withholding Information from Patients (Therapeutic Privilege)," Report of the Council on Ethical and Judicial Affairs No. 2-A-06 (June 2006), http://www.ama-assn.org/ama1/pub/upload/mm/369/ceja_2a06.pdf (accessed February 10, 2008). Also see, e.g., Carlos Henrique Martins Da Silva, "Not Telling the Truth in the Patient–Physician Relationship," *Bioethics* 17, nos. 5–6 (2004): 417–424.

4. Jane Wilson, "To Know or Not to Know: Genetic Ignorance, Autonomy and Paternalism," *Bioethics* 19, nos. 5–6 (2005): 492–504.

5. See, e.g., John Harris and Kirsty Keywood, "Ignorance, Information, and Autonomy," *Theoretical Medicine* 22 (2001): 415–436; Rosamond Rhodes, "Genetic Links, Family Ties, and Social Bonds: Rights and Responsibilities in the Face of Genetic Knowledge," *Journal of Medicine & Philosophy* 23 (1998): 18.

6. See, e.g., Wilson, "To Know or Not to Know."

7. Nicholas Wade, "Genome of DNA Discoverer Is Deciphered," *New York Times*, sec. A, June 1, 2007.

deadly disease. The image of a trans-Atlantic traveler with XDR-TB entering the United States at the Canadian border, despite warnings to customs agents, riveted the American public in the spring of 2007.[8] Although on one variant of this story the traveler apparently knew of his disease (but, he claimed, not of its communicability to others), imagine the possibility of deliberately un-knowing travelers carrying lethal microbes—every day, sitting beside each other on crowded buses, trains, subways, or airplanes.

Pieces of this traveler's story as it was originally reported reveal its poten-tial ethical complexity.[9] Initially, as the story went, the traveler knew he had TB, but on his account did not know that it was a resistant strain. He wanted to get married and to have a honeymoon abroad. He said that when he left on his travels, he did not believe he posed a communication risk, because his sputum samples were microscopically negative—but he advanced the date of his trip before he received a follow up letter from health officials informing him that he should not travel. When finally tracked down in Italy by the U.S. Centers for Disease Control and Prevention (CDC), he evaded a specific no-fly travel ban so that he could get back to the United States. At least by initial reports, he thought his only options were to stay in Italy—away from family and, he feared, without adequate medical treatment—or to charter a plane at the prohibitive cost of $100,000. So he flew back to Canada on commercial flights, via a roundabout route, and slipped over the U.S. border by land.

From the perspective of a person faced with a potentially life-threatening illness, the TB traveler's reactions are not surprising. Desperate for familiar surroundings, loved ones, protection or care, anyone might respond as this patient did, with potentially horrific results for everyone else. This individual–patient perspective must be part of a nuanced ethical account of this case, as the PVV perspective reminds us: a full moral picture must take into account the victim's need for home and treatment.

Traveling home, the man with TB, eventually identified as a young Atlanta lawyer, Andrew Speaker, sat next to a passenger who later asked, "How many other people can do this or will do this? It's hard to think about what this means for the future of air travel."[10] This comment points to another aspect of the PVV perspective, that the man with TB was also a traveler, who got TB from somewhere and who, if cured, might want once again to travel in the relative

---

8. John Schwartz, "Tangle of Conflicting Accounts in TB Patient's 12-Day Odyssey," *New York Times*, sec. A, June 2, 2007. For a subsequent account of the Speaker story, and an argument that it revealed inadequacies in U.S. quarantine authority, see Howard Markel, Lawrence O. Gostin, and David P. Fidler, "Extensively Drug-Resistant Tuberculosis: An Isolation Order, Public Health Pow-ers, and a Global Crisis," *Journal of the American Medical Association* 298, no. 1 (July 4, 2007): 83–86.

9. Ibid.
10. Ibid.

security of not being reinfected. As a sick person, however, his concern was the immediacy of his own need, a perspective from which his mad rush to return home seemed the only reasonable thing to do. But from the immediacy of his situation as victim he forgot that he might also want to be safe from dangerously ill travelers who might be vectors. Our PVV analysis reminds him that the seat on the plane next to him is *his* seat, too. The need to protect everyone—himself included and not just others—must be recognized as a concern of his as well. It is not merely a concern of others, to be imposed on him as a constraint—although from the immediacy of his situation as victim, this is exactly how it might seem. At the same time his victimhood also reminds us that strategies to protect others must be accompanied by genuine support for his victim-side. We shall return to this interplay in later chapters, when we discuss mandated treatment for TB and whether rapid tests for HIV should be mandatory during pregnancy.

In comparison, the tensions in this victim/vector duality are less apparent where genetic information is at issue. With genetic information, the patient who refuses testing for BRCA-1 has decided that she does not want to know whether she is at risk for breast cancer, and thus that she won't acquire the information that would enable her to tell family members who might have the same genetic condition. She has been confronted with the immediate possibility that the information might be beneficial to her but also might be harmful and she has decided not to have it, even though it might be beneficial for other family members to have it. In this, she is comparable to many who could have information that might be significantly beneficial to others but who choose not to acquire or share that information, including those with infectious conditions. Her knowing or not knowing whether she has the gene does not affect whether she transmits the gene to others who are already born; they, too, already have the gene or not. We will explore these issues in the specific context of reproduction in Chapter 11. But the person with a contagious infectious disease can transmit to persons who currently exist; hence her knowing or not knowing her infectious status may make a difference to whether this occurs.

With information about infectious status, by contrast, the patient refusing to know his HIV status is deciding *only* from the perspective of himself as victim that he does not want to know about his own status, that he would rather remain ignorant in light of whatever interventions might (or might not) be available—and thus that he does not want the information that would enable him to tell anyone else. He has not been confronted with the possibility that he might be on the receiving end of other vectors, so to speak, and might want to know of the risk from vectors to him as well as of his own risks to himself. Our PVV perspective reminds him that he is at risk from other vectors, although he does not know what that risk might be. The immediacy of victimhood—is the knowledge worth it to me in my circumstances as victim?—conceals the duality of his circumstances from him, a duality that our PVV perspective brings to light. In deciding whether to be told the truth, he should try to keep in mind the full range of victim/vector considerations, not just the immediate issues he sees as victim. A parallel duality of reasons emerges in considering another staple of the bioethics literature, informed consent.

Informed Consent and the Refusal of a Spinal Tap

Respect for autonomy, it is said, requires that consent be fully informed—and that competent patients not be given treatment without it. Consider the person who refuses a spinal tap to rule out meningitis.[11] What issues come to the fore in understanding whether the consent has been informed and the refusal should be respected?

Informed consent, as traditionally presented, requires that a patient have a reasonable understanding of his or her condition, the therapeutic alternatives (including no treatment), and the consequences of these alternatives. Patients should understand and be able to apply their values to the situation at hand in order to reach a well-considered decision. When patients do not have the ability to understand and act as required for informed consent, they lack decision-making capacity and a surrogate must be called on to help in making the decisions for them. Some writers on informed consent suggest a sliding scale for competence, with insistence on a higher standard if more is at stake for the patient.[12] Decisions to refuse interventions that are clearly life-sustaining would require the highest standard for competence on this account.

Suppose the patient refusing a spinal tap—let us assume that she is competent, informed, and acting voluntarily—has been told and clearly understands that the test could yield a diagnosis that is potentially lifesaving. She understands that the likelihood that she actually has meningitis is fairly low but also that it is a very serious disease if she does have it. Just the same, she refuses: perhaps she is afraid of the risks of the procedure (which, though infrequent, include persistent headache, possible paralysis, and other serious side effects), perhaps she dislikes the thought of a long needle being inserted directly into her spine, perhaps she has religious scruples, or perhaps she refuses without explanation at all. In any of these cases, she is within her legal rights to refuse, at least assuming that she has decision-making capacity.

---

11. The example is from Jonsen, Siegler, and Winslade, *Clinical Ethics*, (New York: Macmillan, 1982) 18–20, 172.

12. See, e.g., James Drane, "The Many Faces of Competency," *Hastings Center Report* 15, no. 4 (1985): 17–21; Allen Buchanan and Dan Brock, *Deciding for Others* (Cambridge: Cambridge University Press, 1989).

But meningitis is a serious, life-threatening and potentially communicable disease—so, the traditional bioethics analysis continues, should we insist on her consent, or should she be compelled to undergo this diagnostic procedure and if it is positive, receive therapy? Perhaps a sliding scale of competence can help out, with the tide turning against refusal if she seems unable to explain her reasoning or if her reasoning is just plain bizarre. But judgments of incompetence may not always be available to license intervention, so the analysis ends in an apparent stalemate. Better communication, efforts to improve patients' trust so that situations like this do not arise, and perhaps calling on family or friends to help her make a wiser decision are the principal tools in bioethics' toolbox at this point.

From the PVV perspective, however, there might be more. In their presentation of this meningitis case, which we mentioned in Chapter 4, Jonson, Siegler, and Winslade asked whether the patient should be discharged against medical advice back to a college dormitory if she succeeds in avoiding the tap. This question begins to hint at the PVV perspective, because it asks whether the situation would be viewed by her dorm mates in the same way it is viewed by the patient herself. If she did not know whether she is herself or her dorm mate, she might see the importance of incorporating a broader range of information in the consent process.[13] If the consent process is viewed as about her values, risks and benefits, the consent process is typically about the risks and benefits for *her*. The process stops short of encouraging her to think about her effects on others—or their effects on her. But when she works through the process of applying her values to assess her alternatives, she might want to take into account the effects of her situation on those about whom she cares deeply. To be sure, she might not care about her dorm mates or want to take them into account—but to the extent that the informed consent process has not brought information about effects on her dorm mates into play, her deliberation has been truncated, even in her situation of actual victimhood. We will have more to say about how to expand the process of informed consent in the context of research ethics in Chapter 10.

There is more to say about the spinal tap situation from the PVV perspective of not knowing whether one is a victim in the immediacy of deciding whether to refuse the tap, or whether one might be the source or recipient of a case of undiagnosed meningitis. Viewed from this perspective, the patient is always in some sense not only a possibly ill victim and vector but also at risk of becoming a victim and vector from others. This susceptibility is an additional reason that should be made clear to her, as a reason *for her* and not just for her dorm mates. From this perspective, some fears of a potential victim—terror at

---

13. For a very broad view of the history of meningitis transmission, see P. Domingo and N. Barquet, "The First Epidemic of Cerebrospinal Meningitis," *Gesnerus* 51, nos. 3–4 (1994): 280–282.

the thought of a long needle, for example—might seem relatively less serious. She is weighing the terror of the needle not just against whether she has (or does not have) meningitis now but also against whether she might be at risk for meningitis from others who have not been diagnosed. Of course, her reasons for refusal might continue to seem overriding to her; our point is that she needs to weigh those reasons against her situation seen as both a terrified victim *and* a person who is not at all terrified and ill but wants protection from such terrified vectors. For she is both: someone who is currently a victim and someone who is at risk—unknown risk—from others.

Of course, some of the refuser's reasons may continue to seem very strong to her, even when she weighs them against her own protection from vectors. Religious reasons may seem to be of this sort: reasons that go to the very basis of identity and that people would want to hold onto whether or not they put themselves at risk, cast themselves as risks to others, or leave themselves subject to risks from others. We will have more to say about the relative weight to be given such reasons in our discussion of conscientious objection to vaccination. At this juncture, our point is that she has not considered the full range of reasons that should be of concern to her if she has not weighed the situation in terms of the risks she might pose to herself and others, as well as the risks others might pose to her.

Finally, the PVV perspective reminds us of the need to be supportive of the patient as victim while she is being considered as vector: taking her concerns seriously, allowing her to express her fears, handling the process gently and non-coercively, and giving her time and comfortable space to delay the procedure if she continues to refuse it. Some tensions may be intractable in the end: despite everything we do to be supportive of her, she may still insist on walking out without the tap. But the PVV perspective helps us to see these tensions in this enriched way.

Another example, that of a patient with a sexually transmitted disease, helps bring out how attention to our PVV perspective could change physicians' discussions with their patients about the treatment of infectious disease. Consider a physician's narrative:[14]

> *John came to the outpatient clinic and complained of penile discharge and burning with urination. A microscopic examination of his discharge revealed bacteria that appeared to be gonococci. His symptoms and laboratory results led me to conclude that he had gonorrhea, a sexually transmitted infections disease. I presumed that*

---

14. Provided by Dr. Jay A Jacobson, one of the coauthors of this volume.

he acquired his infection from a sexual partner and was in some sense a victim. However, because men may have no symptoms for about a week after they are exposed and infected, it was also possible that John had been a vector during that period if he had unprotected intercourse with another partner. If John, now symptomatic, had not sought treatment but was sexually active with an uninfected partner or partners, he could have been simultaneously a victim and a vector.

I spoke to John about his sexual partners and learned that for the last three months, he had an exclusive relationship with Jane. I ordered an injection of ceftriaxone for John and advised him to refrain from sex for at least one week to avoid transmission and/or reinfection. I also asked John to advise Jane that she was probably infected and should be tested and treated. He agreed to do so.

Three days later, Jane appeared for her appointment. She had no medical complaints and specifically no genital symptoms. She confirmed her three-month exclusive relationship with John, but acknowledged two other male partners in the preceding year. Her examination was entirely normal. However, a specimen sent for rapid testing for gonococcal infection was positive.

I explained to her that she, like many women infected with the gonococcus, had no clinical manifestations of infection but could transmit it to her sexual contacts. I also explained that she probably acquired her infection from one of her male partners. She was quiet for a moment as she recalled them. Then she angrily uttered a name and said, "I'll bet it was him!" She seemed to see herself as a victim, even though she didn't experience any physical signs or symptoms. She felt anger, perhaps because of feeling deceived, betrayed, or exposed to a potentially serious and definitely transmissible infection. After a time, she expressed embarrassment and concern for presumably transmitting the infection to John. These feelings were focused on her role as vector in their relationship.

I arranged to give Jane a shot of ceftriaxone and cautioned her about having sex in the next week in order to avoid reinfection and/or transmission. I also explained, as I had with John, that our laboratory reports all positive tests to the state health department. When the department has sufficient resources, they interview the infected patients, ask for the names of their sexual contacts, and then advise the contacts that they have been intimate with a currently infected individual and could themselves be at risk of infection. Each link in the long chain of transmission could be characterized as victim, vector or most often, both.

Here, the physician is thinking about each patient as both victim and vector, and counseling them on this basis. On our PVV view, this is the physician's obligation to *this* patient, not a matter of the physician balancing his obligations to his patient against his obligations to protect others.

Privacy and Confidentiality in the Context of Infectious Disease

Now consider a standard view of privacy and confidentiality. Protecting privacy, it might be said, requires that patients have the right to refuse to permit incursions into their bodies—from cheek swabs to vaginal searches. Protecting confidentiality requires that people should be able to control how information about them is shared—to keep their medical records from their employers, their mortgage companies, their life insurers, or their governments. When people may have passed dangerous infectious conditions on to others, however, insisting that confidentiality be protected fails to protect others. So, perhaps confidentiality should be overridden, permitting practices such as contact tracing. On the other hand, if known practices of contact tracing destroy the trust that is essential to encouraging people to seek care, perhaps it is overall more protective to protect confidentiality and encourage people to get care, even though some people who might otherwise have received information important to their health go without it. This reasoning is an example of what we have called the "flat, conflictual" view—seeing one person's interests in confidentiality as in conflict with another person's interests in knowing.

Public health, moreover, may require that information be gathered and shared. Without access to people's bodies, public health authorities will be unable to assess the prevalence of an infection. For some prevalence estimates, no identifying information about individuals need ever be collected; an example was the CDC's anonymous blood sampling of pregnant women to gain data on the prevalence of HIV.[15] Research that is aimed to determine what microbial strains are in circulation—for example, whether the H5N1 influenza strain has appeared in a population—similarly does not require collection of any identifying information. Other surveillance activities, such as those using existing data sets, may require that information originally about individual patients be stripped of identifiers, resulting in creation of anonymized or "limited" data sets.[16]

15. T.J. Dondero, Jr., M. Pappaioanou, J.W. Curran, "Monitoring the Levels and Trends of HIV Infection: The Public Health Service's HIV Surveillance Program," *Public Health Reports.* 103, no. 3 (May–June 1988): 213–220.
16. This last is a HIPAA term of art—a data set that has been stripped of much identifying information, but that still contains sufficient information to continue to pose risks of individual identification; such data sets require protections not applied to fully anonymized sets. See 45 C.F.R. (2007) § 164.514(e).

In discussions of these issues, "privacy" and "confidentiality" typically appear as twinned concepts. When they do, as with human twins, they typically appear in order: privacy first, confidentiality second. In this ordering privacy is thought of as protecting some aspect of access to the person: guarding him or her from bodily touching, intimacy, or direct exposure to view.[17] Confidentiality is conceptualized as about passing on information: sharing academic, financial, or health records when permission has not been given to do so. This prioritization of privacy over confidentiality may reflect a number of claims. Privacy may be thought to be the more important value, with direct access such as intrusion into bodily space seen as a worse affront than unauthorized informational spread. Or, protecting confidentiality may be seen as a means to protecting privacy, with safeguards against informational spread seen as a way of protecting people against having the information garnered in the first place. But infectious disease invites challenge about whether privacy should be regarded as the superior twin, or whether what it is that is important to protect with respect to how information about the person is gathered and how it is transferred may vary with the circumstances.[18]

A very rough cut on the distinction between the ideas of privacy and confidentiality starts with the latter: confidentiality is about expectations of control over what happens to information about a person, once the information has been gleaned. Confidentiality is violated if medical records are shared with employers without consent, if bank records are forwarded to potential mortgage companies, or tax returns are leaked to the press. Privacy, it seems, is about something closer: invasions of the body, personal space, or liberty. Privacy is *invaded*, and confidentiality is *breached*; violations of privacy are *invasions*, and violations of confidentiality are *breaches*. Surely, it would seem, the physical body of a person (and perhaps also her personal items and spaces) is more important to her than her information, invasions are worse than breaches, and privacy thus would be the superior twin.

But an impressive contemporary confusion of these two ideas casts doubt on this easy conclusion. The massive recent efforts in U.S. federal law to protect patients' health information are styled "privacy" protections. The Health Insurance Portability and Accountability Act (HIPAA) of 1996 has given rise

---

17. Privacy in this sense might also extend to guarding objects associated with her from view: diaries, suitcases, and other personal spaces, for example, as Michael Selgelid and Matthew Liao have pointed out in discussion to us. However, whether or not intrusions into such spaces are invasions of privacy comparable to invasions of the body are not relevant to our discussion here.

18. For a fuller version of this argument, from which some of the following material is drawn, see Leslie Francis, "Privacy and Confidentiality; the Importance of Context," *Monist* 91(1):53-68 (January 2008); for an overview of HIPAA privacy protections from the patient perspective, see U.S. Department of Health and Human Services, "Medical Privacy—National Standards to Protect the Privacy of Personal Health Information," http://www.hhs.gov/ocr/hipaa/ (accessed January 2007).

to an elaborate set of standards for protecting the "privacy" of patients' medical records.[19] But health records are not the person, although they certainly may contain important personal information.[20] Why the confusion? Congress and the Department of Health and Human Services may just have been inarticulate, or may have cynically called upon a grander-sounding value—privacy—to justify the expensive and burdensome regulatory regime they were putting into place. Neither hypothesis seems to capture the fact that invoking "privacy" to protect health records does not seem at all strange, at least to the non–legally-trained ear as well as to some philosophical ears.[21] Perhaps the idea is that access to medical records really does feel a lot like access to the person: the records may describe someone's physical being in great detail, making him or her easy to visualize (consider: "obese white male" or "pale and wasted"). Or perhaps the idea is that medical records are an especially dangerous and revealing piece of information (consider: "HIV-positive" or "dementia of the Alzheimer's type"). These ideas call attention to the delicate nature of the information at issue, not the mere fact that access to the body was involved in its gathering.

Infectious disease examples, we think, urge contextualizing the picture of privacy as the superior twin. Invasions of privacy and breaches of confidentiality are both of moral concern: sometimes, we prevent the invasion because our primary concern is the breach; sometimes, we prevent the breach because we are worried it will lead to invasions. In some contexts, we protect privacy to protect confidentiality rather than the reverse.[22] Infectious diseases provide many good examples of cases where confidentiality matters more than privacy.

"Invasion" of privacy evokes military images: risks to bodily integrity that are very serious such as torture or sustained surveillance and threats. Where diagnoses of infectious diseases are concerned, however, many invasions seem decoupled from serious threats to physical security. With a required sputum sample to test for tuberculosis, the body is not intruded upon; all that is required is a cough and a spit. The sample, even if demanded without consent, may in fact be the basis for *increased* physical security in the form of appropriate health care—at least, if health care is available. Moreover, effective surveillance activities may enhance protection of everyone—a consideration for

---

19. Standards for Privacy of Individually Identifiable Health Information, 45 CFR Parts 160 and 164 (2007).

20. For a discussion of the confusion between privacy and confidentiality in the HIPAA regulations, see Nicolas P. Terry and Leslie P. Francis, "Ensuring the Privacy and Confidentiality of Electronic Health Records," *Illinois Law Review* 2007: 681–735.

21. See, e.g., W.A. Parent, "Privacy, Morality, and the Law," *Philosophy and Public Affairs* 12, no. 4 (1983): 269–288 (defining privacy as "the condition of not having undocumented personal knowledge about one possessed by others").

22. For a discussion of the importance of confidentiality, see Kenneth Kipnis, "Medical Confidentiality," in *Blackwell Guide to Medical Ethics,* ed. Rosamond Rhodes, Leslie Francis, and Anita Silvers (Oxford: Basil Blackwell, 2006), 104–127.

each of us, even the person required to give the anonymous sample. When readily accessible bodily samples—spit, hair, sweat—are gathered, physical security is not on the line as a result of the invasion. Even when a blood sample is involved, what is done with the information the sample provides may be far more threatening to physical security than the procedure to obtain it. People diagnosed with terrifying infectious diseases have been beaten, imprisoned, or worse. In these cases, security is not threatened by the initial access: it is the failure of confidentiality about what was found. Confidentiality, not privacy, is the superior twin here; we protect against the original access because we fear that we will be unable to protect against the information becoming known, not because it was harmful to obtain the information in the first place.

Some of the most frightening images of invasions of privacy are the use of coercion to extract motives or thoughts, or the no-longer-science-fictional use of brain imaging devices to obtain information about mental states. Yet even here, where liberty especially seems threatened, it is arguable that the problem lies not with access per se, but with what information is gathered and with whom it is shared. An infectious disease analogy would be anonymous remote sensing of body temperatures as a means of gauging infection rates in a population, as for instance in airport surveillance during the SARS outbreak. The idea that someone else knows that there is a feverish person is discomforting, yes—but will it affect how the person goes about living, chilling liberty any more than the physical sensation of being feverish already does? Will the knowledge that there is a fever-sensor affect whether the person with a cold stays home or goes to work? Chills may come, of course—literally as well as figuratively—but the figurative ones are most likely to happen if identity is known, the person is watched, and contacts are traced. To be sure, the knowledge that sensing is occurring may lead people with fevers to think twice about how their behavior affects others, but this is to encourage the person to think in an enriched way about illness—to think about the effects on others of what she is doing, rather than to restrict her liberty in a coercive manner. Limits to individual liberty are unlikely to come from sensing anonymous data and storing it in a data bank, so long as the data are fully anonymous, even if the data are used for such health policy purposes as influenza vaccine distribution. Indeed, from the individual patient perspective it might be a good thing if knowledge that there has been a general rise in human body temperatures in a given region led to increases in the supply of antivirals delivered to that region. If linkage is the problem, confidentiality is the driving value; we protect privacy because we cannot be sure that the fever will not be linked to an identifiable individual once it has been detected.

To be sure, there is the risk that if a rise in temperature is observed in a particular region, society in a state of panic may cordon off an entire region without knowledge of who the affected individuals are. The specter of plague—and modern fears of SARS or a pandemic influenza with a fatality rate as great as apparently that of the current strain of avian flu—suggest that this risk is not entirely far-fetched. Efforts to quarantine a whole society are entirely imaginable. These efforts forget, however, that the PVV perspective is not just about populations, but also about real individuals within populations. Panicked responses such as these are unjustified, as are responses that are overbroad or that fail to take individuals into account.

Privacy is also important to intimacy, in addition to security and liberty: without control over invasions of the body, it may be difficult to establish intimate relationships. It is in part through controlled and selective disclosure of information that people become friends or lovers.[23] Here, too, with infectious disease it is arguable that the principal focus of this account is confidentiality: not whether information has been obtained, but whether and how it gets passed along to others. Consider diagnostic medical tests for sexually transmitted diseases: the fact that one person's physician can perform a needle stick or take a cheek swab to obtain the sample for a diagnosis of HIV does not control a sexual partner's decision to share—or not to share—HIV status information within a relationship. What matters to intimacy is whether the disclosure is made and whether it comes from the person, from the physician, or from someone else such as a public health officer tracing sexual contacts. To be sure, learning one's HIV status can affect intimate relationships, but whether one learns this information is not a matter of access but of whether choices about what is done with the information are respected. Someone might, as we have discussed, choose to keep information confidential even from themselves. Someone might want to bar access to the information in the first place from concern that the information will be inadvertently revealed, or that they will be tempted to ask, or that they will live in horror of the thought that someone knows but they do not. We have already demonstrated how the PVV perspective shows that this reasoning is incomplete if it does not also call to mind the person's own status as potential recipient of infection in addition to the person's current status as victim. Here, our point is that it is far less plausible to live in horror of the fact that there are information bytes about body temperature or sputum sample biology that came originally from access to the person but that are in no way at this point linked or linkable, in a data bank somewhere.

Nonetheless, there might be horror at the thought that one has contributed information to a data bank being put to nefarious purposes such as racial targeting or ethnic cleansing. There are ways in which collections of health data have been put to quite awful usage: consider the image of overall social health

---

23. See, e.g., Thomas Scanlon, "Thomson on Privacy," *Philosophy & Public Affairs* 4, no. 4 (1975): 315–322.

as it functioned in the eugenics movement as a reason for sterilizing supposedly "defective" members of the population. The corrective, however, lies in moral constraints on how data banks are used, not on the existence of the banks themselves. Of course, when there is a realistic possibility of the misuse of data banks, refusal to share information with them, even anonymously, should remain a possibility for patients.

Another very serious risk even of entirely anonymous surveillance is that the data will reveal sufficient information about groups to result in stigmatization. Suppose, for example, that fully anonymous data are collected in a region of the country that is associated with a particular racial or ethnic group. Or suppose that the surveillance takes place at a border where immigrants of a particular ethnicity are known to cross. In such cases, information about the prevalence of an infectious condition might be a flash point for prejudice against new immigrants.[24] The cursory examination on Ellis Island of steerage passengers seeking to enter the United States (first and second class passengers were excluded from the examination, perhaps on the theory that if they could pay for expensive passage they might be insulated from illness[25]) played a role in nativist objections to immigrants. Similar concerns about immigrants into the United States who return to Mexico with HIV acquired while away also fuel stigmatization.[26]

These concerns—misuse and the stigmatization of groups—are very real concerns about the use of anonymized data. But there are ways to protect against them, without insisting on individual informed consent.[27] One important caution is to insist that any surveillance activities be openly disclosed and publicized. Another is to require that communitywide surveillance only be entered into after public discussion and authorization—a kind of community consent. If these protections are absent, the risks of misuse of surveillance would remain real, and even the anonymous collection of data would be morally problematic. There are analogs to this in the idea of community consent to research—an idea we will explore in Chapter 10.

---

24. For a discussion of the stigmatization of immigrants as sources of infectious disease, see Howard Stern and Alexandra Minna Stern, "The Foreignness of Germs: The Persistent Association of Immigrants and Disease in American Society," *Millbank Quarterly* 80, no. 4 (2002): 757–788.

25. This suggestion comes from the Ellis Island website. National Park Service, "Ellis Island: History and Culture," http://www.nps.gov/elis/historyculture/index.htm (accessed December 29, 2007).

26. Marc Lacey, "Mexican Immigrants Carry HIV Home to Unready Rural Areas," *New York Times*, sec. A, July 17, 2007.

27. The suggestions here are drawn from the discussion of the use of anonymized data, without individual consent, in quality improvement activities. See Nancy Dubler, Jeffrey Blustein, Rohit Bhalla, and David Bernard, "Informed Participation: An Alternative Ethical Process for Including Patients in Quality-Improvement Projects," in *Health Care Quality Improvement: Ethical and Regulatory Issues*, ed. Bruce Jennings, Mary Ann Baily, Melissa Bottrell, and Joanne Lynn (Garrison, NY: Hastings Center, 2007), 69–87.

A final difficulty about collecting data without identifiers—or using data that have been deidentified—is that it may not be possible to preserve anonymity. The temptation may be to try to reidentify patients, for treatment or preventive reasons; New York City, for example, has reportedly used surveillance data about diabetic patients to try to improve patients' health.[28] Or, it may not be possible to preserve anonymity and have the information continue to be of any scientific use. These are empirical issues that we cannot fully settle here. Suffice it to say that some surveillance activities—the collection of anonymous blood samples in pregnant women to monitor HIV prevalence, for example—have yielded useful information without any threat to identification.[29]

This discussion of privacy and confidentially can be used to highlight the many levels of the PVV analysis. Suppose, for example, that the CDC seeks comprehensive data about the prevalence (proportion in a population) or the incidence (numbers of new cases in a given time period) of a particular condition. These data can be critical to estimating lifetime risk or risks to members of the population of developing a disease at a given point in time. They can be enormously useful in public health planning, in actuarial calculations of insurance rates, in efforts to assess the efficacy or costs of treatment, or in efforts to judge the relative efficacy of social interventions such as public-interest advertising campaigns. In order to be informative about either prevalence or incidence, data sets need not contain any identifying information; they can be fully anonymized.[30] However, data must be collected from individuals; privacy must be invaded in order to collect the data (whether consensually or not), but confidentiality need not be breached in order for the data to be informative for the CDC.

Similar issues arise in other areas of medicine. Consider for instance whether it might be useful for researchers in tumor genetics to study preserved tissue samples. Patient privacy is implicated when the samples are excised. In some cases, no information about the patient is needed at all for the research to take place— the research can be conducted on the tissue material by itself. In other cases, information about the patient is needed but can be fully anonymized once linked to the tumor sample; for example, it may be necessary to link information about response to chemotherapy during the immediate treatment period. The tumor sample can be sent to the researcher with information such as "no response,"

28. For a critical account of New York City's actions, and "creep" from surveillance to intervention, see Wendy Mariner, "Mission Creep: Public Health Surveillance and Medical Privacy," *Boston University Law Review* 87 (2007): 347–395.

29. Dondero, Pappaioanou, and Curran, "Monitoring."

30. To be sure, there may be practical questions about insuring anonymity, if the data sets contain small numbers or if other information is included that might result in few individuals in particular data cells. As an example of controversy about difficulties with insuring anonymity, see Claire Dyer, "BMA's Patient Confidentiality Rules Are Deemed Unlawful," *British Medical Journal* 319 (1999): 1221.

"partial response," or "complete remission" to a given chemotherapeutic regime. In such cases, confidentiality is not breached when the material is sent with the information—although confidentiality would require protection at the initial stage of linking the tumor sample to the patient's record for the purpose of determining the response. If as a practical matter disclosure of the response carries identifying information—or if identifying information is needed for longer term follow up—confidentiality would of course be implicated as well.

But because of infectious disease's often rapid propagation patterns and capacity for transmission throughout a population, these issues are especially crucial in this area of health concerns. For example, infectious disease researchers might want to know whether there appear to be changes in the DNA of viruses appearing in a population. Samples from infected patients will be needed in order to study virus characteristics. Identifying patient information will be unnecessary; of course, if there are very few patients with the infection in question as a practical matter confidentiality may be difficult to protect. Examples might be monitoring of persons with a given infectious condition to see whether resistant or more lethal strains are appearing in the population. When resistant HIV appeared in New York City, for example, identifying information about the patient at issue was not made known, at least publicly.[31] However, sufficiently informative descriptions appeared in the press to raise serious questions about whether his confidentiality was in fact being protected—whether respect for him as an actual victim and vector was adequately provided.[32]

These are all cases in which the information in question is highly valuable and potentially lifesaving for many people. They are also cases in which collecting the information requires bodily invasion of the type that is considered a clear violation of privacy: disease diagnosis, samples of tumor tissues, or samples of other bodily material such as saliva or blood. If we object to collection of the information because we take privacy to be the primary value, we risk never getting the information at all. As a public policy matter, therefore, it may be important to distinguish privacy and confidentiality, and to be careful in assessing whether our objection is to access or to information becoming inappropriately shared.

Withholding and Withdrawing Care at the End of Life.

In end-of-life decision making, as it has been so extensively explored in bioethics, the emphasis has been on patient autonomy, followed by patient interests. If dying patients want to decline life-sustaining treatment, both conventional

31. Shaoni Bhattacharya, "Multi-Drug-Resistant HIV Strain Raises Alarm," *New Scientist* 16 (February 14, 2005): 15, http://www.newscientist.com/article.ns?id=dn7007 (accessed January 2007).
32. E.g., Associated Press, "Rare Drug-Resistant HIV Hits NYC," *CBS News*.com (February 12, 2005), http://www.cbsnews.com/stories/2005/02/12/health/main673667.shtml (accessed January 2007).

bioethics and the law have asserted, that is their right—directly, if they are competent; indirectly if they are not. Advance planning can be used to try to deal with decision making when illness is too acute to permit reflection; substituted-judgment and best-interests standards are employed when autonomy fails. Controversial issues have focused on cases, for example that of Helga Wanglie,[33] where surrogates sought treatment believed to be futile, or laws like Oregon's Death with Dignity Act,[34] which permits competent terminally ill patients to seek direct assistance from their physicians in dying, and other situations where issues of patient autonomy are primarily at stake.

In end-of-life decision making, infectious disease has never received more than the briefest mention, largely in the context of "allowing to die." Pneumonia was traditionally regarded as "the old man's friend," and whether there was anything special about it as an infectious condition received little attention. But pneumonia in the elderly presents several of the features of infectious disease that we elicited in Chapter 3. Decisions about whether or not to treat need to be made quickly—if treatment is to be effective, there is little or no time for careful consideration of the patient's condition and extensive discussions with family members. And the treatment is not burdensome: just a simple antibiotic. Because treatment is not burdensome, typical advance directive statutes in the United States historically tended to group antibiotics with "comfort care," not to be discontinued unless the patient made a specific request. But because the decisions need to be made relatively quickly, the practice in the United States has been treatment.[35] In the Netherlands, for example, there has been extensive reflection on whether antibiotics should or should not be withheld from dying patients,[36] especially frail, severely demented psychogeriatric patients in nursing homes, for whom pneumonia is the ultimate cause of death in about one-third of all nursing home patients and up to two-thirds of demented patients.[37]

Perhaps most important for our purposes, issues of communicability were simply not considered in discussions of treatment of pneumonia. Thus end-of-life

33. For a report of the case, see Ron E. Cranford, "Helga Wanglie's Ventilator," *Hastings Center Report* 21, no. 4 (1991): 23–24.

34. Oregon Death with Dignity Act, Ore. Rev. Stat. (2007) §§ 127.800 et seq.

35. For a discussion of these issues in the United States, see Thomas Finucane's comment on withholding antibiotics: "If a demented patient with pneumonia dies without receiving antibiotics, this could be either terrible negligence or thoughtful therapeutic restraint," in "Thinking About Life-Sustaining Treatment Late in the Life of a Demented Patient," *Georgia Law Review* 35 (2001): 691–705 (702).

36. Esther-Lee Marcus, A. Mark Clarfield, and Allon E. Moses, "Ethical Issues Relating to the Use of Antimicrobial Therapy in Older Adults," *Clinical Infectious Diseases* 33 (2001): 1697–1705.

37. Jenny T. van der Steen, *Curative or Palliative Treatment of Pneumonia in Psychogeriatric Nursing Home Patients: Development and Evaluation of a Guideline, Decision-Making, and Disease Course* (Wageningen, the Netherlands: Ponsen & Looijen), 1; see also Ibid., "Pneumonia: The Demented Patient's Best Friend?" ch. 8.

decision making was seen as a matter of and for the individual patient only. While the type of pneumonia that is most common in the elderly is not contagious, contagion is at issue in end-of-life decision making in other cases where patients are ill with infectious diseases, bringing with it questions about the impact on others of treatment and palliative care. Consider, for example, a patient dying of Ebola, where efforts to continue treatment or even palliative care might expose caregivers to lethal illness. At present, when outbreaks of Ebola are identified, highly specialized teams are dispatched to the area to provide diagnostic, treatment, and disinfection services. Patients are placed in isolation—comforted by nurses gowned in protective garb, but without contact with family and friends whom they might infect.[38] They may die in a manner or setting not of their own choosing, their autonomy apparently sacrificed to the overall good. This is the conceptualization bioethics has inherited from the examples of chronic, debilitating disease that were at the original core of the field.

From our PVV perspective, however, these patients might also care about themselves as vectors, and about whether their family members and friends may get infected and die. This is not to forget their victimhood—the importance of comfort, of efforts to permit safe communication with loved ones, and of efforts to learn how to provide palliative care when patients are dying of acute, lethal, communicable disease. It is to say that the situation of a dying communicable patient is a complex one *for that patient*, as victim in distress and as vector in interconnection with others.

By comparison, utter shock reverberated in the bioethics community when John Hardwig proposed that the interests of others ought to come to the fore in end-of-life decision making, both in their own right and as part of the interests of the patient. End-of-life decision making, Hardwig argued, ought to give substantial weight to the impact on immediate others, especially spouses and family members who might shoulder substantial burdens of care.[39] The concern that Hardwig's argument violated the autonomy of the individual patient was substantial, but would the outcry have been parallel had the patient wanting continued treatment been dying of a highly infectious communicable disease—say, Ebola or multidrug-resistant TB? Should infection control measures fail or not be available, a still-living patient might be a potential vector to others in a way that a patient who had already died might not be. Although the dying patient presumably will not live to be reinfected by others

---

38. For a moving set of photographs of the process of dealing with an Ebola outbreak, see World Health Organization, "Outbreak of Ebola Haemorrhagic Fever in DRC," October 10, 2007, http://www.who.int/features/2007/ebola_cod/en/index.html (accessed December 29, 2007). See also C.J. Peters, "Arming Ourselves Against the Deadly Filoviruses," *New England Journal of Medicine* 352, no. 25 (June 23, 2005): 2571–2573.
39. John Hardwig, "Is There a Duty to Die?" *Hastings Center Report* 27, no. 2 (1996): 34–42.

and so might not see himself from the vector perspective, there is still something to be made of the vector perspective in this case. Dying patients may care about what happens to close relatives or friends: the way in which their memories and legacies live on. Highly contagious, fatal infectious diseases such as Ebola put these legacies at risk in a starkly focused way. Thinking about his vectorhood, an Ebola patient thus might not want to bring family and friends to death with him. This concern for others as concern for self is far starker than the concerns the patient might have for the eventual financial independence of family members that figured in Hardwig's argument—although it is surely a concern of the same type. It is also—unlike in Hardwig's account—put into the context of larger understanding of the self that the PVV perspective employs, an understanding that also compellingly reminds us of the importance of being creative in doing what we can safely to care for the dying person with a lethal infection. We will have a good deal more to say about triage and dying in later chapters on pandemic planning.

Newer Vintages: Obligations of the Physician

The issues we have discussed so far in this chapter—truth-telling, informed consent, privacy and confidentiality, and decision making at the end of life—were the classic loci of protection of individual patient autonomy. Discussions of these issues pressed physicians to shift from a largely paternalistic approach toward patient care in the direction of an ethic of patients' rights not to be interfered with. Particularly with HIV, and also spurred by increasing concerns about the quality of health care, attention shifted toward physicians' obligations to patients and to others. Here, we take up three examples of this shift to positive duties on the part of physicians: the duty to warn, the duty to treat, and the duty to reduce levels of mistakes. These issues have received much discussion that we will not review here; but we can, we think, suggest some ways in which these discussions have failed to appreciate the full complexity of the PVV perspective, especially the importance of vectorhood.

Duty to warn

In a landmark decision in 1976, the California Supreme Court held that a treating mental health professional has a reasonable duty to warn in cases where it is necessary to prevent imminent harm to others.[40] In the *Tarasoff* case, the patient, Prosenjit Poddar, had told his treating psychologist that he intended to kill Tatiana Tarasoff, who had rejected his romantic advances. Although the

---

40. Tarasoff v. Regents of the University of California, 551 P.2d 334 (Cal. 1976).

psychologist reported the threats to the Berkeley police and Poddar was detained for examination, Tarasoff was never notified of the threats; when Poddar eventually killed her, her family sued. Since the *Tarasoff* decision, many states have adopted some version of the reasonable duty to warn when mental health patients express direct threats to others—over the consistent concerns of mental health professionals that this duty will undermine patients' willingness to seek help.[41]

The *Tarasoff* case involved tort liability; with infectious disease, the standard legal approach has been to require physicians to report listed conditions to public health authorities. It is then the responsibility of the health authorities to engage in any contact tracing. With this process, the physician's breach of confidentiality is a clear legal mandate and approaches to others are the responsibility of others in the public health system. To this extent, physicians have been insulated from direct involvement in the process of warning others—they have no "dirty" hands in breaching confidentiality, because they follow the law while others act. To many, this has seemed a reasonable, if uneasy compromise.

Questions have been raised, however, whether this commitment to confidentiality is adequate, particularly when patients may not understand the full extent of the risks they pose to others and when public health authorities are overstretched to say the least. In the *Reisner* case,[42] the court held that the physician had a duty to counsel his patient—a young woman who had acquired AIDS from a blood transfusion—that she posed risks of transmission to her boyfriend. This case involved a clear failure by the physician to explain her illness to the patient. Extending the duty to warn beyond such discussions with patients has, however, as with the *Tarasoff* case, resulted in concerns that eroding the duty to keep identifiable patient information confidential will break patients' trust and discourage care. Although we think this concern is generally right, we do not think the current practice of relying on the law only is quite right either, when patients pose significant and direct risks of contagion to others. From our PVV perspective, it is important for individual patients to understand both that they are entitled to protection of their confidentiality and that they would want protection if they were at risk of infection from others.

In our discussion of truth-telling, we have suggested that patients should be encouraged to consider whether they would want vectors to know the truth; and in our discussion of informed consent, we suggested that patients should be encouraged to consider the complexity of victimhood and vectorhood in the informed consent process. What is raised here is whether the phy-

---

41. See, e.g., Charles Patrick Ewing, "Tarasoff Reconsidered," *APA Monitor on Psychology* 36, no. 7 (2005): 112, http://www.apa.org/monitor/julaug05/jn.html (accessed April 26, 2008).
42. Reisner v. Regents of the University of California, 31 Cal. App. 4th 1195 (1995).

sician has a positive duty both to his patient and to others to make clear the risks that his patient might pose—that is, to warn the patient about the importance of conveying information about risks to others, and perhaps also to warn those others directly. One way to regard this question is to see the patient as vector and to consider with the patient his effects on others to the extent that they might be of concern to him. He might well want to know whether he is putting his fiancée or his children at risk; the failure to share this information was what was faulty about the physician's conduct in the *Reisner* case. We have already used our PVV analysis to suggest how the physician might counsel the patient on this basis. But, as we have also indicated, in our PVV analysis, the patient is more: *both* immediate victim and vector, as well as someone who is challenged by the unknown possibility of victimhood and vectorhood. In treating the patient, the physician is not treating simply the moment of victimhood; he is treating someone who has the concerns of both victim and vector. One of these concerns is surely confidentiality, but there are other concerns *of the patient* as well, including reducing the overall burden of infectious disease.

What we are urging here might not seem new: in cases of an infectious patient who poses a risk to others, confidentiality must be balanced against these risks to others. But we think it is an important shift in focus. For the general way this situation is presented is that confidentiality is the concern of the immediate patient and is paramount for the treating physician; the physician's decision is then whether any duty to others can override the duty of confidentiality. The decision is generally "yes" if the law mandates but "no" if otherwise. What our shift in focus brings to light is the idea that the balance is a balance of interests for *this immediate patient:* his interest in confidentiality, but also his interests as victim and vector in a web of disease. These other interests are his, just as much as his immediate interest in confidentiality. When the physician discusses with the patient his risks to others and what should be done about them in the immediate situation, the conversation should not be framed as what the patient should do "for others"—but as what the patient should do "for *himself*" in a web of disease relationships with others. If physicians and patients think about situations of dangerous contagion in this way, we surmise, there may be fewer intractable patient/other conflicts—especially if part of the mix is always support for the patient as victim. This is an example of how it is both enormously difficult and critical for physicians and patients alike to try to keep in mind the multiple perspectives of the PVV view.

Duty to Treat—or Not to Treat

Since the recognition of HIV at a time when its mode of transmission was unknown, renewed attention has been paid to the duty of health-care providers to treat patients. Arguments have been made that health-care providers undertake special responsibilities when they enter the field, have special obligations in light of the training they have received, or ought to hold themselves to higher standards than others. Arguments have also been made that heroism is voluntary and that it is morally permissible for health-care providers, as for others, to avoid danger, either generally or when they have special responsibilities to others such as their own families. This literature is extensive, and we will return to the idea that duties to treat generate requirements of compensation for harm incurred, in our discussion of pandemic influenza in Chapter 18. What we want to point out at this juncture is that the discussion of heroism has been less tempered by the recognition that physicians might be vectors, too; and that they have responsibilities to their patients to reduce their own risks of vectorhood if they are to treat patients. Arguments for the duty to treat must also take into account whether there can be a duty *not* to treat—or, at least, a duty not to treat unless the physician has taken reasonable precautions to avoid being the agent of contagion himself.

Because a very high proportion of cases occurred among health-care workers,[43] the SARS outbreak brought the victimhood of physicians, nurses, and other health-care providers into sharp focus. But vectorhood on the part of health-care workers was also an issue. The mechanism of SARS transmission was unknown at first and the reasons for the particularly high rate among health-care workers were unclear; however, it was evident early on that SARS was contagious. Health care workers had been vectors in other outbreaks; for example, the 1918 influenza pandemic and the Ebola outbreak in Uganda in 2001.[44] After all, although dedicated caring by health-care workers is rarely conceptualized in this way, physicians, nurses, and others could themselves become vectors of the very disease they were struggling to treat. Indeed, it was a physician staying at the Monopole Hotel who was apparently the source of the SARS infection inadvertently brought to Toronto by a Scarborough grandmother who had stayed on the same floor of the hotel, a transcontinental transmission that resulted in some 44 deaths in Canada.[45]

Risks of transmission from health-care workers to patients—and attendant efforts to protect workers from being either vectors or victims—should be

43. See, e.g., T.H. Wang K.C. Wei, C.A.Hsiung, S.A.Maloney, R.B. Eidex, D.L. Posey, W.H. Chou, W.Y. Shih, and H.S. Kuo, "Optimizing Severe Acute Respiratory Syndrome Response Strategies: Lessons Learned from Quarantine," *American Journal of Public Health* 97, suppl. 1 (April 2007): S98–S100; Gretchen Reynolds, "Why Were Doctors Afraid to Treat Rebecca McLester?" *New York Times*, sec. 6, April 18, 2004.
44. M. Lamunu, J.J. Lutwama, J. Kamugisha, A. Opio, J. Nambooze, N. Ndayimirije, and S. Okware, "Containing a Haemorrhagic Fever Epidemic: The Ebola Experience in Uganda (October 2000–January 2001)," *International Journal of Infectious Diseases* 8, no. 1 (January 2004): 27–37.
45. Clifford Krauss, "The SARS Epidemic: The Overview: Travelers Urged to Avoid Toronto Because of SARS," *New York Times*, sec. A, April 24, 2003.

among the relevant considerations in analyzing the duty to treat SARS or any other contagious infectious disease. Health-care workers who treat patients without attention to reducing their own risks of disease, hence without attention to their own potential vector status—whether for reasons of economic reward or for reasons of highest altruism—fail in their responsibilities to provide good care to patients. The provider who comes to work tired and sick, without considering risks of transmitting the disease she is carrying to the patient, puts patients at risk. When the provider is at known risk, this failure is in one respect parallel to the failures of providers who do not keep up their technical skills or who become alcohol- or drug-impaired: they risk identifiable harms to patients.

If putting the point this way seems inflammatory, it may be because provider failures to see their own vector status are not generally brought to the forefront of responsibilities to patients, but are thought of along the lines of responsibilities to themselves or their families.[46] But consider the example of immunization for physicians: influenza immunization rates among physicians are estimated to be quite low, and physicians with colds or the flu often go to work like many other people.[47] Yet there is no outcry similar to the outcry that might be expected were a similar proportion of physicians known to be drug or alcohol impaired. Perhaps the parallel is inapt: impaired physicians may be more likely to put patients at risk, and do so by means of how their impairment affects their skills as physicians. The connection between infectious physicians and harms to patients may be more indirect, not intrinsic to the care but resulting from some unrelated feature of the physician. Early on in an epidemic, it is of course very difficult to assess the nature and levels of risk, and both medical and public hysteria often occur. Nevertheless, there are circumstances in which it will be relatively clear that providers are at risk of transmitting diseases to their patients, and this risk should be taken into account in assessing the duty to treat or duty to take precautions or even to refrain from treating. Providers clearly do have a duty to minimize the risks they pose to patients and others infected in turn by those patients. These may include measures as simple as hand washing or precautions against exposure, or more burdensome interventions such as vaccination or the willingness to undergo treatment themselves.[48] Duties to immediate patients may be seen as part of

---

46. This issue is raised by Mariette A. van den Hoven and Marcel F. Verweij, "Should We Promote Influenza Vaccination of Health Care Workers in Nursing Homes? Some Ethical Arguments in Favour of Immunization," *Age and Ageing* 32 (2003): 487–489.

47. Ibid. For guidelines about immunization of health-care workers, see Centers for Disease Control and Prevention, "Immunization of Health-Care Workers: Recommendations of the Advisory Committee on Immunization Practices (ACIP) and the Hospital Infection Control Practices Advisory Committee (HICPAC)," *Mortality and Morbidity Weekly Report* 46, no. RR-18 (December 26, 1997): 1–42.

48. Ariel Berk, "Handwashing Lessens MRSA Risk," *Johns Hopkins Newsletter* (November 15, 2004), http://media.www.jhunewsletter.com/media/storage/paper932/news/2004/11/05/Science/

the physician's more general duty to treat patients safely, a part of the physician/patient relationship. Our PVV view also reminds us that such duties to immediate patients have implications for others who may be infected in turn as a contagious disease is transmitted from one to another, sometimes in a widespread way throughout a population.

As always under our PVV analysis, there is a victim-side to the analysis, too. Providers who may transmit contagious diseases to their patients are themselves either victims or at risk of being victims. The availability of appropriate protective, prophylactic, and therapeutic measures thus matters in dual fashion: both as appropriate support for the provider's ability to deliver safe treatment, and as a response to the provider-victim. These are both current, real-world issues, and issues of future policy as well, as we will see in our discussion of pandemic prioritization in Part IV.

Mistakes

Beyond this nuanced understanding of the duty to treat, there are implications of our PVV analysis for mistakes more generally in the context of infectious disease. Since the publication of the initial data from the Harvard malpractice study,[49] followed by the Institute of Medicine's *To Err Is Human* in 1999,[50] much attention has been devoted to reducing medical error in patient care. The image of the equivalent of a jumbo jet of passengers dying each day in the United States from avoidable medical error has brought health-care delivery systems and individual providers under increasing scrutiny. To the best of our knowledge, however, no separate attention has been paid in the mistakes literature to special characteristics raised by some infectious diseases. When infectious diseases are transmissible, a mistake can multiply; and the multiplication can be as fast-moving as a wild fire. This would suggest a model in which mistakes are broadly construed and physicians are accountable morally (and perhaps even legally) for their mistakes to people beyond their immediate patients. However, uncertainty, particularly in the face of an emerging disease, may be extensive: about disease risks, mode of transmission, and even infectious organism. What counts as a mistake—as well as what can and ought to be done about it—may therefore be more limited in the case of some infectious diseases.

Because, as we have seen in Chapter 3, infectious diseases are characteristically acute, easily diagnosed, simply and effectively treated, and readily prevented,

Hand-Washing.Lessens.Mrsa.Risk-2244064.shtml (accessed December 29, 2007).
49. P.C. Weiler, H.H. Hiatt, J.P. Newhouse, W.G. Johnson, T.A. Brennan, and L.L. Leape, *A Measure of Malpractice* (Cambridge: Harvard University Press, 1993).
50. Linda T. Kohn, Janet M. Corrigan, and Molla S. Donaldson, eds., *To Err Is Human: Building a Safer Health System* (Washington, DC: National Academy Press, 2000).

even though potentially transmissible to others, clinical response to them is typically a success story. However, the acuity with which some infectious diseases occur and progress places special weight on prompt diagnosis, and mistakes here can be deeply problematic. Yet diagnosis is usually most uncertain early in the course of disease. Familiar examples include bacterial meningitis, which early on can mimic a viral upper respiratory infection in infants or young children. Bacterial endocarditis in adults, with its early stages of fever, myalgias and malaise, can resemble the early symptoms of a much more common and less dangerous influenza. Furthermore, the more serious diseases are substantially less common than the milder ones they resemble; physicians in diagnosing infectious disease thus face an ethical challenge involving allocation of resources and weighing prospective benefits and burdens. If physicians use laboratory tests and imaging technology to pursue relatively rare infections with patients who have consistent but not yet characteristic signs and symptoms, they will subject many patients to expensive, intrusive, uncomfortable and sometimes risky measures, from blood tests to spinal taps, but only infrequently identify dangerous disease. Patients who are more familiar with the common, less serious disorders may see additional studies as unnecessary, inconvenient, and possibly harmful.

Yet there are two reasons for physicians to explore more aggressive diagnostic strategies in these cases. For the patient as victim, speed in diagnosis may be especially critical to successful treatment. For the patient as vector, rapid intervention may limit spread. With serious influenza, to take one example, antivirals are ineffective unless they are started within a short time window—no more than 48 hours—and a mistake in diagnosis may mean a missed opportunity both to treat this patient and to reduce the likelihood that she will pass the disease along to others. Small pieces of information may significantly decrease uncertainty and rebalance the cost–benefit ratio in acute infectious diseases. Details about recent travel often raise or exclude some diagnostic possibilities. For example, a vacationer returning from the Caribbean with symptoms suggestive of influenza may actually have dengue fever, a mosquito-born, viral disease that occurs primarily in the tropics. To recognize dengue accurately, the physician must inquire about activities ignored or overlooked during most visits, namely travel history and exposures. Patients also may not appreciate the importance of mentioning travel or a particularly relevant activity that may have taken place a week or more before the onset of symptoms.

The importance of targeted questions and truthful answers is even more evident with infectious diseases in some way linked to social stigma. Doctors may be reluctant to inquire about sexual activity—particularly in patients they have known a long time—because of assumptions that they already know the lifestyles of their long-term patients or out of fear of offending them; a survey of primary care physicians in Canada, for example, found that fewer than 25% routinely asked their patients about sexual practices that increased their risk of acquiring sexually transmitted diseases.[51] With infectious disease, avoiding mistakes thus goes beyond technical competence, to social understanding and communicative skill.

As with diagnosis, the rapidly progressive nature of many infectious diseases precludes, or at least threatens, a treatment strategy that is cost-effective and ethically non-problematic for many non-infectious disorders. That strategy is *watchful waiting*. Watchful waiting, involving the passage of time and repeat observations but no intervention, can clarify whether an elevated blood pressure is a temporary aberration or a sign of chronic hypertension. When treatment may need to begin within a rapidly closing window of opportunity, watchful waiting would be a mistake. Treatment delays in meningitis or endocarditis, for example, may lead to fatal consequences or permanent disabilities.

Another treatment strategy, empiric treatment, may also prove mistaken in infectious disease. Because the microbial agents of infectious diseases are biologically adaptable, they can and do respond to antimicrobial agents in ways that are advantageous to them. Thus, intrinsically resistant organisms may become more prevalent and sensitive organisms may mutate or acquire resistance. This creates unusual therapeutic and ethical problems for clinicians. In an effort to address dangerous infections, even though they may be unusual in a particular patient, physicians may understandably be tempted to use agents that are very broadly active and/or agents that are active against even presently resistant organisms. Examples include using an antifungal drug to treat a patient with pneumonia where such an infection is possible, but highly unlikely. Similarly, when the physician suspects that a patient may have a staphylococcal infection, she knows that up to 5% of these infections may not respond to conventional treatment with beta-lactam antibiotics, but they will respond to vancomycin. If this clinician is driven by immediate concern for her patient and by possibilities, not probabilities, she may make therapeutic choices that are not only more expensive with no benefit likely for the patient, but that may increase the likelihood that the patient will have or transmit an organism that will be harder or even impossible to treat. As we will see in Chapter 13, there is an argument for seeing such use of antibiotics as problematic, even if they do not immediately harm the patient.

These distinctive characteristics of infectious disease, including urgency, treatability, and transmissibility, may affect the range of what counts as a mistake and of physician accountability for mistakes. Errors are compounded in

51. B. Maheux N. Haley, M. Rivard, and A. Gervais, "Do Physicians Assess Lifestyle Health Risks During General Medical Examinations? A Survey of General Practitioners and Obstetrician-Gynecologists in Quebec," *Canadian Medical Association Journal* 160, no. 13 (June 29, 1999): 1830–1834.

infectious disease in a way that is not true of other areas of medicine. A physician's failure to diagnose or properly manage HIV infection or tuberculosis, particularly drug-resistant tuberculosis, can have serious consequences for a large number of people who have been exposed to the patient; it could even be responsible for an epidemic. Curiously, there has been little or no malpractice litigation of this kind; the physician's duty has been limited legally to the patient he is treating. The so-called duty to warn cases have not been extended outside the physician's knowledge of a psychiatric patient's credible threat to harm a specific individual. Certain infectious diseases, when present, easily diagnosed, and treated, would seem to create a similar duty, but, with a few exceptions, have not been understood in this way. The uncertainty surrounding diagnosis and treatment, as well as the difficulties in anticipating who might be the likely next victims, would appear to be explanations. There are circumstances in which these explanations are not persuasive, however: transmission of chicken pox, a highly contagious and easily diagnosed condition, between siblings who share a bedroom, for example. In such cases, it seems inconsistent to limit analysis of the mistake and its consequences to the immediate patient.

Conclusion

In this chapter, we have shown how our PVV perspective sheds new light on some of the most traditional issues in bioethics: truth-telling, confidentiality, informed consent, and withdrawing or withholding treatment at the end of life. We have also explored some newer ethical issues for physicians: the duty to warn, the duty to treat (or not to treat), and the significance of mistakes. Our goal has been to show how arguments for protecting patient autonomy understood as resting in the choices of individual patients—but sometimes in conflict with the interests of others—are flat and conflictual. On this analysis, some conflicts between the patient and others are in the end irresolvable; the best that can be done is to try to mediate or to decide whether autonomy must be overridden.

The PVV perspective, we think, can deepen discussions of these traditional cases. Autonomy can be enriched; from the PVV perspective, it is seen as a matter not only of the pressing concerns of the now-ill patient, but also of the patient as way-station of disease. For ourselves, we may care not only about the immediacy of illness, but also about the possibility that we might be victim or vector, and that the overall pattern of illness in our society or our world might affect our victim/vector status. These perspectives, we know, cannot all be held in mind at once, nor can all tensions among them be fully resolved. The autonomy of the individual patient, now-ill, reflects principally the victim situation—this is a first level perspective that analyses in bioethics often reflect.

The PVV perspective reminds us that there is more even to being a victim—the person who is a victim is also a way-station self and in that sense a vector as well—and that these additional considerations may help at times to surmount at least some of the conflicts that appear when autonomy is more narrowly understood. Our PVV perspective also serves to inform analyses of newer issues such as the nature of mistakes that have too often been limited to considerations affecting the individual patient alone.

9

FROM THE MAGIC MOUNTAIN TO A DYING HOMELESS MAN AND HIS DOG: IMPOSING ISOLATION AND TREATMENT IN TUBERCULOSIS CARE

Tuberculosis (TB) ranks among the most dreaded diseases in human history, and continues to be one of humankind's most frequent killers. While evidence of tuberculosis of the spine has been observed in pre-Columbian and early Egyptian mummies, epidemics of this infectious disease first became a serious problem in the seventeenth century, when urbanization and associated crowding created the ideal circumstances for spread.[1] In the twentieth century, improved living conditions and availability of adequate diagnostic and antibiotic therapies had brought tuberculosis under control for most of the population in developed countries. TB, however, has remained all along a serious problem for those in the developing world and for subpopulations in the developed world that do not have access to adequate health care. The WHO currently estimates that one-third of the world's population is infected with TB and more than a million deaths each year can be attributed to this infection.[2]

Although the development of effective antimicrobial treatment has meant that much tuberculosis has come under control in developed countries, the recent appearance of new, extensively drug-resistant forms of tuberculosis (XDR-TB) pose substantial clinical and ethical dilemmas worldwide.[3] How should highly and dangerously infectious patients be managed? Should they be required to undergo observed therapy? Should they be isolated until they are no longer contagious? The specter of XDR-TB is alarming health-care providers across the world—and it is a real, here-now threat, rather than the might-be threat of pandemic influenza. We frame these dilemmas in light of stories of tuberculosis from nineteenth-century European sanatoria to twenty-first

---

1. D.W. Haas and R.M. Des Pres, "Mycobacterium Tuberculosis," in *Principles and Practice of Infectious Diseases*, ed. G.L. Mandell, J.E. Bennett, and R. Dolin, 4th ed. (New York: Churchill Livingstone, 1995), 2213.
2. C. Dye, S. Scheele, P. Dolin, V. Pathania, M.C. Raviglione, for the WHO Global Surveillance and Monitoring Project, "Global Burden of Tuberculosis: Estimated Incidence, Prevalence, and Mortality by Country," *Journal of the American Medical Association* 282, no. 7 (August 18, 1999): 677–686.
3. M.C. Raviglione and I.M. Smith, "XDR Tuberculosis—Implications for Global Public Health," *New England Journal of Medicine* 356, no. 7 (February 15, 2007): 656–659.

century New York City to the current global threat of XDR-TB, focusing in the end on the real-life clinical dilemma of a dying homeless man and his dog. We conclude this chapter with some reflections on ways in which isolation might permissibly be managed in light of our PVV perspective.

Tuberculosis Pathogenesis, Epidemiology, and Therapy

Tuberculosis is due to infection with the bacterium *Mycobacterium tuberculosis* (MTB).[4] This infection is almost always acquired directly by breathing in small airborne particles of respiratory tract secretions that are generated during coughing, sneezing, singing, or talking by a person who has active pulmonary infection. Although in most people infected with TB the person's immune system controls the infection and he or she does not become infectious to others, the 5 to 10% of people infected who do become infectious are responsible for a continuing worldwide epidemic of tuberculosis. This high level of contagiousness occurs in part because transmission from untreated individuals is sustained over a long period of time. In the 1980s, the Centers for Disease Control and Prevention (CDC) proposed that the time was ripe for eradication of TB in the United States, a goal in principle possible because *Mycobacterium tuberculosis* has only a human reservoir. The subsequent epidemic of TB in HIV patients and the development of multidrug-resistant tuberculosis (MDR-TB) plus the increased importation of the disease by illegal immigrants quashed the CDC's plans. At present, worldwide eradication of TB is a very distant hope.

Tuberculosis often begins quietly and unnoticed, but can progress to a fatal conclusion. The initial infection with *Mycobacterium tuberculosis* may cause a mild and often asymptomatic pneumonia; dissemination of the organism to other body parts may occur at this time. An immune response to TB infection develops over a period of three to eight weeks, usually manifested by development of a positive TB skin test. Most patients control this initial infection, but about 5% of a healthy population do not and develop overt disease with fevers, chills, weight loss, and evidence of progressive pulmonary involvement. These patients are generally infectious and can spread the disease to others. However, most healthy people (95%) after this initial symptomatic episode enter an asymptomatic or latent phase of infection that may last for the rest of their lives. Only about 5% of these people will reactivate their latent infection later in life and develop pulmonary infection that may also be infectious to others. This recrudescence of latent TB is often associated with a decline in general immune status that accompanies old age, malnutrition, cancer chemotherapy,

---

4. A useful contemporary source concerning tuberculosis infection and treatment in the United States is P.M. Small and P.I. Fujiwara, "Management of Tuberculosis in the United States," *New England Journal of Medicine* 345, no. 3 (July 19, 2001): 189–200.

or immunosuppressive therapy for arthritic or other diseases. HIV-infected patients are particularly susceptible to progressive or reactivation TB, with a more than ninefold increased risk of activation of latent TB infection.[5]

Tuberculosis is highly infectious in some situations and its infectivity is far more sustained than that of many other infectious diseases. Patients who are most infectious are those who have lung abscesses or cavities, or who have laryngeal TB. In one outbreak on a U.S. navy vessel, a single sailor with a large TB lung cavity infected 80% of the 66 men who shared his sleeping compartment. In another outbreak, a single patient who was not suspected to have TB infected 10 of 13 health-care workers who were exposed over a period of less than three hours.[6] In tuberculosis, however, transmission can be rapid or may continue over a far longer period of time. The untreated TB patient may remain infectious for many months or even for years because the infection progresses relatively slowly. By comparison, the period of infectivity for measles, influenza, and chickenpox, to take some familiar examples, is usually limited to a few days or weeks during which the patient either overcomes the infection or dies.

Effective therapy for TB first became available with the discovery of streptomycin in the late 1940s and isoniazid in the early 1950s. Since that time, more than a dozen new antimicrobials have been made available for the treatment of TB. It can now be said that all patients who are otherwise well nourished and healthy and who receive the full course of recommended therapy can achieve cure for drug-sensitive strains of TB. However, adequate TB therapy is much more difficult for patients to achieve than is therapy for most other bacterial diseases. While most bacterial infections can be cured with a few days or weeks of single-drug antimicrobial therapy, therapy for TB includes multiple drugs and must be continued for 6 months at a minimum. For patients with multiple organ disease, or with drug resistant TB, therapy must be continued for a year or more to be successful—as well as to minimize the development of disease resistant to a still wider range of drugs.

The current major barrier to achieving successful therapy for TB has been lack of adequate compliance with recommended treatment plans.[7] In an unsupervised environment, as many as 39% of patients were lost to study in a six-month treatment regimen and 49% were lost in a nine-month regimen.[8]

5. C.R. Horsburgh, "Priorities for the Treatment of Latent Tuberculosis Infection in the United States," *New England Journal of Medicine* 350, no. 20 (May 13, 2004): 2060–2067.
6. E.A. Nordell and W.F. Piessens, "Transmission of Tuberculosis," in *Tuberculosis: A Comprehensive International Approach*, ed. L.B.Reichman and E.S. Hershfield, 2nd ed. (New York: Marcel Dekker, 2000), 224.
7. M.D. Iseman, D.L. Cohn, and J.A. Sbarbaro, "Directly Observed Treatment for Tuberculosis—We Can't Afford Not to Try It," *New England Journal of Medicine* 328, no. 8 (February 25, 1993): 576–578.
8. D.L. Combs, R.J. O'Brien, and L.J. Geiter, "USPHS Tuberculosis Short-Course Chemotherapy Trial 21: Effectiveness, Toxicity, and Acceptability," *Annals of Internal Medicine* 112, no. 6 (1990): 397–406.

While it is tempting to attribute lack of compliance to demographic characteristics such as low income and poor education or complicating medical/
social factors such as homelessness, alcoholism, and drug addiction, studies of
diverse populations indicate that patients from all social and economic strata
have high rates of non-adherence to the long and often complicated courses
of therapy for TB and other chronic illnesses.[9] Lack of adherence to a recommended full course of therapy has been shown to be an important cause of
development of antimicrobial-resistant strains of TB.[10] The need to improve
compliance with therapy has been the primary force behind recent aggressive
approaches to the management of TB, such as directly observed therapy (DOT)[11]
and the more coercive approaches used in the New York City outbreak that we
discuss below.[12]

Public health officers in some U.S. cities responded to the challenge of non-
compliance by identifying subgroups of patients who fit into profiles of groups
that had high rates of non-compliance, such as former prisoners, alcoholics
and the homeless. These individuals were then subjected to a program of directly observed therapy, in which a trained clinician observes the patient actually swallow the medicine, making sure it has not been "cheeked" by being
hidden between the tongue and cheek and later spit out, or disposed of in
some other way. DOT is usually conducted daily during the first few months,
and then two to three times a week until the regimen is completed.[13]

Some physicians made DOT routine for all of their patients. In the 1970s,
John Sbarbaro in Denver observed that up to 75% of his patients fit the high-
risk profile, and decided that all patients with TB should be included in the
DOT program.[14] It is not clear that his inclusion of all patients was an attempt
to achieve distributive justice, but his writings do indicate a strong paternalistic leaning. Although he agreed that the public health officer had an obligation to his patients to provide a free, convenient, and patient-friendly health
delivery system, and acknowledged that a strong provider–patient relationship
based on trust was the most important factor in achieving compliance, Sbarbaro argued that the provider had a legal obligation to defend the civil rights of
each individual to remain free of a communicable disease. He further argued

---

9. E. Sumartojo, "When Tuberculosis Treatment Fails: A Social Behavioral Account of Patient
Adherence," *American Review of Respiratory Disease* 147, no. 5 (May 1993): 1311–1320.
10. Small and Fujiwara, "Management of Tuberculosis."
11. R. Bayer and D. Wilkinson, "Directly Observed Therapy for Tuberculosis: History of an Idea,"
Lancet 345 (1995): 1545–1548.
12. T.R. Frieden et al., "The Emergence of Drug-Resistant Tuberculosis in New York City," *New
England Journal of Medicine* 328, no. 8 (February 25, 1993): 521–526.
13. Bayer and Wilkinson, "Directly Observed Therapy for Tuberculosis."
14. J.A. Sbarbaro, "Compliance: Inducements and Enforcements," *Chest* 76, no. 6 (December
1979): 750–756.

that the provider's responsibility to achieve patient compliance was an absolute responsibility that "cannot be ignored or covered over by a pious concern for the afflicted individual." This policy of requiring DOT for all TB patients appeared to be successful in 97% of patients. Sbarbaro was particularly proud that only 3% of the patients enrolled in his program required the imposition of forced quarantine, isolation, or restriction of freedom. He concluded that when patients are made aware of the possibility of imposition of force they quickly comply because "the willingness to invoke force stands as clear evidence of professional strength and conviction, and as if dealing with a firm but understanding parent, patients quickly accept their part of the arrangement— freedom in exchange for cooperation."

While public health officers in some cities adopted universal DOT for TB patients with similar rates of success during the 1970s, and increasing reports of success of DOT programs in India and China appeared in the literature,[15] the federal TB program at the CDC and most state programs did not recommend or adapt universal DOT programs for TB control. For some states, reluctance was based on perceived lack of funding despite studies that DOT programs were cost effective compared to the costs of managing treatment failures. For others, there was concern that such universal DOT programs were too paternalistic and that they violated patient's civil liberties.[16] Even today, civil libertarians may well not agree with Sbarbaro, either about the relative balance of threats and liberty or about the reasonableness of paternalism to patients or the public.[17]

TB Control: Sanatoria, Isolation, and Directly Observed Therapy

Because of the highly infectious nature of some patients and the long period of infectivity of untreated patients, public health officials have for most of the twentieth century focused on TB as an infectious disease in particular need of control. Directly observed therapy, isolation, and even quarantine are all strategies that have been deployed to constrain patients with TB.

The Magic Mountain

In his classic novel *The Magic Mountain*,[18] Thomas Mann used a tuberculosis sanatorium in the Swiss Alps as a symbol of the unreality of European society in the days before World War I. For those in comfortable economic circumstances,

---

15. Bayer and Wilkinson, "Directly Observed Therapy for Tuberculosis."
16. Ibid.
17. See, e.g., George Annas, "Puppy Love: Bioterrorism, Civil Rights, and the Public's Health," *University of Florida Law Review* 55 (2003): 1171–1190.
18. Thomas Mann, *The Magic Mountain*, trans. H.T. Lowe-Porter (London: M. Secker, 1929).

the sanatoria provided places to take rest cures, enjoy the delights of seven meals a day, flirt vicariously, promenade along mountain trails, and engage in endless political debates. At the sanatorium portrayed by Mann, people stayed for months and years, hoping to return to their ordinary lives but trapped in a time warp of apparent illness. Life at the sanatorium was materially comfortable but mesmerizing and enervating. Despite the relative economic privilege of the patients at the sanatorium portrayed by Mann, their physicians subjected them to experimental treatment and psychological manipulation in tyrannical and not clearly altruistic fashion. And, like Europe, the patients were quite literally rotting from within.

In the first half of the twentieth century, before antimicrobial therapy for TB became available, TB control was primarily limited to isolating patients in TB sanatoria. Wealthy patients typically enjoyed sanatoria where the provision of good food and fresh air allowed most to slowly heal and become non-infectious, while poor, less fortunate patients were confined for long periods to dismal inner city sanatoria where death rates were high.[19] Both wealthy and poor, however, were confined, and this meant that active TB cases were, so to speak, kept off the streets and out of environments in which the disease could be passed along.

Some observers have credited the TB control practices of screening, case finding, and subsequent isolation of infectious patients for the continued 3–5% yearly decline in the incidence of new cases over the first half of the twentieth century. Others have concluded that steady improvements in the social factors that influenced the spread of TB such as hygiene, nutrition, and living conditions were most important in reducing disease spread.[20] With the Supreme Court clearly recognizing states' police powers for infectious disease control in *Jacobson v. Massachusetts*,[21] and the general fear of the public about acquiring TB, this authoritarian and coercive approach to the management of TB was adopted by many large U.S. cities with little apparent challenge. In the 1950s, Seattle had one of the most aggressive policies of hospitalizing uncooperative TB patients. As medical writer Barron Lerner pointed out, the Seattle TB hospital was effectively "a jail in every sense of the word."[22] In 1957 the American Civil Liberties Union challenged the practice of hospitalization as form of detention,

---

19. S.M. Rothman, "The Sanitorium Experience: Myths and Realities," in *The Tuberculosis Revival: Individual Rights and Societal Obligations in a Time of Aids*, ed. Nancy N Dubler, Ronald Bayer, Sheldon Landesman, and Amanda White (New York: United Hospital Fund of New York, 1992), 67–73.
20. R. Dubos and J. Dubos, *The White Plague: Tuberculosis, Man and Society* (Boston: Little, Brown, 1952).
21. Jacobson v. Massachusetts, 197 U.S. 11 (1905).
22. B.H. Lerner, *Contagion and Confinement: Controlling Tuberculosis Along the Skid Road* (Baltimore: Johns Hopkins University Press, 1998), 139.

but their arguments failed in court.[23] Public health laws enacted at the turn of the twentieth century thus have played a major role in the management of tuberculosis: most of these laws permitted aggressive and often coercive programs for screening, case finding, reporting, and involuntary commitment to TB sanatoria until the infection healed or the patient died.[24]

Surveillance and isolation laws have been variously applied over the twentieth century in response to local outbreaks of tuberculosis. With the appearance of MDR-TB in recent years, these laws have been vigorously implemented in some cities.[25] Today, however, there is little likelihood of reversion to special institutions for isolating TB patients. Truly unmanageable patients are rare; they are usually placed in locked wards or supervised hospital beds, and city or university hospitals generally are used to take care of this small population.[26]

New York City and Directly Observed Therapy

Shortly after therapy became available in the 1940s and 1950s, TB appeared to be coming under control: the rate of decline of new cases increased to 7% per year with the introduction of effective antimicrobial therapy.[27] By the mid 1980s, the incidence of new cases of TB in the United States had declined to an all time low of less than 22,000 per year, and government TB control officers began talking about eliminating TB from the United States over the next 20 years.

Unfortunately, in the mid-1980s, the trend of continued improvement in the control of TB abruptly reversed. By 1992, the annual incidence of TB in the United States had increased by almost 20% to 26,000 cases. This resurgence of TB has been attributed to multiple factors, including a large reduction in U.S.

23. See George J. Annas, "Control of Tuberculosis—The Law and the Public's Health," *New England Journal of Medicine* 328, no. 8 (February 25, 1993): 585–588. From our PVV perspective, a question to ask about these decisions was what the courts would have decided, had treatment facilities not been available for victims. In Moore v. Draper, 57 So. 2d 648 (Fla. 1952), the Florida Supreme Court upheld a new Florida statute providing for mandatory confinement of patients with transmissible tuberculosis. Interestingly, the Court observed that the state passed the statute only after it had significant available facilities "to properly take care of" these patients, noting that the restriction without the facilities would have been "useless."
24. D.A. Hansell, "The TB and HIV Epidemics: History Learned and Unlearned," *Journal of Law, Medicine & Ethics* 21, nos. 3–4 (Fall-Winter 1993): 376–381.
25. Annas, "Control of Tuberculosis."
26. There is one recent reference to an XDR-TB patient locked in a Phoenix jail for failure to comply with a physician's instructions to wear a face mask in public. C. Kahn, "Man with Drug-Resistant TB Locked Up," *USA Today*, April 2, 2007; P. Sampathkumar, "Dealing with Threat of Drug-Resistant Tuberculosis: Background Information for Interpreting the Andrew Speaker and Related Cases," *Mayo Clinic Proceedings* 82, no. 7 (July 2007): 799–802.
27. Institute of Medicine, *Ending Neglect: The Elimination of Tuberculosis in the United States*, ed. Lawrence Geiter (Washington, DC: National Academy Press, 2000), 23–30.

federal categorical funding for TB control and increases in the social factors which promote the spread of TB such as inner city crowding, homelessness, intravenous and crack drug abuse, the arrival of new immigrants from countries with a high prevalence of TB, and the rapidly increasing epidemic of HIV infection. Mortality rates from TB, which had been quite low, began to approach 40% overall, and were as high as 90% for patients with both AIDS and MDR-TB.[28] Several of these outbreaks occurred in hospitals or HIV care facilities and the spread of MDR-TB to healthy medical staff generated fear throughout the medical community.

In the early 1990s, these factors coalesced in New York City to generate a serious epidemic of TB that involved more than 8,000 new cases over a two-year period. This epidemic was particularly frightening because of the appearance of strains of TB that were resistant to one or more TB drugs.[29] Because noncompliance with therapy was a major factor in the development of such drug resistance, TB control officers in New York City and most other major cities began to enthusiastically support DOT programs as a way to secure better compliance. Nationally recognized TB specialists such as Michael Iseman at National Jewish Hospital in Denver[30] and Paul Farmer at Harvard[31] argued aggressively for expanded use of DOT. In 1995 the National Advisory Council for the Elimination of Tuberculosis recommended that DOT be considered for all TB patients.[32]

New York City, with the largest outbreak of MDR-TB, led the way in adopting a very aggressive public health program to contain the spread of TB. In response to its epidemic, the City in 1994 enacted laws that gave expanded powers to the Commissioner of Public Health to issue orders compelling a person to be examined for suspected TB, to complete treatment, to receive treatment under direct observation, or to be detained for treatment.[33] Patients could be detained for 60 days before judicial review, and in some cases they could be detained until they completed a full course of therapy.[34] This new and higher level of public health coercion was effective, with new TB cases declining by 55% and cases of MDR-TB by 87% between 1992 and 1997. Commentators

28. Frieden et al., "Emergence of Drug-Resistant Tuberculosis."
29. Ibid.
30. Iseman, Cohn, and Sbarbaro, "Directly Observed Treatment for Tuberculosis."
31. P.E. Farmer, J.Y. Kim, C. Mitnick, and R.Timperi, "Responding to Outbreaks of MDRTB: Introducing 'DOTS-Plus,'" in *Tuberculosis: A Comprehensive International Approach*, eds. L.B. Reichman, and E.S. Hershfield, 447–469.
32. Centers for Disease Control and Prevention, "Essential Components of a Tuberculosis Control Program: Recommendations of the Advisory Council for the Elimination of Tuberculosis," *Mortality and Morbidity Weekly Report* 44, no. RR-11 (September 8, 1995): 1–16.
33. M.R. Gasner, K.L. Maw, G.E. Feldman et al., "The Use of Legal Action in New York City to Ensure Treatment of Tuberculosis," *New England Journal of Medicine* 340, no. 5 (February 4, 1999): 359–366.
34. Gasner et al., "The Use of Legal Action."

defended the restrictions on liberty imposed by the program on this basis.[35] Similar programs were implemented in other major cities. By 1998, the incidence of new cases of TB in the United States was again declining at a rate of 7% per year and new cases were at an all time low of 18,361.[36]

However, implementation of this more aggressive public health TB control program in New York City did not go unchallenged, with patients' rights advocacy groups expressing fear that the city health department would unfairly direct legal actions against the poor, homeless, and addicted.[37] A subsequent thorough review of the use of legal actions in New York City to control an outbreak of MDR-TB in the early 1990s reported that regulatory orders were issued to fewer than 4% of the 8,000 patients with TB, and concluded that patients were detained on the basis of their history of TB and lack of compliance with therapy, rather than their social characteristics.[38]

Dissenters to the New York City Tuberculosis Working Group report argued, "It is unethical, illegal, and bad public health policy to detain 'noncompliant' persons before making concerted efforts to address the numerous systemic deficiencies that make adherence to treatment virtually impossible for many New Yorkers."[39] The argument that local governments and societies have a moral obligation to address the social ills that created the problem of TB before they resorted to coercion also came from British ethicists representing a society where public health included a broader responsibility for health care and meeting social needs.[40] Strong arguments for greater respect for patients' rights and autonomy also came from AIDS activist groups in New York who had seen the positive effects of a "voluntarism" approach to managing the HIV epidemic.[41] The practical argument was made that stigmatizing TB as a social disease, violating patients' confidentiality by aggressive screening, case finding, forced therapy, and threats of coercion and detention all tended to encourage patients in groups at high risk of contracting TB to avoid public health screening and care.

Although most civil libertarians who addressed the moral justification of the more coercive public health TB control practices in New York and other

35. E.W. Campion, "Liberty and the Control of Tuberculosis," *New England Journal of Medicine* 340, no. 5 (February 4, 1999): 385–386.

36. Hansell, "History Learned and Unlearned."

37. N.N. Dubler, R. Bayer, S. Landesman, and A. White, *The Tuberculosis Revival: Individual Rights and Societal Obligations in a Time of AIDS* (New York: United Hospital Fund of New York, 1992).

38. Gasner et al., "The Use of Legal Action."

39. Dubler, Bayer, Landesman, and White, *The Tuberculosis Revival.*

40. L. Doyal, "Moral Problems in the Use of Coercion in Dealing with Nonadherence in the Diagnosis and Treatment of Tuberculosis," *Annals of the New York Academies of Sciences* 953 (December 2001): 208–215.

41. Institute of Medicne, *Ending Neglect,* 23–30.

U.S. cities agreed that coercion could be justified in circumstances where the infected patient was proven to be at high risk of infecting others, some raised concerns that the new laws did not set a high enough standard for proof of high risk and effectiveness of the coercive alternative. Coker,[42] using the Siracusa Principles for just restriction of human rights[43] as a standard, concluded that the new statutes and practices in New York failed to satisfy several of the principles. He pointed out that the new statutes had moved from proving necessity by requiring strong evidence that the TB patient was infectious for others, to a policy that allowed a patient to be detained because of a history of noncompliance, even if the patient was not currently infectious. Coker noted that the new statutes did not follow the principle that there be no less intrusive and restrictive means available to achieve the same goal. In his 1993 review of state public health laws, Gostin[44] made several proposals for reform with the goal of achieving a better balance between public health and human rights. In particular, he tried to adapt a lesson from the HIV epidemic, that respect for human rights was required in order to protect the public health. He suggested that many state statutes focused on coercive police powers and too few addressed duties of public health departments to pay for and provide all necessary services. Gostin reasoned that cost of therapy should never be a barrier to obtaining voluntary adherence to TB therapy. He advised that surveillance laws should be exercised only when there was a high likelihood of a person being infected, and only when the individual was unwilling to be examined on a voluntary basis. Gostin expressed particular concern with the lack of confidentiality provisions in many state TB control laws, noting that laws regulating the control of venereal diseases and HIV were more sensitive to the patient's autonomous right to privacy. Regarding treatment, Gostin advised that all patients should be offered a highly individualized plan for voluntary DOT therapy to ensure that all individuals were treated equitably, and to that compulsory therapy was used only as a last resort. Commitment statues, he proposed, should be similar to those in the field of mental health: requiring evidence that the patient was a significant risk to the public and assuring the patient's right to full due process hearing *before* commitment, not after 60 days. When isolation or quarantine was justified, he proposed that it should be done in a hospital or medical care setting providing a high standard of medical care, and not in a jail. Gostin was particularly cautious about use of criminal

---

42. R. Coker, "Just Coercion? Detention of Nonadherent Tuberculosis Patients," *Annals of the New York Academies of Sciences* 953 (December 2001): 216–222.

43. The Urban Institute, "The Siracusa Principles on the Limitation and Derogation Provisions in the International Covenant on Civil and Political Rights," *Human Rights Quarterly* 7 (1985): 3–14.

44. L.O. Gostin, "Controlling the Resurgent Tuberculosis Epidemic: A 50-State Survey of Statutes and Proposals for Reform," *Journal of the American Medical Association* 269, no. 2 (January 13, 1993): 255–261.

penalties, suggesting that threat of criminal punishment ultimately might deter individuals from voluntary participation in public health programs.

Mandating DOT: Current Policies

Based on the sobering experience of the outbreaks of MDR-TB in New York and other major U.S. cities in the early 1990s, and on the general success of more aggressive public health control measures, such as DOT and detention when necessary, the Institute of Medicine Committee on the Elimination of Tuberculosis in 2000 advised that all states should mandate completion of therapy for all patients with active TB.[45] In addition, the Committee encouraged more aggressive programs for screening, case finding, and preventive therapy of patients who have latent tuberculosis (skin test positive, but asymptomatic) and who are at risk of reactivation of their infection as they age. In considering the ethics of tuberculosis elimination, the Committee concluded that although individuals with latent TB infection pose only a potential threat of reactivating their infection and infecting others, the need to protect the public justifies mandatory therapy for these individuals, and that particular emphasis should be given to case finding in homeless shelters and prisons.

Unfortunately, the decline in prevalence of MDR-TB was only temporary; at the beginning of the twenty-first century, disturbing reports appeared of new strains of *mycobacterium tuberculosis* (MTB) that were extensively resistant to almost all of the first- and second-line anti-tuberculosis drugs.[46] By 2004, worldwide surveys indicated that about 20% of all MTB isolates were multiple drug resistant (MDR-TB) and 2% of all MTB isolates were extensively resistant (XDR-TB). Except in TB specialty clinical centers, XDR-TB strains have been virtually untreatable, and mortality rates have been in the range of 30–60%. In an outbreak of XDR-TB in the South African province of KwaZulu Natal among patients with AIDS, 52 of 53 patients died.[47] Public fear of XDR-TB has been fanned by media attention to stories of patients like the Atlanta lawyer, Andrew Speaker. Gostin and other commentators have called for implementation of more extensive public health powers of quarantine and surveillance both in the United States and worldwide.[48]

---

45. Institute of Medicine, *Ending Neglect*, ix.

46. Centers for Disease Control and Prevention, "Emergence of Mycobacterium Tuberculosis with Extensive Resistance to Second-Line Drugs—Worldwide, 2000–2004," *Mortality and Morbidity Weekly Report* 55, no. 11 (March 24, 2006): 301–305.

47. Editorial, "Extreme Tuberculosis," *New York Times*, sec. A, September 14, 2006.

48. Howard Markel, Lawrence O. Gostin, and David P. Fidler, "Extensively Drug-Resistant Tuberculosis: An Isolation Order, Public Health Powers, and a Global Crisis," *Journal of the American Medical Association* 298, no. 1: 83–86 (July 4, 2007).

Standard TB treatment involves the use of three relatively inexpensive first-line drugs now available as generics. MDR-TB requires at least two additional second-line drugs, which are unfortunately more expensive and have increased toxicity. XDR-TB requires additional third-line drugs, some of which have even greater toxicities. Treating XDR-TB in the developing world is extremely difficult, given the lack of diagnostic laboratory resources, the challenges of monitoring for multiple toxicities, and the expense of drugs. Except for the successes of Paul Farmer[49] in treating MDR-TB in Haiti and Peru, few patients in the developing world survive MDR- or XDR-TB.

The emergence of these frightening new TB strains has already led to even more aggressive control measures by public health officials in the United States and internationally. The spread of MDR- and XDR-TB has been particularly associated with eastern European prisons, where crowded conditions and inadequate or intermittent initial therapy led to the development of resistance on a broad scale. The release of prisoners into the general public then confounded the problem considerably, both in the eastern European prison population where the issue was originally described and in the United States. As in the New York City outbreak, co-infection with HIV and TB has also been a complicating factor.

Efforts to reduce what is perceived as a threatening epidemic of TB involve surveillance, case finding, and treatment strategies, including DOT. The effort in surveillance is first to determine what proportion of a population has the condition in question; once prevalence has been generally determined, the effort is then to identify subgroups in which prevalence are highest, and then to develop programs for the delivery of treatment that direct attention to the groups that are mostly likely to perpetuate the epidemic. From this population-wide view, one determinant of success is the reduction in the prevalence rate. While the theoretical goal of any such program is 100% coverage (or whatever is necessary to contain the epidemic), in the 1990s, there was talk about completely eradicating TB from the United States.[50] Such goals are rarely achievable for a variety of political and economic reasons. The measure of success is instead movement toward more complete reduction of prevalence. This approach focuses on overall reduction of disease in a population. What our PVV view brings to light, however, is that in the course of overall disease prevention, individual victims also matter.

A Dying Homeless Man and His Dog

Even if DOT or isolation is justified for MDR- or XDR-TB patients—questions we will revisit at the end of this chapter—that is not the end of the story on

---

49. Farmer, Kim, Mitnick and Timperi, "Responding to Outbreaks of MDRTB."
50. D.A. Enarson, "Why Not the Elimination of Tuberculosis?" *Mayo Clinic Proceedings* 69 (1994): 85–86.

our PVV perspective. Isolated patients are victims as well as vectors—as are any patients with dreadful, untreatable infectious diseases, from Ebola and other hemorrhagic fevers, to TB, to the worst imaginable case of pandemic influenza. In this section of our chapter on compelled therapy, we tell the story of treatment failures that ended with the recognition of the inhumanity of isolation and what humane treatment of such victims might actually mean.[51]

> *August 1998. Mr. K, a 41-year-old divorced, unemployed homeless man, was admitted to the hospital for repair of an inguinal hernia. He had suffered from alcoholism for several years, and had the associated complications of cirrhosis of the liver with ascites, a recent history of bleeding from esophageal variceal veins, and pancreatitis. During surgery he was noted to have chronic inflammation of the abdominal peritoneal tissues, and microscopic examination of these indicated changes diagnostic of tuberculosis of the abdominal cavity. Subsequent culture of these tissues grew Mycobacterium tuberculosis, which was found to be susceptible to all the usual TB antimicrobials, and he was started on the recommended regimen of four anti-tuberculosis drugs for six months to be followed by six months of two-drug therapy. Because there was no evidence of pulmonary involvement, he was deemed to be at little risk of infecting others, and he was discharged from the hospital to an apartment in the community with his rent paid by the community TB control program. Because he fit the community health service profile of a patient at "high risk" of being non-compliant with taking his medications (history of alcoholism and homelessness), Mr. K was enrolled in a tightly monitored program of directly observed therapy. The local health service records showed that each day for the subsequent nine months a TB case worker came to his apartment and documented the observation that he took his daily dose of medications.*
>
> *June 1999. Mr. K was readmitted to the hospital for evaluation of possible reactivation of his tuberculosis. He gave a one-month history of increasing cough and sputum production, fever, chills, and 14 kg weight loss. Chest x-ray was consistent with pulmonary tuberculosis, and microscopic examination of his sputum and cultures were positive for TB. Because his TB had reactivated while presumably on TB therapy, there was high suspicion that his TB organisms had become resistant to some of his TB antimicrobials, and subsequent tests revealed that his organism was now resistant to three of the drugs he had received. This resistance pattern was consistent with the public health designation for multiple-drug-resistant tuberculosis, and he was*

---

51. This narrative was provided by Dr. Charles Smith, one of the co-authors of this volume.

started on four new antimicrobials to which his organism was known to be sensitive. He was again discharged to receive DOT at his apartment, and records indicated that he took all of his medications for the subsequent six months and that his sputum cultures became negative for TB after one month of new therapy. Although the federal Centers for Disease Control recommends that patients with MDR-TB continue therapy for at least one year, his physicians for unclear reasons decided to continue this new therapy for only six months. The last public health department or local hospital records of Mr. K receiving any care were in February 2000.

September 2002. Mr. K presented to the emergency room of a community hospital complaining of severe abdominal pain and with alcohol intoxication. Nursing notes indicated that he was also complaining of bloody sputum. No chest x-ray was taken and the possibility of reactivated TB was not considered by his physician. He received pain medications and after sobering up overnight he was discharged with advice to stop drinking and to obtain further care at a government hospital such as the Veterans Administration hospital.

November 2002. Mr. K was admitted to a government hospital complaining of cough with bloody sputum, fevers, and weakness of two-months duration. His chest x-ray showed new lung cavities consistent with pulmonary TB, and culture of his sputum was positive for TB. Tests of the antimicrobial sensitivities of this organism would not be available for a few weeks, and his physicians, fearing that his organism would still be resistant to multiple antimicrobials, initiated therapy with five new drugs, several of which had high levels of potential toxicity. Because pulmonary TB with lung cavities is among the most infectious types of TB, his physicians placed him on strict respiratory isolation in a single room with filtered air flow to reduce the possible spread of his infection to others in the hospital.

Debate among his caregivers ensued regarding the appropriate duration of his hospital isolation. Some argued for keeping him in isolation until the microscopic examination of his sputum no longer showed TB organisms and then continuing DOT therapy at home, this being the usual recommendation for isolated hospitalized patients with TB. Others argued that his past history of failures of therapy and the presence of cavities and MDR-TB put the patient in a special category that was at high risk of spreading his infection to others in the community. This situation, they argued, required that the patient remain in the hospital under strict supervision until he completed at least one course of therapy and he was declared cured of TB.

Mr. K, in addition to his clinical problems associated with his pulmonary TB, was increasingly distressed by chronic abdominal pain related to his pancreatitis and to TB infection of his abdominal *cavity. The pain required increasing doses of morphine and other painkillers. Toxicities of his new TB drugs also began to complicate his hospital care as he developed stomach bleeding and new seizures. After two months of therapy in isolation, Mr. K became discouraged about his deteriorating health and declared, "I know I am dying, and I would like to go home to be with my dog." His physicians indicated to him that if he did not cooperate by remaining in hospital isolation they would invoke state law and get a court order to detain him in the hospital. In the subsequent week, while this dialogue between the patient and his caregivers continued, social workers brought his dog into the hospital for visits in an attempt to accommodate some of his wishes. Mr. K subsequently developed further seizures with associated aspiration of stomach contents into his lungs, had a respiratory arrest, and died.*

There were many failures, both medical and ethical, in the treatment of Mr. K. He may have been profiled as an alcoholic, homeless man, and this may have affected the treatment he received. The therapy he received was inadequate and may have actually worsened his condition. It is unclear why therapy was discontinued too soon: perhaps because Mr. K was thought unable to benefit from better care, perhaps because his infection was misunderstood, or perhaps because there were economic constraints on the care available to him. He was induced—possibly even coerced—into therapy. No one appears to have fully addressed the social issues that contributed to Mr. K's TB and deteriorating health. Perhaps the worst of the compounded failures in the case of Mr. K, we think, was the failure to try to do everything possible to keep his victimhood in view, even as plans continued to require management of his case to reduce the risks he posed to others. Of course, there were gains for Mr. K. as well as failures: when he was discharged from the hospital, he was given an apartment in the community with his rent paid by the community TB control program, but this too was motivated primarily by the effort to reduce the possibility of transmission—after all, it is difficult to do DOT with someone who is homeless. Only as Mr. K's death neared was consideration given to what seemed to matter most to him as a person—his closeness to his dog. But his ability to be with his dog was achieved imperfectly at best through hospital visits; he was not enabled to be home with the dog on an extended basis. If XDR-TB advances—as it likely will—we will need to take our responsibilities to the victimhood of many more Mr. Ks very seriously.

The public appears to have been adequately protected from disease spread from Mr. K, even as incomplete efforts were made to respect his wishes. Bringing Mr. K's dog to the hospital for visits during the last few days of his life was at least a step toward respecting his wishes—and it was a strategy that protected others. The dog itself would not contract tuberculosis and could not spread it to other humans. Even if the dog's presence might have constituted a risk to other patients, that risk would be slight and avoidable.

What Mr. K wanted most was to die *at home* with his dog, but his non-voluntary, coerced confinement in the hospital continued until he died. This was an extreme constraint; yet, according to some, it was fully justified by the extreme risks Mr. K posed to others, particularly in the light of the many failures in TB control that the United States had already seen. What makes this a hard case is the difficulty in identifying compromises that would have both recognized Mr. K's human situation and his genuine choices, but would also have kept him from infecting others. The case reached this point in large part because of failures that had occurred before the end, failures that our PVV perspective helps us to see. But even at the end, Mr. K's wishes were not realized to the extent they might have been, consistently with protection of others.

Directly Observed Therapy from the PVV Perspective

On a view of patients such as Mr. K as vectors, it is permissible to use a range of methods to encourage therapy that are effective in reducing contagion and, even more importantly, reducing the risk of the development and transmission of drug-resistant disease. Among these methods, two are primary: DOT and, when it is ineffective, isolation of a contagious patient. We start with DOT.

Directly observed therapy, discussed above, is an excellent example of a control mechanism that limits vectorhood but that can be used in a way that is sometimes less, sometimes more respectful of the patient as victim. DOT forced on patients can be physically assaulting; but DOT does not need to be delivered in this way. Instead, it can be delivered in a manner that is respectful of the patient's concerns and needs—that is, in a manner that sees the patient as victim as well as vector. Inducements such as free housing, offered along with DOT, both benefited Mr. K and encouraged him to continue therapy. The DOT process was effective in getting therapy to him and was minimally burdensome, although in Mr. K's case it was apparently discontinued before the time frame necessary for his treatment to have been successful. For a time, DOT benefited Mr. K, and he appears not to have objected to it. Unfortunately, too little attention was given to offering Mr. K a convenient and effective alcohol rehabilitation program and an employment rehabilitation program to resolve his homelessness.

Nor was adequate attention given to Mr. K as victim during his subsequent treatment. Somewhere along the way, the recognition appeared to have been lost that Mr. K was not the one to blame for the failure of his initial treatment.

The responsibility for this outcome was primarily the fault of his physicians for recommending too short a course of therapy; health-care providers involved in his care could have tried to restore his trust by apologizing for the errors. In deciding how long to keep Mr. K in the hospital for therapy of his now-resistant, much more dangerous MDR-TB, providers could have insisted on individualizing his treatment plan, recognizing his human need to go back to his apartment if frequent home visits would be able to encourage his cooperation with the drug therapy prescribed to treat his tuberculosis.

Isolation from the PVV Perspective

Respecting Mr. K as victim is far harder in the case of the more coercive interventions that are not obviously beneficial to him: principally the threats to keep Mr. K isolated and in the hospital for an indefinite period of time. Had Mr. K lived a few weeks longer, hospital personnel were prepared to request a court order to detain him in the hospital to receive maximal therapy for TB. Given the severity of Mr. K's condition—its acuity, lethality, and extremely high transmissibility—those emphasizing risks to the public thought they could not in conscience agree to his request to go home to die.

This proposed intervention saw Mr. K as vector, but not as victim—ill, in pain, and deprived of his primary means of social support, his dog. The intervention emphasized protecting others, but did not consider whether within this constraint there were ways to fulfill Mr. K's wishes. At the end, as it became obvious to Mr. K and his clinicians that his chances of survival were decreasing due to his disseminated TB infection complicated by drug toxicities and his underlying state of poor general health, concern for Mr. K would surely have supported his request to go home to spend his final days with his dog. Being home with his dog was Mr. K's most ardent wish, an autonomous choice to forgo further treatment in favor of saying farewell, so to speak, to his most loved one. Mr. K was alone—he did not have family or friends who might have cared about him or whom he might have put at risk. Just as in the hospital, Mr. K at home could have been provided with appropriate sustenance and supervision to ensure that he did not unwittingly infect others. Yet this alternative was simply not explored in his case.

The moral view we are developing here requires seeing a person with communicable infectious disease as both victim *and* vector. The bioethics view has emphasized one of these views, we have argued, and the public health view the other, but an adequate ethics of infectious disease requires seeing the patient as both. To be sure, the tension between the need to protect the public from contagious diseases and the often conflicting need to care for individual patients in a just and ethical manner has been recognized as a deep moral challenge in infectious disease, and has been a particular focus in tuberculosis control and care. Matthew Wynia,[52] for example, has pointed out that balancing the competing obligations to individual patients with obligations to public health is the sine qua non of medical professional life.

The difficulty is *how*, not *whether*, this balancing act should be understood and achieved. On our view, the balance must be understood as bringing together full views of Mr. K as victim and as vector, no matter how hard it is to achieve this. During Mr. K's terminal hospital admission, a view of this patient as both victim and vector would have required caregivers on the one hand to be respectful of Mr. K's wishes for restored freedom, outside the hospital; and on the other hand to accept his rejection of continuing aggressive care when it became obvious that he was dying. Because the local public health system had appropriately provided housing for this homeless patient, it might have been possible for him to spend his last days at home with his dog under the care of visiting nurses and home care programs. But this approach would also have required a full understanding of and respect for the risks this patient might have for the public at large, and his potential role in an ongoing web of disease transmission. In short, respecting Mr. K's wishes both could and should have been accomplished in a way that was consistent with protecting others.

In considering Mr. K as vector, the physician caring for him during his terminal hospitalization would also have had to understand that this patient was a particular risk to hospital employees who might be exposed to the patient during the first few days of his hospitalization when the patient's infectiousness was greatest. In fact, the physicians and other health-care team members caring for Mr. K did a superb job of identifying all hospital employees who cared for Mr. K before he was placed on respiratory isolation, and before his anti-tuberculosis medications were started. Those individuals who directly cared for Mr. K were fitted with the latest technology in masks and other exposure-reduction gear to reduce the likelihood of acquiring TB infection, and all personnel who might have been exposed were then carefully monitored for evidence of TB infection over the next six months. The local county health-care team responsible for TB control was also immediately alerted that a patient with likely highly infectious MDR-TB had just been identified, and they were assisted in identifying close contacts of the patient in the community who needed to be monitored for recent TB exposure and infection. Had Mr. K survived long enough to be considered for discharge into the community before he completed his therapy, the responsible physician would have required

---

52. M.K. Wynia, "Civic Obligations in Medicine: Does 'Professional' Civil Disobedience Tear, or Repair, the Basic Fabric of Society?" *Virtual Mentor* 6, no. 1, January 2004, http://virtualmentor. ama-assn.org/2004/01/pfor1–0401.html.

proof that the anti-tuberculosis drugs had rendered his sputum culture negative for TB before Mr. K was permitted to be at liberty in the community.

Making the health and welfare of this patient together with the health and welfare of the population as a whole the two central components of care in treating Mr. K can be achieved in part in a number of fairly obvious ways. First, it would be necessary to recognize the critical importance of continuity of care in establishing trust between the physician and the patient and in facilitating the physician's understanding of the many personal, medical, and social factors that complicated this patient's infection. In the four-year course of Mr. K's illness, he was treated in at least three different hospitals and a county TB clinic. While most of the care in the first year of Mr. K's illness was capably directed by an individual physician, in the subsequent three years his care became fragmented between multiple physicians and different health care-systems. Breakdowns in communication between changing caregivers was an important contributor to the wrong decision to stop his therapy for MDR-TB prematurely and for lack of follow up after his therapy was stopped. A fragmented health-care system makes it particularly difficult for individual physicians to give care to homeless and uninsured patients and to provide continuity of care, though continuing, well-supervised care with continuous oversight is essential in controlling TB.

So far, we have unified the treatment of Mr. K as victim and vector by pointing out that in constraining him as vector through DOT or perhaps even isolation, attention must also be paid to Mr. K's humanity as victim. But there is a deeper point here from our PVV perspective as well. There is a sense in which Mr. K has interests in DOT policies as a potential victim of transmission from others. Although he does not have family or friends, and thus there is no reason from his immediate personal circumstances for him to see that he does not want not to be a vector, he has been homeless. He got tuberculosis from other homeless people. If he goes back onto the streets as a homeless person, he will be contributing to the ongoing pattern of transmission among one of the worst off populations in society. Thus, as a homeless person, Mr. K has interests in not contributing to the ongoing web of disease among the homeless.

In the background, as we see Mr. K. as an immediate victim and vector, a third obligation may also be apparent. Physicians caring for Mr. K would also have to have a strong social conscience about societal injustices such as poverty, inadequate diet, homelessness, and lack of free access to health care that contributed to this patient becoming infected with TB and to the failure of the health-care system to make an early diagnosis and provide adequate therapy. In particular, this social conscience should be accompanied by the energy and will to take some responsibility and action for correcting these injustices. The story of Mr. K illustrates the more general argument we will make in Chapter 19 that PVV justifies better health infrastructure and decent primary care as a matter of justice.

The practice of Paul Farmer, M.D., is an example of successful integration of the importance of valuing both care for individual patients and understanding and concern for the importance of environmental, political, and public health policies in protecting the community as well as the individual patient.[53] In addressing the tuberculosis epidemic in Haiti, currently one of the world's poorest countries, Farmer has been credited with exhibiting an unusual degree of commitment to providing maximal possible medical care and emotional support to individual patients, while at the same time exerting tremendous effort to finding the resources needed to improving the quality of diet, housing, and medical care available to these impoverished patients. Farmer was among the first to demonstrate that DOT could be very effective in controlling MDR-TB epidemics in communities suffering from extreme poverty,[54] and his leadership in finding the resources to build and maintain a modern hospital for the care of these patients in Haiti stands as an excellent model for the caring practitioner with a social conscience.

Yet not every TB patient is cared for by a physician alert to social realities or with an active social conscience. From a review of the physician's notes for the emergency room visit of Mr. K in September 2002, it appears that Mr. K's social problems of alcoholism and homelessness were clearly recognized, but the response to this information was negative and hostile—a response that probably contributed to the inadequate evaluation for possible TB and triggered the advice to the patient to continue his care at a "government" hospital next time. Other physicians caring for this patient at that time did clearly acknowledge the important role of these social problems, and they worked with the county health officials to advocate for continued support for his public housing, but not all issues were attended to. The problem of Mr. K's chronic alcoholism did not appear to have been addressed, for example.

Historically, physicians have at times been prime leaders in initiating and effecting changes in the environment, such as improved sanitation and water quality, or in reducing unhealthy practices, such as tobacco use. In recent years, some observers have detected a decline in physicians' involvement with social issues that directly affect their patients' health and have postulated that this may be due to the increasing demands on physicians' time associated with declining reimbursements and managed care.[55] Others, such as the American College of Physicians, have placed the principle of social justice on an equal

53. Tracy Kidder, *Mountains Beyond Mountains: The Quest of Dr. Paul Farmer, A Man Who Would Cure the World* (New York: Random House, 2003), 317.
54. P. Farmer, "The Major Infectious Diseases in the World—To Treat or Not to Treat?" *New England Journal of Medicine* 345, no. 3 (July 19, 2001): 208–210.
55. R.L. Gruen, S.D. Pearson, and T.A. Brennan, "Physician-Citizens—Public Roles and Professional Obligations," *Journal of the American Medical Association* 291, no. 1 (January 7, 2004): 94–98.

footing with the principles of primacy of patient welfare and autonomy.[56] Gruen and co-authors defined the physicians' public role as "advocacy for and participation in improving the aspects of communities that affect the health of individuals."[57] These authors point out that the social contract between physicians and communities expects that physicians and physician associations work to improve the public's health in return for the professional autonomy that physicians enjoy.

In recent years physicians who care for AIDS patients have set a high standard for effective physician involvement in changing societal attitudes and public health practices and laws that affect their patients. As discussed earlier in this chapter, activist AIDS patients and their caring practitioners who were faced with the dual AIDS/MDR-TB epidemic in New York City in the early 1990s coordinated their efforts to develop public health practices and laws that were respectful of individual rights while bringing the epidemic under control.

Postscript: Tuberculosis Worldwide

At the beginning of the new millennium, the hopes expressed by some public health planners that TB could soon be virtually eliminated in the developed world and, with adequate funding, brought under control in developing countries were shattered with the recognition in 2006 that XDR-TB was rapidly appearing in all regions of the world.[58] The CDC's 1989 plan for eliminating tuberculosis in the United States by 2010[59] was a casualty of the times, and the public erupted with fear over cases like the one we discussed in the preceding chapter—the case of Andrew Speaker, the Atlanta lawyer who evaded no-fly restrictions for persons with active TB. The WHO estimates that over 400,000 new cases of MDR-TB are emerging every year due to poor management of drug therapy and control of transmission of resistant strains. While it is more difficult and costly to manage MDR-TB than drug susceptible TB, strict management of MDR-TB patients according to new international standards[60] has been successful in achieving cures

56. American College of Physicians, "Medical Professionalism in the New Millennium: A Physician Charter," *Annals of Internal Medicine* 136, no. 3 (February 5, 2002): 243–246.

57. Gruen, Pearson and Brennan, "Physician-Citizens."

58. World Health Organization, "The Global MDR-TB and XDR-TB Response Plan 2007–2008," http://whqlibdoc.who.int/hq/2007/WHO_HTM_TB_2007.387_eng.pdf (accessed December 29, 2007).

59. Ronald Bayer and Laurence Dupuis, "Tuberculosis, Public Health, and Civil Liberties," in *Ethics and Infectious Disease*, ed. Michael J. Selgelid, Margaret P. Battin, and Charles B. Smith (Oxford: Blackwell, 2005), 120, citing the Centers for Disease Control and Prevention, "A Strategic Plan for the Elimination of Tuberculosis in the United States," *Morbidity and Mortality Weekly Report* 38, suppl. S-3, (1989): 1–23.

60. P.C. Hopewell et al., "International Standards for Tuberculosis Care," *Lancet Infectious Diseases* 6, no. 11 (November 2006): 710–725.

in both developed and developing countries. While the true extent of XDR-TB is not known because facilities for its detection are limited, current estimates are that worldwide, at least 10% of MDR-TB patients now have XDR-TB.[61]

Unfortunately, treatment of XDR-TB is considerably more difficult and expensive than treatment of other forms of TB. While XDR-TB has been treated successfully although with considerable expense, time, and toxicity in developed countries,[62] the likelihood is poor that treatment will be successful in areas of the world lacking access to adequate diagnostic services and very expensive anti-TB drugs. For example, in the South African outbreak of XDR-TB in which 52 of the 53 patients died, the median survival period was only 16 days after diagnosis.[63] The WHO has declared XDR-TB a serious emerging threat to public health, and commented that in some parts of the world TB will have to be managed as it was in the pre-antibiotic era—that is, it will be virtually untreatable.[64]

In responding to this new threat of untreatable TB, the WHO and other public health organizations have published new International Standards for Tuberculosis Care.[65] These standards reveal a remarkable move toward considering the patient as both victim and vector. In recognizing the patient as a victim, they acknowledge that mutual respect between the patient and provider is the key to successful implementation of effective drug treatment and communicable disease control. Standard #9 argues for a patient-centered approach to TB management. Care is to be "tailored to each individual patient's circumstances and to be mutually acceptable to the patient and the provider."[66] When patient adherence becomes a problem, providers are encouraged to not blame the patient, but to search for problems in the health-care delivery system, socioeconomic problems, and unique family and personality problems that need to be addressed to improve compliance. For example, the Standards suggest considering opiate substitution, usually methadone, for injection drug users, expanding access to primary care needs along with TB management, and providing other incentives such as temporary housing and nutritional supplements.

61. Raviglione and Smith, "XDR Tuberculosis."
62. J. Furin, "The Clinical Management of Drug-Resistant Tuberculosis," *Current Opinion in Pulmonary Medicine* 13, no. 3 (May 2007): 212–217.
63. N.R. Gandhi et al., "Extensively Drug-Resistant Tuberculosis as a Cause of Death in Patients Co-Infected with Tuberculosis and HIV in a Rural Area of South Africa," *Lancet* 368, no. 9547 (November 4, 2006): 1575–1580; World Health Organization, "MDR-TB and XDR-TB Response Plan," 3.
64. World Health Organization, "MDR-TB and XDR-TB Response Plan."
65. Tuberculosis Coalition for Technical Assistance, *International Standards for Tuberculosis Care (ISTC)* (The Hague: Tuberculosis Coalition for Technical Assistance, 2006), http://www.who.int/tb/publications/2006/istc_report.pdf (accessed December 29, 2007), 7.
66. Ibid.

In considering the patient as a vector in the XDR-TB era, the new standards increasingly emphasize the importance of strictly observed DOT in achieving a cure and reducing the development of drug resistance. The patient-centered and patient-rights approach described above is designed to improve compliance with DOT. The new Standards, however, for the first time clearly articulate the patient's responsibilities as a vector. In partnership with the patient advocacy group World Care Council, a Patient's Charter for Tuberculosis Care has been integrated into the new Standards.[67] The Charter, in addition to articulating the rights of TB patients, also clearly describes the responsibilities of TB patients. These include the responsibility to conscientiously comply with the agreed treatment plan, to show consideration for the rights of other patients and health-care providers, and the moral responsibility to join in efforts to make the community TB free. This is the first TB patient-centered group that we can document as describing the patient's responsibilities. A new ray of hope emerged in mid-2008 with the development of a much more rapid test for MDR-TB, known as a line probe assay, which detects mutations in bacterial DNA linked to drug resistance. This test takes two days instead of the standard two to three months. It thus enables earlier detection of disease—crucial both for treatment of the ill person and for controlling the possibility that resistant disease might be passed on to others before the patient receives treatment adequate to reduce transmission. It requires only a saliva sample and is remarkably inexpensive as well, at a cost of about $8.[68]

We are encouraged that both the public health managers of TB care and patient advocacy groups have moved toward seeing the patient as both victim *and* vector. Perhaps this movement of both groups toward jointly recognizing their mutual interests can be further nurtured by helping both care providers and patients to better understand our PVV perspective: that patients should be counseled to recognize that they are as vulnerable to being infected by others as others are to being infected by them.

67. World Care Council, *Patients' Charter for Tuberculosis Care*, http://www.worldcarecouncil.org/pdf/PatientsCharterEN2006.pdf (accessed December 29, 2007); see also World Health Organization, "MDR-TB and XDR-TB Response Plan," 5.
68. World Health Organization, "New Rapid Tests for Drug-Resistant TB for Developing Countries," http://www.who.int/mediacentre/news/releases/2008/pr21/en/index.html (accessed July 1, 2008).

10

THE ETHICS OF RESEARCH IN INFECTIOUS DISEASE: EXPERIMENTING ON THIS PATIENT, RISKING HARM TO THAT ONE

Research in infectious disease has produced dramatic advances in the eradication, elimination, or control of infectious disease, but also has been highly controversial. Sir Edward Jenner's use of cowpox to immunize against smallpox, Walter Reed's trials of a yellow fever vaccine, the Tuskegee syphilis study, and the Willowbrook study of the transmission of infectious hepatitis are but a few illustrations of experimentation in infectious disease. That these efforts were tolerated at their time—although most now figure among the notorious examples of the exploitation of human subjects—no doubt testifies to the fear in which the infectious diseases at issue were held. It is now canonical in research ethics that most of these studies were deeply problematic despite the knowledge they in some cases yielded. Nonetheless, the ethical principles and the law governing experimentation with human subjects have failed to appreciate the full force of the significance of infectiousness and communicability for research ethics.

Many questions in the ethics of research are raised by infectious disease. Most obvious in today's world—discussed by Solomon Benatar,[1] Peter A. Singer,[2] Paul Farmer,[3] Thomas Pogge,[4] and Michael Selgelid,[5] among others—is the extent to which current research is skewed away from research on the prevention and treatment of infectious diseases that threaten the majority of the world's population. Much less research than would be ideal has been devoted to the development of vaccines for diseases such as malaria or to inexpensive

---

An earlier version of this chapter appeared as Leslie P. Francis, Margaret P. Battin, Jeffrey R. Botkin, Jay A. Jacobson, and Charles B. Smith, "Infectious Disease and the Ethics of Research: The Moral Significance of Communicability," in *Ethics in Biomedical Research: International Perspectives*, ed. Matti Häyry, Tuija Takala and Peter Herissone-Kelly (Amsterdam and New York: Rodopi, 2007), 135–150.

1. Solomon R. Benatar, "Bioethics: Power and Injustice: IAB Presidential Address," *Bioethics* 17, nos. 5/6 (October 2003): 387–400; Solomon R. Benatar, "Commentary: Justice and Medical Research: A Global Perspective," *Bioethics*, 15, no. 4 (2001): 333–340.
2. Peter A. Singer et al., "Grand Challenges in Global Health: The Ethical, Social and Cultural Program," *PloS Medicine* 4, no. 9 (September 10, 2007): e265.
3. P. Farmer and N.G. Campos, "Rethinking Medical Ethics: A View From Below," *Developing World Bioethics* 4, no. 1 (May 2004): 17–41.
4. Thomas Pogge, "World Poverty and Human Rights," *Ethics & International Affairs* 19, no. 1 (2005): 1–7.
5. Michael J. Selgelid, "Ethics and Drug Resistance," *Bioethics* 21, no. 4 (May 2007): 218–229.

modalities for treating common killers of the young, such as infantile diarrhea. Claims of racism in infectious disease research are not limited to the example of Tuskegee, but extend to more contemporary examples of AIDS research and research with directly observed therapy for tuberculosis.[6] Pharmaceutical companies' protection of their intellectual property, together with their drug pricing policies, raise pressing ethical questions.[7]

Also obvious are the dangers of research with pathogens. Laboratories may be difficult to protect, or may be protected imperfectly. Concerns remain that infectious agents stored in poorly guarded laboratories are attractive targets for bioterrorists. Research with pathogens, moreover, may lead to the creation of new infectious agents that are difficult to control—the all-too-realistic stuff of science fiction thrillers. Researchers who want to create XXDR-TB—a super-drug-resistant strain of tuberculosis—may be all too able to do so, without any regulation, in the United States or in other countries of the world today.

In this chapter, we give a brief sketch of a range of issues infectious disease raises for the ethics of research, beginning with two aspects of informed consent: the *who* and the *what* of consent. We view our argument for third party and community consent as an example of how concern for the research subject as not only victim but also as vector might require broadening standard accounts of the ethics of research and human subject protection—whether the issue is self-experimentation or experimentation on others.

Contagion and the *Who* and the *What* of Informed Consent

Our PVV analysis, we think, sheds new light on one core issue in research ethics, the who and what of informed consent, and perhaps broader light on research ethics more generally. Even when research is otherwise justifiable on scientific grounds, where research involves the possibility of communication of disease, informed consent should not be understood solely as a matter of the consent of the individual subject. Others might be infected, put at risk of infection, or left unprotected from these risks. These third parties have interests that may be directly affected by the research. If the subject in research involving communicable infectious disease is seen as victim, his informed consent is what is required; but if he is seen as vector, implications for third parties also must be considered. Yet these third party issues are largely ignored by current policies about informed consent, in criticisms of problematic examples in the history of medical research, and by current research practice. If research policies or practices attend to such issues at all, they do so principally

---

6. Harriet A. Washington, *Medical Apartheid: The Dark History of Medical Experimentation on Black Americans from Colonial Times to the Present* (New York: Doubleday, 2006), 326–327.
7. These questions have been pressed by Thomas Pogge, among others.

through the direct subject—for example, through a consent process that warns the direct subject about the risks of communicability. This focus on the direct subject is inadequate in a significant range of cases of research involving communicable infectious disease.

We begin our argument by explaining how third parties who are at foreseeable and direct risk of contagion when research with human subjects involves a communicable agent are in some respects analogous to direct subjects of the research. Although they are not *subjects* in the sense that data is being collected about them, they are indirect *participants* in the research in that the research puts them at risk—or fails to shield them from risk—in the same way direct subjects are put at risk. We have chosen the term *indirect participants* to describe these affected third parties, in contrast to *indirect subjects*, a term that implies they are fully subjects, or *indirect objects*, a term that ignores agency. The role of indirect participants as both unwitting victims and autonomous agents with respect to the research is ethically relevant, and failure to consider it is ethically problematic.

Moreover, when the research involves risks that are comparable to the experiences people would otherwise have, and that are only minimal risk, the approach should be to inform the research subject about the risks and to recommend that the research subject inform others about the risks. Researchers need not inform third parties directly if the risks posed by the research to them are minimal. An increased risk of contracting a disease with significant morbidity or mortality would not fall into this category. Finally, when the study involves more than minimal risk and is not commensurate with the experiences of ordinary life, what further contact with indirect participants is required is contingent on whether the indirect participant can readily avoid the risk. If the risk is readily avoidable, for example by abstaining from sexual contact, then informing indirect participants of the risk is sufficient. The indirect participant can then choose whether to take the risk. Such action to inform the indirect participant requires the consent of the direct subject, who is not only potential vector but also potential victim. If the direct subject refuses to permit the indirect participant to be informed, the direct subject should not participate in the research. If the risk is not readily avoidable by the indirect participant, researchers should be required to obtain informed consent from indirect participants—who are potential victims—before direct subjects can ethically participate in the research. An example of research falling into this category would be testing a new live-virus vaccine for a serious disease, where there is a significant possibility of viral shedding that might infect other members of the subject's household.

These claims raise a host of questions about informed consent. For example, what constitutes ethical informed consent if a household member at risk is a child, an adult with disabilities, or a patient with dementia? Will consent of the direct subject be sufficient? Which individuals compose the population of indirect participants? What constitutes ethical practice if research poses risks to entire communities? What are the parallels between research with infectious agents and other research involving subjects who may be dangerous to others—violent subjects, for example—but not because they are contagious?

Current Informed Consent Policies and Contagiousness

Guidelines for research involving human subjects uniformly fail to address adequately whether research involving the possibility of communicable conditions requires attention to indirect participant information or consent. Current guidelines typically first analyze whether the research is permissible based on its scientific merit and risk/benefit ratio, and then establish standards for inclusion of subjects, minimization of risks to subjects, and informed consent. The recommended analyses of scientific merit and risk/benefit ratio address the research overall rather than the situations of individual subjects. The inclusion standards and informed consent protocols consider risks to individual direct subjects. The requirement of informed consent protects individual direct subjects—but these subjects only—from involuntary participation in research. The *World Medical Association Declaration of Helsinki*, the *United States Federal Regulations Governing Research with Human Subjects*, and the *Guidelines of the Infectious Diseases Society of America* all fit this pattern.

The *World Medical Organization Declaration of Helsinki* specifies that research must meet criteria of scientific and ethical adequacy. The most general requirement specifies caution about risks in research design: "Appropriate caution must be exercised in the conduct of research which may affect the environment, and the welfare of animals used for research must be respected."[8] With respect to inclusion of any human subjects in the research at all, the Declaration requires "careful assessment of predictable risks and burdens in comparison with foreseeable benefits to the subject or to others."[9]

Addressing the inclusion of individual subjects, the Declaration shifts focus, prohibiting their involvement in research unless the "importance of the objective outweighs the inherent risks and burdens to the subject,"[10] without mention of risks or benefits to others. Informed consent is required from "each

8. "Declaration of Helsinki: Ethical Principles for Medical Research Involving Human Subjects," http://www.wma.net/e/policy/b3.htm (accessed November 2007), sec. B.12. For a discussion of recent controversies about the *Declaration,* involving the *Declaration's* tight restrictions on the use of placebos in research and requirements that subjects be provided with access to therapy after participation, see Howard Wolinsky, "The Battle of Helsinki: Two Troublesome Paragraphs in the Declaration of Helsinki are Causing a Furore over Medical Research Ethics," *EMBO reports* 7, no. 7 (2006): 670–672.

9. World Medical Association, "Declaration of Helsinki," sec. B.16.

10. World Medical Association, "Declaration of Helsinki," sec. B.18.

potential subject." Required information researchers must supply to subjects includes the aims, methods, sources of funding, any possible conflicts of interest, institutional affiliations of the researcher, the anticipated benefits and potential risks of the study, and the discomfort it may entail.[11] This list does not include specific mention of risks to others. Instead, the Declaration directs attention only to population risk/benefit analysis in determining the permissibility of the research overall, and to risks to direct subjects in determining the permissibility of their individual inclusion in the research.

The *United States Federal Regulations Governing Research with Human Subjects* describe risks and benefits to be considered in determining whether research is acceptable. The regulations require that "risks to subjects [be] minimized" by "sound research design" and procedures "which do not unnecessarily expose subjects to risk."[12] Research risks must be "reasonable in relation to anticipated benefits, if any, to subjects, and the importance of the knowledge that may reasonably be expected to result."[13]

Under the regulations, Institutional Review Boards (IRBs) must review research with human subjects. As defined by the regulations, "human subject" includes any living human being about whom data are obtained through intervention or interaction or about whom identifiable private information is collected.[14] Taken literally, this definition would seem to encompass research that involves the researcher him or herself, and not just research involving others. IRB review considers only risks and benefits that may result from the research and not risks and benefits of therapies subjects would receive outside of the research. Possible long-range effects of applying knowledge gained in the research (for example, the possible effects of the research on public policy) are not within IRB responsibility.[15] The regulations require the informed consent process to include "a description of any reasonably foreseeable risks or discomforts to the subject" and "a description of any benefits to the subject or to others that may reasonably be expected from the research."[16] Notably, this list specifically mentions both risks and benefits to direct subjects. With regard to others, including indirect participants, the list mentions benefits but not risks.

In 1993, the Infectious Disease Society of America published guidelines for ethical conduct. The guidelines for ethics in research specified that all research involving human subjects must be subject to IRB review. They charged IRBs to "provide a framework for sound scientific work, while at the same time acting as advocates of the rights of patients, human subjects, and experimental animals

---

11. World Medical Association, "Declaration of Helsinki," sec. B.22.

12. 45 C.F.R. (2007) § 46.111(a)(1)(i) (2007).

13. 45 C.F.R. (2007) § 46.111(a)(2) (2007).

14. 45 C.F.R. (2007) § 46.102(f) (2007).

15. 45 C.F.R. (2007) § 46.111(a)(2).

16. 45 C.F.R. (2007) §§ 46.116(a)(2), (3).

and of the public welfare."[17] The guidelines did not explain who might be regarded as experimental subjects or address whether researchers should consider informed consent from indirect participants. The guidelines' silence on these matters might stem from their original purpose, responding to clear abuses of direct subjects in research studies such as the Tuskegee syphilis study.

Historical Examples of Ignoring Contagion—Tuskegee and Willowbrook

Some of the most (in)famous examples of research with human subjects have involved infectious diseases. They are well known in the annals of bioethics. We document here, however, that those aspects of these studies that were particularly relevant to infectious disease were not at the forefront of the criticism.

Coincidence alone may not explain why research projects involving infectious disease have been among the more notorious examples of ethically problematic research, and why the principle of informed consent was so often violated. Some researchers may have held the importance of protecting the public health to provide an overriding justification that eclipsed the ethical importance of informed consent in research. Critics have viewed this research history as abusive of direct study subjects.[18] Noteworthy is that criticism has virtually ignored the issue of informed consent for indirect participants. Concerns about indirect participants may have been swamped by the overwhelming nature of the concerns about the treatment of direct study subjects. But it may also be indicative of the approach to informed consent that we criticize below that researchers and critics have almost exclusively focused on the autonomy of direct subjects while ignoring potential risks to others who may be directly affected by the research. The Tuskegee syphilis study, in which the natural history of syphilis was studied in some 600 African-American men in the south (399 men already diagnosed with syphilis and 201 men recruited as "controls") by leaving them untreated over a 40-year period—preventing them from receiving treatment even after a simple and highly effective form of treatment, penicillin, had become available—fits this paradigm of criticism.[19] The most widely read history of the study, James Jones's *Bad Blood*, describes Nurse Rivers, the nurse who played a long-term role in the study, as going to the homes of study participants and providing general health care to

---

17. Infectious Diseases Society of America, "Guidelines for Ethical Conduct by Members and Fellows," *Journal of Infectious Diseases* 167, no. 1 (1993): 257–258.
18. See, e.g., Julie Rosenbaum and Ken Sepkowitz, "Infectious Disease Experimentation Involving Human Volunteers," *Clinical Infectious Diseases* 34 (April 1, 2002): 963–971; J. David Smith and Alison L. Mitchell, "Sacrifices for the Miracle: The Polio Vaccine Research and Children with Mental Retardation," *Mental Retardation* 39, no. 5 (2001): 405–409.
19. Centers for Disease Control and Prevention, "U.S. Public Health Service Syphilis Study at Tuskegee," http://www.cdc.gov/tuskegee/timeline.htm (accessed November 2007).

their families. Nurse Rivers was viewed by participants in the study as providing health care to them and to their families; Jones is quite rightly severely
critical of this duplicity. Yet Jones's description contains no mention of the
ethical issues raised by the possibility of transmission of syphilis or of the possible impact on family members if they contracted the disease.[20] This failure to
consider indirect subjects pervaded the Tuskegee study and its aftermath.

The principal compendium of documents on Tuskegee, Susan Reverby's
Tuskegee's Truths, reflects minimal reference to effects on indirect participants
such as sexual partners—even though, at the time the study was initiated, one
justification for study of latent syphilis was the risk that patients might infect
others. It is now known that latent syphilis is not readily transmissible, although untreated infections may be transmissible by pregnant women to their
babies for up to four years.[21] However, it is unclear whether researchers initiated the Tuskegee study with this concern in mind, or whether they worried
about the implications of confusion among subjects about whether they were
receiving treatment for their disease. The Public Health Service, in deciding to
observe the natural history of the disease in those with latent infection, had
assumed it was dealing with subjects who would otherwise not be treated. Initial testing indicated lower rates of infection in Macon County, Alabama than
had been anticipated at the time the study site was chosen—at 20% instead of
35%. Participants were told they were receiving "treatment" and so understandably might not have anticipated their risks to others. They were not informed of these risks of contagion, nor were they given information about
risks to their sexual partners.[22] Moreover, it was clearly known during the early
stages of the study, even before the development of penicillin, that treatment
of syphilis was possible—although long and arduous, involving arsenicals and
other chemicals—and would with one or two treatments greatly reduce the
risks of transmission. Indeed, in 1938 the then Surgeon General Thomas Parran
referred to treatment of syphilis as in effect "chemical quarantine."[23]

The study was not designed to track or report whether subjects infected
others.[24] Transmission of congenital syphilis to offspring was not considered. Jean
Heller, the reporter who broke the story about the study, labeled the subjects as

---

20. James Jones, *Bad Blood* (New York: Free Press, 1993).
21. See Centers for Disease Control and Prevention, "Sexually Transmitted Diseases: Surveillance
2006," www.cdc.gov/std/stats/syphilis.htm (accessed November 2007).
22. Susan Reverby, ed., *Tuskegee's Truths: Rethinking the Tuskegee Syphilis Study* (Chapel Hill:
University of North Carolina Press, 2000), esp. Part IV; and Allen M. Brandt, "Racism and
Research: The Case of the Tuskegee Syphilis Experiment," in *Tuskegee's Truths*, ed. Reverby, 15–33
(20, 21, 23).
23. Thomas Parran, "Syphilis: A Public Health Problem," *Science* 87, no. 2251 (1938): 147–152.
24. Thomas Benedek, "The 'Tuskegee Study' of Syphilis: Analysis of Moral versus Methodologic
Aspects," in *Tuskegee's Truths*, ed. Reverby, 213–235 (230).

the "victims" of the study.[25] The Ad Hoc Study Panel appointed by the U.S. Department of Health, Education, and Welfare to investigate the study concluded, in 1973, that researchers had wrongfully failed to inform subjects about their being risks to others. They drew no further conclusions about wrongs to third parties.[26] The initial settlement of the class action lawsuit brought on behalf of study victims did not include wives or children—although two years later the settlement was amended to add all wives, widows and offspring of the direct subjects.[27] Neither U.S. Congressional inquiries nor President Bill Clinton's apology on behalf of the nation referred to potential third party indirect victims of disease itself, although the President's apology, like the settlement, extended to wives and children generally.[28] Fairchild and Bayer's recent critique similarly focuses on the direct subject:

> [t]hree critical features that characterize the nature of the consistent research abuses that occurred over the course of forty years. The study involved, first, deceptions regarding the very existence and nature of the inquiry into which individuals were lured. As such, it deprived those seeking care of the right to choose whether or not to serve as research subjects. Second, it entailed an exploitation of social vulnerability to recruit and retain research subjects. Finally, Tuskegee researchers made a willful effort to deprive subjects of access to appropriate and available medical care, which changed over time, as a way of furthering the study's goals.[29]

The third party concerns that were raised in the initial criticisms of Tuskegee focused on the general public health effects of the study, and not on the possibility of harms done to indirect participants. Allan Brandt wrote, for example, "the entire health of a community was jeopardized by leaving a communicable disease untreated."[30] This public health concern, while laudable, is a different concern from the one we raise here. We are concerned that researchers violated the autonomy of indirect participants because they did not consider risks to them, even when these risks were unknown, and did not afford them—in the study design or in subsequent apologies—the choice whether or

25. Jean Heller, "Syphilis Victims in U.S. Study Went Untreated for 40 Years," in *Tuskegee's Truths*, ed. Reverby, 116–118.

26. Tuskegee Syphilis Study Ad Hoc Advisory Panel to the Assistant Secretary for Health and Scientific Affairs, "Selections from the Final Report," in *Tuskegee's Truths*, ed. Reverby, 157–181.

27. Centers for Disease Control and Prevention, Tuskegee Timeline, available at http://www.cdc.gov/tuskegee/timeline.htm (accessed April 26, 2008).

28. William J. Clinton, "Remarks by the President in Apology for Study Done in Tuskegee," in *Tuskegee's Truths*, ed. Reverby, 574–577.

29. Amy L. Fairchild and Ronald Bayer, "Uses and Abuses of Tuskegee," in *Tuskegee's Truths*, ed. Reverby, 589–604 (590).

30. Allen M. Brandt, "Racism and Research: The Case of the Tuskegee Syphilis Experiment," in *Tuskegee's Truths*, ed. Reverby, 15–33 (28).

not to undertake exposure to the study's risks. To be sure, contemporary presentations of Tuskegee reference the possibility that at least 40 wives and 19 children of the men in the study were infected with syphilis,[31] but this is a much later development.

The much-criticized Willowbrook research is a similar example. The research used children who were residents of a treatment facility for individuals with developmental disabilities to study the transmission of infectious hepatitis. The research was initiated because the infection rate among residents at the facility was high. The investigators reasoned that infectious hepatitis was "mild and relatively benign" in children in comparison to adults.[32] Reflecting back on the study, its author concluded that it had been justified by the infection rates among patients and employees in comparison to what were judged minimal additional risks to subjects.[33] The study design isolated children who received the artificial hepatitis infection from exposure to other infectious diseases common in the institution.[34] Informed consent was required from the parents of the children involved. The extensive criticism of the Willowbrook study design and consent process does not appear to have addressed risks of transmission to the parents or siblings of the children, or staff of the institution, or the need to involve them on their own behalf in the informed consent process.[35]

Historical Examples of Uncertain Attention to Contagion: The Case of Self-Experimentation

Perhaps because of the salience of infectious disease in the past, there have been impressive historical examples of researchers who began their experiments with themselves. John Hunter, in the late eighteenth century, sought to understand venereal disease by means of self-inoculation with pus from a patient infected with gonorrhea. Hunter apparently died of syphilis—and reportedly conducted his experiment without discussing it with his wife.[36] Toward the end

31. See, for example, CNN's interactive web site about the Tuskegee study, http://www.cnn.com/HEALTH/9705/16/nfm.tuskegee/index.html (accessed April 26, 2008).
32. Saul Krugman, Joan P. Giles, and Jack Hammond, "Infectious Hepatitis: Evidence for Two Distinctive Clinical, Epidemiological, and Immunological Types of Infection," *Journal of the American Medical Association*, 200 (1967): 365–373. Republished as a "Landmark Article," *Journal of the American Medical Association* 252, no. 3 (1984): 393–401.
33. Saul Krugman, "The Willowbrook Hepatitis Studies Revisited: Ethical Aspects," *Reviews of Infectious Disease* 8, no. 1 (1986): 157–162 (157).
34. Ibid., 159.
35. E.g., Stephen Goldby, "Letter: Experiments at the Willowbrook State School," *Lancet* (April 10, 1971): 749.
36. Lawrence K. Altman, *Who Goes First? The Story of Self-Experimentation in Medicine*, 2nd ed. (Berkeley: University of California Press, 1998): 7–8.

of the nineteenth century, Daniel Carreon established—at the cost of his own life—that verruga peruana, a skin disease prevalent in the Andes, and Oroya fever, a potentially deadly blood disease, were caused by the same agent. Surely in such circumstances consent of the research subject is as informed as it could ever be, but questions still remain about the permissibility of such research. Should infectious disease researchers start with themselves as trial subjects and should they consider the risks to others in their decision to undertake such experiments? Or, should infectious disease researchers be required both to protect themselves and to ensure that their family and acquaintances give informed consent to the research?

Perhaps historical figures such as Hunter were motivated by the well-reasoned belief that their research would not only protect others but also protect themselves and their families. If so, blanket condemnation of self-experimentation might warrant rethinking, because it would reflect a paternalistic judgment that the experimenter should not be able to act on his own informed judgment. Such condemnation of self-experimentation as paternalistic, however, does not extend to cases in which the experimenter puts family or other contacts at risk, as Hunter may have done in his experiments with venereal disease.[37]

Infectious disease researchers may also have believed in the safety of their activities—both for their subjects and for society in general. Jenner did not believe that cowpox was unsafe when he experimented on the son of a local farmer; on the contrary, he thought it would be protective. But the fact remains that he made the judgment about safety *for the boy and for others with whom the boy might come in contact.* For the boy, the issue is whether these are the kinds of risks a researcher may permissibly impose on a child with parental consent—particularly in circumstances in which the child's best interests may be balanced against the interests of many in the discovery of an inoculant against smallpox. Jenner is widely admired for the experiment that ushered in modern immunization and has saved countless millions of lives, but what if the boy had died? Questions of safety for society include issues about what risks are permissible (what about the possibility that an infectious agent might escape?) and how to assess these risks (by researchers? by institutional review boards? through widespread public discussion—almost a form of democratic informed consent?). They also raise the issue of whether the decision by a researcher to undertake even self-experimentation with infectious agents imposes an impermissible risk of transmission on the community. Are the types of concerns about safety raised by infectious disease concerns that in some cases require a community informed consent? Walter Reed is perhaps the

---

37. This concern is raised by Altman—as well as the question of whether Hunter really experimented on himself or possibly contracted venereal disease from some other source. Altman, *Who Goes First*, 7–8.

most flagrant example of a researcher who substituted his own judgment for that of others: despite reports of his heroism, he apparently never experimented on himself, replicated experiments that should have been taken more seriously, and permitted his associates to participate in studies that put them at risk of death, in circumstances in which it is arguable that their consent was pressured if not coerced.[38]

Contemporary standards for research ethics make no distinction between self-experimentation and experimentation in which the researchers involve others as human subjects.[39] The U.S. federal regulatory regime contains no discussion of any special issues that may be raised by self-experimentation. Perhaps this is as it should be, guaranteeing protection to researchers and non-researchers alike. However, there remains the risk that researchers may not see self-experimentation as research that really involves human subjects, and thus may fail to bring such research within the purview of IRB review. To the extent that this occurs—and we know of no data about the extent to which this is an actual rather than a merely hypothetical problem—issues of risks to indirect subjects or communities may pass unexamined in studies where the researcher is the sole human subject.

Historical Examples of Considering Contagion: The Common Cold and Polio Vaccine

Several other historical examples of research placed communicability at the center of concern. Research involving transmission of the common cold and research on the polio vaccine are noteworthy examples.

Early research involving transmission of the common cold considered the risks of transmission in the study design. Studies performed at the Common Cold Research Unit in Britain during World War II attempted to ascertain whether colds were transmitted via nasal secretions and whether exposure to freezing temperatures was a risk factor. Conducted at an isolated research facility, these research designs minimized the risk of external transmission while guarding against contamination of treatment groups. Later studies, addressing the efficiency of manual transmission and issues such as the effect of colds on memory, did not feature the two-week isolation characteristic of the British experiments.[40]

Researchers developing polio vaccines considered the risk of contracting polio to the person receiving the vaccination. With the killed-virus vaccine,

---

38. Ibid., ch. 6, recounts the Reed story in chilling detail.
39. See 45 C.F.R. (2007) § 46.102(f). This reading of the federal regulations was confirmed by AAHRPP (Association for the Accreditation of Human Research Protection Programs) in conversation with John Stillman, Director, University of Utah Institutional Review Board. John Stillman, correspondence with the authors, November 2007.
40. Rosenbaum and Sepkowitz, "Infectious Disease Experimentation," 965, 967.

IPV, the concerns were that the vaccine was imperfectly killed or would prove ineffective. The risk of imperfectly manufactured research material became quickly apparent when vaccine produced by Cutter Laboratories proved to contain live virus that resulted in a number of cases of polio.[41]

With the live-virus vaccine, OPV, there is viral shedding from the vaccinated person. This has the advantage of increasing population immunity but the disadvantage of risking infection both to the vaccinated patient and to those who come into contact with the vaccinated patient. Discussions of the ethics of using OPV were well aware of these risks. Jonas Salk persistently championed IPV because of its lower third party risk profile. In 1979, arguing for the use of IPV, Salk pointed out that from 1969 until 1977 in the United States there were 24 cases of OPV-associated paralytic polio among vaccine recipients, 47 cases among direct contacts of vaccinees, and 16 among indirect contacts.[42] Advocates of OPV argued that OPV would produce higher levels of population immunity and thus fewer cases of paralytic polio overall than IPV.[43] A 1977 report by the Institute of Medicine Committee for the Study of Poliomyelitis Vaccines concluded that OPV was the preferred method of immunization but that IPV should continue to be offered to people with heightened susceptibility to infection and people who prefer IPV and are prepared to make a commitment to the required full schedule of vaccinations. About informed consent, the report concluded that documents should be "as brief as possible, while conveying sufficient, accurate information on the benefits, risks, and other special characteristics of the vaccines." The report also recommended that the U.S. federal government assume the responsibility to compensate people with vaccine-associated poliomyelitis, including contact cases.[44]

These discussions did not, however, attend to the problems of informed consent for indirect participants at risk of contagion. The fact that many of the subjects were children whose parents were asked to consent on their behalf may complicate this assessment, because the parents would become aware of the risks as they consented to inclusion of their children in the research.[45] Still, we note that there were no indications that parents were asked to consent on behalf of their other children who might be subject to exposure and were not receiving vaccine, or that there were discussions of third party risks in the informed consent process. This assessment might also be complicated by the

41. Allan M. Brandt, "Polio, Politics, Publicity, and Duplicity: Ethical Aspects in the Development of the Salk Vaccine," *Connecticut Medicine* 43, no. 9 (1979): 581–590 (587).
42. Jonas Salk, "Immunization Against Poliomyelitis: Risk/Benefit/Cost in a Changing Context," *Developments in Biological Standardization* 43 (1979): 151–157.
43. E.g., Alan R. Hinman, Jeffrey P. Koplan, Walter A. Orenstein, and Edward W. Brink, "Decision Analysis and Polio Immunization Policy," *American Journal of Public Health* 78, no. 3 (1988): 301–303.
44. Elena O. Nightingale, "Recommendations for a National Policy on Poliomyelitis Vaccination," *New England Journal of Medicine* 297, no. 5 (1977): 249–253 (253).
45. Brandt, "Polio, Politics, Publicity, and Duplicity."

assumption that the background risk of contracting polio was quite high in any event, especially for children.

The first example of direct attention to the problems of research ethics raised by indirect subjects in polio vaccination was Deber and Goel's 1990 analysis. Deber and Goel pointed to the ethical difference between polio cases that occur to persons who lack immunity, polio cases that involve people who have consented to vaccination, and polio cases resulting from transmission by direct or indirect contact with those who have been vaccinated. Cases in this last category, they contended, involve a kind of involuntary immunization without consent for persons who are susceptible precisely because they have chosen not to be immunized in the first place.[46]

These issues are ongoing in contemporary public health debates about polio eradication.[47] According to a report from WHO, in the past 10 years there have been approximately 200 cases of polio resulting from vaccination in areas of the world with large populations who had not been vaccinated and thus who were at risk for disease—a figure that of course pales by comparison to the number of wild-virus cases of polio annually.[48] Similar controversy may be emerging over the development of a vaccine against avian flu, although the science of flu vaccine is evolving rapidly, as we discuss in Part IV.[49] Concern about risks to immediate contacts also played a role in controversy over recent efforts to immunize first responders against smallpox. The Institute of Medicine has advised caution in extending the immunization program until risks can be evaluated further, including risks to contacts.[50]

Contemporary Examples of Ignoring Contagion

Many contemporary examples of research involve contagious conditions. A principal source of contagion for indirect participants occurs when the experiment is testing a method to prevent infection that proves ineffective. In other

---

46. Raisa B. Deber and Goel Vivek, "Using Explicit Decision Rules to Manage Issues of Justice, Risk, and Ethics in Decision Analysis: When Is It Not Rational to Maximize Expected Utility," *Medical Decision Making* 10, no. 3 (1990): 181–194 (192).

47. E.g., Leslie Roberts, "Health Workers Scramble to Contain African Epidemic," *Science* 305 (July 2004): 24–25; Leslie Roberts, "Two Steps Forward, One Step Back in Polio Fight," *Science* 304 (May 2004): 1096; Leslie Roberts, "Fighting Polio Block by Block, Shack by Shack," *Science* 303 (March 2004): 1965–1966; Leslie Roberts, "The Exit Strategy," *Science* 303 (March 2004): 1969–1971.

48. WHO, "Vaccine-Derived Polioviruses," http://www.polioeradication.org/content/fixed/opvcessation/ opvc_vdpv.asp (accessed February 10, 2008).

49. Keith Bradsher and Lawrence K Altman, "A War and a Mystery: Confronting Avian Flu," *New York Times*, sec. 4, October 12, 2004.

50. Elizabeth Olson, "Panel Urges Shift of Focus in Preparing for Smallpox," *New York Times*, sec. A, August 12, 2003; Institute of Medicine, Board on Health Promotion and Disease Prevention, "Letter Report #3," May 27, 2003.

cases, the research features an intervention that may increase risks of contagion, or the research introduces a new possibility of infection and subsequent contagion. Yet examination of selected examples of current practice evidences little attention to information or consent from anticipated third parties.

Trials of a vaccine against herpes simplex and trials of short-course antiretroviral therapy provide examples of contemporary studies where researchers have not included indirect participants in the consent process. Investigators have addressed third party risks specifically in studies of xenotransplantation. Another example of high profile research where risks of infection and transmission have been raised, but which we do not consider here, is gene therapy, where the mechanism of delivery is a viral vector. Here also the concern apparently has been for direct subjects, not for their direct contacts who might be regarded as indirect participants.[51]

GlaxoSmithKline has sponsored several clinical trials of the safety and efficacy of a vaccine against the herpes simplex virus. The trials enrolled over 400 adult women at risk of contracting herpes, in over 80 study centers on four continents (Africa, Australia, Europe, and North America).[52] The consent form detailed an extended list of risks, including risks of the injection and of blood draws that would be required to test levels of immunity. The consent form explains in detail that the vaccine contains bovine derivatives and has been manufactured to avoid any risk of variant Creutzfeldt-Jacob Disease (vCJD, also called "mad cow disease"). Boldface type cautions participants to avoid pregnancy, as the effects of the vaccine on a fetus are unknown. In an open label study, which offered active vaccine to patients who had received placebo in an earlier trial, patients were informed that 73% of women receiving vaccine in the earlier study had been effectively immunized against herpes simplex. Disclosures reminded participants that the vaccine was still experimental and that they might receive no benefit from study participation. However, the consent form contained no mention of sexual partners or of the risk that if the vaccine proved ineffective and the subjects acquired herpes infection, they might pass the infection on to others.

Participants in this study were at background risk of contracting herpes and transmitting it to their partners, regardless of study participation. Participation in the study offered them a possibility of protection as a result of the vaccination that they would not otherwise have had. Their sexual partners, it might seem, were not at any greater risk from the study than they otherwise

---

51. E.g., Catherine S. Manno et al., "AAV-Mediated Factor IX Gene Transfer to Skeletal Muscle in Patients with Severe Hemophilia B," *Blood* 101, no. 8 (April 15, 2003): 2963–2972.

52. Consent form, Protocol # 208141/037 (HSV-037) (December, 2001), on file with the University of Utah Institutional Review Board.

would have been, and may even have been at reduced risk, so any discussion of risks to them is arguably unnecessary.

This argument has two related replies. First, research studies are held to higher standards than the background risks that might have occurred regardless of research participation. Risk/benefit ratios must be acceptable and risks to subjects must be minimized if possible. We contend that this minimization of risks should apply not only to direct subjects but also to those who might be immediately affected by their participation and thus are indirect participants in the research. Second, participants in the study may have believed that they were receiving protection, when in fact they were not. Believing they had received adequate protection, they might have been less careful to guard both themselves and their partners against risks of contagion. These concerns, we contend, at a minimum require including in the consent form the reminder that the vaccine might not be effective—and that *if* it is not, participants *as well as* their partners may be at risk of infection.

To take another example, trials of short-course anti-retroviral therapy to reduce the likelihood of transmission of HIV from pregnant women to their fetuses have been highly controversial. Participants in these trials have been HIV-positive women in areas of the world where access to anti-retroviral therapy is limited or non-existent. Because short-course therapy initially appeared economically feasible whereas optimal therapy did not, the trials were designed to determine whether short course therapy reduced vertical transmission rates.

At least 15 trials have compared vertical transmission rates in patients receiving the short-course therapy against vertical transmission rates in patients receiving placebo.[53] Defenders of the trials argued that the researchers' duty of care to subjects did not extend beyond the best standard of care available in the subjects' circumstances. Critics argued that because there was an alternative to placebo—the standard of care available in the developed world—the studies violated clinical equipoise and were clearly morally wrong, comparable to Tuskegee in observing seriously ill patients for whom treatment was possible.[54]

Bioethicists have raised many serious ethical issues about these trials. Alex John London, for example, has argued that the concept of "equipoise" is ambiguous between a narrow physiological concept and a broader concept of efficacy in social context.[55] Solomon Benatar has argued for sweeping reforms in the

53. E.g., Paquita De Zulueta, "Randomized Placebo-Controlled Trials and HIV-Infected Pregnant Women in Developing Countries: Ethical Imperialism or Unethical Exploitation?" *Bioethics* 15, no. 4 (2001): 289–311 (292).
54. Marcia Angell, "The Ethics of Clinical Research in the Third World," *New England Journal of Medicine* 337, no. 12 (2001): 847–849.
55. Alex John London, "Equipoise and International Human-Subjects Research," *Bioethics* 15, no. 4 (2001): 312–332.

understanding of ethics in international research, in the context of international justice in health care.[56] Many discussions have highlighted coercion and exploitation of vulnerable populations.[57] When attention has been turned to informed consent from study subjects, the principal suggestion has been involvement of families or communities in the consent process. This suggestion has rested on several grounds. Family and community support is an important protection against exploitation. The societies in which the studies have taken place frequently are communitarian in structure, and do not see consent as an individualized process.[58] The studies themselves may have effects on the communities in which they take place.

Concerns also surfaced about the risks of short-course anti-retroviral therapy to the women involved. One risk is that if anti-retroviral therapy becomes available, later treatment efforts may prove less efficacious for women who have received the short-course therapy. Another is that the short-course therapy may alter the course of the subjects' disease, generating increased viral load or more resistant viral strains. Either of these risks are direct risks to the study subjects. But given levels of heterosexual transmission of HIV, they are also risks to the subjects' sexual partners.[59] Yet we have found *no* criticisms of the HIV trials that mention the unacknowledged increased risks to partners or to communities as an ethical issue in the studies. Where we did find mention of family members, the focus was not on risks to them, but embedded in familial or communal informed consent models, where the concern was the role of the family or community, or the vulnerability of the subjects not the possibility of spread of resistant disease in the community.[60]

Unlike the studies that are silent regarding third party risks, protocols studying xenotransplantation have undergone extensive scrutiny for the safety of both individual participants and the public. Perhaps the difference stems from a perception that transplanting tissues or even organs from animals to humans is new and strange, and from fears of species-jumping infections of unknown character. Margaret A. Clark, for example, argues that patients receiving xenotransplants should be required to consent to take precautions against transmission of bodily fluids. She also argues—a view we share—that they and their intimates must receive information about transmission risks. She suggests that population consent should be sought where there are significant public health risks, but

56. Solomon R. Benatar, "Commentary: Justice and Medical Research: A Global Perspective."
57. E.g., Keymanthri Moodley, "Vaccine Trial Participation in South Africa—An Ethical Assessment," *Journal of Medicine and Philosophy* 27, no. 2 (2002): 197–215; De Zulueta, "Randomised Placebo-Controlled Trials."
58. Moodley, "Vaccine Trial Participation."
59. Thomas C. Quinn et al., "Viral Load and Heterosexual Transmission of Human Immunodeficiency Virus Type 1," *New England Journal of Medicine* 342, no. 13 (March 30, 2000): 921–929.
60. E.g., De Zulueta, "Randomised Placebo-Controlled Trials," 303.

does not otherwise raise the possibility of indirect participant consent where direct risks to third parties are apparent.[61]

Considering the Risks to Indirect Participants

In both the historical and contemporary examples we have discussed, participation of direct subjects in the research creates potential risks for their immediate contacts, such as family members or sexual partners, and sometimes for the public at large. Risks to individual subjects and to society overall have been addressed in public policy requirements, in study design and approval, and in criticism of studies. Research practices are considered unethical if they include direct subjects into studies without informing them of the risks they face and thus without providing information relevant to decisions about participation. Close contacts of such subjects—sexual partners or family members in particular—may be exposed to risks by the participation of direct subjects. Yet these risks to indirect participants have been virtually ignored. Indeed, the failure to consider such third party risks extends even to inattention to providing information about risks of infectiousness to study subjects themselves. This gap in policy and practice, we contend, represents a failure to respect the autonomy of these third parties as potential victims that is analogous to the failure to respect the autonomy of the direct subjects. In response to these concerns, we suggest several changes in current policy.

A first change is attention to risks to indirect participants in study design. Risks of third-party transmission should be explicitly considered in the design of studies. This cannot be accomplished by ensuring that the study has a risk/benefit ratio that is favorable overall. Ethical study design requires not only minimization of risks to subjects, but also minimization of risks to indirect participants. Careful study design may reduce the likelihood of creating indirect participants through strategies such as isolating the direct subject until the likelihood of contagion has passed. Otherwise, people may be subject to risks of the study that might have been avoided in the study design, even though they are not themselves subjects of the research. In some studies involving contagious conditions, however, design features such as these may not be feasible. For example, research with OPV created immunized subjects who continued to shed potentially infectious virus for extended time periods.[62]

A second change is the process of informed consent with direct subjects. When applicable, the informed consent process should include information

---

61. Margaret A. Clark, "This Little Piggy Went to Market: The Xenotranplantation and Xenozoonose Debate," *Journal of Law, Medicine & Ethics* 27, no. 2 (1999): 137–152 (141).
62. E.g., Alan W. Dove and Vincent R. Racaniello, "The Polio Eradication Effort: Should Vaccine Eradication Be Next?" *Science* 277, no. 5372 (1997): 779–780.

about risks of contagion. Issues addressed with direct subjects should include risks of contagion that might result from their participation in the study. Subjects in prevention studies, for example, should be warned that if the method of prevention fails and they become infected, they might pose a risk of contagion to others. In studies that may raise subjects' risks of contagion, such as the trials of short-course anti-retroviral therapy, researchers must inform subjects of this possibility so that they may take it into account in deciding whether to participate in the research.

A third change is the requirement in some cases of informed consent on the part of identifiable indirect participants. Current practice relies on direct subjects to provide contacts with information, if information is to be provided at all, as in the herpes or xenotransplantation research. If the risk to indirect participants is substantial and serious, this may be insufficient. Direct subjects may be reluctant to convey the information. They may have understood the risk imperfectly or may be unable to explain what they have understood. In such circumstances, contacts—the indirect participants—may not receive the information they need to protect themselves should the infection risk eventuate. Protecting the indirect participant requires more than providing information to the direct subject.

At a minimum, indirect participants at significant and serious risk should be provided with the information directly, so that they can understand it and act on it themselves; considering them as potential victims with their own choice to make requires no less. If the risk is unavoidable, consideration should also be given to whether respect for indirect participants requires their independent consent to the direct subject's participation in the study. In short, when risks to indirect participants are potentially as great as risks posed to direct subjects of research, our approach recommends that researchers afford respect for the indirect participant that is similar to that afforded to direct subjects. Contacts or family members of a person participating in infectious disease research must be allowed to understand that the direct subject may be both victim and vector of the disease under study.

We recognize that our approach limits choices open to the direct subject. Direct subjects who do not wish indirect participants to be informed about the risks of the study will not be able to participate in the research. An indirect participant's refusal to grant consent would block participation by the study subject. If the indirect participant refuses consent, when consent is required, the direct subject's participation will also be blocked. Even if self-experimentation were regarded as fully permissible, it might still be blocked if the experimenter/subject failed to consider the risks he was taking for himself also constituted risks for others.

However, we think that this strikes a defensible balance. Participation in a research study should not be equated with receiving beneficial therapy despite the standard that encourages subjects to base their decisions about participation on a reasonable assessment of the risks and benefits to them. When subjects participate in research that may directly affect the risks and benefits for others in significant ways but these others are not consulted, the latter are affected by the research without their consent. When the risks are serious and unavoidable, as they might be with transmission of zoonoses from xenotransplants, their informed consent should also be required.

Considering Indirect Participants: How Far to Cast the Net?

Despite the case we have made for considering risks to indirect participants, we also recognize serious issues about the potential range of indirect participants. Spreading the range too far—say, to fourth or fifth parties, the contacts of the contacts of the indirect participants—could strangle infectious disease research, which is important to all of us as victims. We readily admit that we do not have final answers to this question, although we do think analogies can be developed from efforts at community consent to research. Our goal in this chapter has been to direct attention to this significant ethical issue heretofore virtually ignored. We would suggest, however, that respect for involuntarily involved third parties such as sexual partners or family members requires their involvement in the consent process when they are identifiable and at known, direct, and significant risk.

Another difficulty with our proposals is that some indirect participants may not be able to understand information or to give their informed consent. Children and cognitively impaired family members may be both at greater risk of disease transmission and unable to give informed consent. The standard way to handle such issues, with which we agree, is to obtain informed consent on their behalf from these third parties' proxies. We advise special caution, however, when the proxy, for example a parent, also serves as the proposed direct subject of the research. In that case, the proxy/direct subject may not independently represent the best interests of the indirect participant.

At some point, concern with transmission to indirect participants might be anticipated to include the community. Suppose we know that risks of rapid transmission of a serious disease such as SARS or avian flu exist. Research on the development of vaccines for these diseases might have an overall favorable risk/benefit ratio, given the apparent seriousness of the diseases. However, in the community in which the vaccine trial takes place, members of the community might be placed at special risk, depending on the design of the study.

For studies not involving infectiousness, where we know that some community members may be affected by the study but these community members cannot be identified in advance, the model has been community consent. One example is the trial of installing cardiac defibrillators in community settings such as shopping centers.[63] In this trial, there was little possibility to predict who might use the defibrillators or who might need them. The strategy chosen for consent was to involve the community; nearby workers who might be most likely to be on the scene when an emergency occurred and local governments who arguably might represent the population most likely to be at risk of defibrillator need while shopping. We would suggest further exploration of this possibility in the infectious disease context, if research poses such special risks to communities. Efforts to publicize the study and create an "opt out" possibility, as with the study of the use of the blood substitute polyheme in emergency situations, are logistically difficult in the case of a contagious disease if it is hard to predict who might be at risk of disease transmission from the study.

The ethical problem of indirect participation in research is not an entirely novel concept. In the context of genetic information, where participation by some family members can result in the collection of information about identifiable other family members, third party consent has been raised as a possibility when the risks to the third parties are significant.[64] In the case of genetic information, the third parties are subjects in the sense that the research involves the collection of information about them, and they have been regarded as secondary subjects of the research. When studies involve diseases that are infectious and contagious, identifiable contacts may not be subjects in the sense that information about them is acquired through the study. Nonetheless, the risks of their indirect participation may be as substantial and serious to them as the risks of collecting their genetic information. Research subjects are potential vectors; indirect subjects are potential victims. Informed consent and the ethics of research must be informed and broadened by this interrelationship.

63. On file with the University of Utah Institutional Review Board.
64. Jeffrey R. Botkin, "Protecting the Privacy of Family Members in Survey and Pedigree Research," *Journal of the American Medical Association* 285, no. 2 (2001): 207–211.

11

VERTICAL TRANSMISSION OF INFECTIOUS DISEASES AND GENETIC DISORDERS

Both infectious diseases and genetic conditions are transmitted "vertically"—that is, from pregnant woman to the child she bears. This shared characteristic invites us to examine how we think about and respond to different diseases and categories of disease that can be transmitted to our offspring. At times, the law in the United States has compelled prenatal maternal screening for some infectious diseases such as syphilis, but never for inherited genetic diseases such as cystic fibrosis (CF). In this chapter, we use our PVV perspective to explore whether mandatory screening is more permissible in the case of infectious than genetic transmission, at least where effective treatment is available for the pregnant woman.

We also want to use this chapter to continue to deflate ideas of "exceptionalism," for both genetic testing and infectious disease. Particularly because of the potential implications of genetic information for family members, some commentators have argued that genetic information should be given special ethical protection.[1] Legal policy has followed suit, with a number of states enacting specific laws about genetic testing and the information gathered by genetic tests.[2] Review of research with human subjects may also single out genetic

An earlier version of this chapter appeared as Jay A. Jacobson, Margaret P. Battin, Jeffrey Botkin, Leslie P. Francis, James O. Mason, Charles B. Smith, "Vertical Transmission of Infectious Disease and Genetic Disorders," in *Ethics, Prevention, and Public Health*, ed. Angus Dawson and Marcel Verweij (Oxford: Clarendon Press, 2007), 145–159.

1. Secretary's Advisory Committee on Genetic Testing, "Enhancing the Oversight of Genetic Tests: Recommendations of the SACGT" (Bethesda, MD: National Institutes of Health, 2000), http://www4.od.nih.gov/oba/sacgt/reports/oversight_report.pdf (accessed December 31, 2007).

2. Over 30 states have statutes that provide some degree of special protection for genetic privacy and EU member countries follow the extensive protections in the EU privacy directive. See Nancy J. King, Sukanya Pillay, and Gail A. Lasprogata, "Workplace Privacy and Discrimination Issues Related to Genetic Data: A Comparative Law Study of the European Union and the United States," *American Business Law Journal* 43 (2006): 79–171, 146 n. 224; Deborah Hellman, "What Makes Genetic Discrimination Exceptional?" *American Journal of Law & Medicine* 29 (2003): 77–116; Mark A. Hall and Stephen S. Rich, "Genetic Privacy Laws and Patients' Fear of Discrimination by Health Insurers: The View from Genetic Counselors," *Journal of Law, Medicine & Ethics* 28 (2000): 245–255. As this book went to press, the Genetic Information Non-Discrimination Act of 2007–2008 (GINA) became law in the United States, see http://www.genome.gov/24519851 (accessed June 25, 2008).

information for special scrutiny.[3] We are not "exceptionalists" about infectious disease, neither the diseases discussed in this chapter nor, as we have seen in Chapter 5, HIV/AIDS, nor will we be arguing for what has been called genetic exceptionalism.[4] Instead, our view is that it is important to pay attention to the characteristics of different diseases, and even to differences among diseases of the same type. A rapidly progressive infectious disease, for example, poses challenges for deliberative decision making that a chronic condition does not; adult onset genetic conditions raise different issues about the risks and benefits of prenatal diagnosis than do conditions such as Tay-Sachs that are manifest shortly after birth and lead relatively rapidly to death.

The theoretical structures of bioethics must be able to handle these differences. Our point in this volume is not that infectious disease is always special— it sometimes is not. Rather, because infectious disease cases were not at the forefront of bioethics during its theoretical development, characteristics that are especially apparent in some infectious diseases (but also in some non-infectious diseases) went underappreciated as the field developed. Our aim in this volume is to correct such a "one size fits all" bioethics, understanding how features such as disease transmission must be incorporated into theoretical paradigms and function, perhaps differently, in various disease contexts. When we examine the policies that have developed in the actual case of two vertically transmitted diseases, one infectious and one genetic—syphilis and cystic fibrosis—we find clear differences between the policies that have emerged. In this chapter, we first consider whether there is an adequate rationale for these differences. We argue, based on our PVV view, that while there appear to be differences between the two cases, and the arguments for preventing vertical infectious transmission seem to be stronger than the arguments for intervention to prevent vertical genetic transmission, it is not actually clear whether it is infectiousness per se that is playing the principal role. Rather, the important factor may be the anticipated harms to fetuses/eventual children and their mothers and the available methods for preventing or treating those harms. Thus, while we are concerned in this book with transmissible infectious disease, we also want to explore whether there are more similarities between infectious conditions and other forms of transmission than may have generally been recognized. As we explore whether it is the difference between infectious and genetic transmission that is what matters, we may find that the cases at hand are more similar than the policy structures that govern them might

---

3. David S. Diekema and W. Burke, "Ethical Issues Arising from the Participation of Children in Genetic Research," *Journal of Pediatrics* 149, suppl. 1 (July 2006): S34–S38.
4. For criticism of genetic exceptionalism, see M.D. Green, and J.R. Botkin, "'Genetic Exceptionalism' in Medicine: Clarifying the Differences Between Genetic and Nongenetic Tests," *Annals of Internal Medicine* 138 (2003): 571–575; see also Lori Andrews, "A Conceptual Framework for Genetic Policy: Comparing the Medical, Public Health, and Fundamental Rights Models," *Washington University Law Quarterly* 79 (2001): 221–285.

make them appear—and that the insights we have gleaned from infectious disease may be more broadly applicable.

Many examples of infectious diseases and genetic disorders might enable us to explore which ethical paradigm seems most appropriate and how medical care, public policy, and public health law have responded to the risk of vertical transmission—including syphilis, gonorrhea, hepatitis B, rubella, cystic fibrosis, Huntington's disease, phenylketonuria, sickle cell anemia, and Tay-Sachs disease, to name a few. In this chapter, we focus on syphilis as an example of a vertically transmitted infectious disease and cystic fibrosis as a representative genetic disorder, for three reasons. First, each is or has been relatively common. Second, knowledge about their clinical manifestations, methods of diagnosis, and etiology is longstanding.[5] Third, we can examine a substantial body of public policy and written recommendations and practices associated with these examples.[6] We then compare the recent shift in recommendations for maternal screening for HIV—from "opt in" to "opt out" screening, a policy shift we will examine more fully in the next chapter—as an example of how the preventability of identifiable harm is the principal driver in screening recommendations. Our focus on vertical transmission, the key distinguishing feature of genetic disorders, allows us to examine whether vertical transmission merits special consideration or whether there is something else about genetic diseases—or infections—that warrants a special or exceptional approach.

For this and subsequent chapters, a prefatory note about the use of terminology such as "mandatory" or "routine" is helpful. "Mandatory" is the term used to describe legal requirements, but it is misleading. Legal requirements, such as those imposed for school entry, typically permit many exceptions: for medical reasons, religious reasons, other reasons of conscience, or perhaps any reason at all.[7] They thus fall far short of universal "mandates." A medical practice is "routine" when it is recommended as part of standard care, generally without special counseling, although patients may of course request further information and decide to refuse a routine recommendation. A practice is "opt out" if the assumption is that the patient will receive the care, absent a specific choice to refuse. It is "opt in" if the assumption is the reverse: that the patient will not be given the intervention unless there is a specific choice to have it. More recent terminology describes the option presented to the patient as routine as

5. See, e.g., C. Quetel and J. Braddoch, *The History of Syphilis* (Baltimore, MD: Johns Hopkins University Press, 1992); and D.J. Shal, ed., *Cystic fibrosis* (London: BMJ, 1996).
6. See A. Morabia and F.F. Zhang, "History of Medical Screening: From Concepts to Action," *Postgraduate Medical Journal* 80 (2004):463–469; and B.S. Wilfond and E.J. Thomson, "Models of Public Health Genetic Policy Development," in *Genetics and Public Health in the 21st Century*, ed. M.J. Khoury, W. Burke, and E.J. Thomson (New York: Oxford University Press, 2000).
7. We are not the first to make this observation. See, e.g., Sylvia Law, "Human Papillomavirus Vaccination, Private Choice, and Public Health," *U.C. Davis Law Review* 41 (2008): 1731–1772 (1765–1766).

the "default option,"[8] or as a case of "asymmetric paternalism," where options are presented to the patient without limiting freedom of choice but framed in such a way that the patient is likely to accept one rather than another.[9] Thus when interventions such as testing or immunization are described as "mandated," this does not mean that they will be compelled in all cases, without exceptions.

Syphilis

The first recognized outbreak of syphilis occurred in Naples, in 1494, involving Spaniards from Christopher Columbus's crew who participated in the army of Charles VIII of France.[10] Shortly thereafter, people began to realize that the children of mothers with syphilis were adversely affected at birth.

Congenital syphilis is a severe, disabling, and often life threatening condition for the infant. Nearly half of all children infected with syphilis during gestation die shortly before or after birth. Infants who survive develop early and late stage symptoms of syphilis if not treated. Early stage symptoms include irritability, failure to thrive, and non-specific fever. Some infants develop a rash and lesions on the mouth, anus, and genitalia. Some of these lesions may resemble the wart-like lesions of adult syphilis. A small percentage of infants have a watery nasal discharge and a saddle nose deformity resulting from infection in the cartilage of the nose. Bone lesions are common, especially in the upper arm. Later signs appear as tooth abnormalities, bone changes, neurological involvement, blindness, and deafness.[11]

In the early twentieth century in the United States, syphilis was endemic and approximately one million women of childbearing age had the disease.[12] Congenital syphilis was the leading cause of spontaneous abortions and still-births. It was estimated that about 25,000 fetuses per year died before birth and 60,000 infants per year were born with syphilis.[13] Between 40% and 100%

8. SD Halpern, PA Ubel, DA Asch. 2007. Harnessing the Power of Default Options to Improve Health Care. *New England Journal of Medicine* 357(13) (September 27):1340-1344.

9. George Loewenstein, Troyen Brennan, and Kevin G. Volpp. 2007. Asymmetric Paternalism to Improve Health Behaviors. *Journal of the American Medical Association* 298(20)(November 28): 2415-2417.

10. E.C. Tramont, "The Impact of Syphilis on Humankind," *Infectious Disease Clinics of North America* 18 (2004): 101–110.

11. U.S. National Library of Medicine and National Institute of Health, Medline Plus, Medical Encyclopedia, "Congenital Syphilis," www.nlm.nih.gov/medlineplus/ency/article/001344.htm (accessed December 31, 2007).

12. K.L. Acuff and R.R. Faden. "A History of Prenatal and Newborn Screening Programs: Lessons for the Future," in *AIDS, Women and the Next Generation*, ed. R.R. Faden, G. Geller, and M. Powers (New York: Oxford University Press, 1991), ch. 3, (60).

13. Thomas Parran, "Syphilis: A Public Health Problem," *Science* 87, no. 2251 (1938): 147–152 (149).

of the fetuses carried by women with syphilis were infected, depending on the timing of infection. Current data suggest that there is an up to 80% chance that women who have acquired syphilis within four years, but who have not received treatment, will pass the infection to their offspring.[14]

Since 1906, clinicians have been able to identify individuals infected with syphilis by using microscopy, which reveals the infectious agent, *Treponema pallidum*, in primary and cutaneous lesions. A serologic test identifies antibodies to the pathogen during latent infection and secondary or tertiary stages.[15] Individuals may be carriers of this pathogen for years if they are untreated. Since the 1940s, penicillin has been used to effectively treat syphilis in all of its stages. Infants born to infected mothers who received adequate and timely penicillin treatment during pregnancy are at minimal risk of disease.[16]

Numerous strategies are effective in preventing the vertical transmission of syphilis and reducing the consequences to infected fetuses if transmission has occurred. These strategies include premarital testing of men and women, presumably before conception, and treatment of either or both partners who have a positive test. Prenatal testing of pregnant women is another option. Treatment of an infected woman during pregnancy prevents and/or treats infection in the fetus. It also treats the pregnant woman, reducing risks to her health from the disease. Postnatal or newborn screening of infants does not prevent syphilis, but early treatment of infected infants can reduce morbidity.[17] Thus identification of infection in the woman during pregnancy can be very important both for her well-being and for the eventual well-being of her child.

Cystic Fibrosis

The syndrome of cystic fibrosis has been recognized since the Middle Ages, when infants with salty skin where considered "bewitched" because they routinely died an early death. The syndrome was named "cystic fibrosis with bronchiectasis" by Guido Fanconi in 1936. In 1949, Charles Lowe established it as a recessive genetic disorder and, by 1953, a more precise test for sweat chloride, the quantitative version of "salty skin," became available for diagnosis. This enabled better diagnosis and characterization of the clinical syndrome.

---

14. See Centers for Disease Control and Prevention, "Sexually Transmitted Diseases: Surveillance 2006," www.cdc.gov/std/stats/syphilis.htm (accessed November 2007).

15. Michael A. Stoto, Donna A. Almario, and Marie C. McCormick, *Reducing the Odds: Preventing Perinatal Transmission of HIV in the United States* (Washington, DC: National Academy Press, 1999), ch. 2 (26).

16. E.C. Tramont, "Treponenion Pallidum (Syphilis)," in *Principle and Practice of Infectious Diseases*, ed. G.L Mandell, J.E. Bennett, and R. Dolin 2 vols. 6th ed. (Philadelphia: Elsevier, 2005), 2781.

17. D.G. Walker and G.J.A. Walker, "Forgotten but Not Gone: The Continuing Scourge of Congenital Syphilis," *Lancet Infectious Disease* 2 (2002): 432–436.

Cystic fibrosis results from abnormalities in the cystic fibrosis transmembrane conductance regulator (CFTR) gene, a gene responsible for the formation of bodily fluids such as mucus. People with two defective copies of the gene make mucus that is abnormally thick. Symptoms of CF, typically manifest in early infancy and childhood, include recurrent bouts of pneumonia, failure to thrive, and digestive difficulties. Many males with cystic fibrosis are infertile. Before 1990, most children with cystic fibrosis died in childhood. In recent years, with improved treatment methods, median survival of patients with CF has increased to over 36 years.[18] Death is usually from pulmonary complications.

Cystic fibrosis is the most common fatal hereditary disorder affecting Caucasians in the United States. It is most common among Caucasians of Northern or Central European descent, although there are comparable rates among some Pueblo peoples and significant rates among Hispanics. Risk factors include a family history of cystic fibrosis or unexplained infant death. Because cystic fibrosis is an autosomal recessive disorder, a child must receive an abnormal gene from both parents to be affected. The carrier rate for Americans for the single abnormal gene is approximately 1 in 20. There are approximately 12 million carriers in the United States, and the likelihood that two Caucasian carriers will marry and/or mate is approximately 1 in 400. Because the disease is transmitted as an autosomal recessive, 50% of the offspring will be carriers, 25% will inherit neither abnormal gene, and 25% will inherit both abnormal genes and probably develop the disease. This results in an annual incidence of approximately 1 in 1600 births to Caucasians and 1 in 4,000 total births in the United States. Carriers can be identified by a blood test for CFTR gene mutations.[19] There is no curative treatment for cystic fibrosis. However, early recognition and treatment can lengthen survival and improve quality of life. Treatment includes antibiotics, enzymes, vitamins, and bronchodilators. New treatments include replacement of the DNase enzyme with Dornase (Pulmozyme). Although there was initial hope for gene therapy trials, they have not been successful and none were in progress as of the end of 2007. A committee established by the Cystic Fibrosis Foundation issued evidence-based guidelines for CF care in November 2007; plans are to update the guidelines every five years.[20]

Strategies for preventing cystic fibrosis consist of identifying carriers and having those carriers exercise available reproductive choices. Once carrier status has been established (often as a premarital screen), couples can consider

---

18. Flume et al, "Cystic Fibrosis Pulmonary Guidelines," *American Journal of Respiratory and Critical Care Medicine* 176 (November 15, 2007): 957–969.

19. For general information about CF, see U.S. Department of Health and Human Services, National Institutes of Health, and National Heart, Lung and Blood Institute, "Diseases and Conditions Index: What Is Cystic Fibrosis?" http://www.nhlbi.nih.gov/health/dci/Diseases/cf/cf_what.html (accessed December 31, 2007).

20. Flume, "Cystic Fibrosis Pulmonary Guidelines."

options to prevent the birth of a child with CF, including choosing not to have a child, adoption, artificial insemination with sperm from a non-carrier, in vitro fertilization and selective implantation of an unaffected embryo, or abortion of an affected fetus.

Strategies for Testing for These Two Vertically Transmitted Diseases

Syphilis

Although diagnostic tests for syphilis had been available by 1906, the national venereal disease program initially was only poorly developed and syphilis therapy for pregnant women was marginal and difficult to tolerate. Prenatal syphilis testing was not mandated by law due to, as the then U.S. Surgeon General Thomas Parran put it, "onerous treatment options and the stigma of being shown to have the disease."[21] Indeed, even being tested for syphilis was stigmatizing, and many physicians were reluctant to embarrass women in their care by suggesting it. By 1936, however, Parran had established a program for controlling syphilis that included mandatory premarital and prenatal blood tests.[22] By the end of 1945, 36 states had passed prenatal syphilis screening laws.[23] Under these laws, birth certificates had to record whether the test had been done prenatally and if not had to explain why not. Women and physicians could refuse on religious or other grounds. Although these laws were passed before the introduction of antibiotic treatment, they resulted in a rapid decline of congenital transmission through case finding, contact tracing, and the difficult and less effective therapies available at the time. Perhaps the most important aspect of these screening programs was that by making testing routine, they overcame the resistance of physicians to risk offending patients by suggesting a test for syphilis.[24] When the discovery of penicillin in the early 1940s provided a very effective and non-toxic therapy for the disease, the opportunity to virtually wipe out congenital syphilis became apparent, and within a few years government funding for venereal disease clinics was greatly expanded. These programs were not widely challenged by the public, and proved to be remarkably successful in virtually eliminating congenital syphilis. Most U.S. states and public health entities still maintain the policy of routine screening of women for syphilis during pregnancy.[25]

21. Stoto, Almario, and McCormick, *Reducing the Odds* 26, citing Acuff and Faden, "Screening Programs."
22. Ibid., 25.
23. Ibid., 26.
24. Ibid.
25. Centers for Disease Control and Prevention," Epidemic of Congenital Syphilis—Baltimore, 1996–1997," *Morbidity and Mortality Weekly Report* 47 (1998): 904–907.

These control measures were so effective that, as of 2004, fewer than five states continue to require premarital testing because the frequency of positive results is so low. However, 46 of 50 states still require prenatal testing of pregnant women. Seventy-six percent of states that mandate testing require one early test and 26% require a second later test for all or high-risk women.[26] In situations where the test is mandated, written informed consent is not usually solicited. Thirty-three states allow religious exemption from testing and 13 permit refusal for any reason. The test is quite inexpensive, and insurance generally covers the cost of testing if a bill is generated, but many clinics that do this test do not charge for it. By supporting the infrastructure to deliver prenatal screening, state laws indirectly influence practice, and many state ante-partum screening laws also have misdemeanor penalties for violations. Some states offer laboratory testing at reduced or no cost.[27]

Physician practice is influenced not only by state law but also by professional society recommendations. Current guidelines from the American College of Obstetrics and Gynecology (ACOG) and the American Academy of Pediatrics recommend that all women be screened for syphilis at the first prenatal visit; women considered to be at high risk for the disease should be screened again at 32 to 36 weeks gestation.[28]

As a result of these policies—and practices that are in relatively good compliance with them—new syphilis cases in the United States fell to 32,871 in 2002. New primary and secondary syphilis cases had an incidence of 2.4 per 100,000. Prevalence of carriers among women was 1 in 100,000. The total number of cases of congenital syphilis had plummeted to 451, for a rate of 11.2 cases per 100,000 live births.[29] In 2005, the numbers had fallen to 339 (an incidence of 8.2 cases per 100,000 live births), but a slight increase to 349 (8.5 cases per live birth) occurred in 2006.[30] In the past several years, however, the incidence of syphilis has been increasing among people who engage in high-risk sexual behaviors and those who lack access to care. The CDC has developed a *National Plan to Eliminate Syphilis from the United States*, which involves

26. L.M. Hollier, J. Hill, J.S. Sheffield, and G.D. Wendel, "State Laws Regarding Prenatal Syphilis Screening in the United States," *American Journal of Obstetrics and Gynecology* 184 (2003): 1178–1183.
27. U.S. General Accounting Office, "*Newborn Screening: Characteristics of State Programs,*" Report Number GAO-03-449 (March 2003), http://www.gao.gov/new.items/d03449.pdf (accessed December 31, 2007).
28. American Academy of Pediatrics, *Guidelines for Perinatal Care,* 5th ed. (Elk Grove Village, IL: American College of Obstetricians and Gynecologists, 2002).
29. Centers for Disease Control and Prevention, "Sexually Transmitted Diseases: Syphilis Surveillance Report 2002," www.CDC.GOV/STD/STATS02/Syphilis.htm (accessed December 31, 2007); and Centers for Disease Control and Prevention, "Congenital Syphilis—United States 2002," *Morbidity and Mortality Weekly Report* 53, no. 31 (August 13, 2004): 716–719.
30. Centers for Disease Control and Prevention, "Sexually Transmitted Diseases: Surveillance 2006," http://www.cdc.gov/std/stats/syphilis.htm (accessed December 31, 2007).

among its nine strategies expanded surveillance and community mobilization, intended to control the manifestations of the disease so that it is no longer considered a public health problem.[31] In addition to recommendations to practitioners, medical professional societies also offer guidance to women to prevent vertical transmission of syphilis. They say to women who suspect they may be infected with syphilis and who are pregnant or anticipate becoming pregnant:

> All pregnant women should be tested for syphilis. Pregnant women
> with syphilis are treated right away with penicillin. For women
> with an allergy to penicillin, there is no alternative medicine that
> has proven effective for treatment. Penicillin will prevent passing
> syphilis to the baby, although treatment during the second half
> of pregnancy may not eliminate the risk for premature labor and
> fetal distress.[32]

Cystic Fibrosis

Because there are over 1,300 different mutations of the CFTR gene, development of a genetic test for the disease has been difficult. In 2005, the U.S. Food and Drug Administration approved a blood test for cystic fibrosis, the Tag-It 40 + 4 test, which detects many of the most common mutations and is accurate in diagnosing up to 90% of carriers and affected individuals. The test cannot, however, predict disease severity. Moreover, because the test only identifies the more common mutations, a negative test result does not equal zero disease risk.[33]

Policies regarding cystic fibrosis stand in significant contrast to the policies regarding syphilis. The approach is to offer information and the possibility of choice to patients. None of the states require premarital or prenatal screening for cystic fibrosis. The American College of Obstetricians and Gynecologists now recommends that the carrier-screening test be available to all

31. Centers for Disease Control and Prevention, *The National Plan to Eliminate Syphilis from the United States,* (Atlanta, GA: U.S. Department of Health and Human Services, May 2006), http://www.cdc.gov/stopsyphilis/SEEPlan2006.pdf (accessed December 31, 2007), viii.

32. Women'shealth.gov, http://www.4women.gov/faq/stdsyph.htm#7 (accessed February 12, 2008).

33. Lab Tests Online, "New DNA Test Approved for Cystic Fibrosis Carrier Screening and Diagnosis" (June 24, 2005), http://www.labtestsonline.org/news/cf050624.html (accessed December 31, 2007).

couples who are planning pregnancy or are pregnant.[34] ACOG's information for patients about testing, however, emphasizes that "the decision is yours."[35] Many health-care providers hand out printed material for couples to read; those who may be interested in testing can then discuss it further with their providers. One large health-care organization in California that instituted a program of offering screening to all pregnant women describing themselves or their partners as having white ancestry reported that the program resulted in an approximate 50% reduction in births of affected children.[36] Reported cases of insurance companies attempting to put pressure on pregnant women to undergo testing—or to limit prenatal testing to women who are willing to undergo abortions if the results are positive—have met with intense criticism.[37]

Newborn testing for CF—now widespread—does not prevent vertical transmission, but gives the benefits of early identification of the condition.[38] Rapid diagnosis in the neonate may lead to earlier appropriate treatment, which may be life extending and enhancing. It could also lead indirectly to parental choices, which might prevent or address vertical transmission in subsequent pregnancies.

Syphilis and Cystic Fibrosis Policies Compared

The two vertically transmitted disorders, syphilis and cystic fibrosis, are similar with respect to severity of disease, potential incidence, detectability of cases and carriers, and the absence of curative treatment after vertical transmission occurs. But strategies for prevention differ substantially. An inexpensive safe drug, penicillin, can be used to prevent vertical transmission of syphilis. Only reproductive choices are available to prevent vertical transmission of cystic fibrosis. Available alternatives include avoidance of conception in the first place, the use of methods of artificial reproduction to select or create unaffected embryos, or pregnancy termination. For some couples, these are extremely difficult or ethically unacceptable options.

---

34. American College of Obstetricians and Gynecologists and American College of Medical Genetics, *Preconception and Prenatal Carrier Screening for Cystic Fibrosis: Clinical and Laboratory Guidelines* (Washington, DC: American College of Obstetricians and Gynecologists, 2001).
35. American College of Obstetricians and Gynecologists, *Cystic Fibrosis Carrier Testing: The Decision Is Yours* (Washington, DC: American College of Obstetricians and Gynecologists, 2001), http://www.acog.org/publications/patient_education/cf001.cfm (accessed December 31, 2007).
36. Besty Bates, "Prenatal Screening Halves CF Births: Data from Large Screening Program," *OB.Gyn. News* 38, no. 24 (December 15, 2003): 1–2.
37. Andrews, "Conceptual Framework," 259 n. 291.
38. Thirty-six states and the District of Columbia either now require or are in the process of implementing mandatory newborn screening for CF. Cystic Fibrosis Foundation, "Newborn Screening," http://www.cff.org/AboutCF/Testing/NewbornScreening/#What_states_do_newborn_screening_for_CF? (accessed December 31, 2007).

The types of regulation, policy, and practice applied to syphilis and CF also differ in dramatic ways. Public policy enables and strongly promotes prevention of vertical transmission for syphilis, although when treated it can be a less serious disease than cystic fibrosis. However, policies emphasize parental choice for prevention of cystic fibrosis, although cystic fibrosis almost always results in a shortened lifespan for affected offspring. Thus past and present screening policies for syphilis can be characterized as preconception, prenatal, paternalistic, state mandated, universal, with presumed consent for tests and treatment, widely practiced, and effective. Screening policies for cystic fibrosis can in contrast be characterized as prenatal, postnatal, selective, and voluntary—except, most recently, for newborn testing. Cystic fibrosis screening stresses autonomous, informed, voluntary choices and neutral counseling; syphilis testing is, in effect, mandatory.

The history, professional cultures, and practices of clinicians who do genetic medicine and counseling are different from those who specialize in public health. However, there may be other, perhaps more morally relevant, reasons for the differences in policies. Prenatal testing for syphilis began in an era of paternalism, while screening for cystic fibrosis was not really possible until the advent of genetic diagnosis, already in an era of patient rights and autonomy. There is cheap, easy, effective treatment and prevention for syphilis that is beneficial to both pregnant woman and fetus—which invites universal testing. The nature of the prevention strategies for cystic fibrosis—they are both expensive and morally controversial, especially but not only abortion—may deter government mandates and the wide practice of voluntary testing. Because the chance of vertical transmission in the case of syphilis ranges from 40% to 100%[39] but in the case of cystic fibrosis is only 25%, this conceivably could diminish public pressure and personal preference for prevention, especially if the only preventive measures are avoidance of conception, selective conception via assisted reproductive technology, or abortion—choices that may be expensive or potentially violate strongly held personal or religious positions. The ethical question is whether these differences are great enough to justify the very great differences in policies that have been and remain in place.

Can the Differences be Justified?

The differences between screening practices for syphilis and for cystic fibrosis may rest entirely on historical or other explanations just considered. But we think that they are also morally different, although for reasons that are in part independent of the characteristics of infectious disease. To see this, it may be

---

39. J.F. Bale, "Congenital Infections," *Neurological Clinics of North America* 20, no. 4 (2002): 1039–1060.

helpful to begin with a standard set of six principles developed as guides to effective public health screening, and consider how they might apply to policies governing syphilis and cystic fibrosis. The principles are:

1. Goals are specified and achievable.
2. Natural history is known and intervention effective.
3. Screening tests are without high false positives or negatives.
4. Adequate diagnosis and treatment of true positives is possible.
5. Tests and interventions are acceptable to affected population.
6. Costs of case finding, diagnosis, and intervention are reasonable in relation to benefits and other programs.[40]

With respect to the first principle, the goal would seem to be prevention of congenital syphilis in infants. A seemingly similar goal is possible for cystic fibrosis, but achievable only through expensive and, to some, ethically troubling reproductive choices. For syphilis, the goal may be more specifically stated as the prevention of disease, or a known harm, in an existing fetus, which continues to develop until delivery. For cystic fibrosis, however, at present the achievable goal should be more precisely stated as the prevention not of harm to the fetus, but as prevention of conception or the development of affected fetuses, or more starkly, the prevention of birth of affected infants: it is simply not yet possible to have *this* child without cystic fibrosis.[41] These two goals thus are very different. In syphilis, the primary reason to screen is to prevent harm to a fetus. In cystic fibrosis, although screening may be offered to help parents in preparing for the birth of an affected offspring, the primary reason to screen prenatally is to prevent the birth of a child who has the condition. This different goal for CF is surely more controversial than preventing treatable infection in an identified individual.

With respect to principles two and three, the two disorders are quite similar; in each, the natural history is known, the intervention is effective, and screening tests are without unacceptably high false positives or negatives. However, with respect to principle four, there is adequate diagnosis of both disease and carrier states but while there is simple, cheap, and effective treatment for syphilis, there is less effective treatment for cystic fibrosis. Regarding principle five, the simple, cheap tests and interventions for syphilis do appear

---

40. Stoto, Almario, and McCormick, *Reducing the Odds*, 22–23.
41. For a discussion of what has come to be called the "non-identity" problem, see Jeff McMahan, *The Ethics of Killing* (New York: Oxford University Press, 2002), sec. 8.2. From an impersonal point of view, it may be better for a non-affected child to be born than for an affected child to be born. See, e.g., Laura Purdy, "Genetics and Reproductive Risk: Can Having Children Be Immoral?" in *Bioethics*, ed. Helga Kuhse and Peter Singer (Oxford: Blackwell, 1999), 123–129. From the point of view of an affected child, however, abortion cannot be better; the only alternative to being born with CF is not to be born at all.

to be quite acceptable to the general public and the affected populations. It is still difficult to say on a national level how acceptable the tests and interventions are for cystic fibrosis. However, although they were not asked specifically about syphilis or cystic fibrosis, in an Office of Technology Assessment survey over a decade ago, 83% of Americans said they would take a genetic test before having children, if it would tell them whether their children would likely inherit a fatal genetic disease.[42] In 1992 study of parents of affected children, most families knew that CF could be diagnosed prenatally; of those intending to have more children, 77% had had or were considering prenatal diagnosis. Forty-four percent said they would carry a fetus to term, 28% would abort, and 28% were undecided.[43]

With respect to principle six, case and carrier finding and intervention to prevent vertical transmission has been cost-effective for syphilis, but is, of course, prevalence dependent. Case and carrier finding for cystic fibrosis could be cost effective in the Caucasian population in the United States with its present carrier prevalence, if a significant proportion of informed parents chose strategies that avoid the birth of an affected infant or if it was beneficial for other reasons such as the development of effective and inexpensive treatments. Costs and effectiveness of available treatment are not the only moral considerations at stake, however, and it remains important to ensure that parents are not subtly coerced into testing or into reproductive strategies they would prefer not to undertake.

Thus, we see that with respect to these six principles guiding efficacy of public health screening, intervention strategies for syphilis and cystic fibrosis exhibit critical differences in their specifically achievable goals and the means used to achieve them. This could explain and perhaps justify the differences in public policies that address prevention of these two disorders. From a cost-containment and benefit/burden perspective, although the benefits of two strategies that both prevent the birth of affected infants may be similar, the burdens of preventive strategies for syphilis and cystic fibrosis, both perceived and actual, may nevertheless be quite different.

A second explanation for the difference in policies, not apparent from a reference to principles, is the time and social environment in which each policy was introduced. The period after World War II was a time when it was understandably easy to portray syphilis as the enemy, to laud penicillin as a magic bullet, and to rally public support for a sustained campaign to attack syphilis and to protect its potential victims, especially children. Medical decision making

42. National Institutes of Health, "Genetic Testing for Cystic Fibrosis," *NIH Consensus Statement Online* 15, no. 4 (April 14–16, 1997), http://consensus.nih.gov/1997/1997GeneticTestCysticFibrosis106html. htm (accessed January 1, 2008), 1–37.

43. D.C. Wertz S.R. Janes, J.M. Rosenfield, and R.W. Erbe, "Attitudes Toward the Prenatal Diagnosis of Cystic Fibrosis: Factors in Decision Making Among Affected Families," *American Journal of Human Genetics* 50, no. 5 (1992): 1077–1085 (1077).

at that time would now be described as paternalistic, where physicians generally decided what was best for their patients. It is perhaps no surprise that patients, and even couples about to marry, accepted a near universal mandatory
screening, treatment, and prenatal prevention approach. Currently, there are
widely available tools for carrier and fetal case detection for cystic fibrosis and
legal and biological ways to initiate or terminate pregnancy. These emerged
as medical paternalism was being challenged and displaced by civil rights,
consumers' rights, women's rights, gay rights, and patients' rights, as epito-
mized by the doctrine of informed consent and the current regard for patient
autonomy. Thus, these changes in the social environment, particularly emphasis on individual rights and choice, may be more important in explaining
different strategies than the fact that one type of vertical transmission is infectious and the other is genetic. Neither genetic disease nor infectious disease is
"exceptional"; rather, both the historical and the ethical explanations of differences relate to other factors, particularly ready access to treatment and the availability of methods for preventing transmission. Table 1 presents the contrasts
between syphilis and CF screening.

A Comparison with Prenatal HIV Testing

Until very recently, public health policy for prevention of HIV/AIDS, also a
vertically transmitted infectious disease, looked less like the accepted policy
for syphilis and more like the policy for cystic fibrosis. Despite an incidence of
HIV-infected newborns that rose as high as 2,000 per 100,000, much greater
than that for syphilis (10–100 per 100,000), at least until this writing at the end
of 2007 there was no required premarital or prenatal screening for HIV in the
United States. Indeed, legal requirements in some states such as proof of informed consent and counseling may present barriers for the introduction of
routine or opt out testing practices.[44]

Within the past 15 years, however, it has become clear that prenatal treatment of the pregnant woman can vastly reduce the likelihood of vertical
transmission of HIV.[45] By 2005, the number of HIV-infected infants in the
United States was as low as 111, one-third the number in 1994,[46] a decline

44. Catherine Haanssens, "Legal and Ethical Implications of Opt-Out HIV Testing," *Clinical Infectious Diseases* 45, suppl. 9 (2007): S232–S239. See also A. Saah, "The Epidemiology of HIV and
AIDS in Women," in *HIV, AIDS, and Childbearing,* ed. R.R. Faden and N.E. Kass (New York: Oxford
University Press, 1996), 9–11; and Centers for Disease Control and Prevention, "2002 National STD
Surveillance Report: STDs in Women and Infants," http://www.cdc.gov/std/stats02/women&inf.
htm (accessed January 1, 2008).
45. See, e.g., E. Groginsky, N. Bowdler, and J. Yankowitz, "Update on Vertical HIV Transmission,"
Journal of Reproductive Medicine 43, no. 8 (August 1998): 637–646.
46. U.S. Department of Health and Human Services, Health Resources and Services Administration, "Women's Health USA 2007: HIV in Pregnancy," (Rockville, MD: U.S. Department of Health

TABLE 1 Contrasts Between Syphilis and Cystic Fibrosis Screening

Syphilis	Cystic Fibrosis
Prenatal testing began in an era of paternalism.	Prenatal testing began in an era of autonomy.
There is inexpensive, effective treatment.	There is no preventive treatment for a conceived fetus.
Prevention of transmission is relatively easy.	Prevention of transmission currently involves reproductive strategies that can be expensive or ethically controversial, including avoidance of conception, adoption, selective conception via assisted reproductive technology, and abortion.
The chance of vertical transmission is high, although variable, between 40% and 100 %.	The chance of vertical transmission is 25%.
The goal of screening is to prevent harm to this particular fetus.	Screening may be used to prevent the birth of any affected fetus.
Case and carrier finding is inexpensive and cost effective.	Case and carrier finding could be cost effective if a significant proportion of informed parents chose strategies that avoided the birth of an affected fetus or there were associated benefits such as access to effective treatment. Costs of the test are high.

largely due to increased prophylaxis, treatment, and testing. In 2007, the CDC recommended a policy for routine screening for HIV of all pregnant women and treatment to prevent transmission. While all prior testing for HIV was voluntary ("opt in"), this new policy was presented as routine with an "opt out" option, and thus even so would not have been mandatory.[47] There may continue to be historical reasons for this difference—as we discussed in Chapter 4, HIV continues to be a disease where rights-advocacy shapes policy. And as we shall see in Chapter 12, the availability of effective treatment of HIV for the pregnant woman is also an important factor in assessing the ethical permissibility of any mandatory testing regime.

Conclusion

The observation that there is inconsistency between our treatment of vertically transmitted contagious disease and vertically transmitted genetic disease is descriptive. We have also suggested that there is a principled difference between

and Human Services, 2007), www.mchb.hrsa.gov/whusa_07/healthstatus/maternal/0330hp.htm (accessed January 1, 2008).

47. Centers for Disease Control and Prevention, "Revised Recommendations for HIV Testing of Adults, Adolescents, and Pregnant Women in Health-Care Settings," *Morbidity and Mortality Weekly Report* 55, no. RR14 (September 22, 2006): 1–17.

the two: once a child has been conceived, vertical transmission of genetic disease is currently avoidable only by the decision not to carry on with the pregnancy. With vertically transmitted contagious disease, however, there may be interventions that succeed in treating the child while continuing the pregnancy. Conflicts between the child and the pregnant woman may remain, however, if there are no treatments that will be beneficial to the mother, or if interventions that might benefit the child are potentially risky to the mother. It is at this point that our PVV perspective will come into play in the next chapter, emphasizing what is ethically required in treating the pregnant woman as victim and not only as vector in relation to the child she bears.

Ethical analyses that focus on reproductive liberty of the pregnant (or potentially pregnant) woman would question mandatory testing policies in either case; these are analyses that, in our terms, regard the pregnant woman principally as victim. Analyses that focus solely on the distribution of diseases within a population—that look at populations as a whole rather than individual victims or vectors—would consider instead the costs and efficacy of screening programs and would decide whether they should be mandatory in these terms. Analyses that focus principally on the pregnant woman as vector would consider what can be done to protect the fetus from transmission. In this chapter, we have argued that with contemporary medical technology, the crucial ethical difference between the cases of infectious and genetic transmission lies in what can ultimately be done to prevent transmission to the fetus, that party who would be the victim if transmission occurs. We have addressed specific cases in which effective treatment or means of avoiding birth of an affected child are available for the pregnant woman. In the next chapter, we will explore the permissibility of screening pregnant women for HIV when the only available interventions may be protective of the fetus but may bear particular social and medical risks for the mother, especially those living in developing countries.

12

SHOULD RAPID TESTS FOR HIV INFECTION
NOW BE MANDATORY DURING PREGNANCY OR
IN LABOR?

In the preceding chapter, we explored justifications for the traditional public health requirement that pregnant women be tested for syphilis, and for the contrast between such testing requirements and the regime of voluntary testing for vertical transmission of genetic disease. With respect to HIV/AIDS, by contrast, the voluntary testing regime prevailed until quite recently, because of the special status of HIV/AIDS as a stigmatized disease. In this chapter, we consider whether the current voluntary counseling and subsequent testing (VCT) with opt in consent policy that is used in most developing countries should be retained, or whether HIV testing for pregnant women should now be made routine in clinical practice or even legally required. We argue that "opt out" strategies are justifiable only when the pregnant woman has access to appropriate therapy.[1] Employing our PVV view, we focus in particular on the new rapid tests, now becoming available and in use in many developing world countries, especially when they are used with a pregnant woman who first presents for medical care when already in labor.

An earlier version of this chapter appeared as Charles B. Smith, Margaret P. Battin, Leslie P. Francis, Jay A. Jacobson, "Should Rapid Tests for HIV Infection Now Be Mandatory During Pregnancy? Global Differences in Scarcity and a Dilemma of Technological Advance." *Developing World Bioethics*, special issue on Reproductive Health Ethics: Latin American Perspectives, ed. Deborah Diniz, Florencia Luna, and Juan Guillermo Figueroa, August 2007, vol 7, no. 2: 86-103.

1. Some writers have reached similar conclusions, but their views have focused on testing in pregnancy in general, without particular reference to the type of testing employed or the moment in pregnancy when testing is employed. See Udo Schuklenk and Anita Kleinsmidt, "Rethinking Mandatory HIV Testing During Pregnancy in Areas with High HIV Prevalence Rates: Ethical and Policy Issues," *American Journal of Public Health* 97, no. 7 (July 2007): 1179–1183. McKenna was among the first to address the issue of whether testing pregnant women for HIV should be voluntary or mandatory. See J.J. McKenna, "Where Ignorance Is Not Bliss: A Proposal For Mandatory HIV Testing Of Pregnant Women," *Stanford Law and Policy Review* 7 (1996): 133-157. For a very recent discussion of the CDC's recommendation for opt-out HIV testing of pregnant women in the United States that explores the legal issues raised by the change and argues that opt-out testing is not ethically permissible without linkages to treatment, see Catherine Hanssens, "Legal and Ethical Implications of Opt-Out HIV Testing," *Clinical Infectious Diseases* 45, suppl. 4 (2007): S232–S239.

The basic principle of autonomy—recognized to at least some extent in virtually all cultures and countries—seems to speak for voluntary, not forced testing. But the dramatic changes in testing technology and the much-improved prospects for avoiding transmission of the AIDS virus to the newborn infant now present reasons for requiring testing of all pregnant women. With testing and treatment, the likelihood of an infected woman transmitting human immunodeficiency virus to her infant has dropped from one-third or more to almost zero, and has saved the lives of thousands of infants in the United States alone. Tests for HIV are now quite accurate, specific, sensitive, and can be used for anyone at any time. Some are *rapid*, which means that they bring the benefits of nearly immediate initial results, though positive tests still require confirmation. Thus, in the context of labor, they also raise the possibility of pressured, instantaneous decision making.

The benefits of universal HIV screening of pregnant women and subsequent appropriate treatment and prophylaxis are potentially great in many countries, and could be particularly great in developing countries where HIV infection is of high prevalence and health-care infrastructures are limited. In sub-Saharan Africa alone, as many as 700,000 children each year acquire HIV from their mothers during pregnancy, labor, or breast-feeding.[2] In many developing countries as well as in some sectors of developed countries, many pregnant women have their first contact with the health-care system as they are beginning labor. While the widespread or universal use of the rapid HIV test could greatly facilitate rapid diagnosis and implementation of successful therapy and prophylaxis in time to prevent literally hundreds of thousands of infant infections worldwide,[3] protection for the fetus and mother in terms of prophylaxis during pregnancy and continuing therapy is still very limited in many parts of the world. The 2006 UN Report on the global AIDS epidemic indicated that in 2005 only 20% of people with advanced HIV infection received antiviral therapy and, more disturbing in terms of missed opportunities, only 9% of HIV positive pregnant women received antiviral prophylaxis.[4]

---

2. Carolyn Barry, "The Breast Solution," *Science News* 172, no. 12 (September 22, 2007): 187.
3. Centers for Disease Control and Prevention, "Introduction of Routine HIV Testing in Prenatal Care—Botswana, 2004," *Morbidity and Mortality Weekly Report* 53, no. 46 (November 26, 2004): 1083–1086.
4. Joint United Nations Programme on HIV/AIDS, *2006 Report on the Global AIDS Epidemic*, http://www.unaids.org/en/KnowledgeCentre/HIVData/GlobalReport/default.asp (accessed January 1, 2008). The most recent update of the report, which contains more accurate assessments of the incidence of HIV, does not include new estimates of access to treatment. Joint United Nations Programme on HIV/AIDS, *AIDS Epidemic Update: December 2007*, http://data.unaids.org/pub/EPISlides/2007/2007_epiupdate_en.pdf (accessed January 1, 2008). For a general discussion of the ethical issues raised by limited access to antiretrovirals, see S. Rennie and F. Behets, "AIDS Care and Treatment in Sub-Saharan Africa: Implementation Ethics," *Hastings Center Report* 36, no. 3 (May-June 2006): 23–31.

As of 2007, the most recent figures were that about 28% of HIV-positive people in low and moderate income countries were receiving treatment, indicating slow but still unsatisfactory improvement.[5] Recent estimates of the percent of pregnant women receiving treatment in sub-Saharan Africa vary from 1% in Nigeria to 54% in Botswana, with 11% overall for sub-Saharan Africa. Even in Botswana, however, the gap between the percent of pregnant women receiving testing (almost 95%) and the percent receiving treatment (54%) remained significant.[6] Problems of access to HIV treatment among rural women in India are notable as well.[7] Brazil has been among the leaders in successfully addressing the HIV epidemic[8] with its policy of providing universal access to HIV drugs. Some South American countries such as Argentina and Venezuela provided such therapy to more than 80% of adults with advanced HIV infection, while rates of coverage were only 29% in Paraguay and 37% in Bolivia.

Because of these differences, as we shall show, whether HIV testing in pregnancy, including at the time of delivery, should remain optional or become what has been called "mandatory" is not just a question for physicians, public health officers, and patients in the United States, but a question for all countries. It is a question to be answered in the context of quite different circumstances around the globe. The move from "optional," "voluntary," or "elective" testing may be variously described as the move to "expected," "routine," "required," "mandatory," or "forced"—labels that suggest differing degrees of pressure on the pregnant woman, but that all convey that testing should be done on her. So-called mandatory policies might permit exceptions for severe emotional distress or for religious objections, for example, but public policies would all focus on having all or almost all pregnant women tested.

From our PVV perspective, it is crucial to recognize that a person with a communicable infectious disease is both victim and vector at the same time, a person who is both the recipient of infection from someone else, and a potential infector of another party. An ethically adequate policy in any context must recognize this fact—even in conditions of scarcity or extreme scarcity that make it impossible to satisfy fully our social, legal, and moral obligations to persons in both these roles. Policies mandating HIV testing in pregnant women typically treat the mother as vector and the child to whom she might

5. World Health Organization, *Towards Universal Access: Scaling up Priority HIV/AIDS Interventions in the Health Sector: Progress Report, April 2007* (Geneva: World Health Organization, 2007), http://www.who.int/hiv/mediacentre/universal_access_progress_report_en.pdf (accessed January 1, 2008), 5.

6. World Health Organization, *Towards Universal Access*, 32.

7. C. Chakraborti, "Ethics of Care and HIV: A Case for Rural Women in India," *Developing World Bioethics* 6 (2006):89–94.

8. S. Okie, "Fighting HIV—Lessons from Brazil," *New England Journal of Medicine* 354, no. 19 (May 11, 2006): 1977–1981.

transmit HIV as potential victim, but they sometimes neglect to see that the pregnant woman is also a victim, the recipient of HIV transmission from someone else, a person in medical need. An ethically adequate policy must see her in both these roles.

Controversies over Required Testing for HIV During Pregnancy

Required testing of pregnant women for HIV has a substantial history of controversy. Disputes flared in the United States in the early 1990s with the demonstration that although 30–40% of HIV-infected pregnant women would otherwise pass the infection that causes AIDS on to their newborn children during pregnancy, delivery, or nursing, AZT (zidovudine)—the first antiretroviral drug—offered the potential for preventing maternal/fetal transmission and possibly for controlling the infection in the great majority of cases. In 1994, a large study sponsored by the U.S. National Institutes of Health showed that treatment of HIV-positive pregnant women with oral AZT ante partum, a single dose of AZT intravenously intra partum, and subsequent treatment of the newborn with oral AZT for six weeks, dramatically reduced the acquisition of HIV infection in the newborn from 25% to 8%.[9] The CDC promptly issued national guidelines to physicians to offer voluntary HIV counseling and testing to all pregnant women and to inform them about the benefits of AZT prophylaxis.[10] Yet some public health officials and physicians in the United States and elsewhere argued that *mandatory* screening was necessary to reduce the frequency of transmission and to provide HIV-infected mothers and children the opportunity to receive appropriate care.[11]

However, patient activists and many bioethicists countered that mandatory HIV testing during pregnancy would be a violation of women's autonomy, including their rights to privacy, to confidentiality, and to make their own decisions about how to manage their pregnancy with HIV. These activists and theorists insisted that a voluntary approach to testing would be both more justifiable on ethical grounds and, as a matter of practice, more publicly acceptable.[12] As was the case with most public health policies during the first decade of the

9. Edward M. Connor et al., "Reduction of Maternal-Infant Transmission of Human Immunodeficiency Virus Type 1 with Zidovudine Treatment," *New England Journal of Medicine* 331, no. 18 (November 3, 1994): 1173–1180. Intravenous AZT is now administered continuously intra partum.

10. Centers for Disease Control and Prevention, *Rapid HIV-1 Antibody Testing during Labor and Delivery for Women of Unknown HIV Status: A Practical Guide and Model Protocol* (January 30, 2004), http://www.cdc.gov/hiv/topics/testing/resources/guidelines/rt-labor&delivery.htm (accessed January 1, 2008).

11. C.M. Wilfert, "Mandatory Screening of Pregnant Women for the Human Immunodeficiency Virus," *Clinical Infectious Diseases* 19 (1994): 664–666.

12. McKenna, "Where Ignorance Is Not Bliss."

AIDS epidemic in the United States and in most other countries, patient activists and others supporting an autonomy-based view prevailed, and public health policies for screening of pregnant women for HIV infection emphasized a voluntary approach. Women were to be free to choose whether to be tested or not.

Not all bioethicists worldwide agreed with this view or agreed that a policy of voluntary testing should be permanent. Some predicted that significant changes in the reliability of the testing procedure and in the potential for advanced antiretroviral drugs to prevent maternal/fetal transmission might strengthen the argument for more aggressive or mandatory testing. In 1991, Ruth Faden, Gail Geller, and Madison Powers[13] summarized the deliberations of a working group that assessed the medical and ethical issues surrounding maternal and fetal screening for HIV infection, and concluded that continuation of the voluntary approach to testing was the most appropriate policy—but that "our recommendations could change with advances in diagnostic technologies and medical management." Three years later in 1994, Ronald Bayer[14] argued for the supremacy of maternal rights and voluntary testing over mandatory testing programs, but also predicted that the ethical and political climate would "undoubtedly change" in response to greater evidence that therapy would dramatically extend the lives of HIV-infected women and their children. Two years after that, in 1996, Wilfert and McKenna each argued for mandatory HIV testing of all pregnant women, basing their arguments on the right of the pregnant woman to be aware of her HIV status and then to exercise her right to participate in medical decision making about her pregnancy and health-care options.[15] However, few recognized that this was an international issue and that it might look very different in different national contexts.

In the decade since the 1994 landmark study in the United States showing that maternal/fetal transmission could be reduced, additional studies have further demonstrated the potential benefits of more aggressive screening and therapy for HIV infection. With discovery of additional antiretroviral (ARV) medications, the use of multiple drug prophylaxis during pregnancy and delivery has further reduced the infection rate of newborns in the United States to less than 2%, and general voluntary application of HIV screening during pregnancy in the United States has reduced the yearly incidence of infected

---

13. Working Group on HIV Testing of Pregnant Women and Newborns, "HIV Infection, Pregnant Women, and Newborns: A Policy Proposal for Information and Testing," in *AIDS, Women and the Next Generation*, ed. R.R. Faden, G. Geller, M. Powers (New York: Oxford University Press, 1991), ch. 14 (331).

14. R. Bayer, "Ethical Challenges Posed by Zidovudine Treatment to Reduce Vertical Transmission of HIV," *New England Journal of Medicine* 331, no. 18 (November 3, 1994): 1223–1225.

15. Wilfert. "Mandatory Screening of Pregnant Women"; McKenna, "Where Ignorance Is Not Bliss."

newborns from several thousand to a few hundred in recent years.[16] As we have noted before, according to the 2006 UN Report on AIDS,[17] implementation of routine testing for HIV infection during pregnancy, either by the traditional or rapid techniques, and subsequent offering of preventive ARV therapy has been more slowly implemented by developing countries: in 2005 only 9% of HIV-positive pregnant women received preventive therapy. Nevertheless, the percentage of maternal to child transmission of HIV declined worldwide by more than 10% between 2001 and 2005.[18] These results are encouraging, but not good enough.

Advances in detecting and treating HIV infection during pregnancy achieved in the past 10 years have significant implications for the balance between voluntary and mandatory testing for HIV during pregnancy. A number of studies in both developed and undeveloped countries have clearly proven that diagnosing HIV infection during pregnancy, together with instituting single or multi-drug anti-ARV therapy, has been extremely successful in reducing the transmission of HIV to the fetus—even when the patient appears for the first time during labor.[19] Multiple ARV drug therapy to the mother and child during and immediately after labor can reduce the maternal to child transfer of HIV to less than 3%. However, in situations where adequate HIV therapy for the infected mother is not yet available, the social and medical costs of diagnosing HIV infection in the mother may greatly outweigh benefits to her. Thus while new techniques for rapid testing may make virtually immediate diagnosis possible, in ethical terms they may yield seemingly troubling results.[20]

This is a worldwide issue. The ethical challenge here is of greatest urgency not so much in the United States or other developed countries with ample resources for treating HIV infections, but in the poorer, less well funded countries around the globe—especially where current AIDS initiatives may be in fullest swing, in part because they are the areas in which rapid-test methods of

16. Roger Chou et al., "Prenatal Screening for HIV: A Review of the Evidence for the US Preventive Services Task Force," *Annals of Internal Medicine* 143, no. 1 (July 5, 2005): 38–54.
17. Joint United Nations Programme on HIV/AIDS, *2006 Report*.
18. Ibid.
19. Chou, "Prenatal Screening for HIV"; J. McIntyre, "Preventing Mother-to-Child Transmission of HIV: Successes and Failures," *BJOG: An International Journal of Obstetrics and Gynecology* 112, no. 9 (September 2005): 1196–1203.
20. A parallel phenomenon exists as HIV-infected mothers in some areas of the world face difficulty in their attempt to formula feed to avoid post-natal HIV transmission to their babies when replacement feeding is typically unsafe and stigmatized and breastfeeding is economically advantageous, biologically beneficial, and culturally appropriate. For an excellent discussion of these issues, see F. Fletcher, P. Ndebele, and M. Kelley, "To Nourish Her Young: Ethical Dilemmas Associated with HIV-Infected Mothers and Infant-Feeding," manuscript in progress; and Faith Fletcher and Paul Ndebele, "The Infant-Feeding Dilemma of an HIV-Infected Mother in Southern Africa," paper presented at the annual meeting of the American Society for Bioethics and Humanities, 2006.

diagnosis are best suited for field sites and are more likely than traditional ones to be in use. Yet it will also be an issue, as we will see, in the United States.

Rapid Testing for HIV: OraQuick and Other Tests

One of the great triumphs of modern medicine was the rapid identification in 1984 of the virus causing the AIDS syndrome, and only one year later, the development of a sensitive serologic test for HIV. This initial enzyme-linked immunoassay (ELISA) was highly sensitive, identifying more than 99% of HIV-positive sera, and it was very effective in excluding HIV infection from blood products in developed countries. Unfortunately, the ELISA test was not highly specific; that is, it had a relatively high rate of false positives, particularly when used in populations with a low prevalence of HIV, such as blood donors. The emotional trauma to blood donors and others who were falsely labeled as HIV positive soon led to the addition of the second, more specific Western Blot test to confirm HIV infection. This dual testing, using the initial screening ELISA test and then the subsequent Western Blot confirmation test, have remained the "gold standard" for HIV screening in the United States for the past 20 years. The dual testing system does have the disadvantage of relative slowness—a specimen needs to be sent to the lab, to be included in a batch run, and results returned, requiring a minimum of 24 hours for each test and a possible overall time of one to two weeks for results. The dual method also requires that tests be conducted in a relatively well-equipped and hence expensive laboratory, excluding field testing at the site of care. But the advantages of the traditional method are considerable: levels of sensitivity and specificity that exceed 99%, and in the United States, a federal quality control system that has maintained a high level of reliability.[21]

In the past few years, several new alternatives to the ELISA/Western Blot dual testing system have become available that have at least three substantial advantages: they provide very rapid results; they can be performed by clinical staff with minimal training; and they do not require expensive equipment, refrigeration, or a reliable power supply. The OraQuick rapid HIV antibody test, for example, is capable of using finger stick, whole blood, plasma, or oral fluids as test samples; the sample is mixed with test fluid, the testing dipstick device is inserted into the fluid, and no further laboratory processing or machinery is necessary. Speed of results is of particular significance: OraQuick's results are available after 20 minutes. The test can be performed by clinical or office staff after brief training and the results can be easily read. It is the OraQuick

---

21. There is some dispute concerning false positives with the OraQuick test. See A.A. Wright and I.T. Katz, "Home Testing for HIV," *New England Journal of Medicine* 354, no. 5 (February 2, 2006): 437–440.

test is 99.3% sensitive[22] for HIV-1 and 99.98% specific for whole blood samples, and nearly as specific using oral samples, 99.89%.[23] Current U.S. recommendations are that negative tests do not need to be confirmed; however, positive tests should be confirmed by the traditional dual ELISA/Western Blot method, or by use of a different approved rapid test.[24] The tests do not detect infections acquired within three to six months, because it takes that long for antibodies to appear in the blood, so retesting is recommended if there is a possibility of recent exposure.[25] A number of rapid tests for HIV are now commercially available;[26] all are of high specificity and sensitivity,[27] and many of these tests can be purchased through the WHO bulk purchasing program and are increasingly available in developing countries.

Although the new rapid tests were initially more expensive than the traditional tests, prices have lowered with increasing competition; for example, OraQuick test kits currently sell for $12 to $17 in the United States.[28] In developing countries in Africa and the Caribbean, where resources are often not available to set up expensive central laboratories, the rapid tests are now considerably less expensive and much more easily applied in rural clinics than the standard test.[29] To be sure, because the rapid tests are performed at multiple office sites, it is more difficult to maintain control of quality. This problem may grow as these tests become available over-the-counter to patients;[30] recent reports of false positives using the OraQuick test in some U.S. cities may have

22. LG Wesolowski, DA MacKellar, SN Facente et al. "Post-marketing surveillance of OraQuick whole blood and oral fluid rapid HIV testing," *AIDS* 20(12)(August 1, 2006): 1661–1666.
23. B.M. Branson, "Rapid Tests for HIV Antibody," *AIDS Reviews* 2 (2000): 76–83.
24. Centers for Disease Control and Prevention, "Notice to Readers: Approval of a New Rapid Test for HIV Antibody," *Morbidity and Mortality Weekly Report* 51, no. 46 (November 22, 2002): 1051–1052.
25. U.S. Food and Drug Administration, "OraQuick Rapid HIV-1 Antibody Test: Frequently Asked Questions (FAQs)," http://www.fda.gov/cber/faq/oraqckfaq.htm (accessed January 3, 2008).
26. Program for Appropriate Technology in Health (PATH), "Rapid Tests for HIV: Commercially Available Rapid Tests for HIV," http://www.rapid-diagnostics.org/rti-hiv-com.htm (accessed January 3, 2008).
27. World Health Organization, *HIV Assays: Operational Characteristics Report 14 / Simple/Rapid tests* (Geneva: World Health Organization, 2004), http://www.who.int/diagnostics_laboratory/publications/hiv_assays_rep_14.pdf (accessed January 3, 2008).
28. A.A. Wright and I.T. Katz, "Home Testing for HIV," *New England Journal of Medicine* 354, no. 5 (February 2, 2006): 437–440.
29. Centers for Disease Control and Prevention, "HIV Testing in Prenatal Care—Botswana"; C.J. Palmer et al., "Field Evaluation of the Determine Rapid Human Immunodeficiency Virus Diagnostic Test in Honduras and the Dominican Republic," *Journal of Clinical Microbiology* 37, no. 11 (November 1999): 3698–3700.
30. U.S. Food and Drug Administration, "Testing Yourself for HIV-1, the Virus That Causes AIDS," www.fda.gov/cber/infosheets/hiv-home2.htm (accessed January 3, 2008); see also Wright and Katz, "Home Testing for HIV."

been due to technical errors by poorly trained users.[31] Despite these problems, the rapid tests remain in general far more suitable for use in developing countries than the traditional dual tests.

Rapid Testing for Pregnant Women in Labor

Although arguments for making HIV testing routine or mandatory have often focused on special populations where prophylactic use of advanced ARV drugs would be effective in preventing new HIV infections—for instance, to identify the HIV status of potential source patients who may have infected health-care workers as a result of needle stick injuries, to identify the HIV status of sexual contacts in rape, or to recommend treatment after unexpected unprotected sexual encounters—routine or mandatory testing has been particularly vigorously advocated during pregnancy. As in the needlestick or rape cases, it can be argued, the potential transmittor cannot be allowed to refuse testing when the health and indeed life of the transmittee may be at stake, but this is particularly important when the transmittee is an infant otherwise unable to seek testing on its own. Thus, just as the development of rapid testing makes it possible to institute immediate ARV therapy for the needlestick or rape victim if the source tests positive, so rapid testing in pregnancy makes it possible to provide immediate preventative treatment for the child. It also makes it possible to avoid treatment if the source is negative—something especially important in conditions such as pregnancy, where risks and side effects may be substantial. Especially in high-prevalence areas, rapid tests thus may make it possible to make ideal clinical decisions virtually immediately—especially, as supporters stress, a decision that might save the child.

Rapid testing also has greater capacity than the dual method, it is argued, for bringing HIV-infected patients into the health-care system where they can be counseled and treated. Early trials of the rapid test have been conducted in screening of high-risk populations, such as visitors to hospital emergency rooms in neighborhoods with relatively high prevalence of HIV infection. In a demonstration project at four U.S. emergency room sites in 2002, 60% of patients accepted rapid testing and 98% received their results, a marked increase over the 70% who return after two weeks to receive results with traditional testing. Of those tested, 2.5% were new positives, and 80% of these were ultimately enrolled in HIV treatment and care programs.[32] These early successes using rapid testing have encouraged some public health officials in the United States to propose expanded screening programs of high-risk populations,

---

31. Wright and Katz. "Home Testing for HIV."
32. B.M. Branson, "Rapid HIV Testing: 2005 Update, Routine HIV Screening for Emergency Department Patients," www.cdc.gov/hiv/topics/testing/resources/slidesets/pdf/USCA_Branson. pdf (accessed January 3, 2008), slide no. 34.

while others have proposed or renewed proposals that HIV testing become a routine part of the health evaluation and care of the entire U.S. population.[33] This too has been seen to speak for routine or mandatory testing, when it would ensure that an HIV-infected mother seek care for herself and her child.

Pregnancy that has proceeded to labor offers a particularly compelling case for mandatory rapid testing. The standard tests for HIV that require more than 24 hours at a minimum to provide a result for each component, and often as long as two weeks for complete results, are not useful in screening women for HIV infection during labor. However, prevention studies in developing countries, where pregnant women commonly first present during labor, indicate that rapid testing combined with AZT and multiple ARV therapy during labor can be quite effective in reducing HIV transmission to the newborn.[34] The same is true in the United States. Although antenatal care is highly recommended and practiced for most pregnant women in the United States, a significant percent of women in poor neighborhoods and those without health-care insurance appear for the first time while in labor. In rural areas of developing countries, presentation for the first time during labor is even more common.

In a recent CDC-sponsored multicenter study in areas of high prevalence,[35] a rapid HIV test was offered to 5,700 women who first presented for care while in labor and who had not been previously tested for HIV. Eighty-four percent of these women consented to the rapid test, and results became available to the patient and provider an average of 66 minutes after consent. HIV infection was detected in 34 women, and 18 of these received ARV prophylaxis before delivery and within 33 minutes of receipt of the test result. All of the infants of HIV-infected mothers received ARV prophylaxis immediately after delivery, and only one infant was subsequently shown to have been infected during or immediately after delivery.

With such results, has the ethical situation concerning mandated HIV testing in pregnancy changed, or changed enough to justify a reversal of the policy? The experience of many countries speaks to this issue. Were Faden, Geller, and Powers, as well as Bayer, right, that the moment would come to move from a voluntary to a routine or mandatory testing policy, presumably everywhere that it is practically and politically feasible to do so, indeed, anywhere in the world? Is that moment here?

Our PVV view suggests that the answer is neither yes nor no. The reasons that support mandatory testing, as well as the concerns about it, apply differently

33. S.A. Bozzette, "Routine Screening for HIV Infection—Timely and Cost-Effective," *New England Journal of Medicine* 352, no. 6 (February 10, 2005): 620–621.
34. T.E. Taha et al., "Nevirapine and Zidovudine at Birth to Reduce Perinatal Transmission of HIV in an African Setting: A Randomized Controlled Trial," *Journal of the American Medical Association* 292, no. 2 (July 14, 2004): 202–209.
35. M. Bulterys et al., "Rapid HIV-1 Testing During Labor: A Multicenter Study," *Journal of the American Medical Association* 292, no. 2 (July 14, 2004): 219–223.

in situations in which the mother is at risk of harm than in situations in which the principal sequela of testing for her will be access to therapy. We think medical advances speak for routine or mandatory testing, ideally early in pregnancy (perhaps with exceptions for severe emotional distress or religious objection) in developed countries where adequate HIV treatment is available to both the mother and the child. However, the social and economic realities in many developing countries where access to adequate, ongoing HIV treatment is not currently available argue for a more flexible testing policy that still leaves the option of personal choice to refuse testing or therapy. This is for complex reasons of regard for the mother as victim, as we shall see. Moreover, it remains important to assure that women are not pressured into testing—a potential risk given the rapidity of the testing process. Above all, we recognize that the answer is not as simple as we might hope—not in the United States or anywhere else.

It is particularly important to see *why* HIV testing in pregnancy cannot ethically be made mandatory in many developing countries and in some situations in the United States as well, even when inexpensive, highly reliable, state-of-the-art rapid testing is already available. This is not simply a matter of scarcity of resources and the fact that adequate treatment may not be available; it is because of the way scarcity of resources in specific situations plays off the roles of transmittor and transmittee, vector and victim, of this potentially deadly infection.

Three Illustrative Cases

To help put the ethical question that is posed here in focus, and to show why it is not easy to answer questions about mandatory testing during pregnancy in a general way, consider three patients in three differing countries of the world—the United States, Kenya, and Peru.

Case 1. Anne: An American Woman Presenting Early in Pregnancy

> Anne was a 34-year-old married professional woman living in the United States, with one previous child, who visited her obstetrician in her 10th week of pregnancy. The obstetrician told her that his routine for all of his pregnant patients was to test for HIV infection. She expressed surprise that he would consider the possibility that she could be HIV infected and was anxious about the test. He indicated (in accord with current Centers for Disease Control policy) that she could opt out of having the test by signing a release form, but strongly encouraged her to have the test because it

was a routine test in his office. She expressed anxiety about waiting for test results, even the normal three days, and he then offered the possibility of rapid testing with results in twenty minutes. She agreed to the rapid test.

Half an hour later she was called back into the physician's office. With a distressed look on his face, the physician told her that the initial HIV test and confirmation using an alternative rapid test were positive and there was no doubt that she was infected with HIV. The physician immediately referred her to a professional HIV counselor who spent the next hour with the patient discussing the implications of this diagnosis for her and for her pregnancy. They discussed how to share this news with her husband, whether he might become abusive, the need for him to be tested, and the availability of further counseling for them as a couple to help deal with this frightening diagnosis. They discussed the option for an abortion, and the recent information that with current treatment with ARV drugs, the possibility of her delivering an infant infected with HIV has dropped to somewhere in the range of 1-2%.

Her husband also tested positive for HIV, and they began joint meetings with a counselor to discuss their options for managing her pregnancy and their infections. The significant issue that seemed to confront them was that of abortion, but after considerable reflection they concluded that they very much wanted to have the child, and were encouraged that with modern therapy with multiple ARV's they had a high likelihood of both being relatively healthy for the next 10 to 20 years so that they could provide for the child. They were both employed and had excellent health insurance that covered the costs of HIV treatment. Anne received multiple ARV therapy during the second half of her pregnancy, which greatly reduced her viral load and the chances that the virus would be transmitted during gestation, and the child received ARV therapy for several weeks after delivery. At one year of age the child was HIV antibody negative indicating that the virus had not been transmitted during or after pregnancy. Both parents were receiving state-of-the-art therapy for their infection, and were healthy and working.

Although rapid testing is not characteristically used in prenatal care, especially not while the patient is actually waiting, Anne's situation is representative of the circumstances of many pregnant women who live in countries with advanced health-care systems: she is fully insured, she is well informed about HIV and its impact on pregnancy, and she will have continuing access to ARV therapy.

Case 2. Bwita: A Kenyan Woman Presenting During Labor

*Bwita was a 20-year-old married Kenyan woman who
presented to a small rural obstetric clinic in active labor.
The clinic staff informed her that as part of a grant making
HIV prophylaxis available in some of the most threatened
areas of Africa, it had become possible to do a rapid HIV test for
women during pregnancy. She could opt out of this test, she was
told, but it was strongly recommended so the child might be
protected from acquiring HIV infection. Bwita was well aware
that the rates of HIV infection in this area of Kenya were extremely
high and that effective drug treatment had been generally
unavailable, but she was encouraged to think that there might be
treatment available for her child. Although she was in active labor
and distressed about the possibility of being HIV infected, she
agreed to the test.*

*A rapid test for HIV was performed and within 30 minutes of
her admission, the result was returned as positive. Bwita was told of
this result by a clinic nurse and advised that she could greatly
reduce the likelihood of transmission to her child during delivery if
she agreed to being immediately treated with an antiretroviral drug
and to having her child receive the same drug for several days after
delivery. She agreed to the immediate therapy for herself and for her
infant. The child was delivered healthy and remained so a year
later, a successful outcome.*

*Bwita herself, however, became increasingly symptomatic over
the next several months. In an effort to spread scarce AIDS-
prevention resources as widely as possible, the grant that had
been made available to the local clinic was funded—in accord
with current WHO recommendations—only for single-drug
antiretroviral therapy to prevent mother-to-child transmission
of HIV. This recommendation was considered affordable in a
situation of such scarcity—the Kenya government annual
per capita expenditure on health care is less than US$10—and
because it was cost-effective. Single-drug therapy is able to save
some 80%–90% of infants born to HIV-positive mothers. Bwita
could receive follow up with the same low-cost drug when she
developed AIDS, but the local clinic was not funded to treat
presymptomatic HIV-positive patients with multiple, high-cost
ARV drugs as would have been the case in a fully funded clinic
in a more prosperous nation. The child remained healthy, but no
therapy beyond the single drug she had been given during labor and
delivery was available for Bwita. Although such an outcome is less*

*common than was once thought and sometimes resolves on its own,
Bwita's virus had developed resistance to this single ARV
drug as a result of the brief exposure during delivery, and
her symptoms of AIDS did not improve when the single-drug
therapy was made available to her on an ongoing basis.
One year after her diagnosis, she developed overwhelming
pneumonia and died. Her family continued to care for her now
parentless infant.*

Bwita's situation is unfortunately representative of the situation in many countries where AIDS programs are being introduced but are as yet unable to provide adequate HIV therapy due to funding constraints and poor health-care delivery infrastructure. Indeed, this mismatch between diagnosis and treatment is typical of countries where efforts to control AIDS are at their highest pitch.

Case 3. Consuela: A Peruvian Woman Presenting During Labor

*Consuela was a 20-year-old married woman who lived in a small
village on the eastern slopes of the Andes in Peru, a village that can
only be reached on foot or on horseback. At the advice of the local
midwife, who sensed that the delivery might be difficult, Consuela
and her husband made the arduous trip to the regional clinic in a
town some 50 miles away in her 35th week of pregnancy and
presented in active labor. The clinic staff informed her that it was
their routine to do an HIV test on all women during pregnancy, and
that she could opt out of this test, but it was strongly recommended
so the child might be protected from acquiring HIV infection.
Although she was in active labor, extraordinarily tired from the
journey, and distressed about the possibility of being HIV infected,
she agreed to the test. The rapid test for HIV was performed and
within 30 minutes of her admission, the result was returned as
positive.*

*Consuela was told of this result by an HIV counselor at the
clinic and advised that she could greatly reduce the likelihood of
her child becoming infected with HIV during delivery if she
agreed to being immediately treated with an antiretroviral drug
and to having her child receive the same drug for several days
after delivery. Still in active labor and in increasing discomfort,*

she agreed to the immediate therapy for herself and for her
infant. Her husband agreed, but was too angry to allow
himself to be tested. A healthy child was delivered, and
subsequent testing revealed that the child had escaped
HIV infection.

However, no modern health care was available in Consuela's
village, and she had no way of obtaining antiretroviral drugs.
Indeed, she barely understood the nature of the virus for which
they had tested her or what they had done for her child. When
she shared the information that she was HIV positive with her
husband, he became physically violent, beat her repeatedly and
then left the home and their village—a perhaps not surprising
result in a country that leads the world in domestic violence.
Consuela's family allowed her and the baby to move into their
crowded dwelling, but she became something of a social pariah to
the other villagers, unfamiliar as they were with HIV. Although she
had received modern ARV therapy during delivery in the clinic,
she received no further treatment in her village. Over the next
year, she developed the symptoms of AIDS with weight loss and
recurrent infections. Two years after her diagnosis during delivery,
Consuela died.

Consuela's situation is representative of that of many women in remote areas of less developed countries, where HIV treatment is simply not available on an ongoing basis. Consuela's situation is not merely one of disadvantage under distributive scarcity, but one of complete lack of access to modern health care altogether—except for her single contact during delivery.

The Ethical Implications of "Routine" or "Mandatory" Testing During Pregnancy

In each of these illustrative cases, representing the varied situations in which pregnant women find themselves around the world, the health-care facilities in which Anne, Bwita, and Consuela are delivering their babies have policies of offering HIV screening utilizing a rapid test from which results are available in 30 minutes or less. In all three, the policy is quasi-mandatory; although the patient is told that she can opt out, doing the test is announced as "routine," the default option, or what she gets if she does not object. All are essentially pressured to consent, although two of the patients are already in labor and thus perhaps not in a position for careful reflection. In each of the three cases, the routine-test policy was effective in preventing transmission from mother to child.

The Case for "Routine" or "Mandatory" HIV Testing

The most common arguments supporting more aggressive HIV screening during pregnancy are based on the rights of the fetus to be protected from infection and on the interests of society to reduce the spread of HIV in the community,[36] the latter presumably applying to the mother more than the infant, who without treatment will die before reaching an age at which he or she would be likely to transmit the disease.

There are, however, other ethical arguments supporting more aggressive HIV testing during pregnancy. McKenna bases her argument on the right of the pregnant woman to be aware of her HIV status and then to exercise her right to participate in medical decision making about her pregnancy and health-care options.[37] As illustrated in our Case 1—Anne, an American who presents early in pregnancy—a diagnosis of HIV infection allows the woman to consider abortion, an option that would not be legally possible at a later date during gestation. McKenna argues that a truly informed decision regarding abortion can only be made when the woman knows her HIV status and is adequately informed about the options for managing her own infection and preventing HIV spread to the fetus. Some women might decide that even though the child has a 99% chance of avoiding infection, the burden of motherhood on top of managing her own HIV infection would be intolerable. Yet the desire to bear a child is a powerful force for many women, and the knowledge that early diagnosis and therapy can greatly increase the chances of delivering a healthy child may increase the likelihood of maintaining the pregnancy. Without this knowledge of her HIV status, the woman is denied the right to an informed choice about her options in managing her pregnancy. At the same time, Schuklenk and Kleinschmidt point out that the decision to test may not be truly voluntary unless the woman also has adequate access to abortion should she choose not to continue the pregnancy.[38]

However, information relevant to a decision about whether to continue a pregnancy is not relevant when a woman, like Bwita or Consuela, first presents in labor. Yet it is this very circumstance in which the case for routine or even required use of rapid testing seems to be strongest: when the use of ARVs to

---

36. Thomas R. Frieden, Moupali Das-Douglas, Scott E. Kellerman, and Kelly J. Henning, "Applying Public Health Principles to the HIV Epidemic," *New England Journal of Medicine* 353 (2005): 2397–2402.
37. McKenna, "Where Ignorance Is Not Bliss," n. 8.
38. See Schuklenk and Kleinsmidt, "Rethinking Mandatory HIV Testing."

prevent transmission to the child is urgent. But this is also the case when the possibilities for genuine consent are reduced—when the woman, already in the grip of labor, is in a much less favorable position for considered reflection and voluntary choice making. The pressure for a rapid decision, a rapid test, and rapid institution of therapy before delivery necessarily leads to reduced time for questioning and thoughtful decision making. The ability of a woman who is undergoing the pain and stress of active labor to process information about the rapid test and to make a contemplative decision must certainly be impaired.

These three cases involve something short of fully mandatory testing: they describe the common practice of "routine" use of rapid testing with the official "opt out" approach under which a person could refuse, but is unlikely to do so. The clinician simply says, "I am going to do an HIV test . . . do you have any questions?"[39] To be sure, this approach can in these circumstances be perceived to be coercive and to deny women the time or option to make an informed autonomous decision about testing. The traditional protocol used with the ELISA/Western Blot dual test required detailed counseling about the risks and benefits of testing before the test was offered, and while the current CDC protocol advocates limited counseling before use of the rapid test, this counseling may become less intense and detailed as it becomes a routine with opt out or a mandatory procedure.

The Case Against Routine or Mandatory HIV Testing

In opposition to routine or mandatory testing, others have argued that women should have the right not to know their test results.[40] Their arguments are based on observations in developing countries that, given the choice, as many as 30% of women who are tested by the traditional test fail to return for the results, indicating that many women choose not to know their test results when they are given several days or more to think about this decision.[41] In Chapter 8, when discussing such cases as XDR-TB in airline travel, we considered whether a person may have an obligation to know his or her infectivity status; here a similar issue recurs but in quite a different context. As in vertical transmission of infectious disease generally, including for example syphilis as well as HIV, only a single party—the infant—is likely to be infected, yet there

---

39. R. Bayer and A.L. Fairchild, "Changing the Paradigm for HIV Testing—The End of Exceptionalism," *New England Journal of Medicine* 355, no. 7 (August 17, 2006): 647–649.

40. M. Temmerman, J. Ndinya-Achola, J. Ambani, and P. Piot, "The Right Not to Know HIV-Test Results," *Lancet* 345, no. 8955 (April 15, 1995): 969–970.

41. K. Fylkesnes, A. Haworth, C.Rosensvard, and P.M. Kwapa, "HIV Counseling and Testing: Overemphasizing High Acceptance Rates a Threat to Confidentiality and the Right Not to Know," *AIDS* 13 (1999): 2469–2474.

remains an issue about whether the potential vector has an obligation to become aware of her risks of transmission, assuming testing is available, even though it may exacerbate her situation as victim. After all, even with extensive counseling, the realization that one is HIV infected can be intolerably traumatic, and it is not surprising that some women ultimately decide not to know their HIV status. While studies of suicide rates in HIV infected individuals suggest that an increased rate usually occurs in relation to increased physical symptoms and disability,[42] acute depression and suicide have been associated with learning of a positive HIV test.[43]

Other reasons for not wanting to be tested include fear of the responses of others who learn of a positive result. The potential for social and physical trauma to HIV infected women is particularly large in developing countries. Sociologists studying AIDS in Africa have demonstrated the unfortunate link between a diagnosis of HIV infection in women and subsequent physical abuse by the husband or sexual partner, often followed by abandonment of the woman by her husband and ostracism by the village.[44] A recent WHO study of sexual abuse and HIV infection in 11 countries showed that a prior history of an abusive sexual relationship was highly associated with risk of acquiring HIV. Incidence of such abusive relationships was highly variable, with the lowest rate of 13% found in Japan, while the highest rate of 61% was found in Peru.[45] It is understandable in this setting that many women would prefer to not have the HIV test or to know the result. Recently some rural HIV clinics in Kenya have added women's shelters to their services with the goal of protecting women from violence related to their newly discovered HIV status.[46] The increased risk of violence associated with diagnosis of HIV infection during pregnancy appears to be greater in developing than in developed countries. In one study of violence related to pregnancy in the United States, diagnosis of HIV infection during pregnancy was surprisingly associated with a significantly reduced rate of violence.[47] This fortunate trend in the United States suggests that the social sigma associated with HIV infection may decline over time with

42. F. Starace, "Suicidal Behavior in People Infected with Human Immunodeficiency Virus: A Literature Review," *International Journal of Social Psychiatry* 39 (1993): 64–70.

43. J. Leland, "U.S. Weighs Whether to Open an Era of Rapid H.I.V. Detection in the Home," *New York Times*, sec. A, November 5, 2005.

44. B.O. Ojikutu and V.E. Stone, "Women, Inequality, and the Burden of HIV," *New England Journal of Medicine* 352, no. 7 (February 17, 2005): 649–652.

45. L. Heise, "HIV Disclosure Holds No Added Risk," presented at Microbicides Conference, Cape Town, Africa, April 2006. Published in *The AIDS Reader*, June 2006: 289–290.

46. Charles B. Smith, personal report from Moi Teaching and Referral Hospital, Eldoret, Kenya.

47. L.J. Koenig et al., "Physical and Sexual Violence During Pregnancy and After Delivery: A Prospective Multistate Study of Women with or at Risk of HIV Infection," *American Journal of Public Health* 96, no. 6 (June 2006): 1052–1059.

effective education, better methods to guarantee confidentiality, and the gradual acceptance of HIV testing as a routine health procedure.

Still other arguments against routine or mandatory testing might include respecting the woman's right to refuse treatment for HIV, even if the test result is positive. In the case of tuberculosis, we have argued in Chapter 9, simple acceptance of such treatment refusals fails to do justice to the complexity of the patient's dual status as victim and vector. But perhaps differences in the mechanism of transmission—tuberculosis can be transmitted by a simple cough—warrant differences in approaches to treatment refusals in the two cases, although drawing this conclusion hastily still may fail to provide adequate protection against vectorhood.

Another common argument offered against mandatory testing for HIV infection has been concern that mandatory testing and reporting may have the unintended consequence of causing many patients in high-risk groups to avoid contact with the health-care system, effectively reducing the number of individuals diagnosed and treated for HIV.[48] The AIDS epidemic in the United States and most parts of the world has primarily affected disadvantaged groups and persons of color or minorities, groups that are likely to be more adversely affected by the stigma associated with HIV infection and who are more likely to distrust the public health system.[49] A decision analysis comparing mandatory with voluntary testing concluded that a deterrence rate of 0.5% would be associated with more infant deaths associated with failure to access the prenatal care system than infant deaths caused by failure to diagnose and treat HIV during pregnancy.[50] Experience in the United States with gradually increasing access to and movement toward routine opt out HIV testing programs has not demonstrated that a larger number of individuals are avoiding the health-care system.[51] Indeed, a recent study in Botswana of introduction of routine HIV testing in prenatal care indicated that the routine opt out approach led to an increase from 75% to 90% of women who were tested, and the number of women who came to the clinic after the routine testing was instituted actually increased from 114 to 130 per month.[52]

48. B.O. Taiwo et al., "Cost-Effectiveness of Screening for HIV," *New England Journal of Medicine* 352, no. 20 (May 19, 2005): 2137–2139.
49. J.M. Karon, P.L. Fleming, R.W. Steketee, and K.M. De Cock. "HIV in the United States at the Turn of the Century: An Epidemic in Transition," *American Journal of Public Health* 92, no. 7 (2001): 1060–1068.
50. Inaam A. Nakchband et al., "A Decision Analysis of Mandatory Compared with Voluntary HIV Testing in Pregnant Women," *Annals of Internal Medicine* 128, no. 9 (May 1, 1998): 760–767.
51. Rochelle P. Walensky et al., "Effective HIV Case Identification Through Routine HIV Screening at Urgent Care Centers in Massachusetts," *American Journal of Public Health* 95, no. 1 (January 2005): 71–73.
52. Centers for Disease Control and Prevention, "Introduction of Routine HIV Testing."

Could—and should—this voluntary regime of HIV testing now change, as is recommended? Should HIV testing during pregnancy become more like the syphilis testing during pregnancy we discussed in the preceding chapter—that is, required either by law or as a matter of routine medical practice—with the same intended result, the elimination of vertical transmission of a serious disease from mother to child?

HIV Treatment and Non-Treatment: The Risk of Resistance

The case for mandatory testing in pregnancy rests initially on the interests of the fetus; if diagnosis and treatment are timely, transmission to the child can in most cases be avoided. Protecting the interests of the offspring in being free of a life-threatening disease is of consummate moral importance. However, while the benefits of ARV therapy during pregnancy in preventing transmission of the virus to the child are obvious, concerns remain not only about the safety of these drugs for the pregnant woman and the fetus, but about her potential for development of resistance to ARV drugs. This is not a trivial matter; freeing the mother from the threat of a life-challenging disease is also of consummate moral importance, and this can only happen through the use of effective ARV drugs. For she is victim, too; she cannot simply be regarded as disease vector to the offspring she bears.

Although the issue remains controversial and is the subject of continuing research, initial studies in Africa showed that even a brief exposure of the HIV-infected woman to the single-drug nevirapine ARV therapy during late pregnancy and delivery may lead to development of resistance of the virus to this particular drug, with the effect that her options for effective therapy in her own illness may be reduced.[53] The use of a single dose of nevirapine to prevent maternal/fetal transmission does not jeopardize the possibilities for ARV treatment much later on, but if subsequent therapy is instituted in less than six months—often necessary for immediate treatment of a person discovered to be in an advanced stage of infection, as some women presenting for the first time while in labor are—the problem is much worse.[54] This unfortunate outcome was illustrated in our Case 2—of the Kenya woman, Bwita. Fortunately, more recent studies of dual or multi-drug regimens for prevention of HIV transmission during pregnancy indicate that the development of

---

53. Gonzague Jourdain et al., "Intrapartum Exposure to Nevirapine and Subsequent Maternal Responses to Nevirapine-Based Antiretroviral Therapy," *New England Journal of Medicine* 351, no. 3 (July 15, 2004): 229–240.

54. Shahin Lockman et al, "Response to Antiretroviral Therapy After a Single, Peripartum Dose of Nevirapine," *New England Journal of Medicine* 356, no. 2 (January 11, 2007): 135–147.

resistance is greatly reduced compared to single-drug therapy, and the protective effect on fetal transmission is increased.[55] The development of resistance after multi-drug intrapartum therapy is now regarded as a relatively minor problem in the developed world. However, where single-drug intrapartum therapy is still in use and reliable access to newly developed ARVs cannot be assured, the picture may be quite different. It is not just that funding for rapid test screening, ARVs, and the infrastructure necessary to conduct these programs in developing countries still lags far behind the need;[56] it is that women who receive single-drug ARV treatment during delivery may be worse off in their own prospects for combating the disease. The chance is increased that should they later receive treatment, it will be ineffective due to development of resistance, or that the least expensive and still commonly used single drug nevirapine may be toxic to the mother.[57] In addition, in developed countries where multi-drug therapy is common, toxicity of the newer protease inhibitor anti-HIV drugs may have adverse effects on the pregnancy by increasing the rate of pre-term deliveries.[58] These recent observations provide further need for the woman to be able to make an informed and autonomous decision about the benefits and risks of accepting less than optimal multi-drug ARV therapy to protect the newborn.

Nor is the possibility of single-drug therapy isolated or infrequent; indeed, some policies have had to acknowledge that limited resources may justify less than the best therapy. Although its policy could change now that a single-pill triple therapy dosing format has been approved in the United States, the UNAIDS/WHO, acknowledging that multiple drug prophylaxis was preferred, still noted that in resource poor settings single-drug therapy was associated with health benefits that outweighed the risks of resistance.[59] Such claims are of particular importance in countries with very limited health-care budgets. McKenna was emphatic in linking her demand for mandatory HIV testing during pregnancy with the obligation to provide appropriate therapy to those who test positive; in these developing-world conditions, this demand often

55. Chou et al., "Prenatal Screening for HIV"; McIntyre, "Preventing Mother-to-Child Transmission of HIV."

56. F. Dabis and E.R. Ekpini, "HIV-1/AIDS and Maternal and Child Health in Africa," *Lancet* 359 (2002): 2097–2104.

57. Chou et al., "Prenatal Screening for HIV."

58. R.E. Tuomala and S. Yawetz, "Protease Inhibitor Use During Pregnancy: Is there an Obstetrical Risk?" *Journal of Infectious Diseases* 193 (2006): 1191–1194.

59. Joint United Nations Programme on HIV/AIDS, *Call to Action: Towards an HIV-free and AIDS-free Generation, Prevention of Mother to Child Transmission (PMTCT) High Level Global Partners Forum, Abuja, Nigeria (2005)*, http://www.unfpa.org/upload/lib_pub_file/523_filename_abuja_call-to-action.pdf (accessed January 3, 2008).

goes unsatisfied. Brewer and Heymann[60] have pointed out that the difficulty in meeting the moral obligation to link increased testing with access to appropriate therapy is a critical ethical issue in implementing pregnancy screening programs in developing countries; but they overlook the particularly acute dilemma posed by the new technological possibility of rapid testing for women who do not present for medical care until already in labor—an altogether common situation in much of the developing world. Ideally, it should be the mother who decides, but the circumstances of labor and pressures of rapid testing diminish her ability to choose reflectively. Already in labor and, due to the new technology for rapid testing, discovering her HIV-positive diagnosis for the first time—in less than an hour after she presents—she can hardly be fully informed or in a position to consent or refuse any proposed treatment.

Furthermore, the interests of the infant are at stake as well, and are clearly better protected with mandatory testing requirements and subsequent treatment—regardless of the outcome for the mother. Thus the tradeoff begins to resemble a classic maternal/fetal conflict. However, this dilemma is not easy to resolve, in part because of the timing of the testing when it occurs during labor. But it is also unclear whether it is appropriate to describe the tradeoff as a maternal/*fetal* conflict or a conflict between mother and *infant*. If it is the former, conventional understandings of the relative standings of mother and fetus might apply, as in the usual construal of abortion: where the mother's life is at stake, the interests of the fetus may be submerged. If it is however a live-born child, the case is harder to decide. This tension is set up by the new possibility of rapid testing for HIV—something not possible in labor with earlier, slower dual testing—and because of this, ties even more closely into one of the deepest debates in bioethics.

The dilemma, however, is even more difficult because of the way it might have been settled in some accounts of more conventional bioethics: if the issue concerning a pregnant woman who presents in labor were understood as a maternal/*fetal* conflict, on some accounts it would follow that the woman was entitled to make her own choices: she may choose to favor herself, or choose to favor her forthcoming infant. Furthermore, at least under the usual canons of medical ethics, surrogate decision makers not familiar with her wishes would be morally obligated to decide in her interests. On other accounts, the nearness of the delivery or the potential viability of the child would weigh in the balance against the choices of the pregnant woman. In any case, once the child is delivered, surrogate decision makers would of course decide in favor of

---

60. T.F. Brewer and S.J. Heymann, "The Long Journey to Health Equity," *Journal of the American Medical Association* 292 (2004): 269–271.

treating the child, though this is less effective than treating the child together with the mother during the birth process itself.

Where later multi-drug ARV is assured for the mother, the dilemma between the antenatal health-related interests of the mother and the child is dissolved. But in the developing world, countries initiating aggressive HIV-control programs may be particularly likely to be in the position where the dilemma is acute: to stretch their HIV treatment funds as far as possible, they may end up treating the pregnant woman in the interests of the child but in a way that undercuts the interests of the woman herself.

The Uneven International Picture

Our test cases illustrate the wide differences in availability of adequate ARV therapy for HIV-infected women, and hence the different implications of mandatory testing for each of them. Case 1, Anne, reflects the availability of adequate ARV therapy for most persons in the United States. Case 2, Bwita, illustrates that even in a country where AIDS-prevention programs are being introduced, treatment that protects the child may in effect backfire for the mother. Case 3, Consuela, explores the plight of women who live in rural areas where modern health care is unavailable, but who nevertheless may have access to testing at delivery. Yet while we have been considering women who live in Africa or South America as representative of women who live in the developing world where universal treatment is often not available, such circumstances can also occur in wealthy countries like the United States. Even with an official policy of universal treatment coverage for HIV/AIDS, there are some individuals who slip through the safety net. Consider the case of yet another HIV-positive pregnant young woman:

Case 4. Dolores: A Mexican Woman Living as an Undocumented Immigrant in the United States, Presenting in Labor

> *Dolores was a 20-year-old unemployed married Mexican national who presented to an urban United States emergency room in her 35th week of pregnancy, in active labor. Although she was an undocumented immigrant in the United States, she was given obstetric care because she was in active labor. The clinic staff informed her that it was their routine to do an HIV test on all women during pregnancy, and that although she could opt out of this test it was strongly recommended so the child might be protected from acquiring HIV infection. Although she was in active labor and distressed both about her illegal status, fearing she might be reported*

*to the immigration authorities, and about the possibility of being
HIV infected, she agreed to the test. The rapid test for HIV was
performed and within 60 minutes of her admission, the result was
returned as positive. She was told of this result by an HIV counselor
and advised that she could greatly reduce the likelihood of her child
becoming infected with HIV during delivery if she agreed to being
immediately treated with an antiretroviral drug and to having her
child receive the same drug for several days after delivery. Still in
active labor and in increasing discomfort, she agreed to the
immediate therapy for herself and for her infant. A healthy child
was delivered. One year later the child was negative for antibody
to HIV.*

*Dolores herself, however, had a very difficult time over the
next year. She was not eligible for health care under any federal
or state program in the United States, and although she had
received ARV therapy during delivery, she received no further
treatment. Within the next six months she developed the symptoms
of AIDS with weight loss and recurrent infections. The local
clinic was not adequately funded to provide optimal multi-drug
therapy for undocumented immigrants and she was given the
same lowest cost HIV drug that she had received during the
delivery. Unfortunately, her virus had developed resistance to
this ARV drug as a result of the brief exposure during delivery,
and her symptoms of AIDS did not improve with this therapy.
One year after her diagnosis, she developed overwhelming
pneumonia and died.*

In 2005, Mexico provided coverage for only 71% of patients with advanced
HIV.[61] If Dolores had been diagnosed in her home country of Mexico, she
might well have received adequate therapy, at least if she received her care in a
large city such as Tijuana[62] and was eligible for Mexican Social Security. In a
remote rural area, her likelihood of receiving care would be much reduced.[63]
Depending on her location and specific situation had she remained in Mexico,
Dolores might have been in the same position as Consuela, in Case 3, who was
among the 48% of Peruvians with advanced disease for whom ARV therapy was
unavailable. Or she might have been in the position of Anne, in Case 1, with access

61. Joint United Nations Programme on HIV/AIDS, *2006 Report.*
62. R.M. Viani et al., "Perinatal HIV Counseling and Rapid Testing in Tijuana, Baja California,
Mexico: Seroprevalence and Correlates of HIV Infection," *Journal of Acquired Immune Deficiency
Syndromes* 41, no. 1 (January 1, 2006): 87–92.
63. C. Del Rio and J. Sepulveda, "AIDS in Mexico: Lessons Learned and Implications for Developing
Countries," *AIDS* 16 (2002): 1445–1457.

to full therapy like many in the United States. But emigration or displacement to another country has reduced Dolores's options for treatment dramatically, so that her situation may be more like that of Bwita than Consuela or Anne.

Do Rapid Testing and More Effective Therapy Speak for a Change in Testing Policy?

Does the new possibility of rapid testing, for instance with OraQuick—now cheap and available—speak for a change to mandatory testing? We believe that the answer to this question depends on the socio-economic setting, the prevalence of HIV, and the availability of health care for the women who test positive. In the United States, the encouraging results with rapid screening tests and with more effective ARV therapy during delivery and for both mother and child after delivery have appropriately moved the CDC to become more aggressive in its current recommendations for screening for HIV during pregnancy. For women who present early in pregnancy, the CDC now recommends routine testing by either the rapid or standard methods with the opt out approach. The CDC now also recommends the rapid test be used for HIV screening of pregnant women who initially appear during labor, and that this screening also be a routine procedure with an opt out approach. In this format a woman is informed that HIV screening is routinely done during labor if her HIV status is unknown, but that she has the right to decline testing. While moving toward making HIV testing during pregnancy a routine with the opt out option, the CDC clearly is moving toward implementing mandatory testing in pregnant women.[64]

We agree with the appropriateness of this more aggressive screening policy for pregnant women in the United States who are in the same socio-economic position as our first patient, Anne. She had adequate health insurance and was assured that she would receive appropriate follow up care and the current most recommended ARV therapy. The benefits both to Anne and to her child of testing and therapy far outweighed the risks. This approach thus respects both Anne and her child as victims—as well as reducing the risk that Anne will become a vector. Moreover, as testing becomes more routine, the population as a whole will likely benefit from a decrease in the stigmatization related to HIV testing; identifying a higher percentage of HIV-infected individuals will lead to better control of the spread of the HIV epidemic. Similarly, routine screening for HIV infection during pregnancy should be the policy in other wealthy countries, such as those in most of Europe, where access to adequate therapy is provided to all citizens. Bayer and Fairchild, reassessing the

---

64. Centers for Disease Control and Prevention, "Revised Recommendation for HIV Testing in Adults, Adolescents, and Pregnant Women in Health-Care Settings," *Morbidity and Mortality Weekly Report* 55, no. RR14 (September 22, 2006): 1–17.

issue of personal versus public rights in HIV testing in the United States, imply that an end to HIV exceptionalism, which has recently been proposed by the CDC, can now be better justified in light of improved testing and therapy benefits.[65] When adequate therapy is available, the health-related interests of pregnant woman and child are aligned, although the mother might have other reasons such as religious beliefs for refusing testing.

Thus where therapy is available, the case for requiring testing is strongest. But even in such circumstances it remains important to separate out the rapidity of the test from pressures to undergo it. There is a risk that the immediacy of the test will generate immediate pressures to have it. But informed consent requires that in non-emergent situations the woman should have the opportunity to have the test and its consequences explained to her, so that if she has reasons that would warrant refusal, she has adequate opportunity to voice them and to make sure that they are explored with her. Otherwise, she may be put at risk of abuse or other losses; respect for her as a victim requires protecting her against these.

However, as illustrated by our Case 2 of Bwita, not all pregnant women are as fortunate as Anne in receiving the full benefits of timely HIV diagnosis during pregnancy. In fact, some may be exposed to greater risk in the management of their HIV infection as a result of inadequate single-drug treatment during labor followed by inadequate treatment—albeit treatment—later on. This can happen in Kenya; it can also happen in the United States where AIDS clinics are inadequately or erratically funded, as was Delores's case, Case 4. More broadly, Case 3, Consuela, illustrates the unfortunate socioeconomic situation for most HIV infected women worldwide. With the prominent exception of Brazil, a relatively advanced developing country, a significant percentage of pregnant women in most developing countries do not currently have access to adequate multi-drug ARV therapy for mother and child during delivery or for the course of their HIV illness. In addition, in many developing countries, the stigma and violence associated with a woman's diagnosis of HIV is such that some women decide they are better off not knowing their HIV status. In such circumstances, testing disserves the mother's health-related interests. This conflict provides a reason to support the current voluntary counseling and subsequent testing with opt in consent policy that is used in most developing countries—a reason that would be obviated by the availability of treatment.

Case 4, Dolores, represents the additional plight of women in transnational circumstances—women who might have received continuing therapy in their home countries, but because of displacement, migration, refugee status,

---

65. Bayer and Fairchild, "Changing the Paradigm for HIV Testing."

or for other reasons find themselves in circumstances where they have little or no access to continuing care.

Because they are asked for consent to testing while already in active labor, it is doubtful that Bwita, Consuela, or Dolores could have made a fully informed, reflective decision about whether to receive testing. But inadequate consent, or no consent at all, is not the only reason why mandatory testing would be problematic. After all, presumed consent is accepted in many sorts of emergency settings, and here, because Bwita, Consuela, and Dolores have presented so late in pregnancy, the situation is an "emergency" for their infants. What is problematic is that the decision they are asked to make may be an unfortunate one for themselves. Were testing mandatory, it would favor Anne and all four of the children, but it might come at a serious cost to Bwita, Consuela, and Dolores. Although it is true that a diagnosis of HIV infection was necessary for any of these women to subsequently receive ARV therapy, as Anne and Bwita did, and that their prognosis would have been worse if their infection were not diagnosed until they developed symptomatic AIDS, the social costs of this diagnosis in their particular cultures and the potential adverse effects of inadequate or absent therapy may lead to a net adverse outcome. Furthermore, this dilemma is still worse in the countries where the incidence of HIV is highest—that is, in countries where a pregnant woman has the highest likelihood of already being HIV positive, but where the likelihood of receiving ongoing, lifelong, effective ARV treatment is lowest—that is, in the most underfunded, resource-poor countries. Thus the moral dilemma is most acute in the most health-troubled nations, a product it might be said, of partial but not complete success in the global effort against AIDS.

It is a violation of basic justice to impose policies that make some better off but others substantially worse, at least without a justification for so doing. When mandatory policies cannot be accompanied by treatment, they make patients who are vectors worse off as victims, without the potential benefits of effective therapy. Thus mandatory policies cannot be recommended without substantial misgivings. The initial rationale for considering whether it is time to move from voluntary, opt in testing for HIV in pregnancy to routine, required testing for all pregnant women involved showing that, particularly with the high-reliability rapid tests now available, both parties affected would be better off: the mother would receive earlier and effective treatment for her infection and the child's risk of infection at birth would drop dramatically lower. That is not, however, always the case. The problem of mandatory HIV testing in pregnancy when adequate health care is unavailable is a problem of what has been called "partial compliance" theory,[66] of what justice requires in circumstances of injustice; it is not a problem of what justice might ideally require.

---

66. John Rawls, *A Theory of Justice* (Cambridge: Harvard University Press, 1971), 218–219.

The link between society's decision to mandate HIV testing for pregnant women and society's obligation to guarantee that the HIV-positive woman has access to ARVs and appropriate medical care, made forcefully by McKenna, is crucial here. For the most part, private, federal, and state funding for HIV clinics and programs has provided adequate funding for HIV-infected U.S. citizens, whether under private health insurance, Medicaid or Medicare, or other public programs, especially the Ryan White legislation that funds AIDS care programs, though funding under the latter has not always been sufficient in recent years. People with HIV in the United States in general get treatment, counseling, and other components of care, whether insured or uninsured, and up through 2005 Ryan White federal funds of over $2 billion were generally adequate to cover every U.S. citizen.[67] However, the Ryan White Fund now finds its resources running short; in some places in the United States care is marginal or cannot be offered to all.[68] Furthermore, funding for care for un- documented immigrants in the United States is currently neither adequate nor secure, and subject to strong political pressures as well as regional variability.

For these reasons, we believe that U.S. policy, like that in the developing world, should be flexible in considering the social circumstances of women and availability of follow up care before routine testing and intrapartum treat- ment is applied—that is, it should be flexible in the light of whether a societal obligation to treat can actually be met. For women—such as Consuela, living in a remote village in Peru, or Dolores, a frightened undocumented immigrant hesitant to approach the health-care system—who are unlikely to have access to adequate ARV therapy and medical follow up, extensive counseling and ed- ucation should be provided regarding the potential benefits to the mother and child balanced with realistic discussion of the likelihood and hazards to the mother of inadequate or completely absent therapy. Of course, this is a pious and unrealizable hope if she does not present until already in labor and remains in such jeopardized circumstances.

Ultimately, the success of most public health measures to control conta- gious diseases depends on the maintenance of a high level of trust between the public and public health and government officials who develop and manage control programs; but trust cannot be maintained if it makes some people worse off. The volunteerism approach originally negotiated between AIDS activists and public health officials in the United States has proven to be a compromise

---

67. U.S. Department of Health and Human Services, Health Resources and Services Administra- tion, HIV/AIDS Bureau, "The 2006 Ryan White CARE Act Progress Report," http://hab.hrsa.gov/ publications/careactreport06/careacttoday.htm (accessed January 3, 2008).

68. National Health Policy Forum, "Caring for 'Ryan White': The Fundamentals of HIV/AIDS Treatment Policy," (August 22, 2005), http://nhpf.ags.com/pdfs_bp/BP_RyanWhite_08-22-05.pdf (accessed February 12, 2008); see also Infectious Diseases Society of America, "President's FY 2009 Budget Will Leave Many Infectious Diseases Programs in Shock," http://www.idsociety.org/Con- tent.aspx?id=9772 (accessed February 12, 2008).

that has successfully maintained public trust in the system. The concern we are raising is that a mandatory program for testing all women for HIV during pregnancy, anywhere in the world, would threaten whatever public trust is available because of threats to women's autonomous rights to make decisions about their own health care and that of their offspring in situations in which the interests of some are advanced at the expense of others. Such conflicts between health-related interests would be far less frequent were fully adequate, continuing treatment for HIV available to all. We reluctantly recognize that it is, unfortunately, still not the case that full care is available for all who need it, not only in many developing countries but also in the United States. We also recognize that social issues like spousal abuse may not be resolved by access to adequate treatment.

However, we are encouraged by the latest UN Report on AIDS that in almost all of the more than 150 countries studied, the availability of adequate ARV drug therapy for the mother and the infant is gradually increasing because of steadily increasing funding from wealthy countries and non-governmental agencies, and because of better management of available funds in developing countries. In particular, better-funded multi-drug programs are replacing single-drug programs. These multi-drug programs are less likely to allow the development of resistance in the six months after treatment in labor, and hence to risk making new mothers worse off even as their babies are protected. We look forward to the day when there will be universal access to adequate therapy, and our discussion will no longer be relevant. Before this day, however, universal mandatory testing for HIV in pregnancy remains premature, as there remain circumstances in which consideration for the pregnant woman as victim is inadequate.

13

ANTIMICROBIAL RESISTANCE

In the preceding chapter, we have explored the problem of vertical transmission of infectious disease from the perspective of the pregnant woman as both vector and victim. In this chapter and the next, we take up aspects of patient management that raise specific questions of victimhood and vectorhood: resistance to antimicrobials and then immunization policy. We argue that that these issues have in the main been viewed myopically, with the patient seen from one perspective or the other, but rarely both. With antimicrobial resistance, the problem is more often one of seeing the patient as victim in an overly simple way, so that efforts to curb the development of resistance are regarded as restrictions on good treatment for that patient in order to preserve useful drugs for other future patients. This is not to say that optimal treatment of the patient should be ignored in order to avoid the development of resistance, but it is to say that we need to rethink what such optimal treatment might be—a story with considerable ethical complexity.

Antimicrobial Resistance: An Overview of the Issues

Antimicrobial[1] resistance occurs when an organism that was once susceptible to a given chemical begins to change in a way that reduces or eliminates the responsiveness of the organism to the chemical.[2] Resistance is a natural and recurrent phenomenon: when organisms that are sensitive to an antimicrobial

---

1. In this chapter we will generally use the broad term "antimicrobial" because it includes the more organism-specific terms antibacterial, antiviral, antifungal etc. The term "antibiotic" specifically refers to an antimicrobial that is found in nature and produced by one type of microbe to inhibit others, such as penicillin or streptomycin. Because "antibiotic" is frequently used by non-scientists to refer to a variety of antimicrobials, it is often found in the literature, and we may on occasion use it in our text.

2. For descriptions of the phenomenon of antimicrobial resistance see, e.g., the websites of the World Health Organization, "Drug Resistance," http://www.who.int/topics/drug_resistance/en/ (accessed January 3, 2008), and of the Centers for Disease Control and Prevention, "Get Smart: Know When Antibiotics Work," http://www.cdc.gov/drugresistance/community/faqs.htm#1 (accessed January 3, 2008).

die out, organisms that are not sensitive continue to replicate, passing on their resistant genetic makeup in the process. Because of their ability to pass on resistance genes to other related populations through a process of conjugation whereby plasmids carrying the genes jump organisms, bacteria are especially efficient at enhancing the effects of resistance.[3]

The problem of antimicrobial resistance is serious, immediate, multifaceted, and worldwide. Resistance results in diseases that are more difficult and expensive to treat and that are concomitantly more likely to be passed along as infections persist in their victims. The World Health Organization (WHO) predicts the doomsday of a "post antibiotic" world for some diseases, a world in which resistance has evolved to the extent that no forms of treatment are available. As Selgelid describes the U.S. Office of Technology Assessment's fear, this will result in "plunging humanity back into the conditions that existed in the pre-antibiotic age."[4]

In a report published in 2000, the WHO described in chilling detail the history and prospects for antimicrobial resistance. Shortly after the development in the mid-twentieth century of penicillin, an antibiotic effective against bacteria such as streptococcus and staphylococcus, resistant forms of these bacteria were identified.[5] In the United States in the early years of the twenty-first century, an estimate is that there are nearly 19,000 deaths annually from methicillin resistant staphylococcus aureus (MRSA) and nearly 100,000 cases annually of serious infection.[6] One study of staphylococcus aureus infections occurring while patients are hospitalized reported nearly half involving methicillin-resistant organisms—and significant increases in mortality, morbidity, and hospital costs among these patients.[7] The U.S. Centers for Disease Control and Prevention estimate that about 70% of the agents that cause infections among hospitalized patients are resistant to one or more of the drugs used to treat them.[8]

3. World Health Organization, *World Health Organization Report on Infectious Diseases 2000: Overcoming Antimicrobial Resistance*, http://www.who.int/infectious-disease-report/2000/index.html (accessed January 3, 2008), ch. 3; World Health Organization, "Antimicrobial Resistance," Fact Sheet No. 194 (January 2002), http://www.who.int/mediacentre/factsheets/fs194/en/ (accessed January 3, 2008).
4. Michael J. Selgelid, "Ethics and Drug Resistance," *Bioethics* 21, no. 4 (May 2007): 218–229, citing U.S. Congress, Office of Technology Assessment, *Impacts of Antibiotic-Resistant Bacteria*, OTA-H-629 (Washington, DC: Government Printing Office, 1995), 39.
5. World Health Organization, *Overcoming Antimicrobial Resistance*, ch. 3.
6. R.M. Klevens et al., "Invasive Methicillin-Resistant Staphylococcus Aureus Infections in the United States," *Journal of the American Medical Association* 298, no. 15 (October 17, 2007): 1763–1771.
7. J.J. Engemann et al., "Adverse Clinical and Economic Outcomes Attributable to Methicillin Resistance Among Patients with Staphylococcus Aureus Surgical Site Infection," *Clinical Infectious Diseases* 36, no. 5 (March 1, 2003): 592–598.
8. U.S. Food and Drug Administration, "Facts About Antibiotic Resistance," http://www.fda.gov/oc/opacom/hottopics/antiresist_facts.html (accessed January 3, 2008).

Worldwide, diseases where resistance has become a significant barrier to treatment include tuberculosis, penicillin-resistant pneumococci, enterococcus, cholera, gonorrhea, and the parasitics leishmaniasis and malaria.[9] Typhoid has become resistant to the first line drug chloramphenicol. Shigella dysentery, a diarrheal disease rampant in developing countries, is resistant to the first-line inexpensive antimicrobial co-trimoxazole and is expected to soon become resistant to the more expensive ciprofloxacin.[10] In addition, viruses also can become resistant to antimicrobials—for example, the HIV virus shows remarkable ability to rapidly develop resistance to newly developed drugs. Among the multifaceted causes of resistance, some involve alleged "overuse" in the sense that the antibiotic is being used carelessly, when it will not achieve its intended goal, or when the goal could be achieved in other ways, with little or no cost or effectiveness advantage. Others involve apparent tradeoffs among goals: cheap food, environmental preservation, or human health, to portray some of the goals in the balance very broadly. Still others—which will be the main focus of this chapter—involve decisions about whether to use antibiotics when they may prove effective in the short term for patient care, but may also contribute to the development of overall patterns of resistance: these are the ethically most challenging cases.

One cause of resistance, the extensive use of antibiotics in animal husbandry, is beyond the scope of a discussion of the ethics of infectious disease in health care, but is important nonetheless. The WHO estimates that half of all antibiotic use in the United States and Europe is in agriculture.[11] Significant resistance in food-borne pathogens such as campylobacter or salmonella can be attributed to widespread agricultural use of antibiotics. In response, in 2005 the U.S. Food and Drug Administration ordered that poultry farmers cease using the fluoroquinolone Baytril because of the development of resistant strains of *Campylobacter* bacteria in the intestinal tracts of chickens, bacteria that could then be passed on to humans in imperfectly cooked poultry.[12]

Another factor outside the realm of health care is the use of antimicrobials in ordinary cleaning products in widespread use in the United States, Europe, Japan, and other developed countries. Anti-bacterial soaps, hand wipes, and cleansers have become household staples—almost to the extent that people are thought to

9. World Health Organization, *Overcoming Antibiotic Resistance*, ch. 3.
10. Ibid., ch. 4.
11. World Health Organization, "Use of Antimicrobials Outside Human Medicine and Resultant Antimicrobial Resistance in Humans," Fact Sheet No. 268 (January 2002), http://www.who.int/mediacentre/factsheets/fs268/en/ (accessed January 3, 2008).
12. See, e.g., U.S. Food and Drug Administration, "FDA Announces Final Decision About Veterinary Medicine," news release (July 28, 2005), http://www.fda.gov/bbs/topics/news/2005/new01212.html (accessed January 3, 2008); P. Collignon and F.J. Angulo, "Fluoroquinolone-Resistant *Escherichia Coli*: Food for Thought," *Journal of Infectious Diseases* 194, no. 1 (July 1, 2006): 8–10.

be unwise or even dirty if such products are not in plain view in their homes or offices. These products that contain triclosan, however, may inhibit bacterial growth in a way that leaves more resistant bacteria behind to continue to grow.[13]

Within health care, one factor implicated in resistance is the failure of follow through on treatment regimens. According to the WHO, underuse of antimicrobials is, ironically, as much of a contributor to resistance as overuse.[14] Underuse may be a failure of patients, of physician knowledge about how to use antibiotics, of education about the need to complete courses of treatment, or of social or economic circumstances that make full courses of treatment radically difficult for patients or for their providers. In portraying the dying tuberculosis patient in Chapter 9, we have pointed out how concern for the patient as victim may help in suggesting supportive strategies that are both ethically required and more likely to be successful in avoiding resistance that is attributable to inadequate compliance and follow through with treatment. With these supportive services, we have argued, directly observed, mandated therapy is permissible in light of the patient's dual status. In Chapter 12, we discussed the complex choices facing HIV-positive pregnant women when optimal treatment for HIV is unavailable. Short term antiviral use in the immediate period before delivery reduces the risk of HIV transmission to the fetus, but may increase the possibility for the development of resistant disease in the mother, a problem both for her and for those to whom she might later pass on resistant disease. As better HIV treatment becomes available, this problem may be alleviated correspondingly, but the fact remains that in impoverished areas of the world inadequate and partial access to optimal therapy is a leading contributor to antimicrobial resistance, both for HIV and for other diseases.[15]

Yet another factor in resistance is the behavior of health-care providers. A failure of simple protective measures such as hand washing has been implicated in the transmission of methicillin resistant staphylococcus aureus among hospitalized patients, for example. Hospitalized patients—already weakened and proximate to infectious agents, are a major source of disease spread; hand washing alone could reduce transmission of resistant disease. These measures, we have argued in Chapter 8, are required as part of standard good care to patients. This is perhaps a moral "no brainer": there are no risks and little costs or inconvenience to hand washing—but potentially of great benefit.

Another contributing factor in antimicrobial resistance—physicians' deference to patients' requests for therapeutically inappropriate medications—might be viewed in similar terms. Antimicrobial prescriptions that will not be effective

---

13. See Tara Parker-Pope, "Germ Fighters May Lead to Hardier Germs," *New York Times*, sec. D, October 30, 2007.
14. World Health Organization, "Antimicrobial Resistance."
15. World Health Organization, *Overcoming Antibiotic Resistance*, ch. 3.

against the patient's likely infectious agent—as in a prescription of the antibacterial amoxicillin against a viral infection—are not medical care that benefits the patient. The care is, in medical terms, "not indicated." Efforts to educate both physicians and patients about the importance of avoiding this kind of antibiotic overuse have been partially effective in recent years.[16] In terms of benefits to patients, avoiding such overuse is as much of a "no brainer" as hand washing—but more difficult to achieve in light of advertising and pressures from patients. Research has also scrutinized whether evidence supports the efficacy of some common clinical uses of antibiotics, such as a recent study questioning the use of antibiotics for treatment of acute maxillary sinusitis.[17] But these factors in the development of antibiotic resistance are the easy ones, for they do not represent tradeoffs between good treatment of patients and preservation of valuable antimicrobials for other patients at a later point in time. With hand washing, more appropriate use of antimicrobials, and even directly observed therapy, some of the causes of resistance could be reduced or even eliminated without compromising patient care in any significant way.

But not all of the factors in resistance are so simple. What of cases in which antimicrobial use is beneficial to *this* patient, *now*, but potentially contributes to the overall pattern of the development of resistance? These are the most difficult cases of resistance, and they are our topic in the remainder of this chapter. The standard way to view these cases is as posing a conflict between patients' immediate needs and more long-range concerns that valuable anti-infective agents will gradually lose effectiveness. To the contrary, we believe that our PVV perspective can be used to show that this conflict rests on a partial view of the patient as victim.

Antimicrobial Resistance: Treating *This* Patient Versus Saving Valuable Drugs for Later

Consider some garden-variety, everyday examples for physicians practicing in the developed world today.

Junior's Possible Strep

Junior is brought to the pediatrician by his mother. He is clearly uncomfortable, feverish, and complains of a bad sore throat. The physician performs a rapid test for strep, and the results are negative. Junior's exam is consistent

---

16. See, e.g., Centers for Disease Control and Prevention, *Public Health Action Plan to Combat Antibiotic Resistance: Antimicrobial Resistance Interagency Task Force 2001 Annual Report*, http://www.cdc.gov/drugresistance/actionplan/index.htm (accessed January 3, 2008).

17. Ian G. Williamson et al., "Antibiotics and Topical Nasal Steroid for Treatment of Acute Maxillary Sinusitis," *Journal of the American Medical Association* 298, no. 21 (December 5, 2007): 2487–2496.

with a viral infection; there are no other signs such as a rash that would suggest a more serious condition such as scarlet fever. The usual recommendation in this case would be symptomatic care and instructions to follow up if symptoms have not resolved within several days. The physician is well aware, however, that rapid tests for streptococcal antigens have about a 5–30% false negative rate[18] and he reminds the mother that his routine is to back up each negative rapid strep test with the much more sensitive throat swab for culture for group A streptococci. This practice is recommended by the American Academy of Pediatrics guidelines for managing streptococcal pharyngitis because one of the primary reasons for testing for group A streptococcal pharyngitis is the need to treat the infection and thus reduce the chances of the child developing acute rheumatic fever.[19] He notes that if the culture is positive, he will call the mother and phone in a prescription for penicillin.

Junior's mother, however, is adamant about the need for the follow up test, as well as for immediate treatment for Junior. She, too, is aware of the possibility of a false negative test result. She does not want Junior to endure several days of waiting for the test result—he might, after all, *have* strep, and she recognizes that treatment could be started immediately and discontinued later if the follow up test is negative. There are non-medical reasons for avoiding delays of possibly indicated treatment, too: she is a single parent, and cannot keep Junior home from school for several days while he recovers from his sore throat. Or, Junior has an important math test, soccer game, or chess tournament coming up in two days, and it is critical that he recover from the sore throat in time. Junior chimes in, too: he wants to feel better and get back to school as soon as he can. Junior and his mother see themselves as advocating for Junior: why can't he get the antibiotic that *might* be optimal care for him, even though pediatricians are told to resist such pressures as they contribute to the overall risk of antibiotic resistance?

Emily's Ear Infection

Emily is a three-year-old child who was noted to have the sniffles and be irritable when her mother picked her up at her day-care facility. She woke up several times that evening crying, and the next morning she was noted to have worsening of her runny nose, look flushed, have a dry cough, and for the first

---

18. Sabra L. Katz-Wise, "Rapid Strep Test for Strep Throat," WebMD Medical Reference from Healthwise (August 29, 2006), http://www.webmd.com/a-to-z-guides/rapid-strep-test-for-strep-throat (accessed January 8, 2008).

19. A.L. Bisno, M.A. Gerber, J.M. Gwaltney, Jr., E.L. Kaplan, R.H. Schwartz, and Infectious Diseases Society of America, "Practice Guidelines for the Diagnosis and Management of Group A Streptococcal Pharyngitis," *Clinical Infectious Diseases* 35, no. 2 (July 15, 2002): 113–125; A.L. Bisno, "Acute Pharyngitis," *New England Journal of Medicine* 344, no. 3 (January 18, 2001): 205–211.

time to complain that her ears were hurting. Fortunately her mother, who worked as an emergency room nurse, was not scheduled to work that day, so she decided to take Emily to her pediatrician to be checked for an ear infection. On exam the pediatrician found a child who was in no acute distress as she was playing with toys in the waiting room with a low-grade fever of 101 degrees, a runny nose, and a dry cough with a normal chest exam. Examination of the ears revealed bilateral cloudiness, slight redness, and slight bulging of the ear drums (tympanic membranes). The pediatrician often worked with Emily's mother in covering the emergency room on weekends, so he felt comfortable in discussing with her the latest guidelines for managing ear infections in children.[20] The pediatrician's diagnosis was acute otitis media (AOM) with mild ear pain and low-grade fever (<102 degrees F). He admitted that there was some uncertainty in his diagnosis, as these relatively mild findings and the association with recent onset of the sniffles could indicate that the findings were due to a viral upper respiratory tract infection or they could indicate an acute bacterial infection of the middle ear. In considering whether or not to prescribe antibiotics, the pediatrician and Emily's mother both agreed that antibiotics would be of no value if the infection were due to a virus. The pediatrician also explained that recent clinical trials have shown that mild cases of AOM, such as Emily has, usually resolve in a few days without the use of antibiotics, and that the recent guidelines offer the option of observation rather than immediate administration of antibiotics.[21] The observation option includes giving the parent a written prescription for an antibiotic with the advice that the parent not fill it immediately but closely observe the child for signs of worsening illness over the next 48 to 72 hours. If the child's temperature rises to above 102 degrees F, the ear pain becomes severe, or the child becomes significantly more irritable or lethargic, then the child should be given the prescribed antibiotic. In discussing the advantages of immediate administration of antibiotics versus observation, the pediatrician quoted studies that showed that the antibiotic option provided symptomatic relief by 2–3 days 91% of the time compared to 87% in the observation group, a minor and statistically insignificant difference.[22]

Emily's mother wryly commented that perhaps even a 4% chance of Emily recovering a day earlier might be worth it because she would otherwise have to take a sick day off from her ER job, and the pediatrician commented that he was aware that ER coverage by nurses was currently spotty at best, and she

20. American Academy of Pediatrics and American Academy of Family Physicians, Subcommittee on Management of Acute Otitis Media, "Diagnosis and Management of Acute Otitis Media," *Pediatrics* 113, no. 5 (May 2004): 1451–1465.
21. Ibid.
22. R.M. Rosenfeld, "Clinical Efficacy of Medical Therapy," in *Evidence-Based Otitis Media*, ed. R.M. Rosenfeld, and C.D. Bluestone, 2nd ed. (Hamilton, Ontario: BC Decker, 2003), 199–226.

would be missed. Conversely, the negative side of prescribing an antibiotic included a 16% chance that Emily would develop antibiotic-associated diarrhea and a 2% chance that she would develop an antibiotic-associated skin rash.[23] The pediatrician and Emily's mother also discussed the social or "microbial-environmental" issues related to the increasing prevalence in the community of bacteria resistant to the antibiotics commonly prescribed for treatment of AOM.[24] They agreed that as professionals and as citizens they had some obligation not to contribute to the problem of antimicrobial resistance. However, Emily's mother again wryly noted that Emily is a three-year-old sick kid who may be too young to be expected to contribute to such social goods, and that Emily's father was a lawyer who would not take kindly to Emily's developing complications of her untreated AOM.

George's Possible Staph Infection

George is a patient who has already been hospitalized and who develops a serious bacterial infection. The consulting infectious disease physician thinks that the infectious agent is likely to be staph, but does not know the susceptibility of the organism to particular antibiotic agents. It will take a culture and at least 36 hours to develop this information. The physician also knows that a high percentage of hospital acquired bacterial infections are resistant to first-line antibiotics but susceptible to more expensive, broader spectrum agents— agents that are desirable to use carefully because of their costs, side effects, and the need to avoid the development of organisms resistant to them. In the meantime, the physician has a choice about how to begin treatment of George. George could be started on an antibiotic in common use, nafcillin, which is effective against the most likely infectious agent. The challenge is that an increasing proportion of staph strains (estimates now are upward of 10%) are resistant to this common antibiotic. An alternative is that George could be started on a more powerful, broader spectrum antibacterial, Linezolid, one of the newest generation of antibacterials that remains effective against methicillin-resistant staphylococcus aureus. This approach might avoid the possibility that George will not be given a potentially ineffective drug. Physicians are trying to save this new-generation agent for the cases of genuine resistance, cases

23. R.J. Ruben, "Sequelae of Antibiotic Therapy," in *Evidence-Based Otitis Media*, ed. Rosenfeld and Bluestone, 303–314.
24. Michael E. Pichichero and Janet R. Casey, "Emergence of a Multiresistant Serotype 19A Pneumococcal Strain Not Included in the 7-Valent Conjugate Vaccine as an Otopathogen in Children," *Journal of the American Medical Association* 298, no. 5 (October 17, 2007): 1772–1778; M.H. Samore et al, "High Rates of Multiple Antibiotic Resistance in Streptococcus Pneumoniae from Healthy Children Living in Isolated Rural Communities: Association with Cephalosporin Use and Intrafamilial Transmission," *Pediatrics* 108, no. 4 (October 2001): 856–860.

in which it is clearly needed, because they fear that overuse of the new agent will lead to the development of newer, even more resistant, strains of staphylococci.

In this circumstance, the physician could start by recommending that George be treated with the older agent, nafcillin, and monitored carefully for improvement or worsening of his condition. George is hospitalized, so he can be appropriately monitored. However, the physician also knows that the ordinary course of the infection, even if the chosen antibiotic is effective, is that George is likely to get worse in the short term—so a worsening of his condition cannot be regarded as an indication that the antibiotic is ineffective.

If the consulting physician is a specialist in infectious disease, she will be aware of all of these issues. She will also be aware that the standard practice of physicians who are less familiar with the complexities of this case will be to follow the immediately least risky strategy and start George on the antibiotic that is most likely to be effective in all cases, Linezolid. So she will be aware that resistance to Linezolid is likely to develop in any case because of the overall pattern of prescription practices, and her decisions about how to manage George are unlikely to affect this overall pattern. Risk averse herself, she is concerned about the potential personal and professional consequences for her if she prescribes nafcillin, George has a resistant bacterial strain, and George's condition worsens and eventually results in death. George is, after all, a pretty sick patient, and much is potentially on the line for him.

Antimicrobial Resistance and the Standard View

The standard way to view these cases is that they pose a conflict between the physician's management of *this* patient—the patient before her—and more long-term consequences for patients in general. Viewed in this way, the choice would seem obvious: the physician is treating this patient and should make whatever recommendation is in the patient's interest, leaving aside more general consequences. In Junior's case, this might well be a recommendation against prescribing the antibiotic: there are possible side effects of the treatment for Junior and the reasons that are offered in favor of immediate treatment are not medical ones, although they surely might be important to both Junior and his mother. In Emily's case, the choice is a more balanced one. On the one hand, the antibiotic will be effective; there is a slight chance that faster resolution of the infection might be medically beneficial to her. On the other hand, the antibiotic may have side effects for her. There is, also, the possibility that Emily's mother has relatively immediate medical interests in not having her child, or herself, colonized by a bacterial strain that is resistant to the standard treatment for acute otitis media. After all, AOM tends to recur in children, and Emily may need treatment within the relatively near future for another episode, especially if her mother is also carrying the resistant organism. If this episode of AOM can be managed without an antibiotic, that may preserve effective antibiotic therapy for Emily at another time.

With George, however, the benefits of treatment would seem clear. George is seriously ill, and a wrong choice of antibiotics could prove fatal to him. Without effective treatment now, he may not survive this episode and there will be no benefit to him of practices that maintain effective antibiotics for future patients. Conversely, the benefits to future patients are clear: as we have already recounted, resistant staphylococcus aureus kills almost 19,000 patients per year in the United States, and new effective agents are difficult to develop. So, the standard view: cautious, risk-averse treatment for George apparently lies in conflict with the needs of other patients.

Antimicrobial Resistance and the Tragedy of the Commons

Several recent discussions have moved beyond analyzing antimicrobial resistance as a simple conflict between the individual and the public, to construct it as a "tragedy of the commons" problem.[25] Tragedic commons logic works like this: assume a shared resource, such as common land or ambient air. The traditional example was grazing cows on the village green. Absent regulation, people who use the shared resource get the full benefit of their use but only bear a fractional share of the costs of that use. They get all the milk from their cow— but only bear a fractional share of the cow's grazing costs. It thus seems prudentially rational for each one to continue to use the commons—for each villager to put out another cow to graze. As use increases, the carrying capacity of the commons is eventually reached, then surpassed, and the commons crashes. Individually rational action leads to collective disaster: whether with cows on the village commons, clean air, fisheries, or global climate change.

And so, it seems, with antimicrobials, according to Foster and Grundmann.[26] Each patient, using an antimicrobial as indicated, gets the full benefit of her use. But everyone, collectively, bears the long-range cost of increasing resistance. Thus it would seem prudentially rational to each individual to use antimicrobials as they need them, without regard to shared risks of resistance; but the result is the collectively bad outcome of widespread resistance.

And the tragedy is still worse from the point of view of justice, according to Michael Selgelid.[27] The majority of the antimicrobial overuse occurs in developed countries, among the relatively wealthy, but the costs of resistance are highest among the poor and those in developing countries, who are more likely

25. Garrett Hardin, "The Tragedy of the Commons," *Science* 162 (1968): 1243–1244.
26. Kevin R. Foster and Hajo Grundmann, "Do We Need to Put Society First? The Potential for Tragedy in Antimicrobial Resistance," *PLoS Medicine* 3, no. 2 (January 10, 2006): e29.
27. Selgelid, "Ethics and Drug Resistance."

to become ill with infectious diseases. Newer, broader spectrum antimicrobials that are more effective against resistant pathogens are also more expensive. They, too, are consumed more frequently but perhaps inappropriately by the wealthy. In addition, he contends, pharmaceutical companies have little incentive to develop new antibiotics or to make less expensive ones widely available: there is far more profit to be made elsewhere. The result is a looming commons crash whose bad effects are initially felt most keenly by the poor.

Nor is Hardin's preferred solution to the supposed tragedy of common land available in the case of antimicrobial resistance.[28] Hardin's view was that by privatization, individuals could be forced to bear the full costs of their decisions about land use: if each individual is making decisions about putting more cows on his own land, each individual will have to consider the full costs of maintaining that land. With antimicrobial use, however, individuals apparently can never be made to bear the full cost of their use: they are either treated and get well, or are treated and do not get well—but in using antimicrobials they impose the increased risk of resistance as a negative externality on others.[29] So, Foster and Grundmann conclude that the only reasonable solution is a regulatory one in which some people are asked to bear burdens for the overall good of preserving antimicrobial effectiveness. They conclude that this will involve "brave policy decisions," which should be made based on the best evidence about costs to individual patients, the social costs of resistant pathogens, and the potential for investments into new antimicrobials and better infection control practices.[30]

Selgelid takes this analysis a step further, to argue against distribution of health care through market mechanisms. Market distribution, he contends, contributes to the problem of resistance in two critical ways. The wealthy overconsume, in part because of the enticements of pharmaceutical advertising. The poor underconsume, unable to get or pay for full courses of medication even when some is available. Selgelid is surely right about many of the problems of market-driven health care. But, like Foster and Grundmann, he leaves us with hard policy choices. Recognizing maldistributions in the market will not obviate the apparent underlying problem that gets tragedic logic operating: it really does

---

28. There are many criticisms of Hardin's analysis of individual rationality and the commons logic. One is that communities in fact work out shared norms of understanding that regulate risks of commons overuse. See, e.g., Robert C. Ellickson, *Order Without Law: How Neighbors Settle Disputes* (Cambridge: Harvard University Press, 1991); Elinor Ostrom, *Governing the Commons: The Evolution of Institutions for Collective Action* (Cambridge: Cambridge University Press, 1990); Carol Rose, "The Comedy of the Commons: Custom, Commerce, and Inherently Public Property," *University of Chicago Law Review* 53 (1986): 711–781.
29. This point is made by Selgelid, "Ethics and Drug Resistance," 226. A negative externality is a cost that is not taken into account in a market transaction, such as pollution costs that are not figured into the market price of gasoline.
30. Foster and Grundmann, "Potential for Tragedy in Antimicrobial Resistance."

seem to be individually rational for people to use antimicrobials that are effective against the organisms they harbor. There is thus an irony in Selgelid's view. Although improved distribution of health care might counter the problems of underuse that he details, better access to health care might actually *increase* effective antimicrobial use—and thus increase the risks of resistance that are inherent even in reasonable use of antibiotic agents. However, Selgelid does not mention the possibility of internalizing the costs of antibiotic resistance into transactions between consumers and pharmaceutical companies or health-care providers.

We suggest for further exploration a potential solution to the problem Selgelid has raised. This is to develop a strategy for internalizing the costs of antimicrobial resistance by including in the price of drugs at least some of the costs of developing new antimicrobials to cope with the anticipated possibilities of the development of resistant organisms. There are several different ways such a surcharge might be calculated. One way to mirror the actual economics of the situation would be to take the average historical cost of developing a next-generation antimicrobial, divided by the anticipated number of uses of current-generation antimicrobials, and add that figure as a surcharge to each use of the current antimicrobial.

A far simpler way would be to add a fixed amount, say a $1 surcharge to every course of a first-generation antimicrobial, and a slightly larger surcharge— say, $2—to every course of a second-generation antimicrobial. Funds generated in this way could be used to support antimicrobial research either by the government directly or through grants and contracts; as an example of this kind of strategy, the WHO presently funds a variety of projects under the Initiative for Vaccine Research.[31] To the objection that this strategy imposes costs on those in need—those who are using the antimicrobial—there are several answers. If insurance pays for the drug—as is largely done in the United States today and in most publicly funded health-care systems—these costs are actually shared. Moreover, there are benefits to the patient of having next generation antimicrobials in the process of development—after all, as we discuss below, he or she might need them. To concerns that this strategy might not prove practical, we would note the analogous surcharge on vaccines in the United States, used to fund the federal program that provides compensation for vaccine-related injuries.[32]

However, these attempts to internalize externalities of antimicrobial use may alleviate, but not fully resolve, the problem. If there are delays in drug development, or if organisms become resistant to any known drugs for a period

31. Initiative for Vaccine Research, http://www.who.int/vaccine_research/en/ (accessed February 12, 2008).
32. National Vaccine Injury Compensation Program, http://www.hrsa.gov/vaccinecompensation/ (accessed February 12, 2008). The current surcharge on vaccines is $.75/dose.

of time, or if it is not scientifically understood how to develop yet a new drug, the problem of resistance will remain.

At first glance, application of tragedic commons logic to resistance thus seems ironclad: individually, it is in each person's interests to use antimicrobials, and collectively the result may be the equivalent of an antimicrobial "crash": resistance. The crash may be mitigated to some extent by new drug development, and it surely can at least be postponed by more careful use. Yet it would appear that the underlying tragedic logic remains. Or does it? We think that there are several reasons for doubting both the picture of antimicrobial resistance as a conflict between the individual and others, and as beset ultimately by tragedic logic.

Antimicrobial Resistance and Individual Rationality

For the tragedic logic to unfold as Hardin describes, it must be individually rational for people to continue to increase their use of the commons—that is, to continue to put out yet another cow to graze on the already crowded field. If it is not individually rational for them to do so—if, for example, it is not beneficial for them to put more cows onto the commons until the carrying capacity of the commons is reached—then the tragedy will not get off the ground, or at least the tragedic logic will not play out all the way to a final crash. Hardin applied tragedy of the commons logic to population policy, arguing that because it was individually rational for people to choose to have children, and because they got the individual benefit of the children while bearing only a fractional cost of their children's imposition on the earth (education costs, food costs, carbon footprint, and so on), eventually population growth would lead to a crash of the earth-commons. Stephen Gardiner, however, has pointed out that this argument assumes that it is individually rational for people to continue to have more children, an assumption that is quite likely belied by the data.[33] In fact, as economic circumstances improve, and as children are more likely to survive to adulthood, birth rates characteristically fall dramatically in what is known as the epidemiological transition. These data suggest that people do not continue to prefer to add children to the commons—that is, that there is a point at which it is no longer individually beneficial for them to do so—thus, the tragedic logic may not unfold to the full extent that Hardin suggests.

A parallel point might be made about antimicrobial resistance. It is not always true that more use of antimicrobials is better than less, even in cases in which the antimicrobial might be indicated in the sense that it would be effective against the organism in question. More may not be better than less, even in

---

33. Stephen Gardiner, "The Real Tragedy of the Commons," *Philosophy & Public Affairs* 30 (2001): 387–416.

cases that might be regarded as medically indicated use. Antimicrobials can have side effects, and in each individual decision about whether to use a particular agent to treat a given condition, these side effects play into the decision about whether the antimicrobial should be used. For example, if the use of an antibiotic to treat a baby's ear infection results in significant diarrhea and painful diaper rash, it may not be rational to use the agent even if it treats the ear infection successfully—provided, of course, that the infection will resolve on its own without sequelae. For individuals who expect to have repeated episodes of illness, it may be beneficial to employ watchful waiting to see if a condition normally resolves on its own, as a way to avoid letting themselves becoming infected with resistant strains. Emily's ear infection is a possible example: if antibiotics are given frequently to treat her infections that would otherwise resolve on their own without health consequences to her, she is at greater risk of being colonized with resistant organisms—and thus to harbor a more difficult-to-treat infection that is less likely to resolve either on its own or with now-inadequate antibiotic treatment.

The observation that there may be more circumstances than initially appear in which it might not be individually rational to use antibiotics does not, however, fully obviate tragedic possibilities. If the cases in which use is rational are sufficient to generate resistance, it will still occur, only perhaps a bit more slowly. And, as Gardiner argues concerning population policy, the problems this generates may be even more intractable, because they are intergenerational.

Antimicrobial Use and Passing the Buck

Gardiner follows up the population policy example to identify another tragedic problem. It is individually rational for people to have more children to some extent. That extent is significant enough eventually to prove unsustainable. However, the costs of that ultimate unsustainability are not borne by present generations. The costs are instead borne by future generations. Thus there is no reason in individual rationality for people having children today not to pass the buck to people having children tomorrow. The "real" tragedy of the commons, Gardiner contends, is a problem of intergenerational justice, not a problem of collective action today.[34] It is a problem of people today having no individual reason *now* to avoid harming other people *later*, independent of course, of their reasons not to harm their own identifiable descendents.

Something similar may be at work with antimicrobial resistance, if it develops over a sufficiently extended time period. Patients now considering whether to use antimicrobials might be like Gardiner's people now considering whether to have children: in each case, they will get the benefits, but any later costs will

---

34. Gardiner, "The Real Tragedy of the Commons."

be borne by future generations. No regulatory strategy can be imposed that will give people today reciprocal benefits from future people, to offset sacrifices being made today. With antimicrobial resistance, a parallel point might be made about distance in location, analogous to Gardiner's point about distance in time: resistant cholera or tuberculosis may seem to be a problem for India or Russia and not the United States, with no reciprocal benefits to be achieved by addressing resistance far across the globe. But this analogy is suspect not only on ethical grounds but factually as well: some microbes replicate and in the process evolve so rapidly that they virtually always outdistance efforts to control them. HIV is perhaps the most conspicuous example: the HIV virus replicates and evolves a million times as rapidly as the cells it infects,[35] thus not only making effective treatment difficult—a problem that increases the likelihood of resistance if complex schedules of drug administration are not rigorously kept—but also posing continuing problems for vaccine development.[36] The buck is not passed only to future generations or to remote populations on the other side of the globe; the buck is also passed to people right here and right now.

The PVV Perspective and Antimicrobial Resistance

Thus the facts about how antimicrobial resistance develops do not really support analyzing it as either a tragedy of the commons or as a tragedy distant in time or place. The PVV perspective can help reveal the ethical implications of the fact that resistance is not beset exactly by either of these forms of tragic logic—or even by the simpler logic of a tradeoff between the individual patient and others. It is beset by deep problems of carelessness and injustice, but addressing these problems also is in the interests of everyone together as victims and vectors.

Tragedic logic projects that individually rational activities, together or over time, will mount up to a crisis of unsustainability. The development of this crisis is insidious: before use increases too greatly, people continue undisturbed in their enjoyment of land use, child-bearing, fishing, emissions-spewing, or other activities with effects that will eventually accumulate. Once use mounts up, damage begins to snowball, and crash becomes inevitable. Beforehand, however, people act with apparently relative impunity, despite hand-wringing in the sustainability literature about, for example, whether intense storms, especially hot summers, or unusual weather patterns are harbingers of the cumulative bad effects of climate change to come, whether fishing is really

---

35. Michael Specter, "Annals of Science: 'Darwin' Surprise," *New Yorker*, December 3, 2007, 64–73.
36. Robert Steinbrook, "One Step Forward, Two Steps Back—Will There Even Be an AIDS Vaccine?" *New England Journal of Medicine* 257, no. 26 (December 27, 2007): 2653–2655.

244 Health Care Dilemmas Through the Lens of Infectious Disease

over-fishing, or whether urban-sprawl land use patterns will eventually commandeer all the arable land.

Antimicrobial resistance, unlike these cumulative sustainability problems, grows in pockets. Long before any tipping point at which the percentage of resistant cases of a particular disease far outstrips the percentage of non-resistant cases, there are cases of resistant disease. Resistant disease can develop as soon as microbes first change in ways that enable them to elude antimicrobials directed against them, sometimes in just a matter of days. Furthermore, resistance is not an isolated or uncharacteristic phenomenon, but is ever present in ordinary antimicrobial use; in the words of the World Health Organization, it is a "natural biological phenomenon."[37] In 2007, the public press voiced considerable concern over the seemingly new epidemic of methicillin resistant staphylococcus aureus, but of course there were cases of MRSA long before it began to represent such a high percentage of patients with staph infections that the public became alarmed.

In short, increased use of antimicrobials will increase the frequency of resistance, as will misuses such as failing to take a full course of a prescription. Yet once a resistant strain develops in a susceptible patient, from whatever cause, there is the possibility of resistant disease. Resistance, therefore, is not exactly a problem in which people can be reassured that they are safe until the carrying capacity of the commons is outstripped. This is probably a good thing: we cannot remain too complacent, because the reality of resistance already confronts us here and now. But to respond appropriately—that is, both effectively and ethically—we must understand what sort of problem antimicrobial resistance is, and it is here that our PVV view is, we think, useful. Even in its early stages, resistance is not like the classic problem of the commons; it is, rather, a problem in which there will be patches of commons destruction—a dying patch of land, as it were, with dying cows scattered on it here and there. Nor is it a problem of people who now act in ways that put people at risk later or far away: to carry on the analogy of cows on the commons, the dead land and dying cows are right out there in patches of present-day fields. There is deep uncertainty about who is at risk and when, and how much time may elapse before resistance flares out of control. No individual now knows whether he or she may face familiar or newly resistant organisms. Selgelid makes this point also in arguing that a failure of the wealthy to attend to resistance "may come back to haunt us all—rich and poor alike,"[38] though it is not just a failure of the wealthy alone. This is the uncertainty revealed by the PVV perspective, the uncertainty of the way-station self who can never quite know what is passing through or what is occurring within one's own body; this is part of what it

37. World Health Organization, *Overcoming Antimicrobial Resistance*, preface.
38. Selgelid, "Ethics and Drug Resistance," 221.

means to say that the way-station self lives in theoretically deep uncertainty. Here, the "way-station" metaphor must be understood in a more specific sense: these may be organisms that have been transmitted from one person to another within a population, but resistance develops *within*, not between, the individuals they infect—though those resistant strains can then be passed along to others in the "way-station" way.

Balancing the possibility of antimicrobial resistance is thus a choice for each person *now*. It is a choice within lives, not only a choice across lives. Each person must weigh the benefits *for themselves* of the antimicrobial, against the unknown risk of becoming infected by a resistant organism. Individual choices about antimicrobial use thus weigh risks *for that individual*. It is also a choice across lives. Resistant disease is an all-or-nothing risk, albeit a risk of an uncertain magnitude; but it is also a fractional share of the cost as on the commons analogy, because the resistant organism that develops in one person may also spread throughout a population. The tradeoffs with antimicrobial resistance occur within lives now, but also between lives now and lives in the future. This is as true across the globe: it only takes one traveler with resistant disease to spread resistant organisms far and wide.[39]

With this deep uncertainty of the way-station self in mind, let us return to the three cases discussed above. *Junior*'s reasons for wanting the antibiotic for his strep throat are important to Junior, but they are not health-related reasons. From a purely health-related perspective, Junior, or his parent for him, must weigh the limited health benefits of antibiotic use for him now, against the possibility that he might become infected with resistant strains of streptococcus or staphylococcus. These infectious might be deadly, but there is no way of knowing whether Junior's wrestling team or his football team is likely to become infected with any of them. Junior has longer-range health-related interests in having effective antibiotics to treat staph infections of his wrestling team, in his college dormitory, or in the hospital treating him for a compound leg fracture. Junior's choice lies between these quite serious health-related reasons—unlikely but unpredictable and serious if they occur—and other concerns such as a test or a soccer game, concerns that Junior knows are his right now, but that might be relatively episodic or deeply important. Junior should weigh his decision in these terms: would it be prudential for him to take this slight but unknown risk of serious disease or death at some unknown time in order to take the test or play the game? Sometimes the answer will be "yes," but many more times the answer may be "no." Furthermore, Junior has interests in health-care practices that will encourage him and other patients to think

---

39. The World Health Organization recounts an example of two outbreaks of MRSA that traveled from a small village in North India to Canada. World Health Organization, *Overcoming Antibiotic Resistance*, ch. 3.

about his decision in this way: otherwise, no matter what Junior decides, overall patterns of antibiotic use may intensify the risks of resistance.

Our point is that the physician should consider both the positive and negative health consequences of the antibiotic, as well as the very real health risks of resistance, as issues involving Junior's interests along with all the other interests of Junior or his parent. The standard recommendation in a case like Junior's strep infection should be against antibiotic use, except in the few cases in which Junior can advance a very strong reason to avoid the small risk that he has disease that will not resolve on its own. Of course, proper follow up is also important here—the more sensitive test to be sure that Junior does not have strep, to avoid the possible dangerous risk of scarlet fever. The reasoning here is akin to a shift in the extent and burden of persuasion: it is on Junior to advance a very strong reason that the antibiotic is in his interests. If the decision is pressed in this way, there will be fewer cases in which it is prudential over the longer run for Junior to receive the antibiotic. There may be some such cases: a high school championship game, a mother who will lose her job with one more day of missed work, or an SAT test at the very time Junior needs a decent score to apply to college. But these cases will be far fewer than the day–to–day cases in which Junior or his mother want the antibiotic because they think, wrongly, that they will benefit from the antibiotic at no cost to themselves or to others. Physician practices of exploring these issues with their patients can be expected to lower, although not to eliminate entirely, uses of antibiotics in cases such as Junior's.

Emily has a health related reason to take the antibiotic for her ear infection. This reason may not be very strong, however, unless her symptoms worsen within the next 72 hours. A trial of watchful waiting may not be very risky to her, in comparison to the risks to her if she were to get another infection and find it to be resistant to available antibiotics. Indeed, with patients who are susceptible to recurrent ear infections, the risk of developing resistant infection with antibiotic use over time is actually a known risk[40]—not even a matter of uncertainty about what Emily is likely to catch the next time. The physician should explore these issues with Emily's mother, and also explore her ability to understand the need to return for a follow up visit if the infection does not resolve and the likelihood that she will do so. If patients are encouraged to choose watchful waiting when it is not overly risky to them, overall use will decline, so the probability of resistant strains will also be smaller.

George has a potentially life-threatening infection. Antibiotic use in his case may be life-saving, right now. George is also in a class of patients—hospitalized patients acquiring nosocomial infections—where the risks of both having

---

40. Samore et al., "High Rates of Multiple Antibiotic Resistance."

and transmitting resistant disease are quite high. For George, the decision seems clear: use the antibiotic that is most likely to be effective in treating what is in the judgment of George's physician the likely range of infectious possibilities. But even here, there is more to say. Although the balance quite likely favors the use of the broader spectrum antibiotic in George's case, George too has interests in hospital policies that will reduce the likelihood of drug resistance. He has interests in hospital surveillance and in practices such as hand washing—practices that are performed imperfectly at best in today's hospitals. He has interests, too, in the development of next-generation antibiotics, and so in the small surcharge we have proposed adding to the cost of his drug use.

Conclusion

In this chapter, we have argued that it is too simple to view antimicrobial resistance as a conflict between treating this patient, now, and saving effective agents for later use. Nor is it a problem of inevitable clash between actions that are individually rational and collectively irrational. From the PVV perspective, as a matter of patient care in the developed world, it is partly a problem of prudence, of considering apparent short-term benefits against unknown but serious risks for oneself now and oneself in the future; and it is also a collective problem, because the resistance one engenders in one's own way-station body may also affect others. Recasting decisions about antibiotic use, and the process of decision making between physician and patient in this way, we think, has the potential to reduce the extent to which the use of antibiotics in patient care contributes to resistance. Our suggested surcharge on antimicrobial use to promote the development of new agents has the potential to support important research initiatives.

We should not forget, however, that the use of antimicrobials in appropriate patient care is only one part of the picture. By far the greater causes of resistance are not the individual decisions about patient care that we have detailed here—especially if patient care decisions are made as we suggest. Conceptualizing patient care decisions as the PVV perspective suggests will reduce the overall level of risk, but will pale if other sources of resistance are not addressed. Agricultural use and problems of poverty and injustice that lead to underuse also must be addressed. Our PVV perspective—that we are all in this together—reminds us that these are issues for each of us as well.

14

IMMUNIZATION AND THE HPV VACCINE

Discussions of immunization in public health and the law typically pit public health positions against protection of individual civil liberties. But viewing the problem of immunization in terms of a conflict between individual rights and public health is too simple. This conflictual view focuses on the "real world" situation of known victims and vectors. The person who knows she or those with whom she comes in contact are likely to be victims of disease wants the individual protection that vaccination can provide, or perhaps also the overall protection that vaccines can bring. The person who knows he is likely to be identified as a vector and perhaps coerced into immunization, wants his liberty protected, but may also not want to pose risks to family or friends. The victim/vector perspective, however, moves beyond these conflictual positions in ordinary life to justifications for reducing the overall burden of disease that speak to each as protector and protected. Any decision maker—a competent adult, the parent of an infant or an adolescent, an adolescent along with the parent, or a policymaker—ethically must take into account the consequences to both victims and vectors of decisions that are made about immunization.[1]

This chapter develops the implications of the PVV perspective for immunization decisions in light of a particularly contentious, current immunization issue: the proposal to make human papillomavirus (HPV) immunization a school-entry requirement for young women. Much of the controversy arises because HPV vaccines are ineffective against a particular type of HPV virus once chronic infection has occurred with that type: for maximum efficacy, they must be administered *before* first infection with HPV, and hence before first sexual contact. [2]

---

1. For a sketch of this picture of compulsory vaccination as a conflict between individual liberty and the duty to prevent harm to others, see Stephen Holland, *Public Health Ethics* (Cambridge: Polity Press, 2007), 139–142.

2. The Future II Study Group, "Quadrivalent HPV Vaccine Against Human Papillomavirus to Prevent High-Grade Cervical Lesions," *New England Journal of Medicine* 356, no. 19 (May 10, 2007): 1915–1927. There is evidence that once infection has occurred, vaccination is not effective as therapy against any given virus type. A. Hildesheim, R. Herrero, S. Wacholder et al., "Effect of Human Papillomavirus 16/18 L1 Viruslike Particle Vaccination Among Young Women With Preexisting Infection," *Journal of the American Medical Association* 298, no. 7 (August 15, 2007): 743–753.

The PVV Perspective and Immunization: A Sketch

At the first level of the PVV perspective—that of the individual patient—people will find themselves in many different situations with respect to immunization. Some will be concerned that they are likely victims and want to be immunized. In the developed world, immunization will in general be available, although costs or access to health care may be a problem. In the developing world, immunization is far less likely to be available, and alternative methods of protection like voluntary abstinence or routine cervical screening are often less practicable, whether for religious or cultural reasons, lack of health-care infrastructure, or poverty. Individuals also may tolerate, accept, or welcome immunizations for the primary purpose of preventing themselves from becoming vectors of infections that primarily injure their spouses or other loved ones. This may occur at a social level as well. A well-established example of this dynamic involves immunization of all children, male and female, with rubella vaccine, with the ultimate goal of protecting pregnant women against this fetus-damaging infection.

Not everyone can welcome vaccination, however: for some few people, immunization is medically contraindicated, if they are allergic to the immunizing agent or the vehicle within which the agent is cultured or delivered.[3] Those with family members or other intimates who are immune-compromised may be advised against vaccinations that pose even slight risks of disease. For others, immunization may be forbidden on religious or other conscientious grounds. Still others may refuse available immunization on a variety of personal grounds: unaffordable expense, unpredictable health risks, fear of needle sticks, mistaken scientific understanding about the risks and benefits of immunization, or just vague concerns about medical interventions.

From our second-level, population perspective, the principal concern about immunization is whether sufficient levels have been achieved to reduce the overall risks of disease in a population—the "herd effect." Herd immunity is the

---

3. This is a general issue in vaccine policy. For example, some are allergic to the influenza vaccines cultured in an egg medium or to the gelatin base of the vaccine against chickenpox. Centers for Disease Control and Prevention, Possible Side Effects From Vaccines. (www.cdcgov/vacccines/vac-gen/side-effects.htm) Others may be advised to avoid vaccination with a live agent because household members, family members, or close companions are immune compromised and might be jeopardized by live agent shedding. An unfortunate few may suffer unpredictable and serious allergic reactions to vaccinations (this does not include claims about autism, for which there is no accepted support)—for example, from 1990 to 2007, a total of 857 successful non-autism claims were filed under the U.S. National Vaccine Compensation Program, for a total compensation amount of $725,710,851. These people, who have good reasons as either victims or vectors not to be immunized themselves, may be especially concerned that enough other people around them are immunized to create a protective "herd" effect.

population-level consequence of acquired immunity among some individuals that can reduce the risk of acquiring infection among susceptible individuals. The herd effect achieved by immunization for a given disease depends on the efficacy and coverage of the vaccine as well as the transmissibility of the infection.[4] However, immunization rates may vary greatly among population groups: for example, religious sub-populations may have low immunization rates; so may minority groups or immigrant populations, whether from inadequate access to care or fears of the health-care establishment. And, of course, immunization rates vary widely across the globe. The population perspective thus brings issues of distributive justice in access to care into sharp focus, as we will explore further in Chapter 19.

The third level—both individual and the population perspectives—holds some but fails to hold other important features of immunization in full view. This aspect of the PVV perspective, the hypothetical, Rawlsian-influenced view, asks how immunization would be regarded by those who did not know their actual situations of victim or vectorhood—but who know that they are in some sense always potentially or actually victims and vectors to each other. From this perspective, each person would want to be protected from infectious disease however this can be best achieved—whether by personal vaccination or by reliance on herd effects.

This multi-perspective analysis has implications for discussions between physicians and their patients about vaccination as well as for vaccine policy. Perhaps the most difficult issue in both clinical medicine and in public policy is whether people should be permitted, prohibited, or discouraged from conscientious (or, for that matter, any) objection to vaccine.[5] People who do not know their individual preferences would want public policies that consider what is required to achieve herd effects, especially for their children who cannot choose on their own, but also for themselves. If herd effects can be achieved compatibly with some allowance for individual choice, people who do not know their own views would also want to try to respect such choices. Our hypothetical view asks whether it is important to insist that reasons for refusal be especially significant—reaching perhaps to the individual's most deeply held values, or to values most closely linked to identity. Such values would be regarded as most worthy of respect—and, if refusals of conscience were limited to them, would be less likely to compromise herd effects. Nonetheless, as a practical matter respecting *any* reason for refusal, however frivolous,

4. T.J. John and R. Samuel, "Herd Immunity and Herd Effect: New Insights and Definitions," *European Journal of Epidemiology* 16, no. 7 (2000): 601–606.
5. For a discussion of the emotional objections to mandatory vaccination, see R. Alta Charo, "Politics, Parents, and Prophylaxis—Mandating HPV Vaccination in the United States," *New England Journal of Medicine* 356, no. 19 (May 10, 2007): 1905–1908.

may be important in preserving trust in vaccination programs established by state authority.[6]

To approach these questions let us look in detail at the debate over "mandating" HPV vaccine. HPV vaccine is a particularly good case for discussion in that it raises both personal and social values issues. Because it is expensive and because the disease it prevents, cervical cancer, affects some population groups more frequently than others, it raises serious questions of justice. It also raises sensitive issues about religious and principled objections to immunization, about public information and misinformation, and about adolescent sexuality.

The Long History of Human Immunization

From a public health perspective, mandating immunization against serious childhood infections before entry into schools has proven a very effective policy that has been generally accepted in developed countries.[7] The near-elimination of polio, diphtheria, tetanus, and pertussis and the great reduction of measles, mumps, and rubella virus infections in more affluent countries can clearly be attributed to this public health policy.[8] However, vocal minorities in the United States and in Europe oppose mandatory immunization policies for multiple reasons.

The first attempts to immunize humans against infectious disease probably took place more than 1,000 years ago in China, India, and Egypt where the practice of transferring pus from smallpox skin lesions to the skin of susceptible individuals induced a local skin infection that was felt to protect against the often fatal generalized infection.[9] In the early eighteenth century, some practitioners in Europe and later in the new colonies adapted this practice, called variolation, in attempts to control large epidemics of smallpox in the major cities. These early efforts to control smallpox should come as no surprise: smallpox decimated populations, left many scarred or blinded, and at its

---

6. J.L. Schwartz, A.L. Caplan, R.R. Faden, and J. Sugarman, "Lessons from the Failure of Human Papillomavirus Vaccine State Requirements," *Clinical Pharmacology and Therapeutics* 82, no. 6 (December 2007): 760–763 (762).

7. W.A. Orenstein and A.R. Hinman, "The Immunization System in the United States—The Role of School Immunization Laws," *Vaccine* 17, suppl. 3 (October 29, 1999): S19–S24.

8. S.W. Roush, T.V. Murphy, and the Vaccine-Preventable Disease Table Working Group, "Historical Comparisons of Morbidity and Mortality for Vaccine-Preventable Diseases in the United States," *Journal of the American Medical Association* 298, no. 18 (November 14, 2007): 2155–2163.

9. For an excellent and detailed review of the history of smallpox vaccines see Arthur Allen, *Vaccine* (New York: W.W. Norton, 2007), 25–111. See also F. Fenner, D.A. Henderson, I. Arita, Z. Jezek, and I.D. Ladnyi, eds., "Early Efforts at Control: Variolation, Vaccination, and Isolation and Quarantine," in *Smallpox and Its Eradication* (Geneva: World Health Organization, 1988), 245–276.

height, killed millions of people each year. No respecter of status, smallpox killed world leaders from Joseph I of Austria to Louis XV of France.[10]

Like vaccine opposition today, early opposition to variolation was based both on scientific and religious/ethical grounds. Not all individuals who were inoculated in the skin with smallpox virus developed a limited local infection; some developed the generalized and often fatal disease. In addition, the inoculation of non-sterile pus from a sick individual to a healthy person sometimes led to a fatal cellulitis or a local tetanus infection. The practice of variolation thus represented early attempts by public officials to ask individuals to accept discomfort and some risk for the greater goal of protecting the community, an ethical argument that continues today as justification for public immunization programs. In addition, some observant practitioners believed (probably correctly) that the practice of variolation might have actually contributed to greater spread of the epidemic. On religious as well as ethical grounds, the practice of making oneself sick by injecting evil humors and filth was felt to be unnatural. It was argued that God determined when and how one became ill and died and that self-induced illness or attempts to interfere with God's will was a sin.

The modern era of immunization was initiated with the development of a vaccine against smallpox. In 1796, the British physician Edward Jenner tested the folk legend that milkmaids who acquired cowpox sores on their hands were resistant to smallpox by purposely inoculating a child with the cowpox virus and then later challenging him with the smallpox virus. The cowpox vaccine, later named vaccinia, was rapidly acknowledged both in Europe and the new world as one of the greatest advances in medical history. Where smallpox vaccination became routine, epidemics became less common, and the worldwide use of a cowpox-derived vaccine ultimately led to the worldwide eradication of smallpox in the late twentieth century—a truly remarkable scientific and public health success.[11]

Despite the ultimate success of the smallpox eradication program in saving millions of lives from one of the world's greatest infectious scourges, opposition to vaccinia immunization programs remained vigorous through the last two centuries. It has continued into the twenty-first century, as fear has arisen that the smallpox virus might be reintroduced into the population as an agent of bioterrorism or warfare and vaccination of health-care workers has been recommended.[12] Opposition has familiarly been centered on scientific, religious,

---

10. World Health Organization, "Fact Sheet: Smallpox," http://www.who.int/mediacentre/factsheets/smallpox/en/ (accessed January 5, 2008).
11. World Health Organization, "Global Eradication of Smallpox," *Bulletin of the World Health Organization* 58 (1980): 161–163.
12. S.A. Bozette et al, "A Model for a Smallpox Vaccination Policy," *New England Journal of Medicine* 348, no. 5 (January 30, 2003): 416–425.

ethical, and political grounds. Scientifically, the vaccinia vaccine, like almost all other vaccines developed in modern times, carries with it a low frequency of side effects; however, some of these can be fatal.[13] A small percentage of people receiving the vaccine may develop spread of the vaccinia virus from the usual local skin lesion to a generalized infection of the skin, and rarely the brain and other vital organs with a fatal outcome. Throughout the two-century history of use of the vaccinia virus, opponents of the vaccine have focused on these rare side effects and argued that healthy individuals could not ethically be put at risk of these side effects against their will; proponents have instead insisted that the overall program has been effective in protecting the community.

In countering public apathy or outright antipathy to being vaccinated against smallpox, governments and public health officials in the nineteenth century gradually evolved increasingly coercive laws and policies to enforce immunization, particularly in the cities where epidemics were most damaging. The first mandatory vaccination law, passed in England in 1840, allowed for the taking of personal property or goods from families who refused vaccination.[14] In the United States, vaccination implementation was organized by the cities and states, with Massachusetts passing the first compulsory vaccination law in 1809 and New York implementing the first required vaccination for school admission in 1860.[15] Enforcement of the laws was inconsistent, however, generally increasing in response to current epidemics particularly in the cities, and languishing between epidemics. In some cities enforcement accelerated to the degree that citizens were captured by physical force and immunized. As has frequently occurred during epidemics of infectious diseases, foreigners, immigrants, minority groups, and the poor were targeted as major causes of disease and singled out for coercive immunization practices, raising ethical concerns of justice.

The first major legal challenge to the compulsory vaccination laws in the United States did not occur until the turn of the twentieth century, when Jacobson challenged Massachusetts' smallpox immunization law.[16] Jacobson, a local church pastor, argued that it was "the inherent right of every free man to

---

13. M. Lane, F.L. Ruben, J.M. Neff, and J.D. Millar, "Complications of Smallpox Vaccination: 1968 National Surveillance in the United States," *New England Journal of Medicine* 281 (1969): 1201–1208.

14. See Allen, *Vaccine*, 60.

15. See Orenstein and Hinman, "Immunization System in the United States."

16. W.E. Parmet, R.A. Goodman, and A. Farber, "Individual Rights Versus the Public's Health—100 Years after Jacobson v. Massachusetts," *New England Journal of Medicine* 352, no. 7 (February 17, 2005): 652–654. See also Wendy E. Parmet, "Public Health and Constitutional Law: Recognizing the Relationship," *Journal of Health Care Law & Policy* 10 (2007): 13–24 (arguing that injecting health law into constitutional law helps us to see that issues are not just individual rights against the social good, but what we all want as part of our common fate); Wendy E. Parmet, "Unprepared: Why Health Law Fails to Prepare Us for a Pandemic," *Journal of Health & Biomedical Law.* 2 (2006): 157–193 (arguing that

care for his own body and health in such a way as to him seems best."[17] Jacobson's argument, reflecting individual rights issues raised during the eighteenth and nineteenth centuries, is remarkably consistent with arguments used in the twenty-first century in defense of the autonomous rights of patients to make decisions about their health care. The case ultimately went to the U.S. Supreme Court, which determined that the state had the right to require immunization of an individual in order to protect the public from an epidemic disease. Even so, the Court did set limits: the police power may not be "exercised in particular circumstances and in reference to particular persons in such an arbitrary, unreasonable manner, or might go so far beyond what was reasonably required for the safety of the public, as to authorize or compel the courts to interfere for the protection of such persons."[18] The landmark *Jacobson* decision and subsequent Supreme Court support for school immunization laws in 1922[19] have subsequently empowered national, state, and local governments to enforce a variety of laws and regulations that mandate the use of vaccines to protect the public health.

In Europe in recent years, a variety of methods have been used to encourage the immunization of children, including fines for parents who fail to immunize their children (Belgium and Italy), tax breaks and monetary rewards for those who comply (Austria), and monetary rewards to physicians who have high immunization rates among their patients (UK).[20] The most common and most successful policy, however, has been the requirement that children present proof of immunization for school admission. Ten years after the *Jacobson* decision, only 30% of states in the United States had compulsory immunization laws and as late as 1969, only half of the states had such laws. Public health surveys in the mid-1970s revealed that nationally child immunization programs were failing to reach as many as 40% of children, and rates of measles and other preventable diseases were rising.[21] In response, President Jimmy Carter in 1977 greatly increased funding for childhood immunization and charged the CDC with achieving 90% immunization coverage. States were encouraged to pass immunization laws, and within six years, all 50 states had laws that required immunization for school admission. As expected, child immunization rates approached 90% by the early 1980s. As a result, rates of polio

health law at its outset failed to have infectious disease at the forefront—diagnosing a problem parallel to our diagnosis of the development of the field of bioethics).

17. Jacobson v. Massachusetts, 197 U.S. 11, 26 (1905).
18. Jacobson v. Massachusetts, 197 U.S. 11, 26, 28 (1905).
19. Zucht v. King, 260 U.S. 174 (1922).
20. N.E. Moran, D. Shickle, C. Munthe et al., "Are Compulsory Immunization and Incentives to Immunize Effective Ways to Achieve Herd Immunity in Europe?" in *Ethics and Infectious Disease*, ed. Michael J. Selgelid, Margaret P. Battin, and Charles B. Smith (Oxford: Blackwell, 2006), ch. 14.
21. See Orenstein and Hinman, "Immunization System in the United States."

and measles rapidly declined and public health officials began to talk about eradicating these infections by the new millennium.

Despite their great successes, compulsory immunization policies have also been marked by mistrust, stemming initially from the very real risks of fledgling efforts at vaccine development, as well as from religious concerns. Mistrust has been compounded by policies directed against particular groups, such as immigrants. As we have seen, these concerns have an extensive historical basis, although in the contemporary world of careful vaccine testing, they may be more attenuated than popular opinion recognizes. Disputes over the new HPV vaccine have flared against this long background.

The Epidemiology of HPV: Virus, Warts, and Cancer

Human papillomavirus, a common virus that causes genital warts and cervical and other cancers, is the most common sexually transmitted disease in the United States and worldwide.[22] There are over 100 different genetically unique sub-types of this virus; and infection with the HPV virus is widespread, especially in younger women.

The HPV prevalence numbers are sobering. A recent U.S. study of active HPV infection in more than 2,000 women as determined by the presence of HPV DNA in vaginal swabs indicated an overall prevalence of 27% in women between ages 14 and 59. Young women between the ages of 14 and 19 had a prevalence of 25%, and the peak prevalence of 45% was detected in 20–24-year-old women.[23] These observations indicate that more than 24 million women in the United States between ages 14 and 59 are currently infected with HPV. Serological studies reveal that nearly 80% of women have antibodies to one or more types of HPV by age 50, indicating that they have been infected at one time.

Most HPV infections are of short duration and not associated with illness. However, some infections can become chronic (as measured by the persistence of virus DNA for four months or more), and it is these that lead to cervical intraepithelial neoplasia (CIN grades 1, 2 and 3)—abnormal lesions of the cervix that if left untreated eventually evolve into cancer of the cervix. While many of the 100 different strains of HPV are known to be oncogenic and have been associated with cervical and other cancers, strains 16 and 18 in particular

---

22. D. Saslow et al., "American Cancer Society Guideline for Human Papillomavirus (HPV) Vaccine Use to Prevent Cervical Cancer and Its Precursors," *CA A Cancer Journal for Clinicians.* no. 1 (January—February 2007): 7–28. See also Nubia Muñoz, F. Xavier Bosch, Silvia de Sanjosé et al., "Epidemiological Classification of Human Papillomavirus Types Associated with Cervical Cancer," *New England Journal of Medicine* 348, no. 6 (2003): 518–527.

23. E.F. Dunne et al., "Prevalence of HPV Infection Among Females in the United States," *Journal of the American Medical Association* 297 (2007): 813–819.

account for 70% of cervical cancers in the United States. In the U.S., types 16 and 18 are also the principal causes of other genital cancers such as cancer of the vulva, vagina and penis, and in cancer of the anus. HPV has also been implicated in 20% of cancers of the head and neck, and a recent study of oral-pharyngeal cancers indicated that HPV type 16 infection was an important etiologic factor.[24]

The high prevalence of HPV infection correlates with the relatively high incidence of cervical cancer in women in the United States. In 2006 it was estimated that nearly 10,000 cases of cervical cancer would be detected in the United States, and an estimated 3,700 women would die of cervical cancer. The oncogenic role of HPV is actually far greater than these figures reveal: the rate of diagnosis and mortality from cervical cancer in the United States and in other developed countries would be much higher were it not for the availability of Papanicolaou (Pap) cervical cytology screening for, and surgical removal of, early precancerous lesions of the cervix. The American College of Obstetricians and Gynecologists recommends Pap tests annually for women under 30 who are sexually active, and every 2–3 years for women over 30 who have had three negative tests in a row.[25] For those who are regularly tested, the risk of dying from cervical cancer is quite low. However, the fact that there are still some 10,000 cases and 3,700 deaths annually from cervical cancer in the United States indicates that some women are unable for a variety of reasons to benefit from screening programs—whether because they do not have access to screening, do not seek screening, or have objections to screening—and that an effective HPV vaccine would thus provide additional benefit. Moreover, in the United States today non-Hispanic black women have a prevalence of HPV infection that is nearly twice that of non-Hispanic white women and an associated increased risk of cervical cancer.[26]

Because Pap screening currently requires a robust health-care system, more successful programs have been limited to developed countries. Yet HPV is an endemic global phenomenon. In the developing world where Pap smears for detecting cervical cancer are not available, cervical cancer is the most common cancer in women, and every year more than 250,000 women worldwide die from this disease.[27] When the global health burden of all HPV associated cancers (cervical, genital, etc.) is calculated, 5.2% of all cancers worldwide can be attributed to HPV infection, and the attributable burden in developing countries is 7.7%, considerably greater than the 2.2% burden in developed

24. G D'Souza et al., "Case–Control Study of Human Papillomavirus and Oropharyngeal Cancer," *New England Journal of Medicine* 356, no. 19 (May 10, 2007): 1944–1956.
25. American College of Obstetricians and Gynecologists, *Special Procedures: The PAP Test* (Washington, DC: American College of Obstetricians and Gynecologists, 2003), http://www.acog.org/publications/patient_education/bp085.cfm (accessed January 5, 2008).
26. See Dunne et al., "Prevalence of HPV Infection."
27. Jan M. Agosti and Sue J. Goldie, "Introducing HPV Vaccine in Developing Countries—Key Challenges and Issues," *New England Journal of Medicine* 356, no. 19 (May 10, 2007): 1908–1910.

countries.[28] These increased rates of cervical cancer are due to multiple factors, including increased rates of STDs and the lack of cervical cancer screening programs that have been very successful in reducing the death rates from these cancers in the developed world.[29]

Under a grant from the Gates Foundation, the Alliance for Cervical Cancer Prevention is currently exploring use of new, relatively inexpensive tests for screening for cervical cancers in developing countries, in particular the visual inspection of the cervix with acetic acid (as in vinegar) and rapid-test DNA screens, together with cryotherapy that freezes away a lesion. Their preliminary results indicate that this combination may be the most effective currently available method of secondary prevention of cervical cancer in low-resource settings.[30] The possibility that HPV vaccines may be the most effective way to reduce cervical cancer in developing countries is also being seriously considered.[31] Where regular screening presents an available, if imperfect alternative to vaccine, the question remains open whether it presents a cost-effective and, for our purposes here, a morally preferable alternative to mandatory (whether compulsory, or routine with opt out provisions) vaccination policies.[32] Difficult decisions will have to be made by national and international public health funding programs about how much of their limited funds should be spent on HPV immunization programs. The HPV vaccine will be in competition for funds with established childhood immunization programs and rapidly expanding programs for early diagnosis and therapy for HIV, though these questions of distributive justice do not exhaust the moral issues involved.

Epidemiologic studies of the prevalence of HPV in men indicate that while males are usually asymptomatic carriers (and vectors) of the cancer-associated strains of HPV, infected males do have increased risk of penile cancer and gay men are at increased risk of HPV-related anal cancers. The recent observation that oropharyngeal cancers are highly associated with HPV strain 16 also observed that this cancer was much more prevalent in males (86%) than in females.

---

28. D.M. Parkin, "The Global Health Burden of Infection-Associated Cancers in the Year 2002," *International Journal of Cancer* 118 (2006): 3030–3044.

29. M. Schiffman and P.E. Castle, "The Promise of Global Cervical Cancer Prevention," *New England Journal of Medicine* 353, no. 20 (November 17, 2005): 2101–2104.

30. J. Bradely, "Delivering, Safe, Effective and Acceptable Cervical Cancer Prevention Services in Low Resource Settings," presentation at 2006 XVIII FIGO World Congress of Gynecology and Obstetrics, http://www.alliance-cxca.org (accessed January 5, 2008). New methods of screening for cervical cancer may also be available soon in developed countries. A molecular screening method is currently being studied; it reportedly has higher sensitivity but lower specificity than Pap tests and so may be used in complement with them. See, Carolyn D. Runowicz, "Molecular Screening for Cervical Cancer— Time to Give up Pap Tests?" *New England Journal of Medicine* 357, no. 16 (2008): 1650–1652.

31. The Gates Foundation has funded demonstration projects introducing HPV vaccine in India, Peru, Uganda, and Vietnam. Program for Appropriate Technology in Health (PATH), "PATH to Pave the Way for Cervical Cancer Vaccines in the Developing World," news release (June 5, 2006), http://path.org/news/pro60606-cervical_cancer_vaccine.php (accessed January 5, 2008).

32. Agosti and Goldie, "Introducing HPV Vaccine."

While sexual exposure was also an important risk factor, in this report, sex with a same-sex partner was not a risk factor.[33]

Two additional types of HPV, specifically 6 and 11, are the primary causes of human genital warts. Both men and women are susceptible to HPV-induced genital warts. The annual prevalence is approximately 1% of the sexually active population, and approximately 1.4 million people in the United States currently have genital warts.[34] While genital warts are generally considered benign in that they rarely evolve into cancers, they are very bothersome to those afflicted, and are a cause of frequent visits to physicians for treatment—treatment that often needs to be repeated multiple times. HPV strains 6 and 11 have also been associated with neonatal laryngeal papillomatosis, wart-like growths in the larynx of newborns that can cause respiratory obstruction.

As with some, but not all, other sexually transmitted infections, direct skin-to-skin physical contact such as vaginal or rectal intercourse is necessary for transmission of the HPV virus. The risk factors for acquiring HPV infection include the number of different sexual partners and the frequency of sexual exposures: one exposure is sufficient for transmission, but with multiple partners, the likelihood of exposure increases, as does the likelihood of exposure to multiple types of the virus. The aforementioned prevalence study indicated that women who had only one lifetime sexual partner had a relatively low risk of infection (11.5%) compared to women who had six or more lifetime partners (35%), and particularly to women who in the past year had six or more partners (56%).[35] A more recent large study of the risk of women acquiring HPV infection indicated that the one-year cumulative incidence of first HPV infection was 28.5% with a single male partner, indicating that "monogamy" or avoidance of multiple sexual partners was not an effective preventive practice.[36] Any sense of security against HPV on the part of a woman who is sexually active would thus appear misguided. The documented occurrence of cervical cancer in women who have limited their sexual exposure to other women has led to studies of the prevalence of HPV infection in women who have sex with women. A meta-analysis of these studies indicated that HPV can be sexually transmitted between women, but that this is not as common as in heterosexual exposures.[37] Circumcision among men has been associated with a significant

33. D'Souza et al., "Case–Control Study."
34. J.M. Partridge and L.A. Koutsky, "Genital Human Papillomavirus Infection in Men," *Lancet Infectious Diseases* 6, no. 1 (January 2006): 21–31.
35. Dunne et al, "Prevalence of HPV Infection."
36. R.L.Winer, Q.F. Feng, J.P. Hughes et al., "Risk of Female Human Papillomavirus Acquisition Associated with First Male Sex Partner," *Journal of Infectious Disease* 197 (January 15, 2008): 279–282.
37. J.M. Marrazzo, K. Stine, and L.A. Koufsky. "Genital Human Papillomavirus Infection in Women who have Sex with Women: A Review," *American Journal of Obstetrics and Gynecology* 183, no. 3 (September 2000): 770–774.

reduction in the prevalence of HPV infection and a corresponding reduction in the prevalence of cervical cancer in their sexual partners.[38] However, condom use provides only partial protection against HPV infection and associated warts or pre-cancerous lesions,[39] and "safe sex" is not sex that is safe from HPV.

The HPV Vaccines: Safety and Efficacy

In June 2006, the U.S. Food Drug Administration (FDA) approved Merck's Gardasil, the first effective HPV vaccine, for use in females ages 9 to 26.[40] A similar vaccine developed by GlaxoSmithKline (Cevarix) is currently under FDA review, but had not received approval as of April 2008. Both vaccines are highly immunogenic, with good titers of antibodies to the antigens used in the vaccines appearing in both males and females; these antibodies appear to persist for at least five years. Early data show that for the virus types included in the vaccines, there has been nearly 100% reduction in persistent HPV infection and in development of dysplastic or pre-cancerous lesions of the cervix.

The current HPV vaccines include only 4 of the 100 plus types of HPV, but do include those associated with the most widespread pathology in the United States. Gardasil includes types 16 and 18, which account for 70% of cervical cancers in the United States, as well as types 6 and 11, the primary causes of human genital warts. The GlaxoSmithKline vaccine includes only types 16 and 18.[41] Recent studies suggest that there may also be significant cross-protection against other cancer producing types of HPV.[42]

Vaccine Safety

Based on current information, the two HPV vaccines have an acceptable safety record. Because the vaccine antigen is a virus product produced in another non-infectious biologic system (yeast or a benign virus), there is no fear that a failure to inactivate the vaccine virus would result in a vaccine-related infection.

---

38. Castellsagué et al., "Male Circumcision, Penile Human Papillomavirus Infection, and Cervical Cancer in Female Partners," *New England Journal of Medicine* 346, no. 15 (April 11, 2002): 1105–1112.

39. L.E. Manhart and L.A. Koutsky, "Do Condoms Prevent Genital HPV Infection, External Genital Warts, or Cervical Neoplasia? A Meta-Analysis," *Sexually Transmitted Diseases* 29, no. 11 (2002): 725–735.

40. U.S. Food and Drug Administration, "FDA Licenses New Vaccine for Prevention of Cervical Cancer and Other Diseases in Females Caused by Human Papillomavirus," news release (June 8, 2006), http://www.fda.gov/bbs/topics/NEWS/2006/NEW01385.html (accessed January 5, 2008); Saslow et al., "Guideline for Human Papillomavirus (HPV) Vaccine."

41. See Saslow et al., "Guideline for Human Papillomavirus (HPV) Vaccine."

42. B.M. Kuehn, "Benefits of Newer Vaccines Lauded," *Journal of the American Medical Association* 298, no. 18 (November 14, 2007): 2123–2125.

After five years of observation, side effects such as transient redness, pain and swelling at the vaccine site, and occasional fainting have been minimal and generally similar to those associated with other non-infectious virus antigen vaccines such as the Salk inactivated polio vaccine. Such inactivated products, properly manufactured, pose no transmission risks to third parties, such as occur with the Sabin live polio vaccine (as well as the poorly manufactured batches of the Salk vaccine) and the smallpox vaccines. No one can get HPV from the HPV vaccine.

A concern is that the small number of individuals receiving the vaccine before FDA approval (fewer than 25,000) and the relatively short observation period for detecting uncommon side effects may have failed to identify serious side effects that may not be detectable until the number of vaccine recipients exceeds 100,000.[43] For example, Guillain-Barré Syndrome (GBS), a disease characterized by transient paralysis, has been associated with some batches of the inactivated influenza virus vaccine, and only post-marketing surveillance detected this complication.[44] As of mid-October 2006, Merck claimed that over 750,000 doses of Gardasil had been distributed, and the CDC- and FDA-managed Vaccine Adverse Events Reporting System (VAERS) passive surveillance system for reporting adverse events had not revealed any new or disturbing complications. Two cases of GBS have followed administration of Gardasil together with the meningococcal vaccine,[45] however; and it is too early to determine if this complication will be more common after the HPV vaccine than the 1.36/100,000 overall yearly incidence of this condition.[46] Although risks of the vaccine appear very minimal, they cannot be ruled out entirely at this point in time.

Another safety concern that has been raised about the HPV vaccine is that it may create a false sense of security among those receiving it and their sexual partners. There have been no surveys of adolescents about the effect that a vaccine against HPV might have on their sexual behaviors. Some surveys of adolescents' opinions about the effects of a possible vaccine against the HIV virus have suggested that increases in high-risk behaviors such as more promiscuous sex and use of intravenous drugs would follow assurances that a vaccine would protect them against AIDS.[47] Similarly, there are reports that

43. L.O. Gostin and C.D. DeAngelis, "Mandatory HPV Vaccination: Public Health vs Private Wealth," *Journal of the American Medical Association* 297, no. 17 (May 2, 2007): 1921–1923.
44. A.H. Ropper and M. Victor, "Influenza Vaccination and the Guillain-Barré Syndrome," *New England Journal of Medicine* 339, no. 25 (December 17, 1998): 1845–1846.
45. Centers for Disease Control and Prevention, *ACIP Meeting Minutes October 25–26, 2006: Update on the Quadrivalent HPV Vaccine*, http://www.cdc.gov/vaccines/recs/acip/downloads/min-oct06.pdf (accessed January 5, 2008), 46.
46. A. Chio, D. Cocito, and M. Leone, "Guillain-Barré Syndrome: A Prospective, Population-Based Incidence and Outcome Survey," *Neurology* 60 (2003): 1146–1150.
47. P.M. Webb, G.D. Zimet, R. Mays, and J.D. Fortenberry, "HIV Immunization: Acceptability and Anticipated Effects on Sexual Behavior Among Adolescents," *Journal of Adolescent Health* 25 (1999): 320–322.

availability of new drugs that slow the progression of HIV infection to AIDS has been associated with increases in risky behaviors.[48] Some believe that increases in risky behaviors following HPV vaccination would be unlikely because most people do not have a fear of HPV that is as great as the fear of HIV that has been a significant factor in altering sexual practices.[49] Public concerns about the safety of the new HPV vaccines may be related to recent acceleration of the FDA approval process for new drugs and vaccines.[50] Patient activist groups representing those with HIV/AIDS and cancer have been very effective in the past decade in challenging the FDA to shorten the review process, and to be less stringent about requirements for proof of efficacy and safety in approving potentially life-saving new drugs. Women's activist groups have been particularly forceful in pushing for more rapid approval of treatments for the cancers—such as breast and cervical—that affect women.

Recent examples of post-marketing detection of serious side effects of FDA-approved drugs such as the arthritis drug Vioxx (associated heart problems) have led to the subsequent withdrawal of marketed drugs.[51] Some of these adverse events were known to the pharmaceutical manufacturer but were not disclosed in a timely manner to the FDA.[52] There is also concern among some that Merck's aggressive lobbying and marketing of Gardasil inappropriately influenced the FDA to rush to approval before adequate safety data were collected, as well as state legislators to support including HPV vaccine in the vaccine programs required for school entry.[53]

Efficacy and Cost Effectiveness

Efficacy of the HPV vaccines is well established; trials have shown that both vaccines are nearly 100% effective against persistent infection with the targeted types of HPV viruses and related precancerous lesions[54]—a level of efficacy that is sim-

---

48. D.E. Ostrow et al., "Attitudes Towards Highly Active Antiretroviral Therapy Are Associated with Sexual Risk Taking Among HIV-Infected and Uninfected Homosexual Men," *AIDS* 16, no. 5 (2002): 775–780.

49. G.D. Zimet et al., "Chapter 24: Psychosocial Aspects of Vaccine Acceptability," *Vaccine* 24, suppl. 3 (August 21, 2006): S201–S209.

50. B.M. Psaty and R.A. Charo, "FDA Responds to Institute of Medicine Drug Safety Recommendations—In Part," *Journal of the American Medical Association* 297, no. 17 (May 2, 2007): 1917–1920.

51. R. Horton, "Vioxx, the Implosion of Merck, and Aftershocks at the FDA," *Lancet* 364, no. 9450 (December 4–10, 2004): 1995–1996.

52. Alex Berenson, "Evidence in Vioxx Suits Shows Intervention by Merck Officials," *New York Times* sect. 1, April 24, 2005.

53. Adriane Fugh-Berman, "Cervical Cancer Vaccines and Industry Influence," *Bioethics Forum* (March 15, 2007), http://www.bioethicsforum.org/Merck-Gardasil-pharmaceutical-marketing.asp (accessed January 5, 2008).

54. See Saslow et al., "Guideline for Human Papillomavirus (HPV) Vaccine."

ilar to or better than other well-established vaccines such as polio and measles. However, as we have said, HPV vaccines are ineffective against a given HPV type once chronic infection with that virus type has occurred; thus for maximum efficacy, HPV vaccines must be administered *before* first infection with HPV virus types included in the vaccine.[55] For this reason, administration is recommended for girls and very young women, before first sexual contact. Nonetheless, because the vaccine may provide only partial protection against the additional 30% of cancer-producing HPV types besides those directly covered, for full protection cervical screening will continue to be necessary despite vaccination.

The cost of Gardasil has been a source of concern for public health planners from the start. The most expensive vaccine ever marketed,[56] Gardasil is a potential source of considerable earnings for Merck.[57] The vaccine currently markets for $120 per injection or $360 for the full series.[58] The full immunization schedule not only requires three injections but the added cost of visits to physician offices, so the total cost for protective immunization will usually exceed $400. For example, the Utah State Health Department currently charges more than $500 for the full HPV immunization series. As of 2007, several health insurance companies had agreed to cover the cost of HPV vaccine and it is likely that in time public pressure and cost-effectiveness studies will lead more to follow. The CDC has approved the HPV vaccine for inclusion in the Vaccines for Children (VFC) program; thus children without health insurance who are eligible for Medicaid funding will likely receive free HPV vaccine.

The cost of any vaccine can be weighed against the likelihood that it will prevent illness or death: the cheaper the vaccine and the more serious and prevalent the disease, the higher a vaccine's cost-effectiveness; the more expensive a vaccine and the rarer the disease, the lower its cost-effectiveness. Cost-effectiveness studies reported to date for the HPV vaccine have varied from $1,500 to almost $60,000 per quality adjusted life year (QALY) saved, the variability depending on who is included in the immunization program and which costs and benefits are included in the analysis. This range of cost per QALY places the HPV vaccine within the range of the more expensive currently recommended vaccines (pneumococcal vaccine for children $21,000—$80,000 and meningococcal vaccine $58,000 per QALY). At the very low end of these figures, a recent study by Merck analysts estimated that a policy of vaccinating 12-year-old girls with Gardasil would reduce cervical cancer due

55. Future II Study Group, "Quadrivalent HPV Vaccine."
56. Schwartz, Caplan, Faden, and Sugarman, "Lessons from the Failure."
57. Gardasil had earnings of $1.14 billion for the first three quarters of 2007. Associated Press, "2 Drug Makers' Profits Soar; One Runs Afoul of Wall St.," *New York Times* sec. C, October 23, 2007.
58. Schwartz, Caplan, Faden, and Sugarman, "Lessons from the Failure."

to HPV strains in the vaccine by 78%, at an incremental cost of $4,666 per QALY.[59]

Although as effective, the HPV vaccine is not as *cost*-effective as diptheria-pertussis-tetanus vaccine (DPT), hepatitis B vaccine, or varicella (chickenpox) vaccine, which are said to be overall cost saving.[60] Where the HPV vaccine will rank in priority with other immunization programs with limited budgets will ultimately depend on more consistent cost-effectiveness studies and political and ethical considerations, as well as any pricing changes.[61] It will also depend on comparative cost-effectiveness analyses of alternatives, such as regular Pap test or other methods of screening. At present, some analyses suggest that screening may be more cost effective than HPV vaccine in countries with limited resources, although this assessment may change as vaccine pricing changes.[62]

The CDC and Professional Societies

Within a month of FDA approval, the new HPV vaccine was recommended by the CDC Advisory Committee on Immunization Practices (ACIP) for females between the ages of 11 and 26.[63] Most independent professional societies—including the American Academy of Family Physicians,[64] the American Academy of Pediatrics,[65] the Infectious Diseases Society of America,[66] the American College of

59. E.H. Elbasha, E.J. Dasbach, and R.P. Insinga, "Model for Assessing Human Papillomavirus Vaccination Strategies," *Emerging Infectious Diseases* 13, no. 1 (January 2007): 28–41.
60. Center on the Evaluation of Value and Risk in Health, *The Cost-Effectiveness Analysis Registry: Cost-Utility Analyses Published in 2002 and 2003* (Boston: Tufts-New England Medical Center, ICRHPS), http://160.109.101.132/cearegistry/data/docs/PhaseIIIACompleteLeagueTable.pdf (accessed January 5, 2008). See also Sue J. Goldie, Michele Kohli, Daniel Grima et al., "Projected Clinical Benefits and Cost-effectiveness of the Human Papillomavirus 16/18 Vaccine," *Journal of the National Cancer Institute* 96, no. 3 (2004): 604–615.
61. As the number of recommended vaccines has risen, costs of immunization have risen greatly; in the United States, considerable gaps have been reported in financial coverage of vaccines for uninsured children. Grace M. Lee, Jeanne M. Santoli, Claire Hannan et al., "Gaps in Vaccine Financing for Underinsured Children in the United States," *Journal of the American Medical Association* 298, no. 6 (August 8, 2007): 638–643.
62. Agosti and Goldie, "Introducing HPV Vaccine."
63. Centers for Disease Control and Prevention, "Quadrivalent Human Papillomavirus Vaccine: Recommendations of the Advisory Committee on Immunization Practices (ACIP)," *Mortality and Morbidity Weekly Report* 56, no. RR02 (March 23, 2007): 1–24; Centers for Disease Control and Prevention, "National Vaccination Coverage Among Adolescents Aged 13–17 years—United States, 2006," *Mortality and Morbidity Weekly Report* 56, no. 34 (August 1, 2007): 885–888.
64. American Academy of Family Physicians, "AFFP Policy Statement Regarding Consideration of the Mandated Use of HPV for School Attendance" (February 7, 2007), http://www.aafp.org/online/en/home/clinical/immunizationres/mandatedhpv.html (accessed January 5, 2008).
65. American Academy of Pediatrics Committee on Infectious Diseases, "Recommended Immunization Schedules for Children and Adolescents—United States, 2007," *Pediatrics* 119, no. 1 (January 2007): 207–208.
66. Infectious Diseases Society of America, "Statement on the Human Papillomavirus (HPV) Vaccine," http://www.idsociety.org/Content.aspx?id=6532 (accessed January 5, 2008).

Obstetricians and Gynecologists,[67] and the American Cancer Society[68]—have recommended HPV vaccination of pre-teen girls be implemented as a routine office practice. Indicative of the tensions generated by the vaccine's introduction is that these medical advisory bodies all left decisions about the method for implementation, such as requiring immunization for admission to middle or junior high schools, to the states. The American Academy of Family Physicians specifically advised against mandating the vaccine for school admissions because of its cost, while other groups did not address the school requirement issue.

Disputes over HPV Vaccines

Soon after FDA approval, citing the impressive safety and efficacy data, a *New York Times* editorial advocated inclusion of HPV vaccine with other vaccines required for school entry.[69] With the help of Merck's extensive lobbying, the governor of Texas issued an executive order mandating the HPV vaccine for girls entering middle schools, normally ages 12 to 14. But the Texas mandate was short-lived: amid controversy, the Texas Legislature promptly approved a bill that would nullify the governor's order.[70] Similar controversies erupted in other states such as Michigan and Virginia, as legislatures proposed that the HPV vaccine be required for school admission, while conservative lobbyists opposed the legislative proposals.[71]

At the center of these controversies were the price of the vaccine and the lobbying by Merck in support of requiring the vaccine for middle- or high-school girls. A few months after the introduction of Gardasil in 2006, Jason L. Schwartz of the Ethics of Vaccines Project at the University of Pennsylvania, commenting on a *Business Week* prediction that Merck might triple its vaccine revenues to reach $6 billion by 2010,[72] suggested that the explosive growth of the vaccine business in the United States underscores a period ahead in which ethical considerations will demand much more attention.[73] Adriane Fugh-Berman, writing in the *Hastings Center Report*'s Bioethics Forum, was also concerned

67. K. Ault, "Vaccines for the Prevention of Human Papillomavirus-Related Diseases: A Review," *Obstetrical & Gynecological Survey* 61, no. 6, suppl. 1 (June 2006): S26–S31.

68. See Saslow et al., "Guideline for Human Papillomavirus (HPV) Vaccine."

69. Editorial, "A Vaccine to Save Women's Lives," *New York Times*, sec. A, February 6, 2007.

70. Dan Frosch, "Texas House Rejects Order by Governor on Vaccines," *New York Times*, sec. A, March 14, 2007. See also Schwartz, Caplan, Faden, and Sugarman, "Lessons from the Failure," 761.

71. Schwartz, Caplan, Faden, and Sugarman, "Lessons from the Failure."

72. Jason L. Schwartz, "Gardasil: Profile of Merck Vaccines President; Feature on Early HPV–Cancer Link Proponent," University of Pennsylvania, Center for Bioethics (January 3, 2007), http://www.vaccineethics.org/2007/01/gardasil-profile-of-merck-vaccines.html (accessed January 5, 2008).

73. Arlene Weintraub, "Making Her Mark at Merck," *Business Week* (January 8, 2007), http://www.businessweek.com/magazine/content/07_02/b4016074.htm?chan=top±news_top±news±index_technology (accessed January 5, 2008).

about Merck's influence.[74] Merck has been accused of initiating the most aggressive lobbying campaign in the history of vaccine marketing, with money going to the governor of Texas and legislators in several states. Merck's decision to route a large portion of its lobbying money through the Women in Government group of women legislators proved particularly effective in informing state legislators, as well as in recruiting women to support this vaccine directed against a common woman's cancer. In addition, Merck attempted to encourage insurance coverage for their HPV vaccine, with remarkable success in the first six months after FDA approval. For example, a bill was introduced to the Colorado Legislature to require insurers to pay for the vaccine.[75] As these lobbying and marketing practices were identified by the press and criticized in editorials and by the public, Merck reduced its lobbying efforts, realizing that these practices might in the long term impede trust and acceptance of the HPV vaccine.[76]

Other challenges to mandatory immunization policies came from libertarian groups espousing individual rights who generally oppose all mandatory immunization programs,[77] defenders of autonomy, and religious and conservative groups who were concerned that acceptance of this vaccine against a sexually transmitted disease would imply that their daughters either were or were going to be sexually promiscuous.[78] Among those objecting to mandatory programs, medical ethicists Bernard Lo[79] and Michael Zimmerman[80] each editorialized that

---

74. Fugh-Berman, "Cervical Cancer Vaccines."

75. Steven K. Paulson, "Bill Would Require Insurers to Pay for HPV Vaccine," Associated Press (March 8, 2007), http://cbs4denver.com/politics/Colorado.news.Denver.2.557108.html (accessed January 5, 2008).

76. Merck's lobbying also took place against a background of mistrust in government programs in general. In U.S. health care, the Tuskegee syphilis study has fostered mistrust; see Susan Reverby, ed., *Tuskegee's Truths: Rethinking the Tuskegee Syphilis Study* (Chapel Hill: University of North Carolina Press, 2000). So have concerns that the government has lied to the public about the need to resuscitate the smallpox vaccination program; see V.W. Sidel, R.M. Gould, and H.W. Cohen, "Bioterrorism Preparedness: Cooptation of Public Health?" *Medicine and Global Survival* 7, no. 2 (2002): 82–89. Examples of governments lying to the public about vaccines include the overt decision of the government of India to not tell the public about the risk of acquiring a polio-like paralysis following the oral Sabin vaccine, a risk that, although small (1 in 500,000), is real; see Y. Paul and A. Dawson, "Some Ethical Issues Arising from Polio Eradication Programmes in India," in *Ethics and Infectious Disease*, eds. Michael J. Selgelid, Margaret P. Battin, and Charles B. Smith (Oxford: Blackwell, 2006), ch. 16.

77. M.A. Fumento, "A Merck-y Business. The Case Against Mandatory HPV Vaccinations," *Weekly Standard* 12, no. 25, March 12, 2007.

78. Rob Stein, "Cervical Cancer Vaccine Gets Injected with a Social Issue. Some Fear a Shot for Teens Would Encourage Sex," *Washington Post*, sec. A, October 31, 2005. For a discussion of the role of such cultural factors in opposition to HPV vaccination, see Editorial, "Rolling Out HPV Vaccines Worldwide," *Lancet* 367, no. 9528 (June 24, 2006): 2034.

79. B. Lo, "HPV Vaccine and Adolescents' Sexual Activity," *British Medical Journal* 332, no. 7550 (May 13, 2006): 1106–1107.

80. M. Zimmerman, "Ethical Analysis of HPV Vaccine Policy Options," *Vaccine* 24 (2006): 4812–4820.

HPV vaccine was different from previous vaccines because behaviors that led to human papillomavirus infections were under the control of individuals and thus should not be required for school entry. The extent of freedom-of-choice opposition, however, was sometimes distorted in the press. For instance, the Center for Bioethics at the University of Pennsylvania's Ethics of Vaccines project notes a headline released by a group at the University of Michigan C.S. Mott Children's Hospital, "Majority of U.S. Parents Not in Favor of State HPV Vaccine Mandates," reporting data showing 26% of parents disagreeing with an HPV mandate, 44% agreeing, and 30% "neutral"—thus the headline could equally well have read "76% of Parents Not Opposed to HPV Mandate."[81]

Although generally opposing requiring the vaccine for school entry, most conservative and religion-based health advisory groups have been generally supportive of development and marketing of the HPV vaccine and education of the public about the risks of sexually transmitted diseases. The Christian Medical and Dental Association's policy statement early in 2007 supported the development and administration of vaccines intended to lessen the incidence and consequences of sexually transmitted diseases, and reflected encouragement that the HPV vaccine will reduce the incidence of cervical cancer and genital warts. However, it emphasized that the best advice for sexual health is abstinence before marriage and faithfulness within marriage, and did not address immunization requirements.[82] The Medical Institute for Sexual Health similarly supports the routine use of the HPV vaccine and believes that all adolescent females should be vaccinated, but emphatically opposes mandatory vaccination, believing that timing of vaccination should be decided by each girl's parents in consultation with her doctor.[83]

Focus on the Family, a Christian organization, takes the same view as the Christian Medical and Dental Association, in advocating widespread availability of the HPV vaccine but opposing mandatory immunization.[84] However, Focus on the Family, like Zimmerman and Lo, particularly emphasizes the differences between infectious diseases that can be acquired by just sitting in the classroom—for example varicella (chickenpox)—and HPV, which is spread by sexual activity. The idea that HPV infection is linked with promiscuity is a

81. Jason L. Schwartz, "Gardasil: CDC Response on Safety/Efficacy; Survey on Parental Support for Mandates," University of Pennsylvania, Center for Bioethics (June 15, 2007), http://www.vaccineethics.org/2007_06_01_archive.html (accessed January 5, 2008).
82. Christian Medical and Dental Associations, *Position Statement: Human Papilloma Virus Vaccine*, (Pheonix, AZ: Christian Medical and Dental Associations, January 26, 2007), http://www.cmda.org/AM/Template.cfm?Section=Ethics_and_Position_Statements&Template=/CM/ContentDisplay.cfm&ContentID=4293 (accessed January 5, 2008).
83. The Medical Institute for Sexual Health, "The Medical Institute's Statement on Mandatory HPV Vaccination" (February 2007), http://www.medinstitute.org/content.php?name=HPVVaccineStatement (accessed January 6, 2008).
84. Focus on the Family, "Focus on the Family Position Statement: Human Papillomavirus Vaccines," http://www.family.org/socialissues/A000000357.cfm (accessed January 6, 2008).

common reason for many to oppose requiring the vaccine, even when they fail to object to vaccination for Hepatitis B, another sexually transmitted infection. As the *New York Times* medical columnist Denise Grady opined, "vital discussion about a vaccine has been clouded by promiscuity concerns."[85] In a recent thoughtful review of this issue, Charo concludes that the "opposition seems to be based on the concern that to recognize the reality of teenage sexual activity is implicitly to endorse it."[86]

Even such historically liberal institutions as Harvard University have entered the debate about compulsory vaccination for a sexually transmitted disease. The Seneca, a Harvard women's club, partnered with 13 other women's groups to establish the Harvard HPV Vaccine Awareness Campaign to encourage all undergraduates to get the immunization and to pressure the University Health Services to offer it for free. However, in a debate sponsored by these women's groups, the Harvard Debate Society concluded that HPV vaccine should not be mandatory.[87]

Safety concerns also were among the issues raised by those who opposed the campaign for rapid adoption of mandatory immunization. The National Vaccine Information Center has raised questions about whether there is sufficient evidence to conclude that it is safe to administer Gardasil at the same time as other vaccines, particularly meningococcal vaccine.[88] However, safety concerns are sometimes distorted by public misperception or by the press For example, a news item from JudicialWatch.org, described by the University of Pennsylvania Center for Bioethics' Ethics of Vaccines project as a "breathless press release,"[89] claimed that there were three deaths related to the HPV vaccine, but the CDC vaccine Q&A, *HPV Vaccine—Questions and Answers for the Public,* issued in June 2007, explains clearly why the deaths had other explanations.[90]

Less than a year after FDA approval of Gardasil, requiring HPV vaccine for school entry had become an increasingly unpopular issue; many state legislatures refused to adopt the requirements; and in March 2007 Merck, in the face of increasingly unfavorable press, announced that it was pulling back its lobbying campaign.[91] As of October 2007, 41 states and the District of Columbia

---

85. Denise Grady, "A Vital Discussion, Clouded," *New York Times,* sec. F, March 6, 2007.

86. Charo, "Politics, Parents, and Prophylaxis."

87. Marissa C. Lopez, "Society Debated HPV Vaccine," *The Harvard Crimson, Online Edition* (March 7, 2007), http://www.thecrimson.com/article.aspx?ref=517523 (accessed January 6, 2008).

88. National Vaccine Information Center, "NVIC Letter to ACIP Chairman Regarding HPV VAERS Reports" (August 14, 2007), http://www.909shot.com/Diseases/HPV/D.Morse_in_PDF_2%5B1%5D.pdf (accessed January 6, 2008).

89. Schwartz, "Gardasil: CDC Response on Safety/Efficacy."

90. Centers for Disease Control and Prevention, "HPV Vaccine—Questions & Answers for the Public" (June 28, 2007), http://www.cdc.gov/vaccines/vpd-vac/hpv/hpv-vacsafe-effic.htm (accessed January 6, 2008).

91. Associated Press, "Drugmaker Stops Lobbying Efforts for STD Shots: Merck Criticized by Parents and Doctors for Pushing Cervical Cancer Vaccine" (February 20, 2007), http://www.msnbc.msn.com/id/17246920/ (accessed January 6, 2008).

had introduced legislation to require, fund, or educate the public about the HPV vaccine, and 17 states had enacted this legislation.[92] Only two states, Virginia and New Jersey, had enacted legislation that requires HPV immunization for school entry. Several other states have provided significant funding for a voluntary immunization program, including New Hampshire and South Dakota. Utah enacted legislation establishing an education program, but rejected a proposal to provide specific funding for HPV vaccine. Interestingly, a local businessman then donated $1 million to provide vaccine for the needy, explaining, "God put me on this earth to cure cancer, not to judge others."[93]

Victims, Vectors, and Requiring HPV Immunization

From the PVV perspective, a too-narrow understanding of victimhood and vectorhood has hampered the debates about HPV immunization. Arguments for school-entry requirements, while properly calling attention to the importance of protecting young women, have taken inadequate account of the multiplicity of victimhood. They have also ignored the role of both young women and young men as vectors of HPV.

Safety, Efficacy, and Cost-Effectiveness

Powerful arguments in favor of immunization requirements are the safety, efficacy, and cost-effectiveness of the vaccine. Safety and efficacy are crucial issues for both victims and vectors: unsafe vaccines put people or perhaps others with whom they come in contact at risk, and ineffective vaccines do so with little benefit. We have already presented the highly favorable safety and efficacy profile of the HPV vaccine as it appears to date. Nonetheless, protection of potential victims of vaccination requires that the data about safety should continue to be carefully and openly monitored by impartial bodies such as the FDA. To enhance trust, results of this monitoring should be public.

In addition, if low-probability risks of the vaccine do come to light, the vaccine should be added to the program providing compensation for those who have been injured by vaccination. In Chapter 18, we will develop arguments for compensation when people are subject to constraints to protect others against transmission of infectious disease, and are harmed as a result. Our examples there are constraints in a pandemic, but similar arguments apply when people are harmed by vaccination as well—especially when the rationale for the vaccination is largely to create herd effects that are beneficial to

---

92. National Conference of State Legislatures, "HPV Vaccine Legislation 2007," http://ncsl.org/programs/health/hpvvaccine.htm (accessed January 6, 2008).

93. David Sundwall, M.D., personal communication; see also Carey Hamilton, "Cervical Cancer Battle Gets a $1 Million Jolt," *Salt Lake Tribune*, April 5, 2007.

others, as it might be if HPV vaccination requirements were extended to males as well as females. Although created in large part to encourage vaccine manufacturers faced with liability claims for injury to stay in business, the U.S. National Vaccine Injury and Compensation Program, established in 1988, also speaks to the idea that it is only fair for the government to compensate individuals who suffer complications of a vaccine program designed for the common good. Vaccines are covered by the compensation fund if they are required; HPV vaccine is not currently covered by the program, but should be if vaccination becomes required for school entry.[94]

With respect to efficacy, too, there are important issues to monitor about the HPV vaccine. The vaccine is highly effective against 70% of viral types causing potentially oncogenic HPV infection in the United States—but less effective against the other 30% of oncogenic types. The risk that victims may believe that they are fully protected because they have been vaccinated—and that they are also shielded against vectorhood as a result—remains. This is not an argument *against* requiring vaccination, but *for* continued vigilance to ensure that vaccination is not misunderstood by anyone potentially at risk.

Typically, cost-effectiveness considerations are population-, rather than individual-based: they average the cost (or rather, price) of a vaccine (or any medication) over its impact on the health of the population using it to determine its priority in the list of public health programs vying for limited funds. One particular challenge to the cost-effectiveness of HPV vaccine is that at present it cannot replace the standard method of cervical cancer screening with Pap smears. Another challenge is the very high price of the currently available vaccine. As a result, cost-effectiveness considerations may at present counsel against public funding for the vaccine in circumstances where funding is quite limited. Nonetheless, as previously noted, the U.S. CDC has included the HPV vaccine in its Vaccine for Children program, some states and several foreign countries, including Australia and Mexico, have allocated state money to pay for the vaccine.[95]

Moreover, reliance on cost-effectiveness considerations in vaccination policies raises additional questions from a nuanced PVV perspective. Such decisions do not attend to the individual characteristics or identity of users of the vaccine, or to whether this specific individual would or would not have been infected by the virus in the absence of vaccination. If cost effectiveness decisions are made across a population, moreover, inadequate attention may be paid to distributions within population subgroups. For example, in the United States,

---

94. HRSA, "National Vaccine Injury Compensation Program, Strategic Plan" (April 2006), http://www.hrsa.gov/vaccinecompensation/strategic_plan.htm (accessed February 12, 2008).
95. *HPV Today*, "Approaches to the Use of HPV Vaccines: Interview with Ian Fraser," *HPV Today* 10 (February 2007), www.hpvtoday.com (accessed January 6, 2008), 3.

regular screening for cervical cancer is widely available across the population considered as a whole, but may not be readily available within subgroups with particular challenges to access to health care, especially minority women. Finally, any vaccine requirement that is not accompanied by public or charitable dollars for those who could not pay is surely unjust; indeed, as we shall argue in Chapter 19, the PVV perspective supports funding vaccine initiatives.

Autonomy, Accurate Information, and Differences in Values

A particularly potent ethical argument against compulsory immunization is individuals' autonomous rights to make their own decisions about their health care. This is the argument that Jacobson made in his failed challenge to Massachusetts smallpox immunization laws.[96]

Respect for patient choice is less warranted when the choices are based on inadequate information: potential victims would not want to respect the poorly reasoned choices of others that might have significant adverse effects on their own health. Thus in the debates about requiring HPV vaccine, little weight should be given to concerns that are based on inaccurate information. Public mistrust of the accuracy of safety and efficacy data about Gardasil may be unwarranted, but is hardly irrational in light of Merck's marketing campaign and the recent history of inadequate disclosure of adverse drug experiences. If the move toward mandatory immunization continues, it will be especially important to address issues of mistrust with careful and impartial analysis of data. Otherwise, it will be troubling to people as potential victims of the vaccine to be subject to requirements where risks are not fully disclosed.

An important reason to respect autonomy is that people have different views about fundamental values. Some value health more than others do; some place religious values above all worldly concerns. In a survey of childhood fatalities from religion-motivated medical neglect, several cases of deaths due to childhood vaccine-preventable infections such as measles, pertussis, and diphtheria were documented.[97] Religious, conscientious, and philosophical beliefs are the basis for some individuals not to want to accept vaccines for themselves or for their children. While no church policies mandate members' health-care decisions, Christian Scientists believe in prayer rather than medical treatment.[98] Similarly, some people, apart from organized religious doctrine, philosophically believe that many modern medical practices, including

96. Parmet, Goodman, and Farber, "Individual Rights Versus the Public's Health."
97. S.M. Asser and R. Swan, "Child Fatalities from Religion-Motivated Medical Neglect," *Pediatrics* 101 (1998): 625–629.
98. Church of Christ, Scientist, "Welcome," http://www.tfccs.com/index.jhtml;jsessionid=PTELN ZDIR24KXKGL4L2SFEQ (accessed February 11, 2008).

use of vaccines, are against the rules of nature, and wish to be absolved from mandatory health-care requirements. Out of respect for those whose religious and philosophical beliefs oppose vaccinations, most state laws or policies mandating immunization for school admissions allow for individual waivers.[99]

In insisting on conscientious refusal of vaccination, an individual patient is seeing the situation from her perspective as likely victim of the disease, but is willing to refuse immunization, because she values something else—for example, spiritual salvation, bodily integrity, or "natural" living—more than the risk of illness. She is not, however, viewing the situation from the perspective of someone else, another person who might be infected because she has not been vaccinated and has become ill. She is not thinking about the person who might want protection from her or what, if anything, she owes him to keep this from happening.

When people refuse immunization, the consequences for others may be minimal, if conscientious refusals occur infrequently. Herd immunity may still be present, so others are not put at risk of disease transmission. If herd immunity exists, potential victims have little to fear from vectors, and thus can tolerate conscientious refusals—to the extent that these refusals do not reach a level that threatens herd immunity. At present, conscientious waivers are generally granted to less than 2% of the vaccine-eligible population,[100] and some public health experts concede this small number of unimmunized individuals would not likely interfere with herd immunity.[101] If, however, waivers rise above a level of protective herd immunity—and this level will vary with the transmissibility of the disease, as well as other factors—failures to immunize do put others at very real risk. Outbreaks of measles and pertussis have been clearly linked to small communities with very high rates of religion-based refusal to be immunized.[102] In some of these cases, the waivers are rescinded and immunizations are again required for school entry to control the local outbreak.

The difficulty of achieving herd immunity in HPV, at least in the near future, also weakens the weight of individual autonomy from the perspective of the victim. HPV infection is currently widespread among the U.S. population and across the globe. Herd immunity is thus quite far from present-day reality. Moreover, immunization requirements that are directed against girls only may not generate the requisite level of protection to provide herd immunity,

99. D.S. Diekema and the Committee on Bioethics, "Responding to Parental Refusals of Immunization of Children," *Pediatrics* 115 (2005): 1428–1431.
100. James G. Hodge and Lawrence O. Gostin, "School Vaccination Requirements: Historical, Social, and Legal Perspectives," *Kentucky Law Journal* 90 (2001–2002): 831–890 (875).
101. Diekema and the Committee on Bioethics, "Responding to Parental Refusals of Immunization."
102. Centers for Disease Control and Prevention, "Outbreak of Measles Among Christian Science Students—Missouri and Indiana, 1994," *Mortality and Morbidity Weekly Report* 43, no. 25 (July 1, 1994): 463–465.

although some experts believe widespread immunization of girls would significantly reduce the prevalence of HPV. Although immunized young women will not transmit HPV to young men, the virus remains transmissible from male to male; unimmunized women thus might also remain vulnerable to infection. In addition, even if vaccination is sufficiently widespread to provide herd immunity protection, it will only do so primarily against the 70% of the cervical cancers in the United States.

HPV vaccine requirements that target girls alone thus are best viewed as victim-protective: they protect immunized young women against acquiring HPV infection and hence the possibility of cervical cancer. Secondarily, they protect against vectorhood in that someone who is immunized against infection will not as an individual become a vector for the types of virus included in the vaccine. Viewed as primarily about the victim, the paramount ethical issue about whether to mandate vaccination is whether paternalistic intervention is justifiable, either for adults or for children. For adults with access to health care, the tradeoff is between protection by vaccination and protection through decision making about sexual relationships as well as regular screening.[103]

Another—but by no means unimportant—concern is the possibility that she (or he) will transmit infection to sexual partners. This is a consideration that has been ignored by some commentators, but that should be pressed when decisions are made about vaccination for adults, but it is by no means a decision about immediate intervention in a life-threatening situation.[104] It is a decision to be weighed against other important values, such as religious commitments, though even here the strength of such commitments may vary.

Unsure of their victim/vector status, people would thus want to be certain that individual decisions about immunization are carefully considered in light of full information and appreciation of vectorhood. Herd effects would not be a compelling reason to favor mandatory immunization if herd effects can be achieved through the vaccination of a sufficient number of others, though this of course raises free-rider problems: not every individual can argue in this way. Where there are serious reasons of conscience, vaccination for adults should remain an individual choice—although one that physicians should explore thoroughly with patients, ensuring that their decisions are informed by their possible status as both victim and vector. Of course, herd effects would be an important reason to favor mandatory immunization with narrowly limited opt out provisions, but any opt out possibilities must be weighed against the likelihood of establishing herd immunity and the seriousness of the disease

---

103. See Lo, "HPV Vaccine"; and Zimmerman, "Ethical Analysis of HPV."
104. Lo, in particular, makes the statement that HPV is not contagious. While we acknowledge that the route of transmission of HPV is different than that of measles and most other common childhood infectious diseases, it is an error to claim that HPV is not a contagious disease. See Lo, "HPV Vaccine."

to be controlled in this way. In clinical practice, physicians should explore these issues thoroughly with patients, ensuring that their decisions are informed by their status as both victim *and* vector.

Parental Choice and Children

Childhood immunization laws have been similarly attacked by parents who claim the right to make health decisions for their children. However, as with the 1905 *Jacobson* decision, the Supreme Court in 1922 decided in favor of the need to protect the community from infectious diseases by requiring vaccines for school admission, despite arguments for parental autonomy rights. Some school immunization requirements are now established in all states—but all have medical exemptions, 48 permit religious exemptions, and 20 permit exemptions on other conscientious grounds.[105] A telephone survey of 1,600 parents in 2000 revealed that while 87% of parents thought that immunizations were important to keeping their children well, 18% were opposed to immunization requirements because "they go against freedom of choice" or "only I know what is best for my child."[106]

The standard view of parental choice with respect to children is that parents do not have the right to engage in medical neglect but do have the right to make a range of reasonable health-care decisions with respect to their children. The question is where HPV vaccination fits within this matrix. The vaccine is not immediately life saving, unlike a blood transfusion in a case of critical blood loss. Conversely, it protects against the risk of a serious, sometimes fatal disease—indeed, one that is sometimes fatal in the United States and the developed world, but is a frequent, major killer of women in the developing world where cervical screening is not widely available. The disease does not typically develop until later in life, but if the vaccine has not been administered before the age of sexual activity, protection may come too late. Thus a strategy that recommends parental choice (and permits parental refusal) up to the point at which the child can choose for herself as an adult, may be ineffective in guaranteeing future freedom from infection. Nonetheless, there are alternative means of protection against infection or against the cancer that may develop: abstinence and regular screenings, though regular screenings are available only to those who have access to health care and typically only in the developed world.

---

105. Linda L. LeFever, "Religious Exemptions from School Immunization: A Sincere Belief or a Legal Loophole?" *Penn State Law Review* 110 (2006): 1047–1067. Updated state vaccination requirements are listed on the website of the National Network for Immunization Information, "Vaccine Information," http://www.immunizationinfo.org/VaccineInfo/index.cfm (accessed January 6, 2008).
106. B.G. Gellin, E.W. Maibach, and E.K. Marcuse, "Do Parents Understand Immunizations? A National Telephone Survey," *Pediatrics* 106 (2000): 1097–1102.

HPV vaccination would seem to be a health-care decision within an "intermediate" zone for parents. It may seem for this reason not to be a decision that is so immediately important to protecting the child from mortality or morbidity that it should be mandated. But it is not a decision with negligible consequences, either, and if it is not made in favor of immunization now, it cannot be reversed later on if sexual contact has taken place and infection has already occurred—a very real possibility given the prevalence rates for HPV infection. From the perspective of their children as victims, parents should thus be pressed to have very strong reasons if they oppose immunization for their children—inchoate beliefs or vague concerns will not suffice, although serious religious objections, rooted in basic values, might. In a context where young women may expect access to health care and the ability to make alternative protective choices such as Pap screening later on, this balance might favor parental choice. In situations in which these alternatives are not available and in which a failure to immunize might truly be life threatening, the balance would tip the other way. On this view, HPV vaccination would seem of a piece with other vaccinations that permit a conscientious opt out on the part of parents, at least in the comparatively privileged conditions of the United States today, though this might look very different, as we will see in a later chapter on justice, in the far less privileged conditions of the developing world. Even in her currently privileged condition, moreover, a girl or her parents may not know whether she will actually have access to adequate screening in the future—and this possibility should also be weighed in favor of vaccination.

In a thoughtful discussion of how physicians should respond to parental refusals of immunization, the American Academy of Pediatrics Committee on Bioethics supports immunization requirements for school entry, but also advocates respect for parents or individuals who refuse immunization.[107] The Committee advises that refusals be accepted when the risks to the patient or the community of a failure to be immunized are low, such as in a community where mass immunization programs have been successful in achieving herd immunity and the prevalence of infection is low (polio in recent years in the United States would be an example). However, when the patient or population is seriously threatened during an epidemic (such as might occur during an avian influenza pandemic or a localized measles outbreak), the Committee recommends that state agencies be involved to override parental discretion on the basis of parental neglect and to more aggressively enforce school immunization requirements. Here, the PVV view reveals a policy that would tip in the direction of prioritizing the risk of vectorhood above that of a child's situation as "victim," but only in cases of emergency where there is rapid onset

---

107. See Diekema and the Committee on Bioethics, "Responding to Parental Refusals."

with no means of alternative protection. However, given that mandatory HPV vaccination policies are predominantly aimed at protecting young women as future victims of cancer, not so much against the infection itself—which, after all, typically resolves without sequelae, this situation would seem unlikely to occur with HPV vaccine.

Sexual Transmission

The HPV vaccine is directed against an infection that is primarily acquired through sexual contact. Some have argued that this makes all the difference in whether the vaccine should be required:[108] the risk of exposure to HPV, like other sexually transmitted diseases, is limited to sexually active individuals, and the degree of sexual exposure influences the risks of acquiring and transmitting infection.[109] While much of the success of public health policies for controlling STDs in the past has been due to targeting surveillance and therapy toward high-risk groups, such as prostitutes and those who have multiple sexual partners, the relatively wide distribution of HPV virus infections among the general sexually active population—with a lifetime prevalence risk of 80%—indicates that focusing vaccine use on high-risk target populations will not be effective in controlling this most common of all sexually transmitted infections. The virus is highly contagious, one acquires infection only by exposure to another infected person, and although transmission is by the sexual route, because the great majority of our population is sexually active, most women (and probably most men) eventually become infected. Indeed, the HPV infection rates greatly exceed the rates of some other feared communicable diseases, such as TB[110] and AIDS. Relying on individual choices about sexual behavior, therefore, is not a realistic strategy to protect either victims or vectors from HPV.

Adolescents

A further complication in parental decision making with respect to HPV vaccine involves adolescents. As adolescents become increasingly capable of understanding complex medical situations and their own values, they have a

---

108. By comparison, the acceptance by the general public of hepatitis B vaccinations for infants and young children of both sexes has not appreciably been influenced by the belief that it is primarily a vaccine against a sexually transmitted disease. However, hepatitis B virus is also acquired through close family contacts and blood exposures; and in 30% of the cases, the route of infection is unknown. See Zimmerman, "Ethical Analysis."
109. See G.P. Garnett, "Role of Herd Immunity in Determining the Effect of Vaccines Against Sexually Transmitted Disease," *Journal of Infectious Diseases* 191, suppl. 1 (2005): S97–S106.
110. P.M. Small and P.I. Fujiwara, "Management of Tuberculosis in the United States," *New England Journal of Medicine* 345 no.3 (July 19, 2001): 189–200.

stake in participating in decisions about their health care. This stake is especially strong where reproductive decisions are at stake.[111] Respect for adolescents as decision-makers thus requires that they be adequately informed and be given an opportunity to exercise voice with respect to their victimhood and vectorhood. If respect for the choices of adolescents is to be recognized, adolescents should be able to say that they would prefer to be vaccinated—and to be protected in that way—even if their parents would refuse on their behalf. On the contrary, they should be permitted to refuse vaccination preferred by parents—but only if they have very strong and carefully considered reasons for so doing. Even when adolescents agree with their parents in refusing vaccination, this refusal should be accompanied by careful information about alternative protective means as well as consequences for disease transmission; otherwise, parental refusals should not be honored, because they would be inadequately protective of their children's eventual ability to protect their own health.

This issue is particularly challenging in that it involves adolescents' decision making not about matters like dress, music preferences, future career choices, or other personal matters; it involves decision making about sex. The HPV vaccine is not the only way to avoid HPV infection; there is another way for an adolescent to protect herself: abstain from sex. But some will see this as utterly unrealistic, given what is known about adolescent sexual behavior: 24% of girls are sexually active by age 15, 40% by age 16, and 70% by age 18.[112] Much data suggest that particularly in sexual matters, adolescent intentions do not match adolescent behavior very well: for example, recent studies have shown that adolescents who take virginity-until-marriage oaths do not actually delay sex much longer (if any) than those who do not.[113]

Justice: Immunizing One Gender to Protect Another?

Finally, there are many questions of justice raised by the HPV vaccine. As we have already indicated, in the United States African-Americans are more frequently the victims of cervical cancer than are whites, and across the globe death rates from cervical cancer are highly associated with poverty and the lack of access to regular health care. These are pressing questions of health justice.

---

111. In the United States, adolescents have the constitutional right to decision making with respect to their reproductive care. Even in the case of abortion, parental notification is only permissible if it does not unduly burden this liberty right. Planned Parenthood of Southeastern Pennsylvania v. Casey, 505 U.S. 833 (1992).

112. Centers for Disease Control and Prevention, "Quadrivalent Human Papillomavirus Vaccine."

113. J.E. Rosenbaum, "Reborn a Virgin: Adolescents Retracting of Virginity Pledges and Sexual Histories," *American Journal of Public Health* 96, no. 6 (2006): 1098–1103.

But there is an additional question of justice raised by HPV: whether only young women should be targeted for the vaccine. In the United States, the current FDA approval and recommendations of advisory councils is for immunization of women beginning at age 11 and extending to age 26 to maximize the receipt of the vaccine before HPV infection becomes common. Initial phase III efficacy and safety studies have been done in women because they are the gender most likely to be victimized by HPV infection. However, preliminary studies in boys indicate that the vaccine is just as effective as in young women in producing antibodies against the HPV virus, suggesting that vaccinated boys will be less likely to become infected with HPV and acquire genital warts, or contract rarer conditions like cancer of the penis or anus. From the perspective of both victim and vector, single-sex mandates for HPV vaccine would seem to be unjust. They fail to protect males as well as unimmunized females as victims. They impose the burden of limiting vectorhood on one sex only—and they do so in a manner that has the possible consequence of undermining any significant possibility of establishing herd immunity. They thus leave conscientiously objecting females in a worse position than they would be were the vaccine mandate imposed on both sexes.

Some countries—Australia, New Zealand, Peru, Mexico—have approved the vaccine for both sexes. Debate in countries like the United States that have not (yet) done so is over the relative value and ethics of restricting mandated immunization programs to females who are the principal victims but equal vectors versus including immunization of males who are occasional victims but equal vectors. Additionally, studies proving the efficacy of the HPV vaccine in preventing cancer in males are needed.

An important factor in the gender debate is the perceived ability of the HPV vaccine to induce effective herd immunity in protecting the community. While no population level studies of the effects of HPV immunizations have been reported to date, epidemiological modeling has predicted that vaccines with such high levels of efficacy as has been documented for HPV vaccine have a good likelihood of reducing the prevalence of HPV infection in the community. Garnett assessed the possible efficacy of limiting HPV immunization to women and concluded that with a high level of immunization of the susceptible female population, males and unimmunized females would likely benefit from induced herd immunity. When immunization acceptance is low, however, he concluded that immunization of both sexes would be needed to achieve some herd immunity.[114]

This conclusion raises the ethical issue of the obligation of the individual to undergo the risks of immunization without significant personal benefit or with lower cost-efficacy, such as is mostly the case with HPV vaccine for males,

---

114. Garnett, "Role of Herd Immunity."

for the benefit of increasing herd immunity in the community. The medical ethicist Inmaculada de Melo-Martin[115] has vigorously argued for HPV immunization of both sexes, pointing out that males should share the burden of immunization because they are often the source of the infection and cervical cancer risk is strongly related to the number of a woman's husband's premarital and extramarital affairs.[116] More practically, she also argues that because cervical cancer often takes the lives of younger women who are still caring for children, the husband reaps considerable benefit from sharing the responsibility for preventing this outcome. A recent survey of knowledge about HPV among Yale University male students indicated that many of these men understood that HPV infection was a cause of serious illness for their female sexual partners, and that they were willing to reduce their sexual exposures to other women to reduce the risk to those they care for.[117] Donald Kennedy, the editor-in-chief of the journal *Science*, has also argued for required preschool immunization of both sexes based on the societal value of achieving herd immunity, and he challenges those who argue for freedom of choice in accepting immunization by noting that these "refuseniks" are essentially "free-riders" who enjoy the benefit of herd immunity while actually spreading harm to the population.[118]

The U.S. rubella vaccine policy of immunizing both sexes provides precedent for immunizing boys who are vectors and not significant victims as compared to women who need to be protected against rubella infection during pregnancy and the associated high risk of fetal abnormalities. Inclusion of the rubella vaccine in the universally adapted measles, mumps, and rubella (MMR) vaccine for children has efficiently provided rubella vaccine to potential male vectors without significant public controversy. Australia, Mexico, and the European Union have all approved HPV vaccine for both sexes, citing prevention of genital warts as one of the indications for including males, as well as acknowledging the possible herd immunity benefit.[119]

Although it is justified as a matter of justice, it is currently not clear how the U.S. public will react to recommendations that both sexes be immunized against HPV. We suspect that the relatively high cost of the HPV vaccine will be a significant argument for not including males in mandated and publicly

---

115. Inmaculada de Melo-Martín, "The Promise of Human Papillomavirus Vaccine Does Not Confer Immunity Against Ethical Reflection," *Oncologist* 11, no. 4 (April 2006): 393–396.

116. F.X. Bosch et al., "Male Sexual Behaviors and Human Papillomavirus DNA: Key Risk Factors for Cervical Cancer in Spain," *Journal of the National Cancer Institute* 88, no. 15 (August 7, 1996): 1060–1067.

117. T.S. McPartland, B.A. Weaver, S. Lee, and L.A. Koutsky, "Men's Perceptions and Knowledge of Human Papillomavirus (HPV) Infection and Cervical Cancer," *Journal of American College Health* 53, no. 5 (March-April, 2005): 225–230.

118. D. Kennedy, "News on Women's Health—Editorial," *Science* 313 (2006): 273.

119. *HPV Today*, "Evaluation of the Quadrivalent HPV Vaccine by the Regulatory Agencies in 2006," *HPV Today* (February 10, 2007), www.hpvtoday.com (accessed January 6, 2008).

funded HPV immunization programs. In Chapter 19, we will develop an argument from our PVV perspective for sharing immunization costs. We have also suggested in this chapter—and will elaborate on this in Chapter 18—the case for compensation when people are harmed by constraints such as immunization requirements that are imposed to protect everyone from ongoing burdens of infectious disease.

Justice: HPV Vaccine as a Global Concern

A final issue of justice requires seeing human papillomavirus not just as a threat to individuals, or to the population of a single country, but as a global epidemic—one that, like TB or HIV, looks quite different in different parts of the world. In developed countries with universal access to health care including routine cervical screening, HPV is a widespread infection but one with comparatively infrequent but serious consequences. In the developing world, in contrast, HPV infection is often life-threatening. Every year, around the globe, 493,000 new cases of cervical cancer are diagnosed, and 274,000 women die of the disease, most of them in the developing world.[120] The HPV vaccines could prevent the vast majority of these cases.

If we are to be sensitive to the full range of ethical issues that the possibility of immunization against HPV raises, it is crucial to see ourselves, as the PVV bids us to do, as part of a *global* web of HPV, in which virtually everyone is at some degree of risk, in which some people are better able to protect themselves than others, and in which the problem is worldwide. This is a fusion of three perspectives within our overall PVV view. It involves every individual's own actual situation as HPV-infected, previously infected, or not infected at all. It involves everyone's role as one individual among not just millions but literally billions of HPV-infected or previously infected men and women around the globe. Most important, it brings into play the third aspect of our PVV view, the hypothetical sense that the capacity to protect oneself from HPV or other endemic viruses could have been different for anyone, wherever they may live, as could their capacity to keep from passing these potentially very damaging viruses along.

---

120. Schwartz, Caplan, Faden, and Sugarman, "Lessons from the Failure," 762.

PART IV: CONSTRAINTS, PANDEMICS, AND WHAT WE OWE EACH OTHER AS VICTIMS AND VECTORS

15

A THOUGHT EXPERIMENT: RAPID-TEST SCREENING FOR INFECTIOUS DISEASE IN AIRPORTS AND PLACES OF PUBLIC CONTACT[1]

Up to this point, we have considered both traditional and novel issues in bioethics from our PVV perspective. In the background, and sometimes under direct consideration, have been some of the forms of coercion historically associated with the prevention of disease spread: shunning, belling, circles of containment, *cordons sanitaires*, required screening, reporting, quarantine and isolation, targeted surveillance, rapid testing, contact tracing, public identification of victims, mandatory immunization, mandatory treatment and directly observed therapy, required precautions such as masks or gloves, biohazard suits, closures of facilities such as bathhouses or swimming pools, travel restrictions such as "no-fly" rules, and school, work, and meeting-place closures. New forms of constraints are surely in the offing, such as mandatory molecular diagnosis or publicly positioned detection and surveillance devices, some of which we are about to explore.

Many of these strategies, including historical, contemporary, and hypothetical ones, have been used in ways that involved substantial violations of ethical principles: constraints on liberty, violations of privacy and confidentiality, failure to secure full informed consent, deception, coercion, and treatment of individuals as objects, rather than as persons in their own right. The fears of pandemic infectious disease, recurring with SARS and avian flu, have generated new attention to the use of constraints in the control of infectious disease. It is now time for us to confront these issues more comprehensively in light of our PVV perspective, both as they pertain to pandemic planning and also as a more general matter. We begin to explore issues about constraints—when they are permissible and what people owe each other when they are

---

1. A version of this chapter is to appear as Margaret P. Battin, Ph.D., Charles B. Smith, M.D., Larry Reimer, M.D., Jay A. Jacobson, M.D., Leslie P. Francis, Ph.D., J.D., "Rapid Tests for Infectious Disease: A Thought Experiment About Universal Use and Public Surveillance," in *Cutting Though the Surface: Philosophical Approaches to Bioethics (Festschrift for Matti Häyry)*, ed. Tuija Takala, Peter Herissone-Kelly, and Søren Holm, Rodopi, 2008.

used—in terms of a thought-experiment about surveillance by means of universal rapid testing for communicable disease.

A warning to the reader: our thought experiment may seem outrageous, at least at the beginning. We mean it to seem so; our goal is to challenge everyone to think about what would be—or what would not be—ethically problematic about the implementation of our thought experiment. Can the ethical difficulties be overcome, or are they insurmountable? And what can be made of them in the light of actual present-day circumstances that are likely to prevail for the realistically foreseeable future, not just in the world of a futuristic thought experiment? Are disagreements over the issues the thought-experiment raises still more pressing if it is understood as a proposal, not a mere conjecture? Because it is certainly possible to envision a world in which surveillance for serious infectious disease is pervasive, we think it important to ask what would—and what would not—be ethically permissible about large-scale surveillance and constraints imposed as a result of what the surveillance reveals.

Universal Rapid-Test Screening

New molecular technologies utilizing polymerase chain reactions, monoclonal antibodies, and recombinant antigens now make possible rapid, inexpensive diagnosis of some infectious diseases in a fraction of earlier testing times. In just 20 minutes, as we've seen in Chapter 12, OraQuick identifies HIV-1 status with 99.3% sensitivity and 99.9% specificity—down from the two-week test and confirmation retest of earlier methods—and has high reliability whether a blood sample or oral fluid swab is used.

Similar rapid tests are available or under development for many other infectious diseases, including, for example, malaria, dengue, meningitis, SARS, and influenza. While molecular rapid tests vary in method, the emphasis is speed and most offer results in much less than an hour, and some new technologies promise results in a very brief period of time.

Rapid diagnosis has long been valuable in many areas of medicine, especially in infectious disease: the gram stain and rapid testing of throat cultures for strep are familiar examples. Infrared thermal scanners were used to screen travelers in airports in Vancouver, Toronto, Singapore, and Hong Kong during the SARS outbreak in 2003. The trained eye of the experienced clinician has until recently been the fastest of all technologies, recognizing measles or the smallpox rash on the spot. It cannot, however, see everything, especially where contagiousness precedes visible symptoms, and the new rapid-test methods may mark both a dramatic technological advance and the emergence of pressing ethical dilemmas. Rapid testing via monoclonal antibody is far more specific than gram stain or the temperature sensors used in airports during the SARS outbreak (a practice said to be reassuring to travelers though not of great efficacy[2]). For purposes of this thought experiment, we imagine being able to detect in any passenger any known, diagnosable communicable infectious disease or the underlying pathogen that passenger might be harboring: HIV, tuberculosis, malaria, polio, cholera, SARS, and the full range of sexually transmitted diseases, even common colds and flu.

But the prospect of widespread rapid screening by molecular methods also presents ethical challenges. In the light of the extraordinary technological advance that rapid tests represent, we begin our discussion of constraints by exploring—in a speculative way—just how far this advance could go if widely applied, and still remain ethically acceptable. The ethical concerns raised by such highly accurate rapid tests include security, liberty and informed consent, privacy, confidentiality, and justice. Could a decent society agree to a policy of universal or near-universal rapid-test screening for any—or all—infectious diseases? Does it matter whether the tests are available for some diseases, but not for others? Does it matter whether the tests are virtually 100% accurate, or whether they have significant false positive or false negative rates? Is the screening permissible only if effective treatments are readily available? The thought experiment we will pose here raises these among other issues.

To be sure, the technologies imagined here are not all now available—though some are—and it may never become possible to develop some of them; but we must also recognize that many important aspects of the thought experiment pursued here may be easily realizable in the near future. After all, surveillance akin to the kind we speculate about here, albeit much more primitive, was not only used in the case of SARS but is a plausible strategy in early warning systems for the emergence of new influenza strains. Although on-entry screening is not currently used to test people arriving in the United States from abroad, even though U.S. law prohibits people with HIV from entering,[3] it clearly could be; if rapid tests were used, admission could conceivably be granted or denied on the spot. Animals entering the United States are currently kept in long-term quarantine, but such policies could conceivably be changed to permit rapid testing of veterinary cases. Screening for methicillin resistant staphylococcus aureus (MRSA) carriage is currently conducted in a number of U.S. hospitals in an attempt to reduce the spread of this organism to other patients. In these and other contexts, surveillance is already in place.

The practical question of our thought experiment is whether the new possibility of rapid, highly reliable testing, used nearly universally in public venues, might lower—or potentially eradicate—the global burden of infectious disease.

---

2. The infrared thermal scanners used in airports during the SARS outbreak reportedly did little to constrain disease spread and were quite costly, but apparently made passengers feel more secure. See, e.g., CP, "Scanners Make Travelers Feel Safe," *London Free Press (Ontario, Canada)*, September 25, 2003, B6.
3. 8 U.S.C. § 1182(1)(A)(1) (2007).

We leave aside for the moment a number of practical and ethical questions to be discussed in later chapters, among them whether eradication or control of all or almost all contagious infectious disease is even possible or desirable; whether control of infectious disease should be confined to serious disease only, or whether comparatively minor conditions like colds and athlete's foot should be included; whether treatment would be available for infectious diseases that are identified; and whether, if treatment were not available, compensation would be possible. These are important questions that have great bearing on the ethical issues we raise, but we set them aside to be discussed in detail in the subsequent chapters of this section, in order to turn immediately to whether the picture imagined in the thought-experiment would so severely violate the basic norms of morality that it could not be tolerated.

A Thought Experiment: Rapid-Test Screening for Transmissible Infectious Disease

So consider a thought experiment. Suppose that molecular rapid testing is available for all known communicable infectious diseases, both those that involve human-to-human transmission and those that are transmitted via an intermediate vector. Testing for at least some conditions is no more invasive than the collection of an oral fluid sample, easily accomplished with a single cotton swab rubbed inside the lip by a person with virtually no training. For others, a simple pinprick for blood is all that is required. Whatever the samples, the new rapid tests are more sensitive and specific than prior testing methods; let us suppose that they are all as good as OraQuick is for HIV, with over 99% sensitivity, nearly 100% specificity. There will be a few cases missed, but virtually no false positives. Also imagine that test-processing units are small, portable, and cheap enough so that they can be used in virtually any setting. Because refrigeration, storage, running water, electricity, and sterile syringes are not necessary, collection and testing can be performed virtually anywhere, in the developed or developing world.

Imagine airports, for instance.[4] Suppose, in this thought experiment, that as passengers check in at the departures desk, they are asked to supply, along with their ticket and passport or picture ID, an oral sample, quickly taken with cotton swab supplied by the airline, or a drop of blood from a tiny, sterile, automated and virtually painless finger-prick. The sample is processed, automatically, on the spot. Between the time of check-in and the time of arrival at the

---

4. The World Health Organization estimates that 2.1 billion passengers take airplane flights every year, bringing with them the risk of infectious disease transmission. World Health Organization, "The World Health Report 2007—A Safer Future: Global Public Health Security in the 21st Century," http://www.who.int/whr/2007/overview/en/index1.html (accessed November 2007).

gate, the test is completed and the result relayed by computer to the gate agents as well as to a national or global disease-surveillance network that keeps track of the incidence of the various infectious diseases. People who are "clean" can board the plane. But anyone with a positive test for TB or SARS, or even just the flu, is detained for a repeat test, using an alternative assay if available—thus reducing the already low probability of a false positive. If the positive result is confirmed, they are denied boarding and referred to the airport health clinic for whatever treatment is available. The same is true for the crew. No one is singled out or profiled for risk; just as with baggage screening, everybody is tested. But nobody boards the plane without a negative test result. In our thought experiment, nobody boards the plane with a disease they could transmit to anybody else—at least, with one that has been identified through the rapid-test procedure.

Surveillance of those who fly in planes captures only a segment of the population, however. Thus let us continue the thought experiment: the rapid-test equipment, yielding results for (let us assume) all known communicable infectious diseases in just 20 minutes or less, can be used not only in airports but in schools, stadiums, hospitals, churches, movie theatres, shopping centers, even local grocery stores. Between the time students enter a school vestibule, for example, and the time they are allowed to stuff their books into their lockers, they are tested; it is straight to the school infirmary for those who have a communicable disease. At hospitals and nursing homes, between the time of check-in at the front desk and the time someone is allowed to visit a friend or make rounds on patients there, everyone is tested—visitors, care workers, and physicians. For people riding trains or using the subway, a short delay would be all that is necessary before they are on their way—or held back, in the interests of keeping them from transmitting disease to others, whether in the confined space of a public vehicle or to whatever contacts they might meet at their destination. Some newer technologies seek to reduce the time required for pathogen identification to 120 seconds,[5] and even more rapid point-of-care nanotechnologies based on embedded network sensing and electronic/photonic interchange might reduce diagnostic time to near instantaneousness, with the results of positive tests reported back literally at close to the speed of light.[6]

The same picture could be true all over the world—there would be no entry into spaces of close human contact without first ensuring that people will

5. Vindhya Kunduru and Shalini Prasad, "Electrokinetic Formation of 'Microbridges' for Detection of Proteins," *Journal of the Association for Laboratory Automation* 12, no 5 (October 2007): 311–317; R.K.K. Reddy et al., "Electrical Immunoassays Toward Clinical Diagnostics: Identification of Vulnerable Cardiovascular Plaque," *Journal of the Association of Laboratory Automation* 13, no. 1 (February 2008): 33-39.
6. Larry R. Dalton, "Theory-Guided Nano-Engineering: A Technology Revolution!" Lecture at the University of Utah, October 24, 2007.

not bring their transmissible diseases with them. In many places—airports, schools, stadiums, tall buildings—people already are screened for weapons, and in some institutions—prisons and the military, for example—broader testing is already mandatory upon entry. Our thought experiment about universal infectious-disease testing is a screening of a related sort, in that it screens people for their potential to cause harm to others.

Of course, airport screening of this sort would not prevent all harm to other people—some potential transmittees would still be subject to the spread of aerosolized diseases like flu while checking in at the departures desk, but no more than they are when they check in for a flight now. They would not wait any longer at the gate than they do now, and so would not experience additional exposures while waiting for test results; everything proceeds as quickly (or slowly) as passenger processing and surveillance does now, but with one extra level of scrutiny. People would be protected from exposure, though, in the closed space of an airliner where aerosolized diseases might be spread, and of course from exposure further down the line by other modes of transmission, such as sexual transmission, waterborne transmission, skin-contact transmission, and so on. Airport screening would in theory prevent all transmission by infected passengers on the plane and all transmission after the plane lands.

Would the cost be too high? The magnitude of inconvenience and violations of liberty this thought experiment suggests seem overwhelming. No easy freedom of movement, no spontaneous travel, no liberty of association—virtually all public movement and contact are potentially constricted in the interests of protecting others. Of course, not all movement and association are restricted—those who are disease-free can still board planes or go to the market or visit their (noninfectious) friends in hospitals, but those who are sick cannot pass through until they no longer test positive. As tests become available that can distinguish between persons who are infected and persons who are contagious, the restriction would need only to extend until the contagious period has passed. The number detained might be lower or higher depending on the prevalence in a specific population, raising questions of justice we explore below. In the first year or so of this thought experiment, detainment might be expected to be frequent and perhaps lengthy or even forever for some, where immediate or effective treatment was not available. In succeeding years both the frequency and length of detainment might be expected to decrease, as various diseases came gradually under control and treatment for them improved.

Continuing our thought experiment in this optimistic vein, the inconvenience of airport screening and potential detainment for someone who tests positive need not always be great. For many diseases, over-the-counter or point-of-care tests could be used in advance, before setting out for the airport or other public place. Inconvenience and financial impact could be reduced: for example, airlines could be required not to penalize passengers by charging higher fares for those forced to change their departure dates in this way, and schools or workplaces required not to flunk students or dock pay for workers with confirmed evidence of communicable disease. Nevertheless, not all costs can be avoided: there will be meetings and weddings missed, vacations canceled, and reunions thwarted. For specific diseases with long-term transmission possibilities—HIV or TB, for instance—proof of ongoing treatment or perhaps an antibody titer could be provided, much as a special permit is required to carry a concealed weapon. But the violation of liberty is often substantial: for diseases with acute phases and high transmission profiles—polio or influenza or measles—people cannot pass through public spaces where screening is required until they are no longer identified as infected or, more precisely, identified as no longer contagious. No excuses and no exceptions: dignitaries and pilots are tested at the airport just as routinely as coach class passengers are. Both ballplayers and their coaches are tested at the stadium just as routinely as the spectators; clergy and their altar attendants are tested at churches, mosques, and synagogues along with all their parishioners. In this thought experiment, universal screening means just that—*universal*—in all places of public congregation and contact. There would be no unrevealed infectious diseases.

Would this be an intolerable invasion of liberty and privacy? A colossal inconvenience and disruption of people's plans? Violation of a basic liberty, the right to freedom of travel? An utterly unacceptable program of state-mandated invasions of the body? Would it invite evasions, circumventions of the system, perhaps bribes for those who wish to avoid testing? Would it function as an effective life sentence for some, those who can never go out in the world because they carry unquenchable infectious disease, while it brings virtually complete freedom from disease for others? Would it carry the potential for enormous injustice, entrenching the already unequal distribution of infectious diseases in the world today?

At first thought, it seems the answer to all these questions is "yes." But consider what such a policy could prevent. Much of the most vivid public worry about the transmission of infectious disease, especially highly contagious emerging diseases like Ebola or SARS, involves intercontinental transmission that is only a single plane trip away. After all, although more recent evidence indicates presence of the HIV virus in the United States as early as 1969,[7]

7. M. Thomas, P. Gilbert et al., "The Emergence of HIV/AIDS in the Americas and Beyond," *Proceedings of the National Academy of Sciences* 104, no. 47 (November 20, 2007): 18566–18570. It had already been known that HIV jumped from West African chimpanzees to humans in 1930 and had been present in an unrecognized outbreak in Africa for many years. The Gilbert et al. study

a dozen years before it was first identified, AIDS was originally believed to have arrived in the United States in 1981 with a single airline steward, Gaetan Dugas, popularly identified as "Patient Zero."[8] In 2003, SARS arrived in Toronto from China by plane: a 78-year-old Scarborough grandmother, Kwan Sui Chu, contracted SARS at the Metropole Hotel in Hong Kong on February 21, 2003, and returned to Toronto two days later, where she infected her son; he entered Scarborough Grace Hospital, which would become the epicenter of the Toronto epidemic.[9] And the story of Andrew Speaker, the patient with alleged XDR-TB who evaded authorities to fly home to the United States after his wedding in Greece in the spring of 2007, frightened many airline travelers. So has the story of a 30-year-old woman infected with XDR-TB who took an American Airlines flight from New Delhi to San Francisco with a stop in Chicago on December 13, 2007: health authorities were said to be searching for "dozens" of airline passengers who may have come in contact with her.[10]

Rapid testing at airports might have prevented occurrences of long-distance transmission of highly infectious diseases. Assuming transmission would not have occurred again later in some other way (though this is of course a substantial assumption)—it might have prevented some 44 SARS deaths in Toronto and nearly half a million AIDS deaths in the United States alone.[11]

---

shows that HIV jumped to Haiti in the mid-1960s, where several variants, mostly dead ends, evolved, but that subtype B jumped from Haiti to the United States in about 1969. It is this subtype that has been responsible for the HIV pandemic in the United States. Ironically, 1969 was approximately the year in which the U.S. Surgeon General may have said that it was time to "close the book on infectious disease."

8. Dugas, a French-Canadian who regularly flew the Paris–London–New York–San Francisco routes, has been described as incredibly attractive, popular, and sexually active, responsible for infecting some 250 men a year even after health officials had urged him to stop; he has been scapegoated as crawling through bathhouses looking for men to infect. Nels P. Highberg, Lecture at American Society for Bioethics and Humanities, October 2007; see also Randy Shilts, *And the Band Played On: Politics, People, and the AIDS Epidemic* (New York: St. Martin's Press, 1987). Although more recent evidence shows evidence of the virus in the United States several years earlier, Dugas was clearly at the center of a group of about 40 gay men who played a major role in the initial outbreak of HIV infection in San Francisco.

9. Philip W. H. Peng, David T. Wong, David Bevan, and Michael Gardam, "Infectious Control and Anaesthesia: Lessons Learned from the Toronto SARS Outbreak," *Canadian Journal of Anesthesia* 50 (2003): 989–997. See also *Toronto Star*, www.thestar.com/static/PDF/030926_sars_h4_h5.pdf (accessed March 23, 2006).

10. Associated Press, "Passengers Flew with Infected Woman," *New York Times*, sec. A, January 4, 2008; Mike Swift, MediaNews, "Travelers Sought in TB Case," *Palo Alto (CA) Daily News* (December 29, 2007), http://www.paloaltodailynews.com/article/2007-12-29-pa-tb (accessed January 22, 2008).

11. The cumulative total of AIDS deaths in the US through December 2000 was 459,518. See Centers for Disease Control and Prevention, "HIV/AIDS Surveillance Supplemental Report: Deaths Among Persons with AIDS Through December 2000," www.cdc.gov/hiv/topics/surveillance/resources/reports/2002supp_vo18no1/table2.htm (accessed January 22, 2008).

Keeping just a few passengers from boarding their planes, whoever they were, could have prevented huge loss of life.

Denying air travel to people with infectious diseases, as this thought experiment would, is not intended just to prevent passengers who might sneeze on their seatmates from giving a cold to others on board. A state or internationally mandated policy of the sort in this thought experiment would prevent any person who is identified as a vector of disease from transmitting it later on in any public place. Such a program would, we can assume, dramatically reduce the spread of infectious disease—not only that transmitted over long distances, like the Scarborough grandmother's unwitting transmittal of SARS from Hong Kong to Toronto, but that passed around at home, as she equally unwittingly infected her son, or in private settings, as Patient Zero (perhaps among others) is said to have infected 250 men a year.

Objections to the Thought Experiment's Universal-Screening Policy

There are many potential objections to this thought experiment, objections that demand extensive response; we will develop a more systematic account of these matters in Chapter 16. We sketch four such objections here: violations of bodily integrity and physical security, violations of liberty and consent, violations of privacy and confidentiality, and violations of justice.

Violations of Bodily Integrity and Physical Security

Bodily integrity and physical security—the understanding that one's body is protected from intrusions and damage inflicted by others—are obvious initial concerns raised by our thought experiment. The rapid tests themselves, however, do not involve major bodily impositions or threaten physical security in any serious way. All they require is a moment's stop for a cheek swab or a finger stick, procedures that are not painful, risky, or undignified.

The significant physical threats from the rapid tests are posed by the consequences of a positive test. People will be detained, at a minimum while waiting for the results of a second test. In order to protect their physical security, the waiting area would need to be designed in such a way as to protect people from diseases that might be transmitted by other positive-testers who are also waiting. Logistically, it may also be very difficult to protect confidentiality under realistic circumstances of rapid testing, as we discuss below. There will thus be a need to assure people that their physical security will not be threatened, if there are substantial risks of it becoming known that they are infected with a serious, communicable disease. These threats will be diminished to the extent that easy, rapid, and successful treatment is available for any detected illness, although there will remain the need to protect people against stigmatization associated with having been treated for a contagious disease.[12] But the risks will need to be considered when diseases are untreatable and potentially dangerous to others.

To the extent that physical security cannot realistically be protected under the thought experiment, however, our PVV perspective suggests that it is at least prima facie impermissible. Our PVV perspective is a reminder that the person being detained is not only a vector, but a victim too. As someone who wants to be protected from diseases from others, he sees that constraints imposed on him—like the constraints of the thought experiment—not only restrict him as vector but benefit him as well in his posture as potential victim of contagious disease. But the constraints do not protect him in this way if they turn him into an object of opprobrium vulnerable to physical harm.

Violations of Liberty and Consent

Imagine the restrictions of liberty—not only the huge inconvenience, but the curtailment of freedom—multiplied by the millions of air passengers who would at one time or another be forced to stay behind. This might well seem to outweigh the gain in preventing the spread of disease: after all, intercontinental transmission of life-threatening potentially epidemic diseases, though it has occurred in cases like HIV and SARS, is comparatively rare. And some violations of liberty would turn out to have been unnecessary: even if the new rapid-test technologies have lower false positive rates than the older, slower tests, if they are administered to huge numbers of passengers—indeed, all passengers and all crew on each and every flight, there may be some number of people mistakenly identified and kept behind.

Of course, false positives are a lesser problem if the screening is set up in areas where the prevalence of the disease is relatively high and thus the ratio of true to false positives would be quite high. The burden they impose, moreover, may be comparatively minor: brief delay until, with an immediate retest, the diagnosis is corrected. To be sure, air travelers might have to build in a few extra minutes to allow for the possibility of a retest, but this would not even be necessary if the testing process were incorporated into the screening lines found at major international airports today, or if a first test could be taken at home before even setting out for the airport. There might be a few remaining false positives on retest, but very few indeed if the test is highly specific. If the test is less specific, a greater number of false positives will be detained and

---

12. Lest this seem far-fetched, consider the case of a schoolteacher who was fired after a recurrence of tuberculosis. School Board of Nassau County, Florida v. Arline, 480 U.S. 273 (1987).

possibly even treated unnecessarily. But like the identification of true positives, this will be a limitation on liberty that is part of the best practice we can design for identifying people who might pass disease onto others. The problem of false positives is a reminder that the practice should be designed in the least restrictive manner possible.

The real question, then, is the ethical acceptability of these restrictions on liberty, whether they apply to true or to false positives. After all, if rapid tests were routinely administered for all known infectious diseases, as we are supposing, there would be very substantial numbers of people correctly identified as infected by one or more disease-causing organisms. Disease-surveillance networks on a national or global scale, making accurate identification of outbreaks possible, would assemble huge amounts of data. To be sure, sophisticated forms of molecular testing or nanoengineering might in the future be able to distinguish between people in communicable phases of specific diseases, people in incubation phases but not yet contagious, people currently undergoing effective treatment for disease, or people who carry antibodies from former exposures but who can no longer transmit the disease. For this thought experiment, however, assume just that it identifies anyone who could pass a disease along to someone else, either directly or through an intermediate vector. People testing positive would be detained and offered treatment if available, barred from their flights and other movement through check points—their liberty sharply curtailed—until no longer infected with a disease they could transmit.

The limitations on liberty that would result are relatively minor if the people testing positive can be treated quickly, cheaply, effectively, and without serious side effects. Ironically, the limitations on liberty that would result may also be relatively minor if a person testing positive has contracted a disease so devastating and so rapidly fatal that he will need immediate hospitalization if he is to survive at all—Ebola or SARS, for example. But where people test positive for less acute but still communicable diseases for which no treatment is available—or for which treatment is burdensome, expensive, or lengthy—the limitations on liberty posed by this experiment are potentially immense. Ethical issues would also arise in chronic conditions where treatment reduces infectiousness but does not eliminate it—for example, HIV, where the viral load is reduced but not reduced to zero by treatment. Of course, people under treatment for certain chronic diseases might, say, carry a certificate showing that they were undergoing treatment and had dramatically reduced infectivity, as is possible though not always the case with reduced viral loads in HIV, or treatment for TB and MDR- or XDR-TB; restrictions also might not be severe where the disease itself is little threat to others through casual contact, like hepatitis B or C. On the contrary, it is likely that in highly infectious and highly lethal diseases, such as the much-feared avian flu, there would be little question about the ethical permissibility of even severe constraints on travel, at least for short periods of time at the onset of an apparent pandemic. The most difficult ethical question is about what to do about people with diseases that are communicable but largely untreatable, such as hepatitis B or C: let them fly, or, in effect, ban them from flying permanently? Ban them from other forms of public contact? In these cases, the potential constraints on liberty are extensive and may last a lifetime. The issues here are whether the degree of surveillance imagined in this thought experiment is too extreme, and whether alternative ways of reducing transmission are morally preferable, such as emphasis on protection for which responsibility is assumed by the potential transmittee rather than emphasis on responsibility assumed by the transmittor for refraining from transmission.

Would the moral costs of this curtailment of liberty be unacceptable? The curtailment of liberty protects everyone as potential victims, limits everyone as potential vectors. Each person is both. If the curtailment of liberty is very limited—an extra minute in the airport, just as one checks in, barely more time-consuming than showing one's picture ID or displaying one's passport—then the benefits for *each* clearly outweigh the burdens, and the curtailment would seem to be one to which people might reasonably assent. Indeed, if knowledge of the screening is widespread—as it surely could be—then people might even be said to have consented to it through their appearance in a public place. But if the curtailment is much greater—the missed trips, the isolation until available treatment is effective, or the consignment to status of disease victim for whom no treatment is available with whatever consequences this entails—far more complex questions arise. In these cases, it seems, those who are identified as ill cannot be helped as victims, but can only be constrained as vectors.

Under such circumstances of constraint, it is no longer obvious that for each person as potential victim and vector that they would be better off in the world of our thought experiment. *If* their disease is serious—so serious that it would seem justified to others to override the liberty of someone who might pass it on—then consideration must be given to what might justify the constraints. The idea of presumed consent is far more tenuous here as well, because the choice might be regarded as imposing a coercive burden on people: either stay home or risk lifelong isolation. One mitigation would be the introduction of various forms of compensation for limits on liberty; we will return to this issue in the later chapters of this section.

Violations of Privacy and Confidentiality

Under this thought experiment, state-mandated screening would be done just in places of public contact, as people move from one location to another. This would also raise substantial privacy and confidentiality issues. Some privacy concerns about state-mandated testing would not arise: invading homes or bedrooms to catch people transmitting HIV or other STDs would not be necessary if carriers of such viruses are identified in routine public screening while people are out in the world somewhere; screening need not catch people in the transmission act. Contact tracing, too, might eventually be avoided, if people with disease are identified before they can engage in activities that put them at risk of infecting others. But other issues of confidentiality will come to the fore.

Suppose, for instance, someone is denied boarding a flight but her partner is not: there may be a deeply embarrassing, now-public fact to explain. The only way to prevent the information that she has not passed the screening test (for whatever reason) from coming to light will be to avoid the test in the first place—that is, by not traveling in any public place. People with a first positive test will be stopped, and will need to wait somewhere for the retest and its results. They will be held out of line, retested, and perhaps then sent away. There may be the need to explain to others why a much-anticipated or highly important trip was postponed. The possibility of "pre-testing" and choosing not to go to the airport at all is not a complete solution: if the pretest is so far ahead of the planned trip that it avoids questions about trip postponement, then it may be insufficiently accurate in predicting a positive result; but if it is very close to the time of departure, it just pushes back the questioning by a few hours or a day or so. Of course, whether violations of confidentiality are severe is a function of the range of conditions tested for: if only serious, stigmatized diseases are included, violations of confidentiality may be severe; if the testing covers a very broad range of conditions—not only syphilis and HIV but colds and athlete's foot, a detained passenger might avoid embarrassment with a simple excuse like "I must be getting a cold." Just the same, challenges to confidentiality still remain as long as there is something the detained passenger must explain—whether to business companions, insurance company representatives who might happen to observe, or a spouse.

Invasions of privacy in the sense we explored in Chapter 8—getting direct access to the body—cannot be avoided in our thought experiment. Some of these incursions may be consensual—agreed to on the spot—or regarded as permissible through a kind of presumed consent. Most will be relatively minor in terms of the physical invasion: only a cheek swab or a finger-stick. Of far more concern is the nature of the information and what is done with it: with rapid tests, others will know that someone has Ebola, or HIV, or tuberculosis, or HPV, or even the seasonal flu.

Of course, breaches of confidentiality—that is, non-consensual transfers of identifying information, as we explained in Chapter 8—could be minimized with strict controls on the nature of information reported to a national or global infectious-disease surveillance network. For example, if contact tracing becomes less necessary because infected people are identified in other ways, surveillance databases could be limited to data that are stripped of identifiers. Violations of confidentiality could also be reduced by strict limits set on the uses to which surveillance information might be put.

Yet privacy and confidentiality as well as liberty would be major concerns for an actual program of this sort. No matter what controls are placed on official transfers of information, "unofficial" breaches of confidentiality are highly likely. By the mere fact that people are sorted—some turned away and others left alone—inferences will be drawn about disease status. The question is whether the ethical liabilities would be worth the gain. Once again, attention will need to be paid to ways of preventing or mitigating the damage attendant on confidentiality violations if the screening envisioned in our thought experiment is to be justified.

Violations of Justice

Is this thought experiment just another version of Ellis Island, or perhaps worse? Ellis Island, in New York harbor in the shadow of the Statue of Liberty, was the gateway—or gatekeeper—to America for many millions. From 1892 when the immigration station opened until it was closed in 1954, over 12 million people entered the United States through Ellis Island. Steerage passengers were subjected to health inspections that lasted from a few hours to days, while first class passengers walked straight through, apparently on the theory that they were less likely to be diseased or to become public charges. Official estimates are that about 2% of those who sought to enter the United States were turned away at Ellis Island; the most common reason for denial of entry was the infectious eye disease, trachoma.[13] In 1907, the peak year for immigration into the United States during the twentieth century, 1.25 million immigrants arrived—and 67.4% of them came through Ellis Island.[14]

Among those denied entry into the United States and to many other nations of the world were people with infectious diseases who, after long and arduous sea-voyages in search of a better life, were cut off at the border—inspected, barred from entry, held in involuntary quarantine, and sometimes shipped back to wherever they came from. Many if not most countries had such regulations, and they were all inhumane in the sense that they thwarted people's most basic dreams and consigned them to a public-health

---

13. This description is drawn from the Ellis Island website. The Statue of Liberty-Ellis Island Foundation, Inc., "Ellis Island—History," http://www.ellisisland.org/genealogy/ellis_island_history.asp (accessed January 22, 2008). See also Alan M. Kraut, "Germs, Genes, and American Efficiency, 1890–1924," *Social Science History*, 12, no. 4 (Winter, 1988): 377–394.
14. Kraut, "Germs, Genes, and American Efficiency," 384.

limbo or worse. The idea was to keep diseases out—tuberculosis, measles, diphtheria, trachoma, typhus, yellow fever, cholera, plague—and the only known way to do that was to keep the people who had these diseases out. Ships reporting cholera deaths were quarantined; for example, in the summer of 1892, the Hamburg-American liner *Moravia* arrived offshore at New York flying the yellow flag, reporting that 22 of 230 passengers had died of cholera during the voyage and were buried at sea. Another 96 died during in quarantine during the following month.[15]

Many countries have practiced and continue to employ exclusionary quarantine at national borders. For example, amid great public fear in the wake of the cholera epidemic of 1832, Canada established a quarantine station at Grosse Île, an island in the St. Lawrence 48 kilometers below Québec City, where ships with immigrants were required to land. By 1847, the migrations of poor and malnourished Irish fleeing the Great Famine were huge, with typhus and dysentery rampant among people packed in unsanitary conditions aboard ships unsuited for such large numbers. During the summer of 1847, some 5,000 immigrants died at sea. Many more died waiting offshore for permission to land. Of those who did land at Grosse Île, about 12,000 immigrants including both sick and well were held in quarantine on the island in grossly inadequate facilities. Many of those who had been well became ill, and many never reached their destination; 5,424 are buried at Grosse Île.[16]

It is tempting to describe these events—now regarded as "one of the saddest pages in Canadian history"[17]—as an immense violation of justice, in that it was not only trying to protect people on shore from disease but involved the imposition of serious constraints as a response to public fears. Along with immigrants who were already ill, many others who were well were confined on ships or kept on Grosse Île, even when it was clear that they would become infected and die. These once-hopeful immigrants suffered and lived as *victims*, but they were perceived by the quarantine authorities—and particularly by the public—as *vectors*. These immigrants had hardly consented to such treatment; they had come to the New World for a better future, but were sent back, or died. This was not because they were trying to enter illegally or had past

15. *New York Times*, "How We Guard Against the Introduction of Cholera: Where the Scourge Originated and How the Government Copes With It When It Gets to These Shores. Dr. Doty Explodes Some Erroneous Beliefs on the Subject of the Dread Disease," *New York Times Sunday Magazine*, July 23, 1911.

16. Parks Canada, "Grosse Île and the Irish Memorial National Historic Site of Canada: Management Plan, A Terrible Toll," www.pc.gc.ca/lhn-nhs/qc/grosseile/docs/plan1/sec3/page2biii_E.asp (accessed January 22, 2008).

17. Parks Canada, "Grosse Île and the Irish Memorial National Historic Site of Canada: Management Plan, The Great Famine," www.pc.gc.ca/lhn-nhs/qc/grosseile/docs/plan1/sec3/page2bi_E.asp (accessed January 22, 2008).

criminal records or for any other reason of policy-governed justice, but because some among them were discovered to have communicable infectious diseases, over which they had no control. They had no real opportunity for informed or voluntary consent before they sailed—except consent to the voyage itself, which likely included knowledge of the barrier of Ellis Island—and no guarantee of just procedure once they arrived. To be sure, some of this can be attributed to the fact that the huge numbers of immigrants completely overwhelmed the border stations; but some of it was due to failure to recognize the ethical issues involved in treating people in these ways. Throughout history, border controls and quarantines, used by many authorities in many different time periods for many different diseases, may have reduced the extent of infectious-disease epidemics, even if they did not prevent them, but almost always at significant human cost.

Now consider our thought experiment about molecular rapid-test screening in airports and other places of public contact. Is it as morally problematic as the crude border controls at Ellis Island, Grosse Île, and elsewhere around the world, or perhaps worse? The invasions and restrictions our thought experiment posits may seem to be far greater: people who test positive for communicable disease cannot board planes, trains, ships, or even the downtown subway, whether in the developed or in the developing world. In the most far-reaching versions, assuming the relevant rapid-test technology can be devised that easily, quickly, cheaply, and accurately identifies those who could pass on infectious disease, not only cannot one visit a hospitalized friend, but one can be prevented from going to a ball game, shopping in a supermarket, going to church, or going to class at school. This is a far more invasive conjecture than the kinds of border controls erected at Ellis Island or Grosse Île: those sieved through hundreds of boatloads of immigrant hopefuls, but this new conjecture would affect virtually *everybody*.

But therein lies an important lesson about the justice of constraints. Ellis Island's and Grosse Île's exclusionary policies had comparatively limited effect and were clearly unjust because they were applied to new immigrants only—sometimes just to steerage-class passengers—but did nothing to identify disease-carriers among people already in the country.[18] As a result, these policies did not work, or work sufficiently to avoid contagion overall, because they did not affect *everybody*. Moreover, they were applied in inegalitarian fashion: some were forced to consent, while others were entirely excused. Nor were people already in the country screened in a universal and repeated way for infectious disease. True, there were extensive public health efforts to control infectious disease and heroic efforts to identify, treat, and prevent disease, but

18. *New York Times*, "How We Guard Against the Introduction of Cholera."

nothing that involved routine, regular, repeated screening of virtually the entire population. Nor would it have been possible, because screening would have had to involve physical assessment by a physician or trained public health official, not a simple sample read cheaply and automatically in 20 minutes or less. Thus the high moral cost of the exclusionary quarantine policies at Ellis Island, Grosse Île, and many other places around the world did not weigh well against these policies' effect in reducing the burden of disease.

The conjecture in the thought experiment we are considering here could also cut the other way: these policies would in the case of some diseases involve only moderate practical and moral costs—imposing modest restrictions of liberty, limited violations of privacy and confidentiality, and minor violations of requirements of informed consent, no greater in being forced to miss a plane to receive immediate treatment than when a flight is canceled or rescheduled by the airline on account of inclement weather. For example, a passenger testing positive for syphilis would be given a single injection of penicillin (albeit in the gluteus maximus) that would cure the condition permanently, on the spot. Treatment for *this* passenger is thus a multiple benefit for many others—not only for this passenger, but also for this passenger's future contacts, and for these contacts' future contacts along multiple potential lines of transmission, including vertical transmission to potential children who now can be born without congenital forms of the disease. And it is a benefit to the community as a whole if it contributes to the elimination of the disease—all this, from a single injection. For the person who was unaware that he or she had this disease, testing that identifies it and guarantees treatment is not the sort of constraint one would seek to avoid; on the contrary, it is a process one should welcome as it brings an unanticipated cure. Other diseases, of course, might involve far more sustained constraints, if a passenger were to test positive for a more difficult-to-treat disease or one for which no treatment is effective. As we will see in the next chapter, there are serious questions about whether current data support the efficacy of screening programs so far, though the thought experiment we are entertaining here is based on the assumption of rapid tests with virtually 100% sensitivity and specificity.

But further issues of justice would still be apparent if universal screening of the sort our thought experiment imagines were carried out on a global scale. Because much infectious disease is more prevalent among those of lower socio-economic status and those in resource-poor countries, the moral costs of inconvenience and limitations of liberty, violations of privacy and confidentiality, and the burdens of coercion, would fall more heavily on already disadvantaged people. This would be injustice in the distribution of burdens, not benefits, but injustice just the same.

But suppose effective treatment were available and provided cost-free for all the diseases that could be detected in such screenings. If so, although the frequency of identified disease might be higher in impoverished areas, the corresponding benefits would be higher as well. More disease would be detected—but more people would also be treated. This is the crucial difference between the people sent back from Ellis Island or the people with serious or potentially fatal infectious diseases left untreated and essentially left to die at the overwhelmingly crowded quarantine station at Grosse Île. By contrast, our thought experiment imagines that those identified with positive tests would not only have the advantage of diagnosis for conditions they might not have recognized, but would be guaranteed access to effective treatment as well. This is a substantial practical benefit, in avoiding the harms of disease, but it is a great moral benefit too, in that it insists on treating the person who tests positive not just as a *vector* and thus a risk to others, but also as a *victim*—a human person in need of and deserving of help. It is a distributive benefit for groups of the least well off, those characteristically most burdened by ill health, and especially by infectious disease. If cheap, rapid, non-invasive tests of high reliability were used to screen in virtually every public circumstance, from airports to schools to public transportation, accompanied by immediate treatment, it would mean inconvenience and real limitation for some time as well as substantial short-term societal expense, but its end result would be to detect and treat many or all forms of human-to-human communicable disease and much of that transmitted through intermediate vectors as well, thus virtually eliminating disease and hence improving the lives of all. Here we see in play the Rawlsian aspect of our PVV view—*especially* for the least well off.

This outcome assumes that treatment exists for any infectious disease identified, that the treatment is effective, that it will be available, and that the treatment does not have serious side effects that might lead a person reasonably to refuse it. It also assumes that there will not be substantial numbers of people with other reasons for refusing treatment, such as religious convictions, discussed in Chapter 14, but we leave that issue aside for now. The likelihood of meeting these assumptions may currently seem less than the likelihood of having the rapid-diagnosis tests, but let us assume for the purposes of this thought experiment that effective therapy does exist and can be provided to everyone. Universal, free, effective treatment would be crucial if a program of universal testing is to achieve its goal, the virtually complete eradication of serious human infectious disease. With this guarantee, the poor, rather than being more greatly disadvantaged by such a scheme, would be its greatest beneficiaries: it is from their shoulders that the burden of infectious disease would be primarily lifted.

There is an irony here: the thought experiment of universal rapid screening is most ethically defensible when free, effective, non-burdensome treatment is fully available—but that is exactly when others can protect themselves if they become infected. When the benefits of the thought experiment are greatest—when it would prevent the spread of the most dangerous or untreatable diseases—its moral permissibility may seem more questionable. What if treatment is not available—whether because the disease is one we do not know how to treat or treat very well (for example, hepatitis C), or because treatment is available but too expensive for governments to provide or for individuals in some circumstances to afford, like treatment for HIV? This distributive picture raises further serious questions of justice for our thought experiment, for the experiment places the primary costs of preventing disease on those who are vectors, rather than on those who are potential victims. If disease prevention is available—say, through vaccination, or education and behavior change—but treatment is not, placing the potentially greater burden of transmission avoidance on the vector may be at least partly, perhaps wholly unjust. The injustice will be graver still if the burdens of staying home to avoid being a vector are greater than the burdens of the disease itself, as may be the case with chronic non-fatal conditions that last for lengthy periods of time.

In the chapters that follow, we will make a start on addressing the problems of how to do justice for those who are constrained as victims or vectors, but who do not appear to benefit in any immediate, personal way from the constraint. Such constraints, we will argue, should at a minimum be supplemented by compensation for those harmed by the surveillance process—this would of course apply to our thought experiment, were it to become policy in the real world. Conversely, if compensation were inadequate, or insufficient to outweigh the violations of justice implicit in our thought experiment, it would be at least prima facie impermissible; that is the issue that remains for further discussion in the real-world circumstances of the chapters to follow.

The Thought Experiment in Practice: A "Decade of Infectious-Disease Inconvenience"?

Call the period our conjecture envisions the "decade of infectious-disease inconvenience." It is a considerable leap to be sure, but let us suppose that if this policy were in force for a decade (say, as we shall imagine in a real-world continuation of this thought experiment in Chapter 20, from 2020–2030), the frequency of true positives would decline, and eventually disappear. Like smallpox, not just one human-affecting communicable disease, but many of them—or at least all of them without sizeable non-human reservoirs—could be wiped from the face of the earth. At the end of the decade, let us suppose, the entire apparatus of universal testing could be downsized, largely dismantled and suspended, kept in readiness and only reinstituted if some unanticipated outbreak were to occur.

Clearly, this conjecture is not science fiction—or only science fiction. Already, a research group headed by Dr. Paul Yager at the University of Washington is working under a $15.4 million Grand Challenges in Global Health grant from the Bill and Melinda Gates Foundation to develop diagnostic tools that can be more easily used in the developing world; their point-of-care diagnostic system anticipates being able to test blood for a range of conditions, including bacterial infections, malnutrition, and HIV-related illnesses. The investigators envision that health-care workers would load a small blood sample onto a disposable test card about the size of a credit card, containing all of the necessary test re-agents; the test card would then be inserted into a device about the size of a handheld computer; it would yield results in about 10 minutes.[19] They do not have universal airport screening for infectious disease in mind, but better diagnosis of multiple conditions in the developing world. Yet we can see the implications of technological developments such as this for the world as a whole, particularly as it confronts the threats of infectious disease.

Perhaps most important to the issue of constraints, in theory at least, a universal rapid-test screening policy would be self-limiting in the end, as the various diseases were gradually brought under full control and at least for some, altogether wiped out. Just as with immunization for diseases like smallpox that have been effectively controlled, testing and immunization for further infectious diseases would eventually no longer be required. Although the possibility of complete disease eradication is greatest where humans are the only host—as in smallpox and polio, though not in some other serious infectious diseases like tetanus or histoplasmosis—the list of human-host-only diseases is nevertheless quite long, and similar testing regimens could be introduced for at least animal populations kept in controlled conditions, like poultry and cattle.

Thus the invasions of liberty, privacy and confidentiality, informed consent, and justice generally involved in this policy would be relatively short-lived, but its gains in the elimination of disease permanent. Perhaps simplistic ways of thinking about these moral issues would be put to rest as well: the individualist picture of one person's interests pitted against, rather than with, those of another, would need reform, and a revised understanding of the sense in which one individual's interests in liberty, privacy, confidentiality, and justice are violated would need to be developed. This would be a new ethical picture, perhaps an ancient dream of public health but new to bioethics, of individuals' common interest in extricating themselves—indeed, each and every one—from the web of infectious disease all human beings share.

No doubt actual social acceptance or rejection of such policies would be a function of fear: if no threat were apparent at the moment, testing and treatment

19. Bill and Melinda Gates Foundation, "Grand Challenges in Global Health Selects 43 Groundbreaking Research Projects for More Than $436 Million in Funding" (June 27, 2005), http://www.gatesfoundation.org/GlobalHealth/BreakthroughScience/GrandChallenges/Announcements/Announce-050627.htm (accessed January 22, 2008).

policies would be resisted, but in or after an outbreak of some disease that is widely feared, like SARS, Ebola, or person-to-person avian flu, such measures might be widely embraced. Mandated treatment might remain more controversial, but universal testing might be quite likely to be embraced, much as airport screenings were embraced in the wake of airliner hijackings—even though a good bit of grumbling about the inconvenience might remain, there might be little disagreement about the principle involved.

Thought Experiment? Or Proposal?

Should this conjecture be regarded as a real proposal? Could a decent society agree to implement a policy of universal rapid-test screening for communicable infectious disease, one that might mean substantial restrictions on some people for some time, even if these conditions were met? Would a decent society also guarantee treatment for people testing positive for infectious disease? Even more, would a decent society require treatment (or isolation) for those who did not want to accept treatment, whether for religious reasons, fear of treatment, or to avoid the side effects of treatment? And what if some of these conditions could be met only partially, or perhaps not at all? In the next chapter we develop a full account of the moral conditions that make the imposition of constraints ethically tolerable, including—but hardly limited to—the kinds of constraints this thought experiment has imagined.

One great benefit of thought experiments is that they help to identify critical but unnoticed assumptions. But the relationship of a thought experiment to an actual proposal is always a matter of controversy. If, in this case, the thought experiment makes overly optimistic assumptions, it may not be useful; but if it helps to identify and address the most pressing ethical issues raised by a possible course of action, it can be invaluable.

If this thought experiment were an actual proposal, it might be seen as deeply troubling, in that its "decade of infectious disease inconvenience" may be painted far too optimistically, both in terms of what real gains in the control of infectious disease could likely be achieved and, particularly important here, what its moral costs might be. Would the universal surveillance—ongoing inspection—of one's particularly intimate bodily circumstances, one's physical health, be intolerable in a way that current surveillance of, say, physical presence at street corners or in subways, or withdrawals at ATMs, is tracked by cameras, is at least tolerated? Is it the surveillance that disturbs, or the diagnosis, or the required treatment, or the subsequent constraints on liberty if no treatment is available but one remains contagious, or all of these?

In the end, this speculation is not just a proposal or a thought experiment; rather, it is an invitation to consider what price we would pay if we had some realistic chance of eliminating infectious disease—which, perhaps, we do: a "decade of infectious-disease inconvenience," we might imagine, for the goal of virtually complete eradication, elimination, or control. Clearly, a real-world proposal for implementation of the thought experiment we have been posing here would be an enormously complex undertaking, as we will explore in Chapter 20, and there would certainly be disagreement over the politics, economics, and social impact of such a program. We have set out here to stimulate discussion of the deeper ethical issues raised by this thought experiment and the basis on which they rest. In the next chapter, we present a fuller ethical account of when constraints are justifiable—and when they are not—based on our PVV perspective. In subsequent chapters, we apply this analysis to a pressing case under contemporary discussion—planning for pandemic influenza.

16

CONSTRAINTS IN THE CONTROL
OF INFECTIOUS DISEASE

The thought experiment that we have just undertaken—that of universal rapid testing for all serious, human-affecting infectious disease—brings constraints to the forefront. But it does so as a hypothetical, not as a real-world case. Today's world, however, may soon present a test case for the permissibility of highly targeted, disease-specific rapid testing in airports, as well as for many other types of constraints: the effort to stop the spread of emerging infectious diseases such as SARS or pandemic influenza. Would universal rapid testing, coupled with prohibitions on travel, isolation for anyone who tests positive, and cordoning off of affected areas, be permissible or justifiable at the first evidence of sustainable human-to-human transmission of the H5N1 virus?[1] After all, the preventive value of new interventions is greater early on in a new outbreak than at any other time, when the possibility of reducing spread is greatest. The pandemic planning literature is at this point vast, but has directed limited attention to this immediate question.[2] Yet given the likely shortages of vaccines and anti-virals in the first stages of a pandemic, reducing spread may be a highest-priority strategy. In this chapter, we present a more general theory about the justification of constraints and then deploy it in subsequent chapters to examine certain critical features of contemporary pandemic planning, including the surveillance and travel restrictions contemplated in our thought experiment.

Reflection on constraints and responses to them must be fully informed by our expanded conception of the individual—the "way-station self." As we argued in Chapter 6, liberal philosophy's traditional notion of the person as an independent, free, tall-standing "individual" is inadequate for dealing with

---

1. Writing Committee of the Second World Health Organization Consultation on Clinical Aspects of Human Infection with Avian Influenza A (H5N1) Virus, "Update on Avian Influenza A (H5N1) Virus Infection in Humans," *New England Journal of Medicine* 358, no. 3 (January 17, 2008): 261–273.
2. An exception is Wendy E. Parmet, "Legal Power and Legal Rights—Isolation and Quarantine in the Case of Drug-Resistant Tuberculosis," *New England Journal of Medicine* 357, no. 5 (Aug. 2, 2007): 433–435.

human reality in the context of infectious disease. Viewed from our naturalized version of the veil of ignorance represented by the "way-station" self, constraints do not simply wrong someone by restricting him yet do right by protecting others. Constraining (and thus from one perspective apparently wronging) given individuals is also doing right to these same individuals, by reducing their vulnerability to the mutual transmission of disease in the interconnected web of human biological/ecological relationships. This is why standard harm-principle analyses of constraints do not work very well for infectious disease.

On the view we develop here, the harm principle needs to go up a layer, so to speak, to a conceptual space in which the issue is not "me against you," but "everyone in this together." To constrain a person in the context of infectious disease is both to harm and to protect, and the one cannot be generally separated from the other. In submitting to or being subjected to constraints like required immunization, restrictions on travel into areas of outbreak, or isolation and treatment, a person is *both* violated *and* enhanced by measures to reduce the overall spread of disease. Our analysis considers what people owe one other from this layer of dual risk and advantage, asking not just what each is willing to bear for their own protection as well as for the protection of others, but how what each is willing to bear affects everyone—and thus, what all should expect of one another. We begin with a description of the most important forms of constraints that have been or are being employed against infectious disease.

Forms of Constraint

Constraints employ a multiplicity of strategies raising different ethical concerns.[3] While the varieties of constraint are myriad, both in the historical past and in current practice, we think they can be grouped into four general categories of primary ethical concern, the categories we deployed in examining our thought experiment in the preceding chapter.

Violations of Bodily Integrity and Physical Security

Consider Boston in November 1901, when the Boston Board of Health ordered "virus squads" to vaccinate men living in cheap boarding houses against smallpox. According to the *Boston Globe*:

> Every imaginable threat from civil suits to cold-blooded murder when they got an
> opportunity to commit it, was made by the writhing, cursing, struggling tramps

---

3. For a good discussion of the history of quarantine and isolation and of the role of due process guarantees, see Michelle A. Daubert, "Comment: Pandemic Fears and Contemporary Quarantine: Protecting Liberty Through a Continuum of Due Process Rights," *Buffalo Law Review* 54 (2007): 1299–1353.

who were operated upon, and a lot of them had to be held down in their cots, one big policeman sitting on their legs, and another on their heads, while the third held the arms, bared for the doctors.[4]

Some constraints involve physical impositions on likely vectors or victims. The least intrusive of these are the kinds of mandated diagnostic tests that require just a moment of time: the breath test or cheek swab envisioned in our thought experiment in the preceding chapter. Stool samples or blood tests are slightly more invasive and time consuming. More invasive and potentially more physically risky are required immunizations. Still more invasive are required treatment and treatment that is directly observed, as with the DOT programs imposed on patients with multidrug-resistant tuberculosis we discussed in Chapter 9.[5] These programs all have the potential to benefit the patient-victim or patient-vector, at least if treatment is available, but not all patients want or can have diagnosis, protection, or treatment. Diagnosis of disease may subject people to additional restrictions, such as the limitations on liberty already discussed. To be sure, if treatment is ready to hand, diagnosis may be a crucial first step in restoring the patient to health or in protecting others, as our discussion of rapid testing of pregnant women for HIV/AIDS in Chapter 12 observed. Nonetheless, imposed treatment may not benefit the patient, or may be highly intrusive to patient dignity, as we saw with our case study of the patient with tuberculosis in Chapter 9. Patients may have religious or other conscientious reasons for refusing treatment, and perceive forced treatment as a serious violation of autonomy. Patients also may fail to understand the need for treatment or may find treatment inconvenient.[6] And, as with diseases such as Ebola, treatment may simply be unavailable.

Some traditional and contemporary constraints subject those on whom they are imposed to increased risk. Quarantine is a particular example: if persons who have been exposed to the disease in question but are not yet ill are herded together in crowded, inadequate conditions with other people who are ill, those who might never have become ill face increased risks of contracting the disease. In what bioethicists would describe as a violation of non-maleficence, or the Hippocratic Oath would identify as a violation of the principle "do no

---

4. "Virus Squad Out," *Boston Globe*, November 18, 1901, 7, cited in Michael Albert, Kristen Ostheimer, and Joel Breman, "The Last Smallpox Epidemic in Boston and the Vaccination Controversy, 1901–1903," *New England Journal of Medicine* 344, no. 5 (February 1, 2001): 375–379. We thank Constance Orzechowski for this and several of the following historical examples.
5. See William F. Paolo, Jr., and Joshua D. Nosanchuk, "Tuberculosis in New York City: Recent Lessons and a Look Ahead," *Lancet Infectious Diseases* 4, no. 5 (2004): 287–293.
6. S. Gupta, D. Berg, F. de Lott, P. Kellner, and C. Driver, "Directly Observed Therapy for Tuberculosis in New York City: Factors Associated with Refusal," *International Journal of Tuberculosis and Lung Disease* 8, no. 4 (2004): 480–485.

harm," infection-control containment practices such as quarantine—particularly in the past—often dramatically increased the risks to people they affected.

Quarantine of the old-fashioned sort involved keeping together everyone suspected of having been exposed to disease, whether or not they actually were infected, and requiring them to stay off in a separate place, away from others whom they might infect, until all danger of disease was apparently past. The term originated in the Venetian practice of keeping an infected ship offshore for 40 days, until disease had burned itself out—that is, until everyone aboard who was susceptible had either died or recovered.[7] Quarantine of this kind may keep disease at bay, if modes of transmission are properly understood, but it herds together people in three different sorts of disease status: the currently ill, the exposed who have contracted infection but are not yet showing signs of disease, and those who are thought to have been exposed but would not have become ill but for continued exposure under conditions of quarantine. This was just what happened to the immigrants quarantined at Grosse Île. Undoubtedly, the conditions of quarantine are typically burdensome to all, independent of their disease status, but the burdens are most severe for those who have not been exposed beforehand but are nonetheless subjected to the quarantine: disease and perhaps death that would not otherwise have occurred but for concentrated exposure to others under quarantine.[8]

Contemporary approaches to quarantine attempt to avoid this risk where possible; for example, the Model State Emergency Health Powers Act requires that individuals who are known to be ill be isolated from individuals who are under quarantine.[9] This principled separation of isolation and quarantine was not realized in the quarantines of ships for cholera at Grosse Île and elsewhere, where people were left on board ship until they either died or survived and the disease effectively burned out. It remains to be seen whether the recommendations in the Model Act will be honored under contemporary circumstances of emergency and fear in an H5N1 influenza pandemic, particularly if facilities for treatment of the ill are insufficient and many must remain in the community.

---

7. For an overview of the history of quarantine, including the isolation of lepers in Roman times and the Venetian practice of keeping ships offshore for 40 days, see NOVA, "The Most Dangerous Woman in America: History of Quarantine," http://www.pbs.org/wgbh/nova/typhoid/quarantine. html (accessed January 24, 2008).

8. For a discussion of the issues of justice raised by quarantine of this form, see Daniel Markovits, "Quarantines and Distributive Justice," *Journal of Law, Medicine & Ethics* 33 (2005): 323–338.

9. Centers for Law and the Public's Health at Georgetown and Johns Hopkins Universities, "The Model State Emergency Health Powers Act," December 21, 2001, sec. 604(b)(2), http://www.publichealthlaw.net/MSEHPA/MSEHPA2.pdf (accessed January 24, 2008).

Violations of Liberty and Consent

Consider San Francisco in 1900:

> *The morning following the death of Chick Gin, a 41-year-old*
> *resident of a dilapidated boardinghouse, just after midnight on*
> *March 6, 1900, the San Francisco Health Department rolled out a*
> *full-scale quarantine of Chinatown—days before laboratory tests*
> *confirmed the initial diagnosis of bubonic plague—preventing the*
> *Chinese residents of the city from leaving the neighborhood, going to*
> *work, or going about their business. In this case, only (as it later*
> *turned out) 4 of the 35,000 residents of Chinatown actually had*
> *plague; the rest of the 35,000 who were quarantined were viewed*
> *as potential vectors, people either already exposed or about to be so.*
> *In the following weeks, the Health Department tried to inspect and*
> *disinfect every home and building in the twelve-block area, throwing*
> *people out of their homes, confiscating and burning personal*
> *property, and beating residents who were uncooperative.*[10] *Chinese*
> *were not permitted to leave the area, though whites could come*
> *and go freely. It was not until a group of businessmen led by*
> *Levi Strauss, founder of the company that made blue jeans,*
> *himself an immigrant, raised the requisite funds that food was*
> *even provided for the quarantined Chinese. The Chinese were*
> *forcibly inoculated with the largely experimental Haffkine vaccine,*
> *which had a number of serious side effects and was not known to be*
> *effective.*

Some measures for the control of infectious disease, such as involuntary
quarantine, are straightforwardly restrictive of liberty. Indeed, many infection-
control strategies limit freedom of movement, such as isolation of patients known
to be ill, home quarantine, *cordons sanitaires* around entire communities, or
circles of containment. There are enormous varieties in how these strategies
work, the harms they may impose, whether they are undertaken consensually,
and the extent and distribution of their effects on liberty. Strategies may be
quite focused, as with isolation that affects only persons known to be ill, or
they may be widespread, as with the quarantine of San Francisco's Chinatown

---

10. Howard Markel, *When Germs Travel: Six Major Epidemics That Have Invaded America and the
Fears They Have Unleashed* (New York: Random House, 2004), 49–77.

in 1900. Strategies may also provide opportunities for people who choose to do so to stay at home—examples include work holidays or school closures that are welcomed by some—although burdensome to others. And some forms of liberty-limiting strategies, like closing facilities or canceling public events, may be even less burdensome at least in the sense that they leave people free to go about their daily lives with the exception of enjoying the banned attraction. Some constraints limiting movement violate autonomy by placing restrictions on the potential victim, others on potential vectors, and still others on both. While some restrictions are trivial or even welcome, like requiring masks and gloves, biohazard suits, and other types of precautions to avoid exposure, other restrictions are more burdensome: for example, cancellations of celebratory events or closures of much-used facilities.[11]

Although limiting liberty, sometimes in very important ways, these constraints may also have the advantage of protecting potential victims from infection. The closure of public swimming pools during polio epidemics, for example, kept away both vectors and potential victims and thus may have provided potential victims with protection—although, as we shall see, evidentiary support for the efficacy of social distancing measures generally is a matter of some dispute. Nonetheless, such closures and constraints may cut deeply into core aspects of personal and community life. Constraints may close off communication with associates, work partners, loved ones; they may thwart plans and goals; they may deprive people of necessities as well as luxuries, and they may destroy intimate aspects of sexual life, as with the denial of permission to marry in states that require premarital testing for sexually transmitted diseases or the closure of bathhouses in San Francisco in response to the outbreak of HIV/AIDS.[12]

Throughout the entire episode of the quarantine of Chinatown, only a very few voices seemed to recognize that the imposition of constraints for the protection of some brings moral obligations to others along with it. Among the few who recognized even a portion of the obligations to victims under constraint were a former U.S. Congressman, James G. MacGuire, who said, "The Chinese are practically prisoners, and we who are their keepers should see that they do not suffer,"[13] and a U.S. district judge, William Morrow, who ruled in favor of the Chinese community's resistance to forcible immunization, limiting the government's ability to enforce compulsory inoculations with untested products or, more generally, to violate a citizen's rights in the name of public health.[14]

11. John Barry, *The Great Influenza* (London: Penguin Books, 2004), 208–209.
12. See, e.g., L. McKusick et al., "Reported Changes in the Sexual Behavior of Men at Risk for AIDS, San Francisco, 1982–84—the AIDS Behavioral Research Project," *Public Health Report* 100, no.6 (1985): 622–629.
13. Markel, *When Germs Travel*, 69, quoting the *San Francisco Examiner*, June 1, 1900, 6.
14. Wong Wai v. Williamson, 103 F. 384, 384 (N.D. Cal. 1900); Jew Ho v. Williamson, 103 F. 10, 23 (N.D. Cal. 1900); Wong Wai v. Williamson, 103 F. 1, 9 (N.D. Cal. 1900). In a case decided soon afterward, Jacobson v. Massachusetts, 197 U.S. 11 (1905), the U.S. Supreme Court held that mandatory

Violations of Privacy and Confidentiality

Consider the limitations imposed in Singapore during the SARS outbreak of 2003. Parliament, relying on a 1970s quarantine law originally intended to protect against malaria, tuberculosis, and cholera, raised the penalty for violating quarantine to as much as $5,800 and six months in prison. People who were quarantined were required to appear regularly before Web cameras installed at their homes and to wear electronic bracelets if they did not appear.[15] These practices violated liberty; they also publicly identified those who were subject to the quarantine and thus violated confidentiality.

Concerns about violations of privacy and confidentiality arise in many infectious-disease control practices. Traditional tactics such as belling or otherwise publicly identifying likely vectors, as well as contemporary practices like contact tracing (even if others are informed that they may have encountered a vector without being told the vector's actual identity), either expose or risk exposing the infectiousness or presumed infectiousness of some persons. Although not limiting liberty directly, these forms of control may have significant effects on the supposed vector. To take a modern (and yet still primitive) example, shunning, job loss, and exclusion from schools have been well documented in the case of identification of persons infected with HIV/AIDS.[16]

Another contemporary form of violation of privacy or confidentiality, or both, is raised by targeted surveillance, which can be accomplished through anonymized data sets, most efficiently of electronic health records.[17] As we discussed in Chapter 8, data sets that have been fully anonymized no longer contain confidential information about identifiable patients. They do, however, require that patient privacy have been intruded upon beforehand in order for information about disease status to be gathered. They also risk stigmatization of groups or populations. If it becomes apparent, for example, that rates of measles are highest among particular ethnic groups,[18] that HIV is more common in specific national or population subgroups (such as the fears

---

immunizations when necessary to protect the public health did not violate the U.S. Constitution. Arguing for Massachusetts, counsel distinguished the California quarantine cases by arguing that the order went further than the statutory authorization and applied in arbitrary fashion to Chinese immigrants only.

15. Wayne Arnold, "In Singapore, 1970's Law Becomes Weapon Against SARS," *New York Times*, sec. F, June 10, 2003.

16. Liza Conyers, K. B. Boomer, and Brian T. McMahon, "Workplace Discrimination and HIV/AIDS: The National EEOC ADA Research Project," *Work* 25, no. 1 (2005): 37–48.

17. For a discussion of such data sets and the issues of privacy and confidentiality they raise, see Nicholas P. Terry and Leslie P. Francis, "Ensuring the Privacy and Confidentiality of Electronic Health Records," *Illinois Law Review* 2007, no. 2: 681–735.

18. See, e.g., L.G. Dales et al., "Measles Epidemic from Failure to Immunize," *Western Journal of Medicine* 159, no. 4 (1993): 455–464 (describing a measles epidemic among unimmunized Hispanic children in California).

in the mid 1980s that culminated in a refusal to grant asylum interviews to HIV-positive Haitians[19]), or that Ebola is endemic in particular areas of the world, the result may be unjustified judgments that everyone from the given ethnic group or geographical region poses a risk and is to be avoided.

Violations of Justice

Historically, constraints have often targeted unpopular groups. Consider a 1904 editorial in *The Lancet*, blaming the spread of smallpox on the homeless:

> What a potent factor in maintaining the prevalence of smallpox is that unemployed and largely unemployable degenerate [person] . . . The fact that this parasite upon the charity and good nature of the community is in his turn a vehicle for the spread of other parasites, both animal and vegetable, is common knowledge but practically no compulsory steps have been taken to curtail seriously the vagrant's movements.[20]

Concerns about violations of justice may be particularly urgent in examining policies governing the control of infectious disease, because, as we pointed out in Chapter 3, among the ethically relevant characteristics of infectious disease is that at least some of it disproportionately affects people in precarious or imperiled socioeconomic circumstances: the poor, the malnourished, refugees, and people who live in crowded conditions. We have already described the unequal treatment of immigrants approaching Ellis Island in New York harbor: first class passengers were waved through without inspection; steerage passengers were detained for medical examination. Barricades were strung around areas of concentrated ethnic populations, as the quarantine of Chinatown illustrates, but less often around high-class residential areas. To be sure, these apparent violations of justice were not without a crude basis: at least for some diseases, rates of infection were higher among the poor. But in many of these historical cases, what may have had some rational basis became wholesale racist or classist stereotyping.

Another potential violation of justice, illustrated in contemporary pandemic planning, is constraints on potential victims' access to preventive or treatment measures. Violations of justice, though often overlooked, occur when prioritization schemes are inadequately grounded or access to prevention or treatment is available not on a principled basis but only in a general free-for-all competition. Some distributive schemas may be well reasoned: for

19. See, e.g., Hiroshi Motomura, "Haitian Asylum Seekers: Interdiction and Immigrants' Rights," *Cornell International Law Journal* 26 (1993): 695–717 (701).

20. "The Spread of Small-Pox by Tramps," *Lancet* 1 (1904):446–447, cited in Albert, Ostheimer, and Breman, "The Last Smallpox Epidemic," 375–379.

example, vaccines or anti-virals that are in short supply may be prioritized in a way that aims to reduce spread or to preserve services essential to public order. Even these prioritization schemes may leave those who otherwise might have had access to supplies without them, and this raises questions of justice that we will discuss in Chapter 19.

Constraints imposed to prevent the spread of transmissible infectious disease thus bring significant moral burdens—of personal security, liberty, privacy and confidentiality, and justice. From the perspective of potential victims, these costs may seem justifiable—indeed, it may seem that no costs are too high, if they are life-saving, to protect from infection by others. But from the perspective of potential vectors who may bear the burdens—indeed, the same people, because each person is at least potentially a vector if he or she is a victim—our PVV view recognizes that constraints require further examination and careful justification.

Protecting the Constrained

Justifications for constraints have been long a concern in public health, although as we explored in Chapter 4, attention to the theoretical bases of the ethics of public health is a more recent phenomenon. General treatments of constraints are found in the United Nations Siracusa Principles, which limit the derogation of rights in times of emergencies.[21]

In addition, in the United States, the requirements of due process strict scrutiny—that there be a fundamental state interest and that any restriction be narrowly tailored—apply when fundamental rights are curtailed. In the context of pandemic planning, many groups have worked, and continue to work, to identify a unifying set of principles to justify constraints, both in the context of infectious disease control and otherwise. Various proposals—though differing dramatically in length—have much in common, and it is heartening that they do.[22] These proposals, however, tend to consist of a list of important values, some emphasizing the individual and others solidarity and

21. United Nations Economic and Social Council, U.N. Sub-Commission on Prevention of Discrimination and Protection of Minorities, *Siracusa Principles on the Limitation and Derogation of Provisions in the International Covenant on Civil and Political Rights*, Annex, UN Doc E/CN.4/1984/4 (1984), http://hei.unige.ch/~clapham/hrdoc/docs/siracusa.html (accessed January 27, 2008).

22. These principles are very helpfully surveyed by James C. Thomas in "Ethical Concerns in Pandemic Influenza Preparation and Responses," in a white paper commissioned by the Southeast Regional Center of Excellence for Emerging Infections and Biodefense, Policy, Ethics and Law Core, http://www.serceb.org/wysiwyg/downloads/pandemic_flu_white_paper.May_25.FORMATTED.pdf (accessed Sept. 2007), 6–9. Thomas surveys sets of principles from working groups in Toronto (2005), a commentator in Canada, New Zealand (2006), WHO (2006), and working groups at Siracusa and Bellagio.

the community, without bringing these values together on a common foundation. We believe that our PVV perspective, bringing together as it does both victimhood and vectorhood, sheds light on how these values can work together in justifying both constraints and their limits.

In pandemic planning literature, the initial and highly influential effort to identify guiding principles was *Stand on Guard for Thee*, a 2005 report from the Pandemic Influenza Working Group at the Joint Centre for Bioethics at the University of Toronto.[23] The Working Group identified the following ten values: individual liberty, protection of public from harm, proportionality, privacy, duty to provide care, reciprocity, equity, trust, solidarity, and stewardship. Another Canadian commentator, Jaro Kotalik, suggested three further values: subsidiarity, the precautionary principle, and transparency.[24] The list of principles identified by the New Zealand National Ethics Advisory Committee includes values in decision making processes (inclusiveness, openness, reasonableness, responsiveness, and responsibleness) and substantive values: harm minimization, respect (*manaakitanga*), fairness, neighborliness (*whanaungatanga*), reciprocity, and unity (*kotahitanga*).[25] A working group on therapeutic and prophylactic measures for the WHO Project on Addressing Ethical Issues in Pandemic Influenza Planning identified three guiding values: efficiency, equity, and accountability, and the WHO working group addressing public health measures identified four values: public health necessity, reasonable and effective means, proportionality, and distributive justice.[26] Following the meetings of these working groups, WHO published a set of ethical considerations for a public health response to pandemic influenza. These considerations are based on the assumption that competing values of individual and community interest must be balanced. Particularly important in this balance are both procedural values such as transparency and public engagement and substantive values such as utility and equity.[27] The ethical framework for the 2007 British planning document rests on "equal concern and respect." Because "everyone matters," and "everyone matters equally," British planning is committed to respect,

23. University of Toronto Joint Centre for Bioethics Pandemic Influenza Working Group, *Stand on Guard for Thee: Ethical Considerations in Preparedness Planning for Pandemic Influenza* (Toronto: University of Toronto Joint Centre for Bioethics, 2005), http://www.utoronto.ca/jcb/home/documents/pandemic.pdf (accessed January 27, 2008).
24. Jaro Kotalik, "Preparing for an Influenza Pandemic: Ethical Issues," *Bioethics* 19, no. 4 (August 2005): 422–431.
25. National Ethics Advisory Committee, *Getting Through Together: Ethical Values for a Pandemic*, (Wellington, New Zealand: Ministry of Health, 2007) 4–5, http://www.neac.health.govt.nz/moh.nsf/pagescm/1090/$File/getting-through-together-ju107.pdf (accessed January 26, 2008).
26. Thomas, *Ethical Concerns*, 8.
27. World Health Organization, *Ethical Considerations in Developing a Public Health Response to Pandemic Influenza* (Geneva: WHO, 2007), http://www.who.int/csr/resources/publications/WHO_CDS_EPR_GIP_2007_2c.pdf (accessed January 21, 2008).

harm minimization, fairness, working together, reciprocity, keeping things in proportion, flexibility, and decision making that is open and transparent, inclusive, accountable, and reasonable.[28]

Our own compact list, presented in Table 1, regards these and the many other pandemic planning documents that have been produced in the past several years as positive contributions to the ethics issues in infectious disease. Yet, we think they frequently are insufficiently systematic. In the following section, we develop a view that incorporates both justifications and limits on constraints, drawn from our understanding of the patient as both victim and vector. Whatever the scope of constraints, specific basic procedural and substantive principles must be observed whenever and to whatever extent constraints are imposed, regardless of whether the measures are precautionary, preventative ones, or the emergency measures to stop the spread of pandemic disease that we will consider here.

One helpful way to organize values on the lists is to distinguish between procedural and substantive considerations. This distinction is important, because procedural requirements may be less ethically problematic. Justifications of procedural requirements can elide at least some conflicts among basic values and they can more readily be observed than substantive guarantees, at least in all but the most disastrous circumstances. In contrast, substantive requirements, when they involve provision of goods rather than observation of procedures, often cannot be satisfied, or cannot be satisfied fully. In some extreme circumstances, substantive requirements can barely be satisfied at all—and yet their claims remain of real moral importance. Not surprisingly, a good deal of the pandemic planning literature has focused primarily on procedural guarantees.

TABLE 1 Procedural Protections and Substantive Guarantees in Constraints

Basic Procedural Requirements

P-1 Important interest, supported by evidence
P-2 Least restrictive alternative
P-3 Transparency and disclosure
P-4 Reconsideration

Basic Substantive Guarantees

S-1 Personal security
S-2 Basic survival and health needs, including prevention and treatment
S-3 Communication
S-4 Equitable allocation of burdens
S-5 Compensation for loss

28. Department of Health, *Responding to Pandemic Influenza: The Ethical Framework for Policy and Planning* (November 22. 2007), http://www.dh.gov.uk/en/Publicationsandstatistics/Publications/PublicationsPolicyAndGuidance/DH_080751 (accessed January 21, 2008), 1.

Constraints: Basic Procedural Requirements

Several basic procedural requirements are crucial in the defense of constraints imposed to control the spread of infectious disease. These requirements are much discussed and have guided many of the public and regulatory approaches to constraints of which we are aware. Despite their familiarity, they are worth emphasizing because what they require has not always been fully recognized and because they are at risk of being subject to pressures in difficult-case scenarios of outbreaks of pandemic disease. The procedures include requirements that constraints be carefully justified and that they be as limited as possible within the terms of the justification. They also include the requirement that the need for the constraint be conveyed openly to those who will experience it. Finally, constraints must be subject to challenge and reconsideration, of either their original justification or ongoing support. Although some of these principles may seem cumbersome in times of panic, each of these principles is demanded from our theoretical perspective of respect for each other—that is, ourselves—as simultaneously victims and vectors.

P-1. Important Interest, Well Supported by Data. Constraints that are imposed to protect us from infectious disease limit liberty. Because liberty is an important human interest, restrictions require justification.[29] Thus, there must be a reason sufficient to support a constraint. This is particularly important in the context of infectious disease, where panic may seem to demand immediate action. An example was the imposition of total quarantine just on the Chinese sector of San Francisco for what turned out to be four cases of plague, without clarity about whether that geographical delineation bore a reasonable relationship to the prevention of disease spread. Even SARS, although it was a lethal disease, may have occasioned fear-driven reactions far out of proportion to actual risks—reactions that were very costly not only to individuals, but to involved economies, especially in Asia.[30]

---

29. See, e.g., Roger Doughty, "The Confidentiality of HIV Related Information: Responding to the Resurgence of Aggressive Public Health Interventions in the AIDS Epidemic," *California Law Review* 82 (1994): 113–184 (121–122); Deborah Jones Merritt, "Communicable Disease and Constitutional Law: Controlling AIDS," *New York University Law Review* 61 (1986): 739–799 (777). Merritt's article shares some of our own view; she argues that equal protection analysis of constraints imposed on patients suspected of HIV should proceed from the point of view of a reasonable voter who does not know whether s/he is infected by the disease.
30. Donald Hanna and Yiping Huang, "The Impact of SARS on Asian Economies," *Asian Economic Papers* 3, no. 1 (2004): 102–112 (102).

From our PVV view, insistence on good reason for the imposition of constraints—on an important interest, well supported by data—matters for victims, for potential victims, and for vectors. Victims do not benefit from carelessly imposed constraints, either immediately, because the constraints will fail, or in the longer run because bad experiences with constraints may lead to their being more difficult to impose when they are genuinely needed. As victims, people care about how they are treated as vectors, too; thus they will not want to see themselves constrained where there is no real purpose served by the constraint.

While extensive data support the use of vaccines and antiviral drugs in preventing or controlling an influenza epidemic, there are surprisingly little data to support the implementation of some of the very expensive and socially disruptive non-pharmaceutical interventions commonly recommended by influenza pandemic planners. In the real world circumstances of an apparently incipient pandemic, there may well be epistemological difficulties in fulfilling the requirement for adequate information, especially when the circumstances appear to require haste. In times of limited knowledge about transmission mechanisms—not only a concern of the past when even understanding of the germ theory of disease was lacking, but even now a concern with newly emerging infectious agents—the requirement of a justification well supported by data is both difficult and critical. In the face of poorly understood disease, the understandable real-life reaction of people who realize that they are potential victims may be panic, fear of perceived vectors, and over-reaction to them. Leaving aside irrational fear, adherence to what has been called the "precautionary principle" may counsel adopting constraints that are more severe than eventually appears warranted: in situations of genuine uncertainty, the principle in its most general form cautions the following: *avoid action or inaction that risks the worst possible outcome.* But what is the worst outcome?—increased mortality because of delay in intervention, or massive economic disruption (and possibly also increased mortality) because of excessive intervention? The difficulties involved in weighing the balance of risks and protections in light of all the uncertainties involved in pandemic planning and assessment underline the importance of the opportunities for reconsideration, along with the substantive guarantees of treatment and compensation, which we address in subsequent chapters.

P-2. Least Restrictive Alternative. The use of the least restrictive alternative demands that wherever constraint is used, it should be the minimum amount, imposed on the smallest number of people necessary to achieve the objective in question. Patients should not be put in hospital isolation if home isolation will suffice. Entire quarters of cities should not be quarantined—as in San Francisco during the plague scare—before there is reliable evidence of disease spread. People should not be sent away for life to an inaccessible location as in the Hawaiian leper colony at Molokai without assessment of their actual risks to the community.[31]

If the disease to be prevented is less serious—if, say, the disease consists only in the inconvenient sneezes of the common cold or a fleeting, albeit itchy, skin rash—intrusions on the privacy or liberty of unwilling vectors are less well justified from the perspective of vectors, much as others might like to avoid these conditions as victims. Likewise, recognition of the possibility that anyone might be either victim or vector counsels against overbroad restrictions or restrictions without empirical support, for example capturing an entire geographical area or ethnic group as did the quarantine of Chinatown in San Francisco.[32]

But these are the easy cases, where interests in protection are not very strong, or where there are readily available, less draconian interventions. More often, there will be difficult comparisons among types of restriction: one may be less restrictive in one way, another in a different way. In pandemic planning, choices such as border surveillance impose greater burdens on privacy, whereas choices such as canceling flights impose greater burdens on liberty. These comparisons are complicated further by the paucity of evidence we have already discussed.

Unfortunately, as with the requirement for justification, in situations of panic—not infrequent in epidemics and pandemics of diseases believed to be rapidly transmissible and highly lethal—this requirement of using the least restrictive alternative is all too often overlooked. Draconian restrictions on behavior, association, travel, and many other facets of ordinary life are sometimes rapidly put in place, far out of proportion to the actual health risks that obtain. Furthermore, some restrictions are imposed not by governmental or regulatory agencies authorized to do so, but by the populace taking matters into its own hands. Consider as sobering examples these restrictions put in place during the 1878 Yellow Fever epidemic in the southern United States:

> *Jackson, Tennessee: Residents placed armed detectives and armed*
> *guards on all routes leading into the city. Railroads were forcibly*
> *stopped and passengers and cargo were removed from the trains and*
> *placed into improvised fever camps.*

---

31. For a chilling description of Molokai, see John Tayman, *The Colony: The Harrowing True Story of the Exiles of Molokai* (New York: Scribner, 2006).
32. See, e.g., Doughty, "Confidentiality of HIV Related Information," 121–22.

> *Jackson, Mississippi: Crowds ripped up the tracks of the Atlanta & Vicksburg Railroad for what they believed to be the company's violation of quarantine laws.*
>
> *Winona, Tennessee: The town's three doctors , the sheriff, and the sheriff's deputies fled, leaving public safety in the hands of armed vigilantes.*
>
> *New Orleans, Louisiana: Mobs grew as local authorities tried to use military force to implement quarantine; quarantine measures were left in the hands of roving bands of armed patrolmen and volunteers, who were loosely directed by local health officials to keep the fever outside the town line.*[33]

These historical examples illustrate how fear and social disintegration may undermine commitment to even relatively limited procedural guarantees—a historical lesson that should not be forgotten today, even though there are many legal and social protections against abuse, at least in the developed world.

P-3. Transparency and Disclosure. Transparency speaks to everyone as both victims and vectors, giving explanations of both reasons for constraints and reasons why constraints may be inappropriate at the present time. Sometimes violated in infectious disease public policy—as when China was less than forthcoming about avian flu,[34] this basic expectation requires fully and candidly explaining the reasons for and mechanisms of a policy; being responsive to arguments that the policy is overbroad or unnecessary; and in other ways making accessible and understandable to people who are constrained or may be constrained in the future what the rationale is for such constraints. Transparency and disclosure require making public those matters covered under P-1 and P-2 above, that there be an important interest where constraint is imposed (P-1), and that the least restrictive alternative is used (P-2).

As contemporary planning for avian flu and other pandemics has unfolded both in the United States and internationally, attention has been paid to the

---

33. Margaret Humphreys, *Yellow Fever and the South* (Rutgers University Press, 1992), 13, cited in Peter Patton, "Quarantine: Historical Lessons Learned," Center for Policing Terrorism, Chemical, Biological, Radiological, and Nuclear Working Group (CPT/CBRN), 2004.
34. Geoffrey York, "Human Bird Flu in China; After Initially Dismissing Their Illnesses, Beijing Admits H5N1 Has Infected People," *Globe & Mail (Canada)*, sec. A1, November 17, 2005.

transparency requirement. Pandemic plans have been widely published; most are available on the Web.[35] Many of these plans include guidance for open communication before, during, and after an epidemic.[36] Experts have been involved in the planning; and public responses have been sought and taken into account. To take just one of myriad examples, the U.S. Department of Health and Human Services published a "Request for Information" seeking public comment on vaccine prioritization in case of a pandemic.[37] In addition, there is considerable reason to think that transparency is important not only as a moral requirement but as a practical one. If people are well educated about the risks of a pandemic and understand the reasons for restrictions, disease spread is likely to be reduced.[38] Just the same, apparent transparency is not always adequate. Policies may not be fully explained, and an openly announced policy still may not be fully understood. Our PVV view encourages analysis of what might be missed even in a relatively transparent policy.

P-4. Reconsideration. The possibility of re-examination when constraints are imposed assures each person that they are taken seriously in their plight. Vectors and victims alike should be able to test justifications for constraints and well as appropriate limits on them. From the perspective of potential victims, people should be able to seek reassurance that they will be protected to the extent feasible. And, from their self-same perspective as potential vectors subject to constraints, they should be able to ask whether the costs imposed on them were or remain reasonable. Avenues of reconsideration are an essential demand, because they offer individuals the reassurance that policies are subject to review and correction if they are found no longer justified or necessary. Reconsideration may include challenges to prioritization rankings, access to treatment like vaccines or antivirals, petitions for release from constraining situations like quarantine or home isolation, requests for exemption from unwanted procedures like mandatory immunization, and so on.

Scrutinizing the present-day pandemic planning process with our PVV view will lead us to recommend that such planning expand its horizons. We have found limited attention in published pandemic plans to the actual construction

35. See, e.g., Lori Uscher-Pines et al., "Priority Setting for Pandemic Influenza: An Analysis of National Preparedness Plans," *PLoS Med* 3, no. 10 (2006): e436.
36. See, e.g., Toronto Public Health, *Toronto Public Health Plan for an Influenza Pandemic* (November 2005, updated March 2006), http://www.toronto.ca/health/pandemicflu/pandemicflu_plan.htm (accessed February 2007), 51.
37. U.S. Department of Health and Human Services, "Request for Information: Guidance for Prioritization of Pre-pandemic and Pandemic Influenza Vaccine," http://aspe.hhs.gov/PIV/RFI/ (accessed February 1, 2007).
38. See, e.g., John M. Drake, Suok Kai Chew, and Stefan Ma, "Societal Learning in Epidemics: Intervention Effectiveness During the 2003 SARS Outbreak in Singapore," *PLoS One* 1 (December 20, 2006): e20; University of Toronto Joint Centre for Bioethics, *Stand on Guard for Thee*, 13.

of methods for re-evaluation and reconsideration of the need for constraints once a pandemic seems to be under way. For example, the U.S. Department of Health and Human Services pandemic plan treats issues such as "international activities, domestic surveillance, public health interventions, the Federal medical response, vaccines, antiviral drugs, and communications."[39] Notably absent from this list is an explicit mechanism for ongoing, real-time reassessment of judgments about the urgency of the threat and the need for response. In practice, public comment is often divisive and sometimes seriously politically polarized, but it is nevertheless morally important that such voices be heard. As our PVV view shows, such voices—the voices of those who are both victims and vectors—might in several senses be the views of every single person.

Constraints: Basic Substantive Guarantees

In addition to procedural protections, a number of substantive guarantees for those subject to infection-preventing constraints are also of importance. These substantive guarantees include protection of personal security, provision of basic survival and health needs, availability of means of communication, attention to whether burdens are distributed equitably, and compensation for identifiable economic losses when compensation would generally be available in similar non-pandemic contexts.

These guarantees involve positive provisions; hence they may be viewed not just as negative rights but also as entitling people to the provision of a good. Positive rights—rights to goods or things—and any concomitant duties to render aid are notorious sources of contention in liberal theory.[40] In what we say below and in our chapter on compensation, positive claims that have been defended in other contexts, such as discussions of the right to a decent minimum of health care, are surely relevant, but we do not attempt to defend them here. Our point is simply that to the extent to which such rights are justified outside of the infectious disease context, they remain claims people have as infectious-disease victims and vectors.

We also recognize that there may be enormous difficulties in meeting these claims in pandemic circumstances, as economies collapse and the means to provide what is morally required are simply unavailable.[41] Of course, localized,

39. U.S. Department of Health and Human Services, "HHS Pandemic Influenza Implementation Plan," http://www.hhs.gov/pandemicflu/implementationplan/intro.htm#bookmark_6 (accessed February 2007).
40. Patricia Smith, *Liberalism and Affirmative Obligation* (New York: Oxford University Press, 1998).
41. For models of the economic costs of influenza epidemics, see Martin I. Meltzer, Nancy J. Cox, and Keiji Fukuda, "The Economic Impact of Pandemic Influenza in the United States: Priorities for Intervention," *Emerging Infectious Diseases* 5, no. 5 (September-October 1999): 659–671.

rapidly controlled episodes—like SARS, for instance—may be small enough in scale so that a society can act to provide those members of its population whom it constrains protections for their physical safety, support for their basic needs, access to communication, and compensation for their actual financial losses, including the costs of quarantine, isolation, lost work time, and other economic losses, without severe strain. Indeed, in general, the society that acts prudently and rapidly to contain a new outbreak before it becomes widespread will in general be much more able to make good on the substantive guarantees it owes as a matter of ethics when it imposes constraints. Yet limited societal resources nonetheless may make satisfying even the most basic of substantive guarantees difficult or impossible. Understanding, then, that background scarcity issues, especially in crises or in already compromised, very poor societies, may affect the actual capacity to satisfy substantive guarantees, we explore their moral importance below.

S-1. *Personal Security.* People identified by others as carriers of disease, and hence as threats to themselves, are often treated with hostility. In all ages, people have been pelted with stones, driven from villages, set on fire, abused by their caregivers, rejected by their partners, or killed in a variety of ways. An anthropologist working in primitive areas of Papua New Guinea reports stories, although unconfirmed, that in some groups people with AIDS or suspected of having AIDS are summarily shot and thrown into the river.[42] In some African areas today, abuse or abandonment by their husbands of women who are diagnosed as HIV-positive is widespread.[43]

A common social response by people who feel threatened toward people they view as threats is to try to destroy the threat by driving them away, harming, or killing them. These may be understandable and even justifiable responses to aggressors of various sorts. But to regard people who have communicable infectious diseases in this way is to regard them as vectors only, and to overlook the fact that they are already victims as well. Infectious vectors are not only aggressors—if they even can be called that—but also people themselves under threat.

Thus a justifiable moral response to infectious disease must include a basic commitment to protecting the personal security of individuals with infectious disease, even if that disease is communicable to others.[44] This may involve the provision of guards, police, fencing, and so on, where the purpose is protection

---

42. Polly Wiessner, personal communication to M. Battin, 2006.
43. B.O. Ojikutu and V.E. Stone, "Women, Inequality, and the Burden of HIV," *New England Journal of Medicine* 352, no. 7 (February 17, 2005): 649–652.
44. Madison Powers and Ruth Faden, *Social Justice: The Moral Foundations of Public Health and Health Policy* (New York: Oxford University Press, 2006).

of the victims, not wholesale segregation. Security protections need not increase the risks of disease transfer if they simply separate the uninfected from feared vectors by isolating likely vectors, though of course security "protections" are sometimes misused. Indeed, security protections for vectors may themselves reduce risks of transmission, if attacks would ironically put people in harm's way. This underscores the importance of distinguishing isolation from quarantine, as well as the need to protect those who are isolated, because they are victims too, not just to protect future victims they might, as vectors, infect.

S-2. Basic Survival and Health Needs, Including Prevention and Treatment. To be imposed in an ethically defensible way, constraints must also attend to the basic survival and health needs of those being constrained. In infectious disease control, it is people who are ill or are at risk of becoming ill who are the ones being constrained. Constraints, to put the point succinctly, may turn vectors into victims, for example, when people with a communicable disease are placed in involuntary quarantine or isolation. This is particularly true if the conditions of quarantine or isolation are primitive, as they were in the Hawaiian leper colony on Molokai: inadequate shelter, unsanitary conditions, little food, no warmth, no care for either the infectious disease or other health- or life-threatening conditions from which the person may be suffering.[45] Even more benign conditions under which constraints are imposed will sometimes exacerbate the harms caused by disease; for example, when being held means delays in receiving usual health care.

Where possible, the imposition of constraints, like involuntary isolation and quarantine, must be accompanied by attempts to secure for the individual being constrained (or at the very least, in crisis situations where the government or other constraining party cannot do so, not to block provision of these by other parties):

1. basic survival needs: water, food, clothing, shelter;
2. prevention and treatment for the infectious disease for which constraints were implemented;
3. relief or amelioration of suffering associated with the infectious disease;
4. treatment for other medical conditions which are exacerbated by the quarantine or other constraint process.

This list is only the beginning of a substantive list of basic health needs. These demands are already recognized as basic expectations in medical care: they are the way we should treat victims in any health-care context. But they

45. Tayman, *True Story of the Exiles of Molokai.*

have sometimes been overlooked, especially in the historical past, in attempts to control infectious disease, especially where the contagious person was seen primarily as a vector and not also as a victim. Yet a vector is also a person whose victimhood may be exacerbated by measures of disease control—and who must be treated with respect as victim, too.

To be sure, satisfying the requirements for basic survival and health needs on this list is not easy. It is made more complex by the need to prevent disease transmission, which in the case of some highly infectious or poorly understood emerging diseases (like Ebola or SARS) may be compromised by attending to even the most basic health-care needs of vectors—taking vital signs, feeding, providing nursing or comfort care—but these vectors are victims too. Even relief of suffering may risk disease transmission, if health-care workers themselves become agents of transmission.[46] Nonetheless, meeting the needs of victims is already recognized as a basic expectation of justice in medical care.[47] The risk is that meeting these needs may be overlooked in attempts to control infectious disease, presumably because the contagious person is seen primarily as a vector and not also as a victim. Curiously, a societal obligation to provide basic health and survival needs to persons involuntarily detained is recognized in criminal contexts, where individuals are also viewed as a threat to society. For example, in the United States, prisoners are entitled to food, clothing, shelter, and health care, but this has not always been fully recognized in disease-control contexts especially where severe constraints have been imposed.

The relief of suffering, the promotion of recovery or cure, and like measures are all basic to treating a person as a victim rather than simply a vector of disease—these are basic commitments of medicine, and obligations of providers to their patients. From the victim perspective, these concerns cannot be ignored, although they have often been forgotten in the most problematic cases of the past. Sometimes these abuses are cases of not meeting basic health needs by not providing health care that is available, like the failure to provide inmates in Russian prisons with effective treatment for tuberculosis. Sometimes it is a failure to provide general health care, as in the banishment of lepers in Hawaii to an area virtually without services. And sometimes it is failure to provide or permit the acquisition of even the most basic necessities for maintaining health, as in the blockade of Chinatown to prevent the spread of

---

46. This has been reported for both SARS and Ebola. See, e.g., Monali Varia et al., "Investigation of a Nosocomial Outbreak of Severe Acute Respiratory Syndrome (SARS) in Toronto, Canada," *Canadian Medical Association Journal* 169, no. 4 (August 19, 2003): 285–292; Margaretha Isaacson et al., "Clinical Aspects of Ebola Virus Disease at the Ngaliema Hospital, Kinshasa, Zaire, 1976," http://www.itg.be/ebola/ebola-12.htm (accessed February 4, 2008).
47. E.g., Powers and Faden, *Social Justice*; Norman Daniels, *Just Health Care* (Cambridge: Cambridge University Press, 1985).

plague that also left people without food, until Levi Strauss intervened. Treatment of people with infectious disease is less likely to be as harsh today, at least in many parts of the world, but it is important to remember how the basic subsistence needs have gone unmet and basic principles of medical care have gone unrecognized in some infectious-disease contexts.

There will be difficult cases in implementing these requirements. Some hard cases are those in which, as we have seen, the society is so poor, or so disastrously affected by a disease outbreak, that it can provide little in the way of tangible support for the people on whom it imposes constraints. Another kind of hard case in honoring the substantive societal obligation to provide support for basic survival and health needs for those constrained arises in what might be called cases of grave illness. In some diseases, palliative care is most likely all that can be offered, though providing even palliative care is a substantive obligation itself. With diseases like Ebola or SARS—where the likelihood of survival is difficult to predict and it is also difficult to know whether treatment will make any difference. The question is still more difficult in diseases in which contact with the victim is highly risky for others. At the end of the day, from a situation of not knowing their status as victims or vectors, people would wish both that comfort care in dying be provided but also that it be accomplished to the extent possible without creating new victims of almost certainly fatal illness. However, this is not an easy choice; there will remain the recognition that victims have had important moral interests overridden, despite the justifiability of the choice made.

S-3. Communication. One of the most troubling aspects of some constraints designed to control infectious disease such as isolation or home quarantine is that they quite literally separate people from one another, sometimes permanently. A patient with Ebola who is isolated not only suffers from illness but also almost surely dies—and, depending on what is done for isolation, may die alone. As a practical matter, methods to foster communication when such constraints are imposed are likely to improve compliance. With mobile phones or photographs transmitted over the Internet, people are at least be able to keep in touch with each other, to ask each other what they think about the way they are treated, to express love and concern, and to console one another. These are modes of communication that, in today's world, are relatively inexpensive, and that in any case do not risk infection transfer.

From our theoretical perspective, there is much further reason to insist on the importance of maintaining and enhancing such modes of communication. They are critical to transparency: communication is needed to explain the reasons for constraints. They are critical to reconsideration: without communication, people may be left unable to question the need for their confinement. Most critical of all, communication reflects respect for the humanity of the victim: his or her need for continued contact despite the risks that he or she as vector might pose. Dying is awful, but dying alone may be even worse.

P-4. Equitable Allocation of Burdens. A fourth substantive guarantee is consideration of whether constraints are distributed equitably.[48] Constraints that affect some people but not others are inequitable to at least that extent. Attention to the need to justify constraints will help to ensure that inequities do not exceed what is necessary. But an additional concern is that the burdens of constraints may fall more heavily on already disadvantaged groups. If, for example, a central city health-care facility is taken over to treat pandemic victims, that closure may bear more heavily on local residents who have depended on the facility than a closure elsewhere might harm people who are more mobile. Reservoirs of infection may be concentrated in impoverished areas, necessitating constraints that are not required elsewhere. Infection control measures such as destruction of domestic animals or quarantine may bear more heavily on those who are already worse off.[49]

If reservoirs of infection are concentrated in already impoverished locations, the burdens of disease prevention may fall more heavily in the first instance on the poor. This may be inevitable, but it should also be the subject of great concern. From their perspective as victims, each must recognize that some are bearing burdens that protect everyone—and that they may be people who are least able to afford the burdens. Although vectors recognize that constraints must be necessary to avoid more extensive victimization, the PVV perspective also demands respect for each individual victim and the sacrifices they make. For anyone, after all, might be a victim too.[50] This victim perspective requires respect for the individuality of victims and thus cares not to exacerbate already existing inequalities. Concerns about equitable burdens will also figure heavily in our following discussion of what compensation may be required for constraints.

S-5. Compensation for Loss. Some of the likely constraints employed in infection control will result in economic damages that would be compensable in other contexts: closure of facilities, slaughter of livestock, or condemnation of property.

---

48. This concern is emphasized in the pandemic planning report from the Toronto Joint Centre for Bioethics, *Stand on Guard for Thee*, 15–16.

49. For a discussion of the burdens imposed on impoverished people by the destruction of domestic animals, particularly poultry, see Ruth R. Faden, Patrick S. Duggan, and Ruth Karron, "Who Pays to Stop a Pandemic," *New York Times*, sec. A (February 9, 2007).

50. An analogous point with respect to justice is made in the disability literature: we all have been (as infants and children) and all quite likely may become once again, dependent on the care of others. See, e.g., Eva Feder Kittay, *Love's Labor: Essays on Women, Equality, and Dependency* (New York: Routledge, 1999).

When property is condemned for public use in the United States, for example, compensation is required as a constitutional matter.[51] This is so whether the condemnation requires destruction of the property or public assumption of ownership. Respect for those who are constrained requires that we at least consider analogies to economic compensation that would be available for other condemnations of property. Otherwise, vectors who are constrained to protect everyone will ironically do worse than those who bear the costs of public benefits in other situations.

As we explore here and in the next chapters, which focus on issues of compensation and deprioritization, it may be impossible to make up all losses to those who are justifiably constrained. Limited social resources, as we said, may make even morally required responses difficult. For example, the government of Uganda was reportedly delayed in compensating the families of the 16 health-care workers who died in the Ebola epidemic in 2000.[52] Where a pandemic is of much larger scale, financial compensation even for actual losses may not be possible. Such a situation might be the case were, for example, pandemic avian flu on the scale of the 1918 flu to break out in the twenty-first century, affecting a quarter of the global population at the very high fatality rates reported so far for avian influenza.

Nevertheless, whether a society is or is not able to satisfy its obligation to provide certain substantive guarantees to those it constrains—protection for physical security, adequate basic necessities like food, shelter, and health care for those who are placed in isolation or quarantine, access to communication, and compensation for loss—respect for each person as victim and vector requires that that society at least be open to the possibility of sharing costs socially rather than leaving them on the individual victims or vectors who incur them.

Conclusion: The Limits on Constraints

Because outbreaks of infectious disease are so often met with fear and panic, insistence on appropriate justification for constraints is an especially important matter. In this chapter, we have used our PVV view to identify a set of limits on constraints imposed in the effort to control the spread of infectious disease, a set of requirements that to some degree overlaps with others that have been proposed by other writers and working groups, but that is grounded in our PVV perspective. The procedural list includes good justification, the least restrictive alternative, transparency, and reconsideration. The substantive

---

51. U.S. Constitution, Amendment 5 (federal government), Amendment 14 (state governments).
52. Charles Wendo, "Caring for the Survivors of Uganda's Ebola Epidemic One Year On," *Lancet* 358 (2001): 1350.

list includes, to the extent possible, personal security, basic survival and health needs, communication, equitable distribution of burdens, and compensation for certain economic and other losses.

In the next chapter, we turn to the application of our principles to specific issues in pandemic planning. These principles, informed by our PVV perspective, help us to identify several critical aspects in which contemporary pandemic planning, particularly as it is practiced in the United States, falls short.

17

PANDEMIC PLANNING: WHAT IS ETHICALLY JUSTIFIED?

In the previous chapter, we defended a set of guarantees that must be met for constraints to be justified. They included both procedural and substantive guarantees:

Procedural guarantees:
P-1 Important interest, supported by evidence
P-2 Least restrictive alternative
P-3 Transparency and disclosure
P-4 Reconsideration
Substantive guarantees:
S-1 Personal Security
S-2 Basic survival and health needs, including prevention and treatment
S-3 Communication
S-4 Equitable allocation of burdens
S-5 Compensation for loss

In this chapter, we consider several important features of today's pandemic planning process with respect to these guarantees. Our focus here is the ethical justification of constraints such as surveillance and travel restrictions, school and workplace closures, and home quarantine and isolation. Our account is based on a snapshot of international, national, and state plans available on the Internet in early 2008. An important caveat is that the science of pandemics and their prevention is rapidly evolving, as antivirals, prepandemic vaccines, and new methods of vaccine manufacture appear on the scene. Pandemic plans, too, are moving targets.[1] Thus, rather than trying to present

---

1. Draft plans are posted on the pandemic flu web site of the U.S. government, http://www.pandemicflu.gov/plan/states/stateplans.html (accessed July 1, 2008). As an example of the rapidity with which the science is developing, in the summer of 2008, a report was published of a new technique for cell-culture manufacture of a vaccine effective against a range of H5N1 strains, Hartmut J. Ehrlich et al., "A Clinical Trial of a Whole-Virus H5N1 Vaccine Manufactured from Cell Culture," *New England Journal of Medicine* 358 (2008): 2573–2584. The technique needs less lead time and is not dependent on egg culture—but does require enhanced biosafety protection in manufacture. Additionally, a prepandemic vaccine manufactured by GlaxoSmithKline has been

quantitative data about plans incorporating specific types of provisions—a number that would be continuously changing—we employ examples of ethically desirable as well as problematic features in pandemic planning.[2] Our goal is to contribute to improvement overall in the planning process.

The question in this chapter is whether the constraints proposed in the current pandemic plans are ethically justified. In the next chapter, we apply our PVV view to analyze the ethical justification of compensation for harms that result from these constraints. Chapter 19 focuses on distributive justice questions raised by pandemic planning—the justice of allocations set out in plans, the justice of the planning process itself, and the more general questions of distributive justice and health security raised by our PVV view. We begin this chapter with a basic account of the features of pandemic influenza that are crucial to understanding the ethical issues it raises.

Influenza: "The Last Great Uncontrolled Plague"

"Epidemic influenza remains the last great uncontrolled plague of mankind," wrote F. M. Davenport,[3] and it is the contagious infectious disease that is also the focus of the most sustained contemporary disaster planning. The 1918 flu pandemic was one of the most devastating episodes of infectious disease in human history. But flu of such pandemic proportions has not been the experience of most people alive today, and "flu" is often taken lightly as a common infection sustained from time to time by nearly everybody, hardly a cause for concern. Thus it is important to distinguish between endemic or "seasonal" influenza and the pandemic influenza that has become the subject of global fear.

Endemic or "Seasonal" Influenza

Infection with influenza viruses is universal; most can recognize the typical acute illness characterized by fever, headache, muscle aches, malaise, and cough that is characteristic of endemic or "seasonal" infection with human strains of influenza viruses. Unlike most common cold viruses, influenza viruses

approved by the European Commission for distribution in the European Union. As an example of a policy shift, Roche, the manufacturer of the anti-viral Tamiflu, is now allowing businesses to pay an annual fee to stockpile Tamiflu reserves sufficient to protect their entire work force and hopefully available within 48 hours, http://www.pandemictoolkit.com/tamiflu-supplyordering/stock-piling-dilemma.aspx (accessed July 1, 2008).
2. A very useful quantitative study of the appearance—and absence—of overt recognition of ethical choices in state pandemic plans is James C. Thomas, Nabarun Dasgupta, and Amanda Martinot, "Ethics in a Pandemic: A Survey of the State Pandemic Influenza Plans," *American Journal of Public Health* 97 (April 2007): S26–S31.
3. F.M. Davenport, "Influenza Viruses," in *Viral Infections of Humans*, ed. A.S. Evans (New York: Plenum Publishing, 1977), 273–296.

tend primarily to infect the lower respiratory tract; hence, the typical cough and the greater systemic symptoms of fever and aches and pains that accompany influenza are often serious enough to keep healthy adults from working for a day or two. Although most otherwise healthy adults and children experience only temporary discomfort from a bout with influenza, each year 10–20% of children and 5% of adults have an influenza-related illness,[4] and the resulting visits to physician offices and emergency rooms and lost work time together can cost several billion U.S. dollars each year.[5] The very young, the very old, and patients with underlying heart and lung disease are most likely to suffer more serious respiratory illnesses, such as pneumonia, often requiring hospitalization and sometimes proving fatal. In fact, one of the most reliable indicators that seasonal influenza is active in a community is a noticeable increase in the rate of pneumonia-associated deaths.[6]

Unlike most other viruses that infect humans, influenza viruses possess a remarkable ability to undergo frequent change and thus to avoid the usual long-standing immunity that follows infections with more stable viruses such as measles or chickenpox. The process of gradual change in the two surface antigens of the virus is called antigenic drift. In most years when endemic or seasonal influenza occurs, the presence of protective antibodies in the majority of the population is sufficiently high or at least cross-reactive with the new virus to protect most individuals. Therefore, large outbreaks or epidemics of influenza are rare, despite the usual antigenic drift of influenza viruses.

Pandemic Influenza

Influenza viruses also have the ability occasionally to experience dramatic changes in their genetics and antigenicity due to reassortment of their fragmented genome—that is, to undergo antigenic shift. While most viruses have a single particle of genome, influenza viruses have a genome divided into eight separate pieces. When two quite different strains of influenza virus infect a single cell, the intracellular mixture of pieces of genome can be reassorted; new offspring viruses may then appear that possess a new combination of genes from each of the original infecting viruses. For example, influenza viruses that

---

4. K.G. Nicholson and J.M. Wood, "Influenza," *Lancet* 362 (2003): 1733–1745.
5. S.C. Schoenbaum, "Economic Impact of Influenza," *American Journal of Medicine* 82, supp. 6A (1987): 26.
6. In the United States during the 2006–2007 flu season, mortality from influenza and pneumonia peaked at 7.7%; in the three preceding years, peaks ranged from 7.8% to 10.4% of all deaths. Centers for Disease Control and Prevention, "2006–07 Influenza Season Summary," http://www.cdc.gov/flu/weekly/weeklyarchives2006-2007/06-07summary.htm (accessed February 6, 2008). See R.C. Baron, et al, "Assessing Trends in Mortality in 121 US Cities, 1970–79, From All Causes and From Pneumonia and Influenza," *Public Health Report* 103 (1988): 120.

usually infect only birds may occasionally infect domestic animals such as pigs or horses. If these domestic animals happen to also be infected with a human strain of influenza, the resulting offspring of this mixed infection may produce a quite new virus that contains some of the genes that cause illness in birds, together with the new ability to infect humans. This scenario has been the cause of the fear that the current widespread epizoonosis of avian influenza H5N1 may acquire the genes necessary for human-to-human infectivity.

When antigenic shift introduces new influenza viruses to a human population that lacks prior experience with the new virus, the environment is laid for a very widespread epidemic—that is, pandemic—of influenza. Such was probably the case when a new strain of influenza with many of the characteristics of avian influenza appeared in 1918 and caused a worldwide epidemic that killed an estimated 50–100 million people across the globe—more people in a year than the plague of the Middle Ages killed in a century and more people in 24 weeks than AIDS has killed in 24 years, according to John Barry.[7] Pandemics of influenza probably due to antigenic shift also occurred in 1957 with influenza A Japan (H2N2) and again in 1968 with influenza A Hong Kong (H3N2).

New strains of influenza are typically named after the site of origin of the virus; recent pandemic viruses all appear to have originated in China or elsewhere in Asia where conditions of crowding and close living with domestic fowl and pigs provide the ideal environment for gene exchange and reassortment among human, domestic fowl, and animal strains of influenza. The more recent pandemics were not as severe as the 1918 pandemic because the viruses were not as pathogenic for humans, and there was probably some cross-protective antibody present in the community. The current strain of avian influenza A, H5N1, is particularly worrisome because it has high pathogenicity for birds as well as for the few humans it has infected—more than 60% mortality reported among confirmed human cases reported to the WHO by the end of January 2008, usually due to pneumonia and respiratory failure.[8] These observations raise the concern that H5N1 has the potential to cause a 1918-like pandemic, should it acquire the ability for efficient human-to-human transmission.

The Pandemic Potential of Avian Influenza

In 1997, an outbreak of the new H5N1 strain of avian influenza virus occurred in the live poultry markets in Hong Kong. Because previous outbreaks of avian influenza in domestic poultry markets have occasionally been associated

---

7. J.M. Barry, *The Great Influenza* (London: Penguin Books, 2004), 5.

8. World Health Organization, "Cumulative Number of Confirmed Human Cases of Avian Influenza A/(H5N1) Reported to WHO" (February 5, 2008), http://www.who.int/csr/disease/avian_influenza/country/cases_table_2008_02_05/en/index.html (accessed February 6, 2008).

with transmission to humans, local public health officials started surveillance for human cases. It became apparent that the H5N1 virus had infected 18 people, 6 of them fatally.[9] Hong Kong officials responded rapidly by culling all poultry in Hong Kong—more than a million domestic chickens, ducks, and geese—and the Hong Kong outbreak appeared to have been effectively controlled.

However, WHO influenza surveillance workers soon detected the H5N1 virus in apparently healthy wild ducks along the coast of China; and the infection slowly spread to other wild migratory ducks, geese, and swans in China. Six years after the initial Hong Kong outbreak, an explosion of outbreaks of the H5N1 virus appeared in poultry markets throughout Southeast Asia; and by 2005 this virus had spread, most likely by migratory waterfowl, to Europe, India, and Africa. The H5N1 virus was of particular concern to veterinary health officials because it was unusually pathogenic and fatal for domestic poultry. It could also cause non-fatal infections in wild birds, with spread via migrations. Vigorous efforts to control the virus included culling more than 250 million domestic poultry and widespread use of vaccines to protect remaining healthy flocks. By 2008, the H5N1 virus was known to be surviving extensively in wild waterfowl populations with regular spread to domestic poultry flocks in Asia, Africa, India, and Europe.[10]

The observation in 1997 that the H5N1 avian influenza virus could also spread to humans with a high mortality rate was prophetic. Beginning with the documented spread of the virus to domestic poultry throughout Asia and other continents in 2004, infections of humans have increasingly been seen, with a total of 359 documented human infections and 226 deaths in 15 countries as of the end of January 2008,[11] a high fatality rate of just over 60% among documented cases. While this very high human mortality rate may be skewed because identification of the virus in patients has most often occurred when patients were already seriously ill and hospitalized, and persons with asymptomatic infections or very mild illness were less likely to be tested, this rate remains extraordinarily high even for hospitalized patients. The high pathogenicity of the H5N1 virus for birds and for the few known infected humans was particularly disturbing to local, national, and international public health officials who saw the potential of this virus to cause a pandemic similar to the 1918 pandemic.

---

9. R.G. Webster and E.A. Govorkova, "H5N1 Influenza—Continuing Evolution and Spread," *New England Journal of Medicine* 355 (2006): 2174–2177.

10. Writing Committee of the Second World Health Organization Consultation on Clinical Aspects of Human Infection with Avian Influenza A (H5N1) Virus, "Update on Avian Influenza A (H5N1) Virus Infection in Humans," *New England Journal of Medicine* 358, no. 3 (January 17, 2008): 261–273.

11. World Health Organization, "Confirmed Human Cases of Avian Influenza A (H5N1)."

For the most serious pandemic of influenza in modern history, the 1918 influenza pandemic, recent genetic analyses of that virus indicate that it was also a virus of primary avian origin, avian influenza A (H1N1). Both the 1918 virus and the current H5N1 virus are unusually pathogenic for mammals and humans with high rates of pneumonia and ultimately fatal infection. The 1918 virus proved to be very contagious, spreading rapidly from human to human. Although the lack of reliable laboratory tests in 1918 made it difficult to assess the true mortality rate, it has been estimated that 8–10% of young adults then living died in that pandemic.[12] Although the present-day H5N1 strain is not currently very efficient in spreading from human to human—as of this writing, there have been only a few documented cases of human-to-human transmission, and then only with prolonged and very close contact[13]—the ability of influenza viruses for antigenic shift leads to concern that efficient human-to-human transmission may ultimately be acquired by the H5N1 virus.

A worldwide pandemic of often fatal influenza requires not only a strain of the virus that is highly infectious and pathogenic for humans, but also a large portion of the population without any previous experience with similar viruses and thus any form of protective antibody. The H5N1 virus appears to have both of these characteristics. If H5N1 also spreads rapidly from human to human, as did the 1918 H1N1 virus, the result could be devastating. These similarities between the H5N1 virus and environment and the 1918 influenza pandemic have led public health officials to project that a similar pandemic in a world now harboring three times as many people could result in more than 300 million deaths worldwide, with associated political unrest and socio-economic devastation.[14] With the recent memory of an outbreak of another highly infectious and fatal virus disease, SARS, there has been a remarkable effort by local, state, federal, and international public health experts to begin planning for a possible avian influenza pandemic.[15]

Pandemic Planning: The Use of Models

Infections with pandemic potential may involve novel agents or occur in a naive population or in new circumstances. Planning thus must be based in part on predictive assumptions about mode and efficiency of spread, expected rates of mortality and morbidity, and the likely efficacy of preventive measures such

---

12. Barry, *The Great Influenza*, 4.
13. K. Ungchusak et al., "Probable Person-to-Person Transmission of Avian Influenza A (H5N1)," *New England Journal of Medicine* 352(2005): 333–340.
14. R.J. Whitley, and A.S. Monto, "Seasonal and Pandemic Influenza Preparedness: A Global Threat," *Journal of Infectious Diseases* 194, supp. 2 (2006): S65–S69.
15. Lawrence O. Gostin, "Public Health Strategies for Pandemic Influenza," *Journal of the American Medical Association* 295 (2006): 1700–1704.

as social distancing, among other assumptions—and may be limited by the availability of data. Avian flu pandemic planning is based on a variety of models that have been developed in order to test potential strategies for preparing in advance for such a catastrophe.[16] The most optimistic scenarios anticipate low transmission rates, modest infection spread, relatively low fatality rates, and the rapid development of a vaccine.

Because the more optimistic scenarios do not present ethical tradeoffs explicitly—on optimistic assumptions, for example, vaccine rationing would not be required—it may be tempting to think that they are not as ethically troubling as the models that vary the assumptions in ways that suggest the need for widespread rationing. Nonetheless, the more optimistic scenarios do raise ethical issues, especially those posed by decisions that risk failing to anticipate the worst. Such optimistic models—were they the only models used in planning—fail to attend to what has been called the "precautionary principle" in environmental planning and other policy choices: the general idea that steps should be taken to avoid apparent threats of serious human harm, although the probabilities of this harm are uncertain or unpredictable.[17] If such steps are not taken, and the harm ensues, some people will be damaged but without social consideration of the ethical issues this raises. Because pandemic plans that model worse case (although perhaps not the worst case) scenarios pose the choices at stake explicitly, rather than as it were letting the chips fall where they may, we focus our discussion on them. But we caution that more optimistic planning assumptions—while hopefully all that will be required—may generate results that are quite similar to the explicit choices envisioned for the more pessimistic scenarios, if the optimism proves to have been ill-founded.

Plans that prepare for a range of "worst case" scenarios pose the ethical challenges of pandemic planning explicitly by modeling a rapidly spreading, global epidemic on the scale of the 1918–1919 flu, but with the even higher mortality rates that characterize current avian influenza in humans.[18] The best-case scenario postulated for U.S. pandemic planning for person-to-person avian flu assumes a minimum 25% increase in the need for inpatient care, ICU beds, and ventilator support.[19] Under the worst-case scenario assumptions, it

---

16. The U.S. federal government has produced software for states to use in modeling pandemics of varying degrees of severity. See Centers for Disease Control and Prevention, "FluAid 2.0," http://www2.cdc.gov/od/fluaid/default.htm (accessed February 6, 2008).

17. For a discussion of the precautionary principle, see Stephen Gardiner, "A Core Precautionary Principle," *Journal of Political Philosophy* 14, no. 1 (2006): 33–60. Gardiner argues that the "precautionary principle" has been interpreted in many different ways, and proposes a version of the principle based on the Rawlsian idea that those actions are just, which maximize the minimum for those affected by the choice at stake.

18. U.S. Department of Health and Human Services, *HHS Pandemic Influenza Plan* (November 2005), http://www.hhs.gov/pandemicflu/plan/pdf/HHSPandemicInfluenzaPlan.pdf (accessed February 6, 2008), 16.

19. Ibid., 16.

is estimated that 30% of the population would become ill and half of these people would seek outpatient care. Depending on the severity of the illness, models predict that from 865,000 to 9.9 million people would need hospital care, from 128,750 to 1.49 million would need ICU care, from 64,750 to 742,500 would require ventilator support, and from 209,000 to 1.9 million would die.[20] Even these assumptions may be too optimistic, depending on the efficiency of spread and the lethality of a pandemic avian influenza; certainly, the mortality figures are too optimistic for the over-60% mortality rate observed to date in patients hospitalized with H5N1 influenza. These assumptions might also be utterly inaccurate for other forms of widespread disease, such as an outbreak of smallpox or an entirely new, devastating pathogen developed in the laboratory and spread by bioterrorism.

Planning Processes and Procedural Guarantees

Because the anticipated needs for preventives, for health care, and for other support in an infectious-disease outbreak are greater than the anticipated supply, at least on the models we are discussing, some process must be put into place for anticipating allocation decisions. The World Health Organization (WHO) plan recommends both international and national measures; it was developed after international consultation and is available on the Internet.[21] European Community guidance is publicly available,[22] as are the plans of European Economic Community nations. Over thirty national plans are on the WHO website;[23] with notable absences of plans from Cambodia, China, Laos, Myanmar, and Vietnam—all nations with early reports of cases of H5N1 in poultry as well as human cases of H5N1.[24] Of Southeast Asian nations, only Singapore, the Republic of Korea, Thailand, and Indonesia have published plans on the WHO website; in addition, only India, Hong Kong, Sri Lanka, and Vietnam

20. Ibid., S3–3.

21. World Health Organization, *WHO Global Influenza Preparedness Plan* (Geneva: World Health Organization, 2005), http://www.who.int/csr/resources/publications/influenza/GIP_2005_5Eweb. pdf (accessed February 7, 2008).

22. Commission of the European Communities, *Communication from the Commission to the Council, the European Parliament, the European Economic and Social Committee and the Committee of the Regions on Pandemic Influenza Preparedness and Response Planning in the European Community*, COM(2005) 607 final, Brussels (November 28, 2005), http://eur-lex.europa.eu/LexUriServ/ site/en/com/2005/com2005_0607en01.pdf (accessed February 7, 2008).

23. World Health Organization, "National Influenza Pandemic Plans," http://www.who.int/csr/ disease/influenza/nationalpandemic/en/index.html (accessed July 1, 2008). A few more, including plans from Hong Kong, India, Sri Lanka, and Vietnam are available on the website of the Canadian organization, PandemicWatch. Mount Sinai Hospital, "PandemicWatch.ca," http://microbi-ology.mtsinai.on.ca/avian/all-pandemic-plans.asp (accessed July 1, 2008).

24. World Health Organization, *H5N1 Influenza: Timeline of Major Events* (January 14, 2008), http://www.who.int/csr/disease/avian_influenza/Timeline_08%2001%2014.pdf (accessed February, 7, 2008).

have plans available on the Canadian site, PandemicWatch. Britain's plan, also available on the Internet, was undergoing widespread public comment in the winter of 2007–2008.[25] In the United States, a template for pandemic planning was developed under the auspices of the Department of Health and Human Services, with state plans guided by that template.[26] State planning processes have attempted to be inclusive, but with varying degrees of actual public input. All state plans are available on the Internet,[27] allowing for widespread public access and comment on the ongoing planning process.

One of the difficulties of the planning process is the potential for "silo"ing: albeit with international and national coordination, planning takes place jurisdiction by jurisdiction. The WHO and other international organizations such as the European Community have worked to coordinate plans, and federal systems such as the United States have developed templates for all subsidiary units to employ. Nonetheless, there are risks of less than ideal coordination among areas where integrated planning might be especially helpful in preventing disease spread; often, there is no clearly-defined mechanism to encourage common planning by unrelated jurisdictions sharing interrelated travel patterns. This is a particular concern for planning in some federalist systems. For example, in the United States, the plans of Missouri and Illinois do not even mention each other—although St. Louis, Missouri, and East St. Louis, Illinois, function as a conurbation and might benefit from shared planning about prevention and treatment.[28] The Michigan plan treats any relation with Canada as a border control activity, despite the interconnections between Detroit and Windsor, Ontario and although Indiana reports cooperation among the Canadian province of Ontario and states along the border.[29] On the other hand, the U.S. CDC has

25. U.K. Department of Health, *Pandemic Flu: A National Framework for Responding to an Influenza Pandemic* (November 2007), http://www.dh.gov.uk/en/Publicationsandstatistics/Publications/PublicationsPolicyAndGuidance/DH_080734 (accessed February 7, 2008).

26. U.S. Department of Health, *HHS Pandemic Influenza Plan.*

27. U.S. Department of Health and Human Services, "PandemicFlu.gov: State Pandemic Plans," http://www.pandemicflu.gov/plan/states/stateplans.html (accessed February 7, 2008).

28. State of Illinois, *Illinois Pandemic Influenza Preparedness and Response Plan*, version 2.05 (October 10, 2006), http://www.idph.state.il.us/pandemic_flu/Illinois%20Pandemic%20Flu%20Plan%20101006%20Final.pdf (accessed July 1, 2008); Missouri Department of Health and Senior Services, *Pandemic Influenza Plan*, working document version 2.0, February 9, 2006, http://www.dhss.mo.gov/PandemicInfluenza/PandemicPlan.pdf (accessed July 1, 2008). The Illinois plan does mention the need to "coordinate" with neighboring jurisdictions during Pandemic Phase 6, but without any indication about what this might mean or how it might be accomplished. By contrast, at least some environmental planning in the United States has long been regional in nature—the Lake Tahoe Regional Authority, for example, was established in 1969 and brings together California and Nevada—although many would contend that coordination of environmental planning in the United States has also been far less than ideal.

29. Michigan Department of Community Health, *Pandemic Influenza Plan*, version 3.1 (May 2007), http://www.michigan.gov/documents/mdch/MDCH_Pandemic_Influenza_v_3.1_final_draft_060107_2_198392_7.pdf (accessed July 5, 2008), 43–46; Indiana State Department of Health, *Pandemic Influenza Plan* (revised October 2006), http://www.in.gov/isdh/files/PandemicInfluenzaPlan.pdf (accessed July 1, 2008), 9.

apparently coordinated a surveillance process for the area around Washington, DC, including the neighboring states of Maryland and Virginia, which contain the major airports of entry to the Washington area.[30] An additional problem is that affected areas of the world, although recognizing the need for transparency about plans, may have limited surveillance capacity and thus limited ability to gather and share information needed for health emergency containment.[31]

How well do pandemic plans measure up to our procedural requirements, P-1 to P-4? At the present time, it seems fair to say that, of the procedural guarantees, transparency (P-3) is the requirement best met with respect to the plans that are available. The initial wave of enthusiasm for pandemic planning in 2005 or 2006, however, has not been followed by a similar wave or plans with greater specificity than the original drafts.[32] The absence of published plans from many nations in Southeast Asia—the primary area of influenza origination— is another concern with respect to transparency.

Published plans are subject to public examination and discussion, although in the United States they typically have not been developed through a full administrative process of notice and comment rule making, much less legislation. As we have already mentioned, Britain sought widespread public comment for its plan in 2007–2008. Many state plans comment on the importance of public participation in plan development and communication in order to increase responsiveness, understanding, and compliance. The basic frameworks of all state plans are public knowledge—and this is a good thing—but it would be even better if plan details were in some cases less sketchy about hard moral choices to be addressed. For example, it is unlikely that people would be able to go online and ascertain which of their local facilities have been designated to treat them should they become ill—although they surely will be able to discover that it is anticipated that demand for treatment will outstrip supply.

As they are formulated, plans attempt to meet the standards of good justification and least restrictive alternative, our P-1 and P-2. Nonetheless, because plans are generated for a range of scenarios, they can attempt to put into place priorities and constraints that are tailored to each set of assumptions, but they cannot anticipate which set of assumptions best predicts what will actually occur. The risk is then that the plan that is actually put into place is a mismatch with what is actually occurring—too draconian, perhaps, for the actual

30. Virginia Department of Health, *Emergency Operations Plan Attachment Pandemic Influenza* (March 2006), http://www.vdh.virginia.gov/PandemicFlu/pdf/DRAFT_Virginia_Pandemic_Influenza_Plan.pdf (accessed July 7, 2008), supp. 9, 1.
31. See, e.g., Socialist Republic of Vietnam, *Vietnam Integrated National Operational Program for Avian and Human Influenza 2006–2010* (May 2006), http://microbiology.mtsinai.on.ca/avian/plans/Vietnam.pdf (accessed July 5 2008), 4, 23–24.
32. E.g., Missouri Department of Health and Senior Services, *Pandemic Influenza Plan*.

emergency, thus imposing unnecessary harms on people erroneously believed to be vectors; or too optimistic about the spread or lethality of the infection, thus failing to provide available protection to victims.

This possibility of a mismatch between the severity of the assumptions employed in the plan and actual events underscores the importance of P-4—the opportunity for reconsideration. Yet in circumstances of panic and the need for quick responses, reconsideration is likely to be difficult to achieve. It is therefore noteworthy if plans do not devote as much explicit attention as might be useful to the actual processes that will be used for ongoing reassessment about the measures that are necessary for control and treatment. The WHO method of addressing this problem is to divide pandemic strategies into stages, and to assign to the Director-General the responsibility of designating pandemic phases and to national governments the responsibility of determining national subdivisions of phases.[33] The WHO also continues to sponsor updates on what is known about the characteristics of H5N1 and the implications for pandemic modeling.[34]

In the United States, the Secretary of Health and Human Services will exercise the responsibility of designating pandemic stages at the federal level.[35] There is certainly need for such federal coordination, and there is also need for ongoing state-by-state, as well as regional, assessment linked to local circumstances, for example of the need for school or workplace closures. Recent federal guidance addresses the need for states to have explicit operating plans.[36] California has built a reconsideration mechanism into its plan, specifically assigning responsibilities for high-level policy decisions to the Directorate of the California Department of Health Services.[37] Indiana has proposed a Technical Advisory Group to the state health commissioner especially to propose policy revisions in the course of a pandemic.[38] North Carolina assigns responsibilities for pandemic management to a State Emergency Response Team.[39] Other state

---

33. World Health Organization, *WHO Global Influenza Preparedness Plan*, 9.

34. See, e.g., Writing Committee of the Second World Health Organization Consultation on Clinical Aspects of Human Infection with Avian Influenza A (H5N1) Virus, "Update on Avian Influenza."

35. U.S. Department of Health and Human Service, *HHS Pandemic Influenza Plan*.

36. U.S. Government, *Federal Guidance to Assist States in Improving State-Level Pandemic Influenza Operating Plans* (March 11, 2008), http://www.health.state.nm.us/flu/FEDERAL%20GUIDANCE%20TO%20ASSIST%20STATES.pdf (accessed July 1, 2008).

37. California Department of Health Services, *Pandemic Influenza Preparedness and Response Plan* (September 8, 2006), http://www.dhs.ca.gov/ps/dcdc/izgroup/pdf/pandemic.pdf (accessed July 7, 2008), 11.

38. Indiana State Department of Health. 2006. *Pandemic Influenza Plan* October. Available at http://www.in.gov/isdh/files/PandemicInfluenzaPlan.pdf (accessed July 5, 2008), 14–15.

39. North Carolina State Laboratory of Public Health, *N.C. Pandemic Influenza Plan* (updated January 2007), http://www.epi.state.nc.us/epi/gcdc/pandemic.html (accessed July 1, 2008), appendix A-1.

plans also assign responsibility for reassessing pandemic stages to designated officials—but without explicitly discussing the moral urgency of effective reconsideration mechanisms.[40]

Outside of the United States, the British plan is especially thoughtful about the need for reconsideration in light of whether actual data conform to predictions used in modeling.[41] Given the likely impact on both victims and vectors (who are, after all, the same people) of a mismatch between modeling and exigent pandemic circumstances, we think the British plan's strategy for reconsideration should be emulated elsewhere. Much is uncertain in pandemic planning, and much is at stake, so ongoing mechanisms for reassessment are essential.

Pandemic Constraints: Procedural and Substantive Ethical Guarantees

Three principal types of constraints have been widely proposed in pandemic plans: surveillance and travel restrictions, event closures and other forms of social distancing, and isolation and home quarantine. Because they are so common, they are our focus here, although surely other types of constraints are possible—such as mandatory wearing of masks in public places. In general, constraints are more likely to be effective early in a pandemic, when it is possible to stop spread before it has become extensive. Yet the irony is that this is just when it may be most difficult to tell if a pandemic is incipient and hence to assess the need for constraints with any certainty at all.

How Influenza Spreads

Some basic knowledge about how influenza spreads is helpful to assessing the likely efficacy of constraints as measures of control. Influenza viruses are spread by multiple routes, including small particle aerosols that reach deep into the lung, large particle aerosols that bring the virus to the upper respiratory airways, and fomites (hands and coughed-on surfaces). While the small particle aerosol route can affect others at some distance (such as others in an airplane), all of these routes are most efficient when there is close person-to-person contact.[42]

---

40. E.g., Florida Department of Health, *Pandemic Influenza Annex* (October 2006), http://www. doh.state.fl.us/rw_Bulletins/flpanfluv104final.pdf (accessed July 7, 2008), 15.

41. U.K. Department of Health, *Pandemic Flu: A National Framework*, 21.

42. An example of the effectiveness of small particle aerosols in spreading influenza is an outbreak on an airplane that sat on the runway for 4.5 hours, 3 hours of which lacked any ventilation of the aircraft. A single passenger with an acute febrile/cough illness (later proven by the laboratory to be infected with influenza), infected 91% of the crew and passengers over this short period

Larger particle aerosols produced by people with influenza when coughing or sneezing usually settle to the ground within a few meters, so that only individuals who are physically very close to the person (such as family members, playmates, and caregivers) are likely to become infected as the larger particles come in contact with the nasal mucosa or the conjunctiva. These particles also settle onto objects and surfaces in the immediate vicinity of the patient—fomites, as explained in Chapter 2—and people can become infected or transmit infection by touching the fomite and then touching their noses or eyes, or in the case of health-care workers, touching other patients. Gloving and frequent handwashing by hospital personnel are common methods used to reduce transmission by large particle aerosols and contaminated fomites.[43] The current spread of the avian H5N1 to humans has generally required very close physical contact such as might occur when physically handling infected birds. The rare cases of human-to-human transmission of H5N1 have also involved close physical contact between family members or medical caregivers and the patient.[44]

Methods of Control and Evidence of Efficacy

Methods for control of influenza are designed to inhibit all three possible means of spread: small particle aerosols, large particle aerosols, and fomites. Negative pressure rooms keep aerosolized particles from going outside the room in which the patient is isolated. Barriers such as surgical masks may prevent inhalation of aerosolized particles. Hand washing and gloving may prevent transmission by touch. So may sanitary measures designed to disinfect fomites. Isolation keeps patients sufficiently far away from others so that transmission of aerosolized particles from one to another cannot occur. To be successful, social distancing methods must keep people sufficiently separated so that aerosolized particles do not spread from infected persons to others and transfer does not occur from one person to another from fomites. Commentators agree that hygienic measures such as hand washing and good sanitation, and barriers such as surgical masks, are of proven efficacy in preventing disease spread.[45]

of time. M.R. Moser et al., "An Outbreak of Influenza Aboard a Commercial Airliner," *American Journal of Epidemiology* 110 (1979): 1–6.

43. C.B. Bridges, M.J. Kuehnert, and C.B. Hall, "Transmission of Influenza: Implications for Control in Health Care Settings," *Clinical Infectious Diseases* 37 (2003): 1094–1101.

44. Writing Committee of the World Health Organization Consultation on Human Influenza A/HS, "Avian Influenza A (H5N1) Infections in Humans," *New England Journal of Medicine* 353 (2005): 1374–1385.

45. E.g., Cochrane Collaboration, "Interventions for the Interruption or Reduction of the Spread of Respiratory Viruses (Review)" (2007), http://www.thecochranelibrary.com (accessed January 30, 2008); World Health Organization Writing Group, "Nonpharmaceutical Interventions for

In a recent policy review addressing pandemic influenza spread, the WHO Writing Group recommended multiple non-pharmaceutical interventions including hand washing, masks and other hygiene barrier measures. They also recommended isolation of patients, quarantine of contacts, and social distancing measures such as closures of schools and discouraging non-essential travel to affected areas.[46] The Writing Group concluded that social distancing may be particularly likely to be effective in rural areas, where there are fewer points of contact among large groups of people, as well as in settings such as college dormitories or military barracks where disease may spread rapidly in close quarters. In addition, it suggested that school closures are especially likely to be helpful in diminishing disease transmission, given the known role of children in passing on communicable diseases, although with the caveat that efficacy may be diminished in urban areas where children are likely to meet elsewhere. The Group noted in their introduction, however, that the evidence base for their recommendations is limited, consisting primarily of historical and contemporary observations rather than controlled studies.[47]

Recently, two historical analyses of the efficacy of public health interventions in U.S. cities during the 1918 influenza pandemic concluded that early implementation of multiple interventions was significantly associated with blunting the epidemic, reducing both peak mortality and mortality overall. However, their data did not allow separate analysis of interventions such as use of isolation and quarantine in comparison to closure of schools.[48] According to one of the studies, coordinated closures of schools and other public events were better than fragmented efforts. For example, Pittsburgh banned public gatherings but did not close schools until a later point in time, and did not fare at all well in reducing mortality.[49] Not surprising, this study also concluded that measures instituted earlier in a pandemic were more effective than ones instituted later, after disease had already become widespread.[50] Critics of the historical studies are concerned that they do not take account of the specific migration patterns occurring in 1918 as World War I was coming to an

Pandemic Influenza, National and Community Measures," *Emerging Infectious Diseases* 12, no. 1 (January 2006): 88–94.

46. World Health Organization Writing Group, "Nonpharmaceutical Interventions."

47. Ibid.

48. R.J. Hatchett, C.E. Mecher, and M. Lipsitch, "Public Health Interventions and Epidemic Intensity During the 1918 Influenza Pandemic," *Proceedings of the National Academy of Sciences of the United States* 104, no. 18 (May 1, 2007): 7582–7587; M.C.J. Bootsma and N.M. Ferguson, "The Effect of Public Health Measures on the 1918 Influenza Pandemic in U.S. Cities," *Proceedings of the National Academy of Sciences of the United States* 104, no. 18 (May 1, 2007): 7588–7593.

49. Markel et al., "Nonpharmaceutical Interventions Implemented by US Cities During the 1918–1919 Influenza Pandemic," *Journal of the American Medical Association* 298, no. 6 (2007): 644–654 (650).

50. Markel et al., "Nonpharmaceutical Interventions," 644.

end, and that the circumstances of 1918 may not be comparable to the more extensive social integration in today's world.[51]

Finally, in the only published critical review of non-pharmaceutical interventions for interruption or reduction of the spread of respiratory viruses, the Cochrane Collaboration concluded that there is a lack of proper evaluations of global and highly resource-intensive measures such as screening at entry ports or social distancing measures such as closing theatres and canceling public meetings. They did find studies that supported the use of hygiene barrier measures such as frequent hand washing and use of masks, gowns, and gloves, as well as several studies that supported the closure of schools and daycare centers because of the important role children play in the transmission of influenza.[52] It is noteworthy that the Cochrane Collaboration employs the rigorous standards of evidence-based medicine—standards that may or may not be appropriate to use in decision making about the possibility of a devastating event of uncertain probability.

A difficulty with the studies reviewed by the Cochrane Collaboration is that they tend to focus on the efficacy of interventions considered one-by-one. Recent modeling suggests that a combination of social distancing and targeted prophylaxis and treatment may be far more effective than any one of the strategies alone. The authors of this modeling study, however, note explicitly that a lack of data hampered development of the models, and recommend further research.[53]

Surveillance, Border Surveillance, and Travel Restrictions

Surveillance and travel restrictions are commonly suggested as methods of disease control. Surveillance attempts to identify occurrences of pathogens or actual disease; border surveillance attempts to identify persons who are carrying disease at political or geographical borders; and travel restrictions are applied to people who are ill, to people who are thought to have been exposed, or to closure of entire areas to movement in or out.

One way to assess these methods is whether any of them meet P-1 and P-2— that is, whether there is sufficient evidence that they support the clearly important interest in disease control and whether they are less restrictive than other, similarly effective alternatives. We should note at the outset that there are difficulties in comparing alternatives in this way. Even if evidence about strategies in particular situations is available, evidence about comparisons may

51. Jacobo Dib, Jr., "Letter: Nonpharmaceutical Interventions Implemented During the 1918–1919 Influenza Pandemic," *Journal of the American Medical Association* 298, no. 19 (2007): 2260.

52. T. Jefferson et al., "Interventions for the Interruption or Reduction of the Spread of Respiratory Viruses," *Cochrane Database of Systemic Reviews* 4 (October 17, 2007): CD006207.

53. M.E. Halloran et al., "Modeling targeted layered containment of an influenza pandemic in the United States," *Proceedings of the National Academy of Science* 105(12): 4639-4644 (March 25, 2008).

be quite limited; and different alternatives may impose restrictions that are also difficult to compare. There are also deep questions about whether paradigms drawn from "evidence-based" medicine (where the randomized clinical trial is the "gold standard") are appropriately used in the context of pandemic planning, given predictive uncertainty and the wide variety of potential pandemic situations.[54] Requiring a very strong evidence base for constraints to be imposed may violate the precautionary principle of attempting to avoid the uncertain probability of very bad outcomes, since it might delay imposition of these constraints far too long for them to be effective.

Other questions we will explore about these constraints are substantive: focusing as they do on efforts to prevent vectors from disease spread, constraints may overlook important protections for victims. This is not to conclude that constraints are unjustified—but that their justification must be weighed against and accompanied by possible protections for victims. PVV's insistence on considering both victims and vectors helps to bring this dual concern into view. Are the constraints accompanied by protection of personal security and the effort to provide people with basic survival needs? Is human-to-human communication provided for those who are constrained? Are the burdens of constraints distributed equitably? Finally—our question for the next chapter—are constraints accompanied by compensation for those who have been harmed by their imposition?

Surveillance. The importance of surveillance in the sense of identifying and reporting cases of disease is crucial in pandemic preparedness: after all, without the early identification of disease, the need for protective measures will go unrecognized until disease has become widespread and difficult to contain. The alternative—a kind of universal precaution against disease spread, without knowing where or even whether there is disease, analogous to the universal precautions now in use for HIV—would appear far more intrusive than surveillance followed by intervention when disease is identified. In general, public health surveillance, based in well established public health law, provides a very high level of protection, even for those individuals whose identity is known to public health officials. Nonetheless, as our discussion of privacy and confidentiality in Chapter 8 developed, there are risks to surveillance for potential victims: most important, that confidentiality may not be protected and that groups may be stigmatized.[55]

Standard public health practices are typically successful in avoiding these risks. However, with the time-pressures and public hysteria that might be generated in

---

54. See, e.g., Cecile Bensimon and Ross Upshur, "Evidence and Effectiveness in Decisionmaking for Quarantine," *American Journal of Public Health* 97 (April 2007): S44–S48.

55. These concerns are emphasized in the recent criticism by the American Civil Liberties Union of contemporary pandemic planning in the United States. George Annas, Wendy K. Mariner, and Wendy E. Parmet, *Pandemic Preparedness: the Need for a Public Health—Not a Law Enforcement/ National Security—Approach* (January 2008), http://www.aclu.org/pdfs/privacy/pemic_report.pdf (accessed January 28, 2008), 28–29.

a widespread pandemic of serious disease, it is important to anticipate any stresses that might be placed on the protections now built into public health surveillance practices. Otherwise, surveillance would cast people as vectors without respect for them as victims. Responding to initial reports of disease outbreaks with fear and coercion, rather than with efforts to provide appropriate treatment and community support likewise would treat people only as vectors rather than as victims of illness. Moreover, there is also the practical point that any such failures to respect victims would run the risk of undermining the trust that is essential to effective surveillance, on the part of individuals, groups, or even nations.

In 2005, the World Health Assembly adopted new International Health Regulations designed to augment surveillance capabilities. Under the regulations, all states parties (that is, all members of the WHO) agree to notify WHO of health events that might create an emergency of international concern. The regulations specify that a single case of some diseases—polio, SARS, smallpox, and pandemic influenza—constitute such an emergency. Political difficulties remain, however, in developing effective enforcement capacity for the regulations.[56] These difficulties include reluctance of countries concerned about overly harsh restrictions, as well as complexities of legal implementation within federalist and other systems.[57]

Various regional arrangements, for example within the European Community, or between the United States, Mexico, and Canada,[58] also augment surveillance capacity. These arrangements are of differing specificity; for example, the Association of Southeast Asian Nations (ASEAN) has a summit declaration of the importance of cooperation, but no specific plans for how this might be carried out.[59] ASEAN cooperation also has extended to stockpiling 500,000 courses of Tamiflu[60]—hardly a supply that would suffice for the vast

56. World Health Organization, *International Health Regulations* (2005), http://www.who.int/csr/ihr/IHRWHA58_3-en.pdf (accessed January 28, 2008); see M.G. Baker and D.P. Fidler, "Global Public Health Surveillance Under New International Health Regulations," *Emerging Infectious Diseases* 12, no. 7 (July 2006): 1058–1065.
57. The United States and China are examples. See Baker and Fidler, "Global Public Health Surveillance"; see also United States of America, "Statement for the record by the Government of the United States of America concerning the World Health Organization's revised International Health Regulations" (May 23, 2005), http://usinfo.state.gov/usinfo/Archive/2005/May/23–321998.html (accessed February 7, 2008). For a general discussion of the issues, including the specific example of SARS in Canada, see Kumanan Wilson, Christopher MacDougall, and Ross Upshur, "The New International Health Regulations and the Federalism Dilemma," *PLoS Medicine* 3, no. 1 (January 2006): e1.
58. This is the Early Warning Infectious Disease Surveillance Project, funded by the United States to enhance surveillance in bordering provinces of Mexico and American states. United States Mexico Border Health Commission, "Early Warning Infectious Disease Surveillance Project," http://www.borderhealth.org/ewids.php?curr=programs (accessed January 24, 2008).
59. Association of Southeast Asian Nations, "East Asia Summit Declaration on Avian Influenza Prevention, Control and Response" (December 2005), http://www.aseansec.org/18101.htm (accessed January 24, 2008).
60. ASEAN Secretariat, "ASEAN Cooperation in Combating Avian Influenza (November 2007)," http://www.cafte.gov.cn/include/linshiwenjian/download/6ASEAN.ppt#256 (accessed January 24, 2008).

population of the region, unless the outbreak were stopped very early on. By contrast, the European Community has longstanding, enforceable require-ments for cooperation, including surveillance.[61]

The WHO also may rely on information from unofficial sources, including nongovernmental organizations (NGOs), if the information is verified.[62] In addi-tion to providing treatment, NGOs such as CARE and Médecins sans Frontières are important sources of information about disease outbreaks.[63] That NGOs play this informational role underlines the importance of support for victims in the development of trust, garnered by NGOs through providing treatment or other social services. It is thus noteworthy that the International Health Regulations specifically address protection of the confidentiality of health data and permit disclosure of identifying information only where necessary to manage a public health risk.[64] The regulations also provide for support from the WHO for nations attempting to develop the public health capacity for surveillance.[65]

Support for public health surveillance capacity, however, is not the same as reassurance that every effort will be made to provide treatment in response to reports of outbreaks of disease. Ideally, we suggest, the WHO surveillance reg-ulations should link reporting of health emergencies to immediate prevention and treatment responses. This strategy increases the likelihood of contain-ment, develops trust, and respects those who are ill as victims in need.

Border Screening and Travel Restrictions. With respect to pandemic planning, the global plan of the WHO attempts to calibrate appropriate responses to different pandemic phases, divided by extent of disease activity as revealed by surveillance.[66] WHO Phase 1 is the interpandemic period in which no new in-fluenza subtypes have been detected; Phase 2 is the period in which new sub-types have been identified in non-human animals but not in humans; Phase 3—the world's current phase—involves new human infections but no or very limited person-to-person transmission; Phase 4 involves highly localized hu-man-to-human transmission; Phase 5 involves larger clusters but still localized human-to-human transmission; and Phase 6 refers to the period of wide-spread pandemic transmission.[67] At no phase does the WHO recommend

---

61. Commission of the European Communities, *Commission Working Document on Community Influenza Preparedness and Response Planning*, COM(2004)201 final, Brussels (March 26, 2004), http://europa.eu/eur-lex/en/com/wdc/2004/com2004_0201en01.pdf (accessed January 24, 2008).

62. World Health Organization, *International Health Regulations*, article 9.

63. For an illustrative example of this, see, e.g., A. Moore and M. Richer, "Re-Emergence of Epi-demic Sleeping Sickness in Southern Sudan," *Tropical Medicine & International Health* 6, no. 5 (2001): 342–347.

64. World Health Organization, *International Health Regulations*, article 45.

65. Ibid., article 13.

66. World Health Organization, *WHO Global Influenza Preparedness Plan*.

67. Ibid., 7.

compulsory intra-national travel restrictions, regarding them as "impractical in most countries but likely to occur voluntarily when risk [is] appreciated by the public."[68] The organization likewise rejects *cordons sanitaires* around entire geographical regions as impractical.[69]

Internationally, the WHO recommends permitting surveillance at borders if needed to promote public trust—but would not encourage the practice due to lack of proven benefit.[70] It does not recommend screening for symptoms, health declarations for at risk travelers, thermal screening, or medical examination at borders—regarding all of these as of unproven efficacy. An exception is the feasibility of entry screening for geographically isolated areas that are infection-free, such as islands. WHO does, however, recommend alerts for travelers, daily self-examination for travelers from at risk areas, and self-reporting of symptoms.[71] These limited recommendations with respect to border surveillance and travel restrictions rest on judgments that most of these interventions are impractical and that there is no evidence that they are of health benefit.[72]

Given the infrequency of pandemic events and the ethical difficulties of conducting randomized trials of such practices as border surveillance, it is not surprising that there is little or no published evidence about border screening measures.[73] "No evidence" in support of border surveillance should not be confused with "the evidence does not support" in the sense that there is actual evidence that the intervention does not work. With border screening, there are simply no studies of the type that meet contemporary evidence-based standards; indeed, it is hard to imagine how such studies could be conducted. There is, however, the WHO Writing Group's assessment that the efforts of some locations to curtail travel during the 1918 pandemic were of uncertain efficacy at best—though, of course, this was almost a century ago and social circumstances are quite different today.[74] The efficacy of border surveillance will also depend crucially on the features of any actual pandemic infection—for example, whether it has a lengthy period between time of infection and detectability in someone subject to border screening.

The draft British plan treats border surveillance in some detail. Britain is, after all, an island; although not particularly remote, it has succeeded in preventing the introduction of rabies into the country. Birds fly, however, and so the model for control of rabies in animal populations is inapplicable to control of avian influenza in wild bird populations. Britain's modeling for human-to-human

---

68. Ibid., 44.
69. Ibid., 44.
70. Ibid., 45.
71. Ibid., 44–45.
72. Ibid.
73. Cochrane Collaboration, "Interventions," 1, 7
74. World Health Organization Writing Group, "Nonpharmaceutical Interventions," 90–91.

transmission of H5N1 originating elsewhere suggests that only complete clo-sure of all borders would prevent influenza spread into the country.[75] Britain estimates that even a 99.9% efficacy rate in border screening would only delay the spread of the virus by about two months.[76] Border screening that is based on the observation of symptoms will let people pass who are infected but who have not yet become overtly ill and thus would be unlikely to meet this effi-cacy rate, so Britain does not include border screening of any kind in its draft plan. Britain does, however, intend to continue to monitor the data and to make plans for rapid implementation of screening at airports and ports if this becomes recommended.[77]

Given what is currently known about how testing works and the incubation period of influenza viruses, even the extremely accurate rapid-test screening hy-pothesized in our thought-experiment in Chapter 15 will not succeed in keeping all infection out of an island nation such as Britain. Influenza has a 1–4 day incu-bation period—that is, a 1–4 day period between an exposure and the appear-ance of symptoms of actual illness. Suppose a traveler is exposed on day 1, travels on day 2, and begins to be symptomatic on day 4. A rapid test administered be-fore the virus has multiplied sufficiently for viral shed to be detectable will not succeed in identifying the traveler as the infectious time bomb he or she might be. In order to keep flu entirely out of an island such as Britain, more than bor-der surveillance would thus be necessary: for example, detaining all travelers for 4 days, until the known incubation period has passed. Apparently this delay be-tween infection and symptomatic disease is one of the major difficulties in devel-oping strategies that are effective in preventing spread of pandemic influenza.[78]

So plans such as Britain's do not propose screening of all entrants at the border. Nor does Hawaii, the United States' island state, plans full port of en-try screening of the type proposed in our thought-experiment. Instead, Hawaii proposes port of entry screening only of people who are reported by airlines to appear ill—that is, only of travelers who are sufficiently symptomatic to have come to the attention of airline personnel.[79] Guam—another island—likewise proposes to institute heightened screening of those displaying symp-toms of illness when there are reports of human-to-human transmission of

75. U.K. Department of Health, *Pandemic Flu*, 24.
76. Ibid.
77. Ibid., 74.
78. C. Fraser, S. Riley, R.M. Anderson, and N.M. Ferguson, "Factors That Make an Infectious Dis-ease Outbreak Controllable," *Proceedings of the National Academy of Sciences* 101 (2004): 6146–6151; see also Baker and Fidler, *Global Public Health Surveillance*.
79. Hawaii State Department of Health, *Hawaii Pandemic Influenza Preparedness & Response Plan*, version 08.1 (January 2008), http://hawaii.gov/health/family-child-health/contagious-disease/pan-demic-flu/fluplan.pdf (accessed July 5, 2008), 15–23. Hawaii estimates that at any given time there are about 300,000 travelers within its shores and that it receives about 2.5 million tourist visits an-nually. Many of these travelers come from Southeast Asia, where new strains of influenza emerge.

H5N1 in areas with direct flights to Guam—but does not propose to close the border to such flights.[80] Guam also entertains the possibility of restricting travel from Guam to areas where there are H5N1 outbreaks—a strategy that might protect Guam's residents from becoming ill elsewhere and bringing disease back with them, but that will not otherwise interrupt transmission.[81] The island nation of Japan also proposes to detain and quarantine at the border suspected cases returning from regions where infection has been identified.[82]

Depending on the circumstances, a delay that buys even a week's time might have major implications in blunting a pandemic and thus in saving lives. Given this recognition, it is noteworthy that Britain's plan—like the plans of other island nations—does not contemplate completely closing borders for a period of time after a pandemic has been identified—the only strategy that Britain believes would succeed in keeping a pandemic out entirely.[83] Britain's current judgment is that "The possible health benefits that may accrue from international travel restrictions or border closures need to be considered in the context of the practicality, proportionality and potential effectiveness of imposing them, and balanced against their wider social and economic consequences."[84] There are clear difficulties about when and for how long to impose a border closure. If a closure is imposed early—before disease is likely to have spread into Britain—it is more likely to be effective. But assuming the disease continues to spread elsewhere, border closure is also more likely to need to be continued for a significant period of time in order to make any difference in what would have been the pattern of pandemic spread without border closure, and thus more likely to generate severe social disruption, including interruption of important lines of supply. If closures are imposed later, they are less likely to be effective because disease may already have spread into Britain.

Nonetheless, Britain's estimate that border surveillance that is 99.9% effective would delay onset of a pandemic for up to two months might still allow for manufacture or distribution of antivirals and for the implementation of a vaccination program, as well as for staffing of triage facilities, and implementation of public information programs. With screening that is 90% effective, Britain anticipates a more modest one-to-two-week delay in the arrival of the

80. Guam Department of Public Health and Social Services, *Guam Pandemic Influenza Plan: Draft* (January 25, 2006), http://www.guamhs.org/pdf/2006/Guam_Pandemic_Influenza_Plan_1–25–2006_DRAFT_.pdf?PHPSESSID=6241a277611dee8a84a88f721f7b2f7d (accessed July 5, 2008), 16–17.

81. Guam Department of Public Health and Social Services, *Guam Pandemic Plan*, 17.

82. Ministry of Health, Labour and Welfare, *Pandemic Influenza Preparedness Action Plan of the Japanese Government* (November 2005), http://www.mhlw.go.jp/english/topics/influenza/pandemic01.html (accessed January 28, 2008).

83. U.K. Department of Health, *Pandemic Flu*, 24.

84. Ibid., 28.

virus.[85] The impact of any such delays, of course, will depend on the speed with which antivirals or vaccines can be made available, as well as on the time to protection by vaccine; even two months' delay, for example, would be minimally helpful if vaccines are not expected to be available for three months and immunity requires several weeks after vaccination to develop, though antivirals might blunt some of the force of the epidemic. The availability of reported new techniques for the rapid manufacture of vaccine would thus make a great difference in whether border surveillance is adequately justified in comparison to other alternatives. Britain appropriately plans to continue to keep the evidence on the benefits of border closures, screening, and travel restrictions under review.

Any effort to test and retain passengers at borders focuses on their status as vectors; to take this approach fails to attend to them as victims, unless attention is paid to their needs for treatment and other forms of support. The specter of a modern Ellis Island—say, the Channel Islands in Britain or one of the Hawaiian Islands put to that purpose as Kaluapapa on the island of Molokai was used to isolate lepers—haunts any proposal for extensive border surveillance. A critical factor, then, if passengers are to be detained at borders for any period of time, whether for full diagnosis or for treatment to be effective, would be to provide support for them, especially facilities for them to stay. Perhaps the most difficult aspect of this would be providing separate facilities, at a minimum for those who are apparently ill—that is, isolation at the border until the patient is no longer contagious. Without such separation, even those who are detained without symptoms until an incubation period has passed would be placed at potential risk of infection from other detainees. The logistics of achieving such separation are not impossible, however, although they are not addressed in any plan of which we are aware. Even a plan such as Hawaii's, which proposes border screening of patients who appear to be ill, lacks any separate discussion about what will be done with identified patients or those with whom they have travelled. Presumably, actually-ill patients will be isolated in a hospital setting, as this is what Hawaii proposes for initially identified cases; but the plan says nothing specific about what is planned.[86] With cancellation of all travel that is not absolutely essential—a likely eventuality if border detention is announced and enforced—airport and possibly also seaport hotels might be sufficient for keeping travelers in comfort but not at greater risk of infection until any incubation period has passed; although attention would need to be paid to the difficulties in staffing such facilities and providing food, needed treatment, and other forms of support.

In sum, the strategy of border screening that is found in some island plans—for example, Japan, Hawaii, and Guam—is based on identifying

---

85. Ibid., 74.
86. Hawaii State Department of Health, *Hawaii Plan*, 36–47.

symptomatic patients for heightened examination once a pandemic is under way elsewhere. This strategy represents a serious effort to deal with the threat, but may in some respects prove an inadequate half-way position. It will miss all those who have been infected but are not symptomatic, as well as those whose symptoms are sufficiently minimal to escape scrutiny. It will also miss those who have been exposed by symptomatic patients during travel—unless what is contemplated is detaining all travelers arriving with a suspected case until the case is disconfirmed. It thus may not be fully effective in delaying pandemic spread for any extended period of time—although if short-term delays matter, as they would if vaccines were likely to be available quickly, the case for it would remain. It also may be too broad, imposing all the burdens of screening on those who display symptoms of illness that may or may not be pandemic in nature. Finally, the screening programs that have been proposed should devote further attention to those detained as victims; plans do not specify where they will be located, whether they will be given treatment, or what will happen to those travelling with them.

"Snow Days" and Social Distancing: Closures and "Stay at Home" Recommendations

In pandemic planning, social distancing is commonly proposed as a method to prevent disease spread. The patriotic parade in Philadelphia during the 1918 influenza epidemic that brought crowds together in circumstances ideal for spread was described by John Barry in sweeping detail as an example of what not to do in pandemic conditions.[87] For Americans born before the mid-1940s, closed swimming pools during polio epidemics remain vivid memories of parental fear and summer heat. There are many forms of social distancing, each with social costs of differing severity and distribution. School closures might include day-care centers, kindergarten, and primary schools only, or middle schools, high schools, and universities. University closures might or might not be associated with permitting students to return home—depending on whether there are concerns that returning students might bring disease along with them. Workplace closures might involve complete shutdowns—as with construction sites—or the implementation of telecommuting. Suspended public gatherings might or might not include sporting events, public transportation restrictions, theatres, parades, rock concerts, and churches.

Plans generally reflect the consensus among commentators that we presented earlier in this chapter that school closures are the most justifiable method of social distancing in preventing disease spread. Hawaii's plan, for

---

87. Barry, *The Great Influenza*, 208–209.

example, cites the limited evidence in support of across-the-board social distancing strategies, but suggests that there is reason to think that school and day-care center closures might be especially helpful.[88] Hawaii also believes that other social distancing methods, for example avoiding non-essential travel and recommending closures of gathering places such as churches might be helpful, depending on the circumstances.[89] Britain believes that school closures could reduce pandemic peaks and the total number of cases by as much as 10%—and could reduce clinical cases in children by up to 50%; it thus believes that any disruptions caused by closures would be more than justified by the numbers of lives saved.[90] Children are, as Britain puts it, "super-spreaders"; and Britain also notes that the disruption in essential services caused by school closures is not likely to be as great as disruptions caused by other types of closures. Massachusetts as of 2006 was waiting for evidence about the role of school closures in reducing spread,[91] but also included school closures, stay at home recommendations, and other "voluntary methods of self-shielding" in its draft community containment plan.[92] Plans reflect more doubt about the efficacy of event closures, however. Britain, for example, believes that mandatory restrictions on public gatherings are unlikely to prove effective.[93] Nonetheless, most plans include provisions for recommending that gatherings be curtailed, or that people be encouraged to stay home, especially if they are in groups at high risk from infection.[94]

Whether voluntary or compulsory, any model that relies on asking people to stay at home and out of public contact as a means to reduce pandemic spread requires extensive public cooperation in order to be effective. Cooperation, in turn, is dependent on adequate communication, both ethically and practically. The U.S. federal plan notes the importance of communicating with the general public: this is to promulgate the plan and its specific details about what facilities are closed, to provide general information how the pandemic is progressing, and to counsel individuals about whether to stay home and where

---

88. Hawaii State Department of Health, *Hawaii Plan*, 38.

89. Ibid., 38–40.

90. U.K. Department of Health, *Pandemic Flu*, 81.

91. Massachusetts Department of Public Health, *Massachusetts Influenza Pandemic Preparedness Plan* (October 2006), http://www.mass.gov/dph/cdc/epii/flu/pandemic_plan_2.pdf (accessed July 5, 2008), 24.

92. Massachusetts Department of Public Health, *Community Disease Control and Prevention: Draft* (October 9, 2006), http://www.mass.gov/dph/cdc/epii/flu/pandemic_plan_public_comments.pdf (accessed February 8, 2008), 8.

93. U.K. Department of Health, *Pandemic Flu*, 80.

94. E.g., Massachusetts Department of Public Health, *Community Disease Control and Prevention*, 8; Minnesota Department of Health, *Mitigation Strategies: Use of Non-Pharmaceutical Interventions* (April 2007), http://www.health.state.mn.us/divs/idepc/diseases/flu/pandemic/plan/npioverview.pdf (accessed January 30, 2008), 15–16

to go in case of illness. Adequate public information is seen as central to such plans, in part for efficiency and in part to prevent panic. Yet information delivery is not a simple matter. For example, the New Mexico plan notes the importance of delivering information in languages other than English.[95] Arizona, New Mexico's neighbor, has developed an extensive set of strategies to communicate with a multiplicity of disadvantaged populations, including Native Americans, people who do not speak English, and people with disabilities.[96] Given the impressive diversity of populations in the United States, Arizona's is an effort to be emulated in other states—a point that the population level of our PVV perspective emphasizes.

Plans typically do not address at all the problem of person-to-person communication, yet enabling people who are staying at home to contact family or friends may be especially important to their emotional well-being—as well as to their willingness to stay home. Adequate phone service or even Internet communication are critical to respecting victims in pandemic planning, but to the best of our observation have not been incorporated into published plans in the United States.

In plans for a number of U.S. states, school and workplace closures are described as "snow days." This old-fashioned, bucolic image invokes cozy days at home, away from school or work responsibilities with time to play in the snow that has impeded transportation.[97] Describing staying at home during a pandemic as a "snow day" is rhetoric that may cloak serious failures to consider the plight of people who stay at home as victims, however. The overt coercion in the "snow day" strategy is that public places or gatherings are closed and thus people cannot go to them. The further hope of the strategy is that people will judge that they will be better off if they self-shield at home rather than risking exposure by going out. The "snow day" strategy of limiting disease transmission is that many fewer people will be in crowded places where disease transmission is likely; it will not work if people simply shift their gathering place, say, from school to church, or from workplace to public transportation and shopping centers.

95. New Mexico Department of Health, *Pandemic Influenza Plan* (April 16, 2007), Suppl. 10, http://www.health.state.nm.us/ohem/documents/supplement10publicinfo.pdf (accessed July 5, 2008).
96. Arizona Department of Health Services, *Demographics and Effective Risk Communication* (April 2005), http://www.azdhs.gov/phs/edc/edrp/es/pdf/adhsspecialpopstudy.pdf (accessed January 30, 2008).
97. See, e.g., Maryland Department of Health and Mental Hygiene, *Draft Pandemic Influenza Plan for Maryland*, version 6.0 (2006), http://bioterrorism.dhmh.state.md.us/docs_and_pdfs/DRAFTFluPlanDec2006Part2.pdf (accessed July 5, 2008), 228; Virginia Department of Health, *Emergency Operations Plan*, supp. 8, 17; see also Global Security.org, *Pandemic Flu Mitigation—Social Distancing*, http://www.globalsecurity.org/security/ops/hsc-scen-3_flu-pandemic-distancing.htm (accessed January 28, 2008).

Expecting people to stay home—even if voluntarily in response to public appeals—carries with it responsibilities to those who do abide by these urgent requests. Even if the constraints are "soft"—that is, recommended and requested rather than required—they fail to respect the person as victim if they ignore basic survival needs such as food and hydration—or medical care for people who become ill, as we discuss in Chapter 19. Plans generally recognize that "snow day" strategies will prove untenable if they do not address these needs. Where they differ initially is over specificity: some plans such as Britain's lay out in great detail the methods they will use to ensure delivery of basic supplies,[98] while others simply note that this is an important issue to be addressed.[99]

With respect to how to provide supplies to people staying at home, the most important ethical difference among plans is over the assignment of responsibilities. Some state plans in the United States, for example, explicitly state that stockpiling home supplies is an individual responsibility and that the public role is educational about how to do this.[100] Some plans direct attention to people who might not be able to provide for themselves—for example, recipients of home-delivered "meals on wheels"—but do not otherwise see essential supplies as a public responsibility.[101] Still other plans rest on the premise that in pandemic circumstances provision of essential supplies is a public matter—not one for individuals alone.[102] On our view, respect for people who stay at home as victims

---

98. See, e.g., U.K. Department of Health, *Pandemic Flu*, ch. 9.

99. The Delaware plan, for example, simply provides that preparing the public for quarantine is an issue to be addressed. Delaware Department of Health and Social Services Division of Public Health, *Delaware Pandemic Influenza Plan* (Final April 2007), http://www.dhss.delaware.gov/dhss/dph/files/depanfluplan.pdf (accessed July 4, 2008), 45.

100. The Indiana and Ohio plans are examples. Indiana State Department of Health, *Pandemic Influenza Plan*, 37; Ohio Department of Health Bureau of Infectious Disease Control Immunization Program, *Influenza Pandemic Response Plan* (version 2.0, September 2005), (version 2.2, September 2005), http://www.odh.ohio.gov/ASSETS/399540667CF446508D5E663610B7396A/ODHFluPlan.pdf (accessed July 1, 2008), appendix H, 58–59. The Texas plan gives detailed instructions to individuals about how to carry out their responsibilities to stockpile essential supplies. Texas Department of State Health Services, *Pandemic Influenza Preparedness Plan* (October 2005), http://www.dshs.state.tx.us/idcu/disease/influenza/pandemic/Draft_PIPP_10_24_web.pdf (accessed February 1, 2008), appendix F, 76–82.

101. For example, the Hawaii plan includes: "establishing a phone bank" with the contact information for American Red Cross services (which include home delivery of "meals and materials"), recognition that people will be more likely to adhere to quarantine requests if "they understand that those in quarantine will be more accessible to receive supplies and necessary health care," and a recommendation that families should be prepared to voluntarily stay home by having an emergency supply kit that includes food, water and medications. Hawaii State Department of Health, *Hawaii Plan*, 6, 37, F-2. As such, the plan recognizes the importance of providing supplies, but appears to provide no public mechanism beyond providing contact information for the American Red Cross and a recommendation that individuals plan by stockpiling essential supplies.

102. For example, the Colorado plan specifically recognizes that "effective isolation or quarantine" requires provision of essential supplies and lists key planning tasks such as establishing procedures for delivery of supplies to those in isolation or quarantine. Colorado Department of Public Health, *Pandemic Influenza*, attachment 7.

generates shared responsibility for making sure that supplies are available; whether or not they are coerced, people are bearing burdens that help to limit the overall burden of disease and should be supported as a result.

School closures, as we have mentioned, are less disruptive of economic activity and basic social services than are workplace or transport closures, at least in the short term. Nonetheless, school closures even of short duration may prove quite costly for people who are dependent on schools or day care in order to work themselves. So are "snow days," for people who lose income. In the next chapter, we will defend compensation for people who lose income because of school or workplace closures, but who are dependent on daily or weekly wages and do not have sick leave. In Chapter 19, we will address the issues of justice raised by very grave gaps in providing care when people are seriously ill but cannot be accommodated in hospital settings. In the final section of this chapter, we take up what is required when people are constrained by home isolation or quarantine because they are ill or have been exposed.

Isolation and Home Quarantine

The most effective method for controlling small particle and airborne spread of influenza is isolation of the patient in a negative pressure environment—a method that, although highly effective, is expected to be available only in a limited number of cases.[103] In the United States, plans typically contemplate instead home isolation for patients who are symptomatic, together with home quarantine of family members they have exposed.[104] The American Medical Association counsels that quarantine should be instituted only when it is scientifically supported and is the least restrictive alternative, and then only with careful attention that it is not arbitrarily targeted to particular groups.[105] Studies of evidentiary support for home isolation or quarantine suggest that these strategies are most likely to be effective early on, as a method for controlling spread from an initial set of cases.[106] Because of the time lag between infection and symptoms, as well as difficulties in identifying mild cases, people who have been exposed are likely to have distributed infection in the community without having been identified as candidates for isolation or quarantine. Britain thus has concluded that as a method to control spread, home isolation and quarantine will become unsustainable after the first several hundred

---

103. Cochrane Collaboration, "Interventions," 8.
104. E.g., North Carolina State Laboratory of Public Health, *N.C. Pandemic Influenza Plan*, appendix I-1, 2; Ohio Department of Health, *Influenza Pandemic Response Plan*, 43.
105. American Medical Association, "Report of the Council on Ethical and Judicial Affairs," CEJA Report 1—I-05, http://www.ama-assn.org/ama1/pub/upload/mm/31/quarantine15726.pdf (accessed February 1, 2008).
106. World Health Organization Writing Group, "Nonpharmaceutical Interventions," 89.

cases—although this is an empirical claim it plans to keep under review.[107] The case for isolation and quarantine outside of the hospital setting, therefore, is weaker once a pandemic has taken hold in widespread fashion.

This way of viewing pandemic circumstances, moreover, treats people who have been exposed primarily as vectors. Several of our substantive requirements, especially personal security (S-1) and basic survival and health needs, including prevention and treatment (S-2) are ignored in plans that simply recommend isolation and quarantine without explicit plans for supporting those who are thus constrained. At least with "soft" stay-at-home strategies, people are not prohibited from going out for food or for other supplies in the way they would be under quarantine. Understanding people under home isolation or quarantine as victims is one of the most critical ethical gaps in many—but not all—pandemic plans.

Suppose that a person is required to stay at home during a pandemic, either because of symptomatic illness (isolation) or exposure (quarantine). Plans need to think carefully about what this will be like for the person and his/her intimates. We have already discussed the issue of essential supplies when constraints are "soft." When constraints are "hard," the case for public responsibility is even stronger: people are being required to stay home, not for their own good, but for the good of others. There is a public responsibility to make sure in return that their basic needs are attended to while they are at home. Some plans in the United States address this issue with care, but others treat it as an individual responsibility—just as though the person were staying at home by their own choice and for their own benefit.[108]

When isolation is accomplished in a hospital in negative pressure rooms, others are carefully protected from the ill patient. With home isolation, however, protection of others is likely to be far more uneven, and many plans fail to address this issue adequately. Even if a patient is not sufficiently ill to require more than home care, there is no guarantee that she will not infect those caring for her or living with her—or that their severity of illness will not be greater than hers. There ought to be clear guidelines in pandemic plans about how people at home will be helped to avoid infecting one another, as well as available supplies such as masks and gloves to aid them in doing so. The Maine plan addresses this concern in detail,[109] but some other plans do

---

107. U.K. Department of Health, *Pandemic Flu*, 75.
108. States are encouraged to see maintaining supplies as an individual responsibility by the Homeland Security Council's 2005 *National Strategy for Pandemic Influenza*, http://www.whitehouse.gov/homeland/pandemic-influenza.html#section6 (accessed February 1, 2008). The *Strategy* does not preclude other sources of support, however.
109. Maine Department of Health and Human Services, *Pandemic Influenza Plan*, www.maine.gov/dhhs/boh/DRAFT%20Pan%20Flu%20Plan%20071205_revised_rb.pdf (accessed July 5, 2008), 27–29.

not. The Indiana plan, for example, unhelpfully provides that patients at home must be isolated from other household members, without explaining how this is to be accomplished or how patients are to be cared for.[110] Without careful attention to protection against within-the-home illness spread, plans are failing to treat home caregivers as potential victims. Furthermore, if exposed caregivers are not quarantined themselves, they may transmit disease to others.

There are some exceptions to this grim picture of the potential plight of victims expected to stay at home, however. Britain will have a government-maintained flu telephone line for treatment recommendations and home delivery of antivirals and other forms of supportive care such as over-the-counter and essential medications. Britain's plan carefully maps out what this will mean for patients.[111] Colorado's plan has an excellent list of what might be needed by those under home quarantine: food and water, shelter, medicines and medical consultations, mental health and psychological support services, other supportive services (e.g., day care), and transportation to medical treatment, if required.[112] Massachusetts plans to employ quarantine only under exigent circumstances: "In the Pandemic Alert Period, especially during Phase 3 or 4 when little or limited person-to-person transmission has been documented, quarantine of contacts should be implemented *only when there is a high probability that the ill patient is infected with a novel influenza strain that may be transmitted to others.*"[113] Massachusetts also has thought very seriously about how to treat people who are under quarantine either as patients or as exposed contacts; the state plans daily (or twice daily) contact by public health workers and available treatment and social supports.[114] Idaho's plan begins with an epigram about the state's experience in 1918: "In October of 1918, some city officials in Southern and Central Idaho decided to close the public schools as a way to prevent the flu from spreading further . . . In the larger towns and cities, such as Twin Falls, the hospital became overcrowded with sick people so they had to find other places to put them. Since the schools and churches were already closed, city officials decided to turn these buildings into makeshift hospitals."[115] Perhaps with this experience in mind, Idaho plans to call on the Red Cross for emergency shelter and delivery of essential supplies.[116] These are

110. Indiana State Department of Health, *Pandemic Influenza Plan*, 12.
111. U.K. Department of Health, *Pandemic Flu*, 104–105.
112. Colorado Department of Public Health, *CDPHE Internal Emergency Response Implementation Plan: Annex U: Disease Outbreak: Appendix 1: Pandemic Influenza Attachment*, http://www.cdphe.state.co.us/epr/Public/InternalResponsePlan/Attachment7.pdf (accessed January 26, 2008), 7–3.
113. Massachusetts Department of Health, *Community Disease Control*, 5 (emphasis in original).
114. Ibid.
115. Idaho Department of Health and Welfare, *Idaho Pandemic Influenza Response* (March 2006), http://www.healthandwelfare.idaho.gov/DesktopModules/Documents/DocumentsView.aspx?tabID=0&ItemID=4523&MId=11634&wversion=Staging (accessed July 5, 2008), vi.
116. Ibid. 19.

good beginnings in thinking about the needs of victims at home, but planners ought ethically to devote far more attention than is apparent to date to the urgency of making supportive services available and to the logistical difficulties in arranging their provision. In short, planners need to devote far more attention to regarding potential vectors as also victims, even while they recognize victims, or potential victims, as also potential vectors.

In Sum: Ongoing Ethical Issues for Pandemic Planning

The pandemic planning process to date has been protean. Yet at least from the information that is publicly available, it is clear that critical ethical issues remain for ongoing attention. Given the uncertainty about the shape a pandemic may take, as well as what constraints may be effective, there is continuing need for structure for coordination and re-examination of plans. Surveillance has been addressed, but also required attention to how the known availability of care for victims may help in both preventing disease spread and addressing the situation of victims in ethical fashion. Social distancing strategies, with the exception of school closures, appear to be of uneven effectiveness, especially if they are implemented later in a pandemic. With both "snow day" closures and home isolation and quarantine, many plans should address the social obligation to provide support for those who have been constrained for the public good. Finally, plans should attend to the public responsibility to protect caregivers when patients are isolated at home.

18

COMPENSATION AND THE VICTIMS
OF CONSTRAINT

During an outbreak of communicable infectious disease like pandemic influenza, as we have just seen, efforts to control transmission almost certainly will mean that some people will be constrained. We turn in this chapter to the issue of compensation when people have been harmed by such constraints, even when the constraints were justified. The imposition of justified constraints does not extinguish obligations to those whose moral claims—for example, to liberty or to health care—are overridden. Constraints typically are designed to reduce vectorhood. Our principle S-5 holds that compensation for loss is required by respect for victimhood, and it is this requirement that we address here. The position we develop is that when people are harmed by constraints that are publicly imposed and that are intended to protect the public, compensation is required as a matter of what we owe each other as enmeshed in a web of infectious disease, when the constraints bear particularly heavily on some individuals and largely benefit others.

Justifying compensation raises many issues, among them why compensation is owed, to whom it is owed, what is owed, and who is obligated to pay the compensation. Here, we start with why people might be owed compensation when they have been harmed because they have been considered possible vectors. We then take up the more difficult issue of why compensation is justified in some cases of pandemic harm, but not in others. Should we, for example, compensate the wealthy air traveler who loses out on a business deal because she is kept off the plane because of her influenza symptoms? What about the day laborer who loses wages because the construction site on which he works is closed by a "snow day"? Should we compensate the family members who are kept at home with a family member who has pandemic influenza and who later become sick themselves, even though it is difficult to tell whether they would have been exposed and become ill anyway? And why should these victims of constraint be compensated, if others who suffer in a pandemic are not: the subsistence farmer whose chickens sicken and die before flocks are

We are grateful to Heidi Malm, Tom May, Saad Omer, and Daniel Salmon for working with us on an earlier version of the material in this chapter.

culled, the workers who go without pay because the construction company has no new contracts, or the people who have not had access to adequate health care earlier in life and are more susceptible to illness as a result?

There may be enormous difficulties in meeting any claims for compensation after a pandemic, as economies collapse and the means to provide what is morally required are simply unavailable.[1] Although localized, rapidly controlled episodes of contagious disease—like the 2003 SARS epidemic, for instance— may be small enough in scale so that a society can respond generously without significant strain, compensating for actual financial losses—the costs of quarantine, isolation, lost work time, and other economic losses, limited social resources nonetheless may make even these responses difficult. For example, the government of Uganda was reportedly long delayed in compensating the families of the 16 health-care workers who died in the Ebola epidemic in 2000.[2] Where a pandemic is of much larger scale, financial compensation even for actual losses may not be possible. Nonetheless, moral claims to compensation are important to recognize; even if they cannot be fully realized, recognizing them not only expresses respect for those who were harmed but reminds us that we ought to do what we can.[3]

Compensation

Discussions of compensation for harms sustained from measures for the control of infectious disease have appeared in the literature, but principally addressed as reciprocity to those who are seen as taking on special risks or responsibilities: health-care workers or their family members who are injured by vaccines,[4] health-care workers who get sick or die in the line of duty,[5] or health-care facilities that bear disproportionate economic burdens in pandemic care.[6] Nevertheless, compensation more generally for losses in the wake of constraints or prioritization schemes has not been part of the pandemic planning debate.

The seminal ethical document in the pandemic planning process, the Toronto Joint Centre for Bioethics' *Stand on Guard for Thee*, is an example of

1. Martin I. Meltzer, Nancy J. Cox, and Keiji Fukuda, "The Economic Impact of Pandemic Influenza in the United States: Priorities for Intervention," *Emerging Infectious Diseases* 5, no. 5 (September–October 1999): 659–671.

2. Charles Wendo, "Caring for the Survivors of Uganda's Ebola Epidemic One Year On," *Lancet* 358 (2001): 1350.

3. Note how important even apologies remain to the U.S. soldiers exchanged as prisoners of war with the Japanese or the indigenes who fought for France in World War II.

4. AAEM/SAEM Smallpox Vaccination Working Group, "Smallpox Vaccination for Emergency Physicians," *Academic Emergency Medicine* 10, no. 6 (June 2003): 681–683.

5. Lynette Reid, "Diminishing Returns? Risk and the Duty to Care in the SARS Epidemic," *Bioethics* 19, no. 4 (2005): 348–361.

6. Vickie J. Williams, "Fluconomics: Preserving Our Hospital Infrastructure During and After a Pandemic," *Yale Journal of Health Policy, Law & Ethics* 7 (2007): 99–152.

this oversight.[7] The Toronto report recommends compensation for health-care workers who incur injury based on the ethical value of reciprocity. With respect to the general public, however, the report states only that governments should have public discussions of what compensation is appropriate for individuals injured by pandemic constraints such as quarantine, as well as what entities might be responsible for any compensation.[8] Subsequent plans have not improved on the statements in *Stand on Guard for Thee*. There is no general discussion of compensation for the constrained in international plans,[9] in the U.S. federal plan, or in any of the U.S. state plans available online for review.[10] In some plans, psychosocial support is considered in relatively detailed fashion, but as the type of support needed during or in the immediate aftermath of a disaster.[11] For example, Virginia's plan has noted the need to address lost wages and business losses during the imposition of social distancing methods such as "snow days."[12] And Mark Rothstein has demonstrated in detail the failure of pandemic planning in the United States—and state or federal law—to address the problem of income support and job security for those required

7. So is the most recently released ethics discussion of which we are aware. See James C. Thomas, *Ethical Concerns in Pandemic Influenza Preparation and Responses*, white paper commissioned by the Southeast Regional Center of Excellence for Emerging Infections and Biodefense, Policy, Ethics and Law Core (SERCEB), http://www.serceb.org/wysiwyg/downloads/pandemic_flu_white_paper.May_25.FORMATTED.pdf (accessed September 2007). Both the Toronto and the SERCEB white paper discussions cite reciprocity as a value. But it is discussed principally in the context of responses to workers who bear special burdens of care during an influenza pandemic, not as a matter of reciprocity to the constrained and deprioritized we discuss here.

8. University of Toronto Joint Centre for Bioethics Pandemic Influenza Working Group, *Stand on Guard for Thee: Ethical Considerations in Preparedness Planning for Pandemic Influenza* (Toronto: University of Toronto Joint Centre for Bioethics, 2005), http://www.utoronto.ca/jcb/home/documents/pandemic.pdf (accessed January 27, 2008), 15. See also Jaro Kotalik, "Preparing for an Influenza Pandemic: Ethical Issues," *Bioethics* 19, no. 4 (August 2005): 422–431.

9. See Lori Uscher-Pines et al., "Priority Setting for Pandemic Influenza: An Analysis of National Preparedness Plans," *PLoS Medicine* 3, no. 10 (2006): e436.

10. The federal plan is U.S. Department of Health and Human Services, *HHS Pandemic Influenza Plan* (November 2005), http://www.hhs.gov/pandemicflu/plan/pdf/HHSPandemicInfluenzaPlan.pdf (accessed February 6, 2008). State plans are also available. See U.S. Department of Health and Human Services, "PandemicFlu.gov: State Pandemic Plans," http://www.pandemicflu.gov/plan/states/stateplans.html (accessed February 7, 2008). This is not to say that discussions have entirely ignored compensation. For example, the Model Health Emergency Health Powers Act provides for compensation when facilities are taken over for use in a pandemic, but not when they are destroyed as a disease risk. Center for Law and the Public's Health at Georgetown and John Hopkins Universities, "The Model State Emergency Health Powers Act" (December 21, 2001), http://www.publichealthlaw.net/MSEHPA/MSEHPA2.pdf (accessed January 24, 2008), sec. 506. Our contention in the subsequent chapter will be that these and other recommendations are inadequate from the point of view of justice.

11. E.g., Kentucky Cabinet for Health and Family Services, *Kentucky Pandemic Influenza Preparedness Plan* (April 2007), http://chfs.ky.gov/NR/rdonlyres/6CD366D2–6726–4ADo–85BB-E83CF769560E/0/KyPandemicInfluenzaPreparednessPlan.pdf (accessed July, 2008), supp. IX.

12. Virginia Department of Health, *Emergency Operations Plan Attachment Pandemic Influenza* (March 2006), http://www.vdh.virginia.gov/PandemicFlu/pdf/DRAFT_Virginia_Pandemic_Influenza_Plan.pdf (accessed July, 2008), supp. 8, 7.

to stay home during a pandemic.[13] But these aside, under our PVV view, the general failure to address compensation is a serious omission: it forgets attention to victimhood, even as constraints attend to vectorhood.

Models of Compensation

The philosophical, legal, and public health literatures contain a number of models of compensation for those who have been constrained to protect others from infectious disease. The models draw from contract law, tort law, and property law. In these models, compensation is usually but not always understood as financial compensation for tangible losses. As we shall develop later in this chapter, however, it is important to remember that some of the most crucial losses of pandemic victims may not be measurable in monetary terms at all.

One model for compensation—contract law—would compensate people based on agreements: for example, insuring health-care workers for the physical risks they encounter on the job. Contract has the disadvantage that it is limited to the scope of agreements that may or may not be regarded as fully voluntary. As the locus of contract law is individual choice, it may not encourage adequate infectious disease policies, for market failure among other reasons. Tort law would pay people for risks imposed negligently by others, but is limited to cases of fault or otherwise unreasonably dangerous products or activities. Neither contract nor tort sees compensation as a public matter, yet our victim/vector perspective suggests that protecting us from infection benefits us all.

The property model of compensation is eminent domain. It would compensate people for resources taken over or perhaps condemned for the public good, such as a health-care facility dedicated to treatment during a pandemic, or possessions burned to eliminate disease reservoirs. It has the advantage of recognizing that the costs of compensation are to be socially shared. But eminent domain, we will argue, also sees recompense in a limited way.

Costs and Losses That Are Candidates for Compensation

A short list of legally imposed demands that are likely to have identifiable economic costs can be drawn from the pandemic planning discussions.[14] From the victim/vector perspective, we contend, the most important factors to consider in whether these costs should be socially shared or whether they should be borne by those who incur them include: their severity, whether they are concentrated

---

13. Mark Rothstein and Meghan Talbott, "Encouraging Compliance with Quarantine: A Proposal to Provide Job Security and Income Replacement," *American Journal of Public Health* 97 (April 2007): S49–S56.
14. This list is drawn from the Haddon matrix. See Daniel J. Barnett et al., "A Systematic Analytic Approach to Pandemic Influenza Preparedness Planning," *PLoS Medicine* 12, no. 2 (December 2005): e359.

on particular individuals or widespread, whether or not they are analogous to other safety costs ordinarily borne by the individual, whether they were reasonably to have been expected, and whether they are imposed primarily to benefit others or also to benefit the individual himself or herself. These concerns are familiar in other contexts: they are the kinds of considerations we generally take into account in deciding whether costs should be socially shared. More general issues of justice in health care, both nationally and internationally, remain in the background of what we say as well, but these are questions that will be addressed in Chapter 19.[15] Here, we will look at compensable items like costs for tests, treatment, protective equipment, travel restrictions, property losses, quarantine, physical risks, and more.

Tests

Costs of tests may include equipment, drugs and reagents, or labor. When testing for infection is mandated, as in the rapid screening involved in our thought-experiment in Chapter 15, we should consider whether these costs should be borne by individuals being tested or be shared socially. Current practice in the United States is to impose costs of tests, like costs of health care generally, on individuals or their insurance. From the victim/vector perspective, however, we recognize that some testing programs may be implemented for the public good rather than principally for treatment of individuals as patients; there is thus an argument for sharing these costs socially that is independent of background arguments about whether the costs of health care are a social matter. As a practical matter as well, from the perspective of ordinary life, testing programs may be more likely to succeed if their costs are borne publicly, because people who do not otherwise have the resources to pay for health care will at least not face economic barriers to testing.

Immunization and Preventive Treatment

Costs of prevention include antivirals, immunization, and any costs associated with adverse reactions to preventive methods. At present in the United States, costs of antivirals such as Tamiflu are currently borne as treatment costs by individual patients. Costs of immunizations, however, are sometimes borne publicly, on the recognition that it is better overall for most to be immunized than for those who cannot pay to avoid immunization. In the United States, these vaccination

---

15. See, e.g., Madison Powers and Ruth Faden, *Social Justice: The Moral Foundations of Public Health and Health Policy* (New York: Oxford University Press, 2006); Norman Daniels and James Sabin, *Setting Limits Fairly: Can We Learn to Share Medical Resources?* (New York: Oxford University Press, 2002); Nancy Kass, "Public Health Ethics: From Foundations and Frameworks to Justice and Global Public Health," Journal of Law, Medicine, and Ethics 32, no. 2 (2004): 232–242.

programs extend even to undocumented immigrants—a sensible (and humane) protective strategy. The federal vaccine compensation program is also available to those who have been injured by required vaccines, as we mentioned in Chapter 14.

Policy decisions to share the costs of immunization reflect practical concerns: that people in poverty will go without immunization and thus pose risks to the rest of us, and that vaccine makers will withdraw from the market if they have to bear the costs of product liability lawsuits when people are injured by vaccination. We think that these policies also are defensible from the victim/vector perspective; from that perspective, we recognize that mechanisms to prevent disease spread both reduce the likelihood that we will be vectors to each other and protect each of us from becoming victims, and so should be supported.

By contrast, the argument to share the costs of antivirals publicly is somewhat less clear. When private individuals use scarce antivirals that they have acquired for themselves, they may protect themselves; but they might also be able to protect themselves in ways that did not consume a scarce good, such as by staying away from areas of likely disease transmission. Allocation of antivirals to health-care workers and providers of other essential services so that they can remain on the job represents a benefit shared by us all in a time of epidemic; the case for socially shared costs from the perspective of "we are all in this together" is much stronger for them.

Protective Equipment

Costs of required protective equipment include everything from the gloves that have become a part of universal precautions against blood-borne illnesses in health care, to equipment donned by people who work with poultry, to the elaborate biohazard suits employed by infectious disease researchers with deadly viruses such as Ebola. Some of this equipment is standard on-the-job safety, no different from the protective goggles worn by metalworkers or the helmets worn on construction sites. Where extraordinary expenses are involved, primarily for the public safety, however, the victim/vector perspective would suggest socially shared costs. As a practical matter, it might also be helpful for costs of protective equipment to be subsidized in impoverished industries where disease transmission is a serious risk and where the costs of protection are high in comparison to economic resources. Poultry raising practices in the developing world are a case in point.

Border Control, Travel Restrictions

Trips may be canceled and other costs may be incurred when borders are closed or travel restrictions or surveillance are in effect. In such cases, people bear costs for their own good, but also for the public good. They have made

investments—purchased tickets, made plans to attend events—on the legitimate expectation that travel was permitted. At least in this respect, direct costs
of canceled travel arguably should be shared socially, along the same lines as
the costs of property destruction, considered below. From the victim/vector
perspective we would consider that compensation is reasonable. Conversely,
people with the resources to travel may be more affluent as a background matter, so the case for compensation is more complex, given competing demands
for resources. Some decisions not to travel may be made individually but not
under state compulsion, such as decisions to stay home in response to travel
advisories. These decisions are surely to be encouraged as a means of reducing
disease spread and are highlighted in many international and national pandemic plans. These decisions primarily benefit the stay-at-home traveler and
are not the result of direct state coercion. Thus arguably compensation should
not be paid for losses associated with such canceled travel. In the interests of
encouraging such conduct that benefits everyone, it is important to ensure
that people do not suffer penalties such as forfeited airfare or trip deposits
when such decisions are made in response to travel advisories. This is the appropriate parallel to people who stay at home during "snow days," and who
should not suffer penalties of lost wages. In contrast, travel plans made after
advisories of an epidemic—decisions to travel to the risk—do not carry the
aspect of legitimacy based on expectations, except of course for those such as
medical personnel who are expected to take the risks.

Closures or Destruction of Property

In order to prevent transmission of infectious disease, it may be important to
destroy property that is a disease reservoir. The massive killing of poultry infected with avian flu is only the most recent illustration. British farmers were
compensated when their herds were destroyed to prevent the spread of hoof and
mouth disease, but the effects on community life overall may have been irre-
mediable.[16] The practical need to offer compensation for culled flocks to poultry farmers in Thailand and other countries has been widely recognized, if not
fully met.[17] From the victim/vector theoretical perspective, such compensation

16. See, e.g., Paul Harris, "The Plague upon Our Village," *Observer*, news, January 20, 2002, 13.
17. See, e.g., Peter Alford, "Bird Flu Financial Help for Jakarta," *Australian*, local, June 26, 2006, 2;
Keith Bradsher, "The Front Lines in the Battle Against Avian Flu are Running Short of Money,"
New York Times, sec. 1, October 9, 2005; Mary Ann Benitez, "One Fifth of Live Poultry Stalls Agree
to Close in Flu Buy-Back," *South China Morning Post*, August 26, 2004, 1; John Aglionby, "Farmers
Count Flu's Bitter Cost," *The Observer*, news, January 25, 2004, 26, reporting promise of the Thai
government to pay farmers for culled stock; Alan Sipress, "Bird Flu Upends Industry, Livelihoods
in Thailand," *Washington Post*, sec. A1, January 25, 2004, reporting that promises of compensation

also seems justifiable, at least to some extent. People may be bearing substantial costs, even entire livelihoods. These costs may not have been reasonably anticipated—although, if they could have been, the case for compensation is undermined; consider by comparison the situation of farmers whose vegetables are destroyed because of *E coli* contamination resulting from known unsafe farming practices. And the costs are borne to protect us all.

Businesses may also be shut down, temporarily or permanently, as infection control measures. Examples include the closure of bathhouses in San Francisco during the HIV/AIDS epidemic, the closures of swimming pools during polio epidemics, and the efforts to close stalls selling live poultry as a means to control avian flu. Some of these closures may be unanticipated and quite costly; the case for compensation in these cases is analogous to the case for compensation in the case of property destruction. Questions about the reach of such compensation are difficult. Lost profits may be enormous and difficult to estimate; these problems must weigh in the balance of whether to compensate and are an important reason for the concerns about the inadequacy of compensatory models we explore below.

Seizures or voluntary requisition of property for use in treating or isolating infectious patients also may cause serious economic loss. Hospitals that are the designated centers for treating patients in epidemic situations may be unable to treat other patients.[18] Large public facilities may become locations for housing either victims or people who have not yet become infected. The property law model for compensation in such cases of "temporary takings" would be the reasonable rental value of the property.

Isolation and Quarantine

The economic costs of lost wages and quarantine loom large as well: lost wages, educational costs and delays (e.g., college tuition for students barred from attending class), and lost business opportunities. The issues here are like those raised by business losses: the losses are focused on the individual, not easily to be anticipated, and for the benefit of us all. If quarantine is short-lived, the losses may be more limited and compensation an easier fiscal matter. Sick leave policies that are designed to encourage infectious workers to stay home are analogous; workers out on sick leave continue to receive pay, although

---

to Thai farmers remain indefinite and Chaanda Chakraborti, "Pandemic Management and Developing World Bioethics: Bird Flu in West Bengal," *Developing World Bioethics*, forthcoming, describing "botched" culling practices and poor crisis management skills in the January 2008 H5N1 outbreak in West Bengal, India, as "particularly glaring" in the case of fixing the compensation rate paid for the birds to be culled.
18. For a thorough discussion of the complex issues involved in compensating hospitals providing care during epidemics, see Williams, "Fluconomics."

they do consume accumulated sick leave days that might be available on other occasions. Decisions to stay home may benefit the individual as well and may be taken more for individual benefit than for overall protection of others; in cases of an individual staying home when it is unwarranted as a matter of infection control but chosen out of fear of exposure, the case for compensation falters.

Historically, quarantines often herded together the ill, the exposed, and those believed to have been exposed. Such practices increased the risks of illness to those who, albeit exposed, might not have become ill but for the proximity to illness under the quarantine. Although more modern methods emphasize isolation—separation of individuals known to be ill from others they might infect—pandemic influenza plans frequently contemplate home quarantine of the ill or the exposed, a practice likely to subject family members to increased risks even when they are accompanied by the protective measures we defended in Chapter 17. In such circumstances, care-giving family members arguably are analogous to other caregivers or essential service workers and thus are owed compensation for their injuries as a response to what they have done to benefit those afflicted with disease. Even though they are at home with family, they bear increased responsibilities for pandemic care or for reducing disease transmission as a benefit for others.

Physical Risks

Infectious diseases pose risks to caregivers: they might get sick or even die from disease. Those who deliver essential services—food, communication workers, sanitation workers, transportation workers, and the like—may also be exposed to risks they would not encounter but for the need to provide these services. When health-care resources are scarce or overwhelmed by a pandemic, patients may not receive care that they otherwise would have received. People who are asked to stay home may be unable to access basic services or receive basic medical supplies. People herded into quarantines may be placed at greater risk of infection than they otherwise would have been; people caring for patients in isolation may be at far greater risk of disease than they would otherwise have been, had other facilities been available for the care of infected patients.

The pandemic planning literature has paid significant attention to the problem of compensating health-care workers and some other essential service workers. This is as it should be: these workers are bearing focused and potentially very high costs, for the benefit of the rest of us. Even if some health-care workers—infectious disease physicians, for example—might have expected to encounter these risks as a matter of career choice, other health-care workers have not: nurses' aides or hospital laundry workers, for example. Those who provide essential services—such as food delivery workers—even more clearly have not anticipated the special risks of exposure to lethal disease as a part of their job choices; these are the sacrifices of victims that arguably have an especially strong case for compensation. However, these arguments for compensating essential service workers do not preclude arguments for compensating others such as family care givers. We would also note that some losses—one's own death, risks to family members—cannot be made up for in full by economic compensation at all.

From this discussion, we can draw several important points about the inadequacy of compensation models. First, compensation suggests economic recompense; but for some losses, economic recompense may be insufficient or utterly inadequate. Death, injury, loss of an entire family—these harms are not subject to economic replacement. Even when material compensation may be adequate, demands on public economic resources may be too great to provide it, especially in times of pandemic where economic resources will be strained or even collapse. Second, some ways of implementing economic compensation—especially contract or tort law—misframe the issue as between private actors rather than as a public concern. The costs of compensation, we have argued, should be shared socially when constraints benefit all. The recipient of compensation might be an entire community rather than individuals only; an example is the effort in HIV/AIDS research to provide health care to communities some of whose members have participated in studies.

An Outline of the Case for Compensation: Response to Social Choices

Summarized, the case for compensation is as follows. The constraints set out in pandemic influenza planning are social choices—that is, they are arrived at by "official" decisions, typically of governmental agencies with public discussion and advice. Even when these choices are well justified, they place some people in situations of greater disadvantage than others, albeit with the goal of benefiting everyone. These choices treat people as members of a population faced with the overall burden of disease, not as individuals who may turn out to be victims of disease. They ask people to bear harms, or increased risks of harms, for the overall good. Such social choices, we hold in this chapter, generate at a minimum obligations of some kind of return for the choice that creates disadvantage.[19] Some of those who are disadvantaged will suffer

---

19. There is one seminal discussion of such general obligations of return in the infectious disease context, arguing that if we expect people to comply with a duty not to infect others, society must reciprocate with commitments to treatment, nondiscrimination, and in some cases compensation. See John Harris and Soren Holm, "Is There a Moral Obligation Not to Infect Others?" *British Medical Journal* 311, no. 7014 (November 4, 1995): 1215–1217.

identifiable harms; a response which views them as individual victims would be to try if possible to compensate them for that harm.

To be sure, it will in some cases be unclear whether the harms people suffer are causally related to the disadvantage: perhaps people who are constrained would have become ill or otherwise been harmed even if they had been in more favored positions. But the case for compensation does not rest on any direct causal chain. It rests on the idea that the social choice to constrain some people, as made in pandemic plans, itself generates obligations to those people—obligations to try to make it up to those people as individuals for the fact that they have been disadvantaged as part of a population's response to threat, when the harm is of a type anticipated in the decision to constrain. Moreover, in some cases it will be hard to know how much to compensate, or to compensate at all—if the result has been the death of an entire family, for example. In what follows, we offer some observations based on our PVV perspective about how pandemic influenza planning might approach these difficult issues about compensation.

Caveats Associated with Partial Compliance Theory

A critical caveat for our argument in this chapter is that pandemic influenza planning must recognize that those harmed by pandemic constraints are likely to be over-represented among those who have already experienced disadvantages in their lives. People who are poor may experience higher risks of exposure to infectious disease because they live in more crowded conditions and have less adequate sanitation. They may be more likely to get sick or to suffer greater levels of mortality and morbidity because they have poorer nutritional status and are more likely to have been exposed to environmental toxins that impair their health status. With jobs that pay hourly wages or that lack benefits such as sick leave or vacation time, poorer people may lose more if they are required to stay at home—and be less able to stay away from possible sources of exposure than others who have resources that enable them to stay at home. If reservoirs of infection are concentrated in impoverished areas, constraints such as quarantine may be imposed on these areas that are not imposed elsewhere. Infection control measures such as destruction of domestic animals also may bear more heavily on those who are already worse off.[20]

---

20. For a discussion of the burdens imposed on impoverished people by the destruction of domestic animals, particularly poultry, see Ruth R. Faden, Patrick S. Duggan, and Ruth Karron, "Who Pays to Stop a Pandemic," *New York Times*, sec. A, February 9, 2007.

Philosophers call theorizing about what justice requires in circumstances of injustice "partial compliance theory."[21] If health care in the United States is a significantly unjust system, in the sense that its benefits and burdens are not fairly apportioned, and health status is to some extent therefore unjustifiably unequal, pandemic planning against this background must be regarded as an exercise in partial compliance theory. Questioning the justice of health care in the United States is beyond the scope of this chapter, but we will discuss it in the next chapter.[22] One of our concerns will be whether understanding pandemic planning as a partial compliance problem has implications for the case for compensation. We contend that it does: if partial compliance theory— doing justice under circumstances of injustice—requires paying special attention to the situations of those who are most vulnerable, for example, then the case for compensation for victims is strengthened still further.

Here, we address primarily clear cases of the types of harm anticipated in pandemic influenza planning constraints we have examined: people who are injured by surveillance; who lose daily wages because they are required to stay at home and do not have jobs that come with sick leave or vacation pay; and who become sick while they are subject to constraints such as quarantine. We recognize that many indirect or more subtle harms may also occur, but they are not our focus here. We assume that the constraints and priorities are themselves just, although they may be superimposed on a background of injustice. We assume as well that the individuals are not themselves culpable in a way that might otherwise deflect claims for compensation. They are just ordinary people, constrained in pandemic circumstances because they or others are ill. If compensation of the constrained can be justified at all, these are the kinds of cases in which the justification will be clearest.

Tort Law, Social Choice, and Reciprocity

Historically the picture of compensation in tort law was that the duty to compensate arose when one person was harmed by the fault of another. This picture

---

21. The term is originally John Rawls's. John Rawls, *A Theory of Justice* (Cambridge: Harvard University Press, 1971). Rawls classifies both naturally caused straitened circumstances such as drought and human injustice together as partial compliance contexts, without separating the two. Arguably, therefore, any pandemic situation is a partial compliance situation in which ideal justice cannot obtain. Rawls leaves unexplored whether natural and social partial compliance contexts require different treatment; our remarks here refer to the background injustice of social circumstances and we leave open whether they are also relevant to natural disasters.

22. We fully recognize that a different kind of response to the issues we raise here would be to urge the United States to make greater strides toward health justice, for example in the form of universal health care. In this chapter, our goal is to make the positive case for compensation; we think this is an important issue in its own right, regardless of one's position about health justice more generally.

insisted that the compensator be at fault and that the harm be attributable to the fault in the legal sense that the harm would not have occurred "but for" the fault.[23] The doctrine of "strict" liability replaced a finding of fault with proof that the product or conduct at issue was unreasonably dangerous but continued to insist on a legally recognized causal relationship between the product's dangerous nature and the harm. "No-fault" schemes such as worker's compensation or some proposals for tort law reform in medical malpractice maintain only the requirement of a causal connection between the source of compensation and the harm.[24] Through this connection, they create incentives to reduce the likelihood of harm by better safety practices even though they do not require a finding of fault per se in the generation of the harm. "Market share" liability attributes responsibility for compensation by market share to manufacturers of products such as diethylstilbestrol (DES) or asbestos that caused harm, without requiring the injured person to trace the harm they sustained causally to a particular manufacturer.[25] These tort law theories all retain a connection between the source and the resulting harm, however attenuated.

Other compensation schemes have been put into place principally for the incentives they create; as with tort law, these schemes generally require a causal relationship between the source and the injury. For example, the need to ensure vaccine availability was a principal driver of the National Childhood Injury Compensation Act's provision of no-fault compensation for children injured by vaccines.[26] The Act requires either demonstration that the injury meets criteria set out in the Vaccine Injury Table[27] or that there was a causal connection between the vaccination and the injury;[28] and that there is not a

---

23. Legal cause is not the same as scientific cause and is a notoriously difficult notion. For an argument that legal cause is a normative concept, see H.L.A. Hart and A.M. Honore, *Causation in the Law* (Oxford: Clarendon, 1962).

24. See, e.g., David M. Studdert and Troyen A. Brennan, "Toward A Workable Model of 'No-Fault' Compensation for Medical Injury in the United States," *American Journal of Law & Medicine* 27 (2001): 225–252; William M. Sage, Kathleen E. Hastings, and Robert A. Berenson, "Enterprise Liability for Medical Malpractice and Health Care Quality Improvement," *American Journal of Law & Medicine* 20(1994): 1–28.

25. See, e.g., Kenneth R. Lepage, "Lead-Based Paint Litigation and the Problem of Causation: Toward a Unified Theory of Market Share Liability," *Boston College Law Review* 37 (1995): 155–182.

26. 42 U.S.C. § 300aa-10 (2007); see Richard J. Webby and Robert G. Webster, "Are We Ready for Pandemic Influenza?" *Science* 302, no. 5650 (2003): 1519–1522.

27. 42 U.S.C. § 300aa-14(c) (2007); 42 C.F.R § 100.3 (2007). The injury table is established by rule and represents side effects and time frames that are generally accepted to reflect a causal relationship between the vaccine and the injury. For a critical discussion of the functioning of the table in this regard, see Lainie Rutkow, Brad Maggy, Joanna Zablotsky, and Thomas R. Oliver, "Balancing Consumer and Industry Interests in Public Health: The National Vaccine Injury Compensation Program and Its Influence During the Last Two Decades," *Penn State Law Review* 111(2007): 681–735.

28. 42 U.S.C. § 300aa-11(c) (2007).

preponderance of the evidence that the injury was due to some other cause.[29] For vaccines received after 1988, compensation is funded by an excise tax of $0.75 on every dose of vaccine administered—thus the costs of compensation are shared among all those receiving vaccine but not among those who choose not to be immunized.[30] Recognizing the risks of immunization, as well as resistance to participation, Section 304 of the Homeland Security Act provides for compensation from the federal government for health-care workers injured by participation in the federal smallpox vaccination program.[31]

Still other compensation structures rest more directly on the idea of reciprocity. When people take on special burdens to benefit society, and suffer harm of a type anticipated from the burden, compensation may be morally required as a response. Programs to compensate soldiers who have been injured in war are an illustration, as are compensation programs for miners suffering from black lung and other diseases. The argument for compensating health-care workers who take risks to care for others and incur burdens is that they have borne a disproportionate burden to protect others and that reciprocity thus requires that society try to make up to them for their losses.[32] Some reciprocity-based compensation schemes require the assumption of the disproportionate burden but no subsequent proof of a causal link between the burden and harm; educational and other benefits for returning soldiers were defended on this, among other, grounds.[33] Programs to compensate health-care workers for pandemic illness appear not to insist on proof that the illness was contracted in caring for patients rather than from other sources of exposure.

By contrast, some compensation programs represent in theory social responses of compassion to a disproportionate harm itself. Examples include state programs to compensate crime victims, the compensation provided after 9/11, disaster relief, and perhaps even "bail-outs" such as responses to the savings and loan or sub-prime mortgage crises. To a significant extent, these latter efforts

---

29. 42 U.S.C. § 300aa-13(1)(B) (2007).

30. Centers for Disease Control and Prevention, "CDC Vaccine Price List," http://www.cdc.gov/vaccines/programs/vfc/cdc-vac-price-list.htm (accessed February 9, 2008). Funding compensation by increasing the costs for those who bear the burden of vaccination—rather than sharing the costs with those who free ride—seems perverse.

31. Centers for Disease Control and Prevention "Guidance for the Healthcare Community Concerning Section 304 of the Homeland Security Act," http://www.bt.cdc.gov/agent/smallpox/vaccination/healthcare-304-guidance.asp (accessed February 9, 2008); for a discussion of the program, see Rutkow, "Balancing Consumer and Industry Interests," 725–729.

32. University of Toronto Joint Centre for Bioethics Pandemic Influenza Working Group, *Stand on Guard for Thee*, 11.

33. See, e.g., Theda Skocpol, *Protecting Soldiers and Mothers: The Political Origins of Social Policy in the United States* (Cambridge: Harvard University Press, 1992); Florence Wagman Roisman, "National Ingratitude: The Egregious Deficiencies of the United States' Housing Programs for Veterans and the 'Public Scandal' of Veterans' Homelessness," *Indiana Law Review* 38 (2005): 103–176.

at relief should be regarded as acts of charity in response to extensive, concentrated, and unanticipated suffering. They may also reflect the idea that social choices—limited investment in policing, inadequate disaster protection programs, or deregulatory decisions—increased the risks of harm and so to some extent there is a shared social responsibility for the harm, albeit one that is indirect. The view of compensation as a matter of what we owe those who have been disadvantaged by social choices that we develop below draws on these familiar strategies.[34]

The "Constrained" in Pandemic Influenza Planning

Constraints, as we have seen throughout this volume, are a time-honored method for attempting to halt infection's spread. Let us rehearse just briefly some of the constraints we have explored. They include restrictions on movement: travel prohibitions, *cordons sanitaires*, quarantine, and isolation.[35] Many state pandemic plans provide for "snow days"—days on which people are required to stay home from work and schools are closed. Pandemic response plans also specifically include restrictions such as quarantine and isolation and recognize the harms that might ensue.[36] Because patients in isolation are known to be infected, they may fail to receive care that otherwise would have been available if there are difficulties in delivering care in the isolated setting. Depending on how they are structured, quarantines may increase risks of exposure and infection to those who have not yet been infected but are included within the quarantine.[37]

Constraints, as we have seen, also include physical intrusions ranging from minimally invasive diagnostic tests (for instance, a cheek swab, as was the example in our thought-experiment in Chapter 15), to blood tests, to required immunizations, to mandated and directly observed treatment such as

---

34. See, e.g., Naomi Seilor, Holly Taylor, and Ruth Faden, "Legal and Ethical Considerations in Government Compensation Plans: A Case Study of Smallpox Immunization," *Indiana Health Law Review* 1 (2004): 1–27. This is the best ethical discussion we have found of the obligation to compensate those who have been harmed by a public health intervention. It relies on a tort law analogy, seeing compensation as owed when harm is caused by governmental action aimed to avert a greater harm. Our suggestion relies on obligations of reciprocity generated by the governmental decision rather than a direct causal link between the government action and the harm.
35. For a good discussion of the history of quarantine and isolation and of the role of due process guarantees, see Michelle A. Daubert, "Comment: Pandemic Fears and Contemporary Quarantine: Protecting Liberty Through a Continuum of Due Process Rights," *Buffalo Law Review* 54 (2007): 1299–1353.
36. E. Vinson, "Managing Bioterrorism Mass Casualties in an Emergency Department: Lessons Learned from a Rural Community Hospital Disaster Drill," *Disaster Management Response* 5, no. 1 (2007): 18–21.
37. Daniel Markovits, "Quarantines and Distributive Justice," *Journal of Law, Medicine & Ethics* 33 (2005): 323–338.

with MDR-TB. The motivation to compel treatment for MDR-TB and XDR-TB patients especially, as we have explored in Chapter 9, is a response to concerns of burgeoning disease spread.[38] Forced prevention, diagnosis or treatment may of course benefit the patient, but it may also have significant and harmful side effects. This can be the case for immediate effects of treatment administered: for example, side effects of anti-tuberculosis drugs can include renal failure and liver toxicity (with a reported incidence rate of 9.2 per 1,000 and a case fatality rate of 4.7%).[39] These can also include more generalized health risks, like the development of drug resistance, and social risks, like that of abuse, as was the issue with mandatory testing of pregnant women for HIV, as we have seen in Chapter 12.

Strong utilitarian reasons promote the provision of compensation in return for the imposition of constraints, if it appears that the promise of compensation increases the likelihood of compliance. Increased compliance has been offered as a reason to provide income replacement and job security for people required to stay home from work during a pandemic.[40] Negative attitudes toward involuntary quarantine in the United States suggest the need to rely on incentives to achieve even minimally protective compliance rates.[41] Employees injured by vaccinations also may be eligible for workers' compensation or for compensation under the program for federal employees—or so the U.S. overall pandemic plan notes.[42]

But the argument for compensation is more than the practical need to create incentives for compliance; it is a moral argument as well. Consider first those who are required to follow the "snow day" strategy of staying home from jobs during a pandemic and who thus lose pay because they have no sick leave or vacation benefits or because they work in jobs such as construction where pay is hourly and telecommuting is not an option.[43] These people are asked to bear a burden—a

---

38. Jacqui Wise, "Southern Africa Is Moving Swiftly to Combat the Threat of XDR-TB," *Bulletin of the World Health Organization* 84, no. 12 (December 2006), http://www.who.int/bulletin/volumes/84/12/news.pdf (accessed February 9, 2008), 924–925.

39. E.J. Forget and D. Menzies, "Adverse Reactions to First-Line Antituberculosis Drugs," *Expert Opinion on Drug Safety* 5, no. 2 (March 2006): 231–249.

40. University of Toronto Joint Centre for Bioethics Pandemic Influenza Working Group, *Stand on Guard for Thee*, 13; Rothstein and Talbott, "Encouraging Compliance."

41. Robert J. Blendon et al., "Attitudes Toward the Use of Quarantine in a Public Health Emergency in Four Countries," *Health Affairs* 25, no. 2 (March-April 2006): w15–w25.

42. U.S. Department of Health and Human Services, *HHS Pandemic Influenza Plan*, E-32. The HHS plan does not note any other available sources of compensation, for example for any injured non-workers.

43. Some pandemic plans explicitly contemplate "snow days," a bucolic euphemism suggesting happy families playing together, rather than the considerable costs of lost wages and others hardships. See, e.g., State of Illinois, *Illinois Pandemic Influenza Preparedness and Response Plan*, version 2.05 (October 10, 2006), http://www.idph.state.il.us/pandemic_flu/Illinois%20Pandemic%20 Flu%20Plan%20101006%20Final.pdf (accessed July 1, 2008), 63; Minnesota Department of Health,

lost wage, losses in liberty, losses in communication, and interference with personal projects and meaningful activities—in the interests of reducing disease spread. Some of the state pandemic plans remind people of the need to keep sufficient supplies on hand;[44] others consider the importance of delivering essential supplies.[45] We have examined all U.S. state pandemic influenza plans published or posted on the Web as of this writing; no plan that we could find proposes compensation for lost wages, although some come close. The Arkansas plan notes that the "community trauma" of a pandemic will include lost wages.[46] A draft Massachusetts plan provides that all necessary support services should be provided for people in home or other quarantine, including mental health services; and notes the possibility that financial support for medical leave will need to be considered.[47]

One objection to this argument might be that it proves too much. For example, our view might be thought to justify compensation for those who voluntarily "self-shield," staying home as a mode of self-protection even if a "snow day" has not been declared, when they have borne the burden of lost wages and benefited the rest of us by not becoming likely vectors of disease transmission. Massachusetts notes in its plan that such self-protective behavior may have a public benefit.[48] Nonetheless, this objection holds, it seems problematic to suggest that people are owed compensation for lost wages in such cases: the decision to stay home was voluntary and quite likely personally beneficial.

It does not follow, however, from our argument that compensation would be owed in such cases of self-shielding—or that it would not be. Whether income security should be provided to voluntary self-shielders as a matter of justice (rather than as a matter of encouraging prudent behavior) is a difficult issue, but it is not the problem we are tackling here.[49] Our argument in this

Pandemic Influenza Plan, Draft, version 2.5 (April 2006), http://www.health.state.mn.us/divs/idepc/diseases/flu/pandemic/plan/mdhpanfluplan.pdf (accessed July 5, 2008), 72. See also the Arkansas plan, developed post-Katrina, recognizes the community trauma of lost wages but does not include a discussion of compensation, Arkansas Department of Health and Human Services, *Arkansas Influenza Pandemic Response Plan* (August 2006), http://www.healthyarkansas.com/pandemic_influenza/pandemic_influenza_plan.pdf (accessed February 9, 2008; link no longer valid), app. 9.
44. E.g., Indiana State Department of Health, *Pandemic Influenza Plan* (October 2006), http://www.in.gov/isdh/files/PandemicInfluenzaPlan.file (accessed July 5, 2008), 37.
45. Arkansas Department of Health and Human Services, *Arkansas Pandemic Response Plan*, 91, app. 2.
46. Ibid., app. 9.
47. Massachusetts Department of Public Health, *Community Disease Control and Prevention: Draft* (October 9, 2006), http://www.mass.gov/dph/cdc/epii/flu/pandemic_plan_public_comments.pdf (accessed February 8, 2008) 19.
48. Ibid., 8.
49. Rothstein and Talbott, "Encouraging Compliance."

chapter rests on the claim that implementation of the social decisions to constrain that have been developed in pandemic plans as a means to benefit everyone are the basis for a duty to compensate in return. In so constraining some, the state is benefiting others—perhaps everyone—by treating people as vectors. In return, it must respond also to what is morally required in the recognition of vectors as victims. Persons who stay home voluntarily have not been disadvantaged by such a social decision to impose constraints on them, even though they may act in ways that benefit both themselves and others. It is also worth noting that people who are able to self-shield may be those who have the resources to enable them to act self-protectively. Nonetheless, as Massachusetts has noted, there may be other reasons to consider encouraging people to stay at home and supporting them when they do, even if mandatory constraints are not imposed.

Restrictions on movement such as isolation or quarantine view patients or potential patients primarily as possible vectors, deflected from transmission by separation from the rest of the population. Yet the constrained are also victims—people who may suffer or die. Isolation raises the possibility that people will not get care at the level they need, a topic we explore further in the next chapter. Quarantine of the exposed in groups subjects those who have been exposed but not infected to increased probability of exposure from other detainees. Home quarantine may make it more difficult for exposed persons to avoid subjecting family members to risks of exposure; that is why respondents in Hong Kong and other societies with experience of SARS preferred other quarantine locations outside of the home.[50] When policies treat the constrained solely as vectors, they ignore this victim-side of their humanity. If the constrained become sick, regard for each of them as a victim requires that we try to make it up to them for what they have lost. This argument does not rely on proof of a causal relationship between the constraint and the harm: patients might have done poorly even without the isolation, or family members might have gotten sick from sources other than the quarantined family member. It relies on the idea that these people have been asked to do something extraordinary—be constrained, at home or elsewhere—because of a social choice to protect everyone, and have suffered the very harm contemplated in the social choice.

Or consider mandated treatment. The argument for compensating healthcare workers who take risks in caring for others and incur burdens is that they have borne a disproportionate burden to protect others; reciprocity thus requires that society try to make up to them for their losses.[51] There is a parallel

---

50. Robert J. Blendon et al., "Attitudes Toward the Use of Quarantine."
51. University of Toronto Joint Centre for Bioethics Pandemic Influenza Working Group, *Stand on Guard for Thee*, 11.

to other people for whom medical interventions are mandated. Required immunization or therapy may have side effects; people who undergo such interventions for the benefit of all are owed compensation when they are harmed. They have borne burdens associated with policies that were put into place to protect everyone–including themselves..

Another, central objection to this argument is that people who are constrained are also benefited. For example, vaccines serve primarily to protect the individual who is vaccinated and secondarily to contribute to the herd effect, which protects others. The difficulty with this reply is that even when constraints are just and the benefits real, the burdens of them do not fall proportionately. A few people who are vaccinated will have severe side effects, or may shed disease from a live vaccine and thus injure family members or friends. The mandatory nature of childhood vaccination, for example, was an important consideration in the creation of the National Vaccine Injury Compensation Program in the United States. Some people who are exposed in a situation of quarantine will die or become gravely ill—when their risks of infection have risen because of the quarantine imposed to benefit everyone. Even though a constraint is ethically justified, this justification is a separate question from whether people who are harmed by the constraint have moral claims that are not extinguished by the justification of the constraint. Even though a constraint is as limited and as carefully justified as possible, it is impossible to ensure that the resulting effects on people will be justly distributed; additional questions of justice are posed by what to do for those who are harmed under constraints.

Anticipating Costs and Losses

There are of course many difficulties in determining who is owed compensation and what they are owed. Harms may be variable and difficult to prove. Some harm—for example, death of an entire immediate family from infection contracted while under quarantine—may apparently defy compensation. And social resources may be very limited if the economy has been shattered by a pandemic.

Nonetheless, several types of likely harms for the constrained are relatively easy to anticipate, especially wages lost due to constraints, costs of medical care for those who become ill while quarantined at home or while caring for others in the home, and income support for children or spouses of those who die after exposure during quarantine. Pandemic influenza planning should be considering these harms and what compensatory responses might be offered to them. Our discussion here sketches out how existing and readily available models might be extended to cover these cases. We employ such extant models on the assumption that it will be simplest to build public policy from existing templates. We also note several important issues in adapting the existing models to the compensation cases we discuss.

Lost Wages

Unemployment compensation is an insurance scheme that provides temporary income support for people who have lost jobs. In the United States, it is funded by a 6.2% employment tax paid on the first $7,000 of wages for covered employees. States administer programs pursuant to federal minimum standards. Benefits are a fractional amount of wages up to a state-specified maximum.[52] Eligibility standards include a minimum time of employment, minimum earnings, and availability for work.

Unemployment compensation provides a reasonable model of compensation for employees who are required to temporarily stay at home. It would provide a guaranteed, known wage amount for individuals who otherwise would not have income support during that period. The chief disanalogy between unemployment compensation and the pandemic "snow day" case is that workers are required to be available for work, despite current unemployment. Unemployment compensation also is not a program available to the self-employed. These major gaps have been addressed when special unemployment compensation is available as part of federal disaster relief—but only partially, as the special relief is just a fraction of the ordinary unemployment compensation amount.[53] Another gap might be the situation of undocumented workers, who presumably are not eligible for unemployment compensation but who might be over-represented among employees who do not have sources of support when they are required to stay at home. These gaps would also need to be adapted to unemployment compensation in pandemic circumstances. An additional issue that has not been addressed for the case of unemployment compensation in disasters is that state compensation amounts vary widely, with levels generally lower in poorer states with more limited tax bases.

At least in theory, pandemic planners can model the likely number of "snow day" stay-at-home requirement under different pandemic scenarios. Planners can thus also calculate tax amounts that might be necessary to provide a reserve fund that would be available should pandemic constraints be imposed. This additional amount could be garnered by a special surcharge on

---

52. Almanac of Policy Issues, "Unemployment Compensation," Almanac of Policy Issues, http://www.policyalmanac.org/social_welfare/archive/unemployment_compensation.shtml (accessed February 9, 2008).
53. See, e.g., Pamela Winston et al., "Federalism After Hurricane Katrina: How Can Social Programs Respond to a Major Disaster?" *Tulane Law Review* 81 (2007): 1219–1261 (1233–1235).

the unemployment compensation tax, or by reliance on general tax revenues, though one disadvantage to relying on a surcharge to the unemployment compensation tax is that the tax is highly regressive and discourages employment of full time, low-cost workers.[54] However, in addition to the social-choice argument we have developed, a primary argument for thinking through the funding of something like an unemployment compensation subsidy is that people are more likely to comply with "snow day" requirements if they can be reassured that they will have some kind of replacement income for the period they are required to stay at home. This factor of general benefit suggests considering use of general tax dollars to augment unemployment compensation for those who lose wages due to pandemic constraints, as well as efforts to expand the compensation program to all workers who lose wages because they are subject to constraints.

Costs of Medical Care for Those Who Become Ill Under Quarantine

Compensation for costs of medical care for those who are constrained may be to some extent a moot issue in pandemic circumstances. People who become ill under influenza quarantine would most likely either have recovered or have died by the time compensation becomes a realistic possibility. The most likely candidates for compensation for medical expenses would be those whose pre-existing conditions are worsened by pandemic constraints. One type of example would be someone initially with planned elective surgery that is delayed due to pandemic quarantine. Another would be someone who has ongoing health consequences from influenza contracted during quarantine.

Health financing systems—Medicare, Medicaid, and private insurance—should be prepared to experience increased claims rates during an immediate post-pandemic period. To the best of our knowledge, this has not been modeled in the pandemic planning process. Another—and quite likely—type of person who might incur increased needs for health care as a result of pandemic constraints would be someone who does not have health insurance and who is dependent on public clinics or emergency rooms that have been given over to treating influenza patients. Our emphasis here is what is owed as a matter of return for constraints, not the more general issues of justice about access to health care in the United States. Nonetheless, if these patients have more complex medical needs that are attributable to planned pandemic structures, they too warrant concern in response to their situation as victims disadvantaged by social choices to protect us all. One way to meet that concern would be to open Medicaid enrollment to such patients on a special or expedited basis.

54. Lawrence H. Summers, "Some Simple Economics of Mandated Benefits," *American Economic Review* 79, no. 2 (1989): 177–183.

A special difficulty that must be addressed in the United States is that since the Personal Responsibility and Work Opportunity Act of 1996, many legal but non-citizen immigrants are not eligible for Medicaid.[55]

Loss of Income Support for Spouses and Children

Workers' compensation has been suggested as a model for pandemic first responders who are injured by vaccinations or illness contracted on the job. Historically, workers' compensation was established as a scheme of administrative compensation that replaced the tort system of compensation with certain, but less generous recoveries. It typically pays for health care and replacement percentage of wages up to a pre-set ceiling. Workers' compensation also may pay a flat rate death benefit, similar to a life insurance payout; amounts may be reduced for nonresident alien beneficiaries in some states.[56] Workers' compensation is funded through employer insurance premiums that are experience-rated; the goal of such experience rating is to create incentives to improve workplace safety.

Even for pandemic responders who are injured on the job, workers' compensation is a problematic compensation model. Pandemic risks are largely not under the employer's control, although some such risks might be reduced by appropriate training, equipment, and risk assessment. General tax revenues rather than experience-rated employer premiums might therefore be a more appropriate funding source.

For the constrained who lose income support, the analogy with workers' compensation is even more inapposite. Perhaps the argument might be that they are in a sense doing a "job"—accepting the constraints or prioritizations, for the general good. But there is no employer to look to as a source of premiums; general tax revenues would seem the likely source. Nevertheless, workers' compensation payment schedules are a useful analogy for compensation amounts. They are settled, modest, and capped. They might thus avoid some of the enormous difficulties of equity that attended the 9/11 compensation process.[57]

---

55. 42 U.S.C § 1396a (2007); Howard F. Chang, "Migration Regulation Goes Local: The Role of States in U.S. Immigration Policy," *New York University Annual Survey of American Law* 58 (2002): 357–370.

56. Adam S. Hersh, "Go Home, Stranger: An Analysis of Unequal Workers' Compensation Death Benefits to Nonresident Alien Beneficiaries," *Florida State University Law Review* 22 (1994): 217–241.

57. Lloyd Dixon and Rachel Kaganoff Stern, *Compensation for Losses from the 9/11 Attacks* (Santa Monica, Calif.: Rand Corporation, 2004), http://www.rand.org/pubs/monographs/2004/RAND_MG264.pdf (accessed February 9, 2008). The principal amounts of 9/11 compensation went to businesses and first responders; questions were also raised about compensation amounts for higher income earners.

Another possible analogy is the bottom-weighted Social Security system, but this has the difficulty that people who die under pandemic constraints may well be over-represented among those who have accumulated limited amounts of Social Security eligibility.

Social Choice and Compensation: A Limited Conclusion

If an influenza pandemic occurs, some people are likely to be constrained. Indeed, this may be the majority of individuals in a population where the threat of epidemic spread is great. To date, pandemic planning has largely considered justifications for compensating health-care workers who shoulder the burdens and risks of care as a matter of reciprocity. It has not as yet attended very thoroughly to possible justifications for compensating the constrained. In this chapter, we have developed social-choice as an initial argument for extending compensation to those constrained under the social choices implemented under pandemic plans, beyond the narrow range of compensation considered in the basic plans. We have also considered what some possible models for compensation might be. The argument from respect for people as victims and vectors is, we think, clearest for the constrained whose losses are the result of identifiable social choices.

Nonetheless, there may be analogous arguments to be made for those who have been disadvantaged by the social choices made in health policy, especially for those who fail to receive health care because of circumstances of injustice. Then, too, what about those who are "deprioritized" to receive vaccination, antivirals, or intensive care in pandemic plans? In the next chapter, we turn to pandemic prioritization and issues of justice raised by our PVV view.

19

PANDEMIC PLANNING AND THE JUSTICE
OF HEALTH-CARE DISTRIBUTION

Pandemic planning poses stark and potentially tragic issues of distributive justice. Who should receive scarce supplies of vaccines or antivirals? Who among the seriously ill should be triaged to home care, admitted to hospitals, or given ventilator support? Some of the pandemic planning process has emphasized efforts to avoid or blunt the impact of scarcity: the development of new, much quicker molecular techniques of vaccine manufacture, stockpiling of antivirals, and increases in hospital "surge capacity" are the primary examples. All plans, however, recognize that under a worst case scenario and perhaps also under fairly bad case scenarios, choice may be inevitable. Some—perhaps many—people will die who might otherwise have lived, had prevention or treatment been available to them.

The triage choices in pandemic planning for the distribution of vaccines and antivirals are open, coordinated, and institutionally adopted. Perhaps this is one reason why they have drawn so much attention. Yet in today's world, vast numbers of deaths occur annually from diseases that could be treated quite easily, were resources only available. For example, the WHO estimates that about 1,000 children die every hour of diseases that are largely preventable or treatable with low-cost interventions.[1] Pneumonia and diarrheal diseases are primary culprits, but so is malaria: one African child dies of malaria every 30 seconds. These deaths are not subsequent to institutionally adopted, written-out prioritizations of the sort found in pandemic planning, decisions that a scarce resource should be given to some who meet carefully chosen criteria but not to others, but they are the result of multiple decisions and non-decisions that have critical distributive justice consequences nonetheless. Because they have so many points of entry—from the legal regime of intellectual property rights over vaccines and pharmaceuticals, to displacement from strife and conditions in crowded refugee camps—identifying these decisions as a matter of distributive justice is a far more protean problem than discussion of pandemic triage. Thus the justice *of*

---

1. World Health Organization, *What Are the Key Health Dangers for Children?* (October 2007), http://www.who.int/features/qa/13/en/index.html (accessed January 26, 2008).

pandemic planning—of the decisions to devote resources to counter a prospective harm in a context of many actual harms—has drawn less ethical attention than the questions of justice *within* pandemic plans.

No doubt there are other explanations for the apparent assumption that devoting considerable resources to pandemic planning is just. There is the thought of a widespread disease with a 60% mortality rate, and there are the descriptions of the 1918 pandemic that make the avian influenza threat seem personally real to people in the developed world in the way that neglected tropical diseases do not. People in the developed world can see themselves dying of pandemic influenza—as members of their grandparents' or great-grandparents' generations died. The proclivity in the United States is to devote resources to saving identified victims but concomitant difficulties in developing policies to deal effectively with the protection of statistical victims are well known among political theorists.[2]

Nonetheless, there are serious questions of justice about the allocation of extensive resources to pandemic threats. Every U.S. state has a coordinated pandemic plan to address a potential emergency—albeit incomplete—but only a handful of states, Massachusetts and Hawaii among them, have made similar coordinated efforts to address the health needs of their share of the estimated 46.5 million residents of the United States without health insurance.[3] In the United States, the initial federal appropriation for influenza planning was $3.8 billion, including $1.8 billion for vaccine development,[4] and the second year's appropriation was $2.3 billion.[5] At the same time, states have reportedly been cutting back on the funding available for the purchase of other vaccines for uninsured or underinsured children in the United States; there are serious gaps in the economic availability of vaccines to disadvantaged children, such as pneumococcal conjugate vaccine and hepatitis A vaccine.[6] As we noted in Chapter 14, the expense of the HPV vaccine may be a barrier to widespread use of this protective against cervical and other cancers. The funding for the entire expansion of the state children's health insurance plan (S-CHIP) vetoed by the President in the fall of 2007 was $35 billion—and this was a proposal that would have extended health insurance availability to approximately 10 million children in the United States.[7] Although ignoring a genuine pandemic risk would surely

2. See Guido Calabresi and Philip Bobbitt, *Tragic Choices* (New York: Norton, 1978).

3. Kaiser Family Foundation, *The Uninsured: A Primer* (October 2007), http://www.kff.org/uninsured/upload/7451-03.pdf (accessed January 26, 2008)

4. Department of Health and Human Services, *Pandemic Planning Update* (March 13, 2006), http://www.pandemicflu.gov/plan/pdf/panflu20060313.pdf (accessed February 6, 2008).

5. Department of Health and Human Services, *Pandemic Planning Update III* (November 2006), http://www.pandemicflu.gov/plan/pdf/panflureport3.pdf (accessed February 6, 2008).

6. Grace M. Lee et al., "Gaps in Vaccine Financing for Underinsured Children in the United States," *Journal of the American Medical Association* 298, no. 6 (August 8, 2007): 638–643.

7. E.g., Sasha Issenberg, "House Fails to Override Veto of SCHIP—Democrats Vow to Continue Pushing a Bill," *Boston Globe*, October 19, 2007, A2.

be unwise as well as problematic from the point of view of justice, questions should also be raised about the justice of how resources have been allocated to pandemic planning. In this chapter, we begin with several of the most important questions of justice *within* pandemic planning: allocation of vaccines and antivirals, as well as allocation of palliative care. We then set questions about the justice *of* pandemic planning within the implications of our PVV view for distributive justice in health care. In a nutshell, the claim we defend is that attention both to justice within pandemic planning and to the justice of pandemic planning point in the same direction: increasing the resources allocated to the provision of a basic minimum of health care, especially primary care, in the United States and elsewhere.

PVV and Distributive Justice

In Chapter 7, we summarized our PVV view thus: Ethical problems in infectious disease should be analyzed, and clinical practices, research agendas, and public policies developed, that always take into account the possibility that a person with communicable infectious disease is both victim and vector.

More specifically, our view moves on three levels. It begins from the perspective of actual, identified victims and vectors: full awareness of the personal human reality of illness or apparent protection from illness—as well as the realization that one is a threat to others and a possible object of constraint. It then continues with a second level, insisting that population-wide patterns are of relevance but must be seen against individual reality, too; to be morally adequate, policies that attend to how populations fare must also hold in view that persons must not be treated as mere data-points. Finally, our PVV view moves to the hypothetical level of the way-station self: a full awareness of both actual and theoretical uncertainty must inform both our moral prescriptions and policies.

For pandemic planning, the PVV perspective has several important implications. We have already speculated that part of what has given pandemic planning impetus in the developed world is that people can identify themselves as potential victims of avian flu—in a manner they cannot imagine they might be victims of Ebola or Rift Valley fever. Although important, this individual-victim perspective is myopic unless other vantage points of PVV are held equally in view, including the first-level, real-life situations of vectors. From the second level of PVV, much planning appropriately attempts to reduce overall risks of disease spread through the allocation of vaccines and other preventives. At the same time, these decisions must not lose sight of the actual situations of disease victims who may find themselves not in priority groups for care, as well as for overall distributive implications in the population. Adequate planning must take into account both distributions within a population and the circumstances of those not favorably affected by a policy. Finally, the uncertainty of the way-station self—that anyone might be either victim or vector or both, if not of this disease then of others—continues to press that these are concerns for *everyone*, not just for those apparently at greatest risk of becoming ill in real-life circumstances. It is here that pandemic planning requires further attention, to the extent that it fails to focus on the development of health infrastructures that decrease pandemic risks, increase the likelihood of disease identification before spread has become extensive, and reduce the overall burden of disease worldwide.

Justice *Within* Pandemic Planning

A predominant focus of attention within pandemic planning in the developed world has been the allocation of vaccines and antivirals. A second focus has been triage of what is called "surge capacity"—the ability to handle a far larger influx of patients than normal, whether due to a pandemic, a natural disaster, or a terrorist attack. From our PVV perspective, the most important missing element in some of these discussions has been attention to the situation of those we call the "deprioritized": victims or potential victims who are low on lists for vaccines, antivirals, or stepped-up treatment. A noteworthy and admirable exception is the recent European emphasis on protecting individuals as victims by making sure that plans are in place for delivery of supplies and needed services, a predominant initiative of pandemic planning in the European Community for 2008–2010.[8] As with our earlier discussions of constraints and compensation in pandemic planning, we should caution that this discussion is based on a snapshot of plans available in early 2008. Planning recommendations change virtually daily. Despite the moving target, we think that our PVV perspective yields enduring insights into how to approach issues of distributive justice within pandemic planning—as well as how pandemic planning may fit within a more general view about global health security.

Allocating Vaccines and Antivirals: Considering Both Vectors and Victims

Vaccines provide immunity to infection from a pathogen; immunity may be partial or complete. To provide protection, vaccines must be administered sufficiently in advance of exposure for immunity to take hold: approximately two weeks in the case of influenza vaccines. Antivirals such as Tamiflu interfere with viral replication and thus reduce the likelihood that exposure will result in infection, as well as mitigating the severity of infection and contagiousness

---

8. European Centre for Disease Prevention and Control, *Technical Report: Pandemic Influenza Preparedness in the EU/EEA* (December 2007), http://ecdc.europa.eu/Health_topics/Pandemic_Influenza/pdf/Pandemic%20prepare%20web%201.pdf (accessed February 4, 2008), 17.

of the host. For maximum effectiveness, antivirals need to be administered either before infection or early in the course of an infection—the earlier the better—before viral replication has taken extensive hold. Prepandemic vaccines, based on viral strains circulating earlier than the pandemic itself, may turn out to be sufficiently close to an actual pandemic virus to be relatively effective against it. If so—and the science of this is developing rapidly—it might be possible to stockpile prepandemic vaccine sufficiently in advance to obviate some of the rationing issues that we discuss below.

Vaccine Prioritization. In the United States, the initial federal framework for the prioritization of vaccines gave first priority to vaccine and antiviral manufacturers, health-care workers, and essential service personnel. Following these groups for priority were people who were thought most likely to suffer adverse outcomes from influenza infection: the elderly, those with co-morbidities, and the very young.[9] This prioritization also recognized that groups at greatest mortality risk might vary with the type of pandemic—after all, in 1918 it was healthy young adults who had the highest death rate from infection—and concomitant need to reassess these prioritizations as more became known about any particular pandemic. The policies reflected in these prioritizations were maintaining public health and medical-care infrastructures, together with protecting the most vulnerable victims. The prioritizations were criticized, however, for being somewhat self-serving—the definition of "essential services" was at best unclear—and for paying inadequate attention to the role of vaccination in preventing potential disease transmission by targeting those who were most likely to be vectors, such as school-age children.[10]

In the fall of 2007, the United States opened revised draft guidance for allocating vaccines to public comment.[11] The draft guidance attempts to introduce both more precision into the definition of categories and to strike a balance among the competing interests of people in different category types. Thus the structure of the guidance is to identify general categories, "levels" of equal priority within categories, and "tiers" of priority within levels for vaccine

---

9. U.S. Department of Health and Human Services, *HHS Pandemic Influenza Plan*, app. D (November 2005), http://www.hhs.gov/pandemicflu/plan/pdf/AppD.pdf (accessed February 6, 2008), D-13.

10. By Tom May (personal communication) and by Mark Rothstein (personal communication).

11. U.S. Federal Government, *Draft Guidance on Allocating and Targeting Pandemic Influenza Vaccine*, http://www.pandemicflu.gov/vaccine/prioritization.html (accessed February 6, 2008). The comment period closed December 31, 2007. As this book went to press, a report was published of a new technique for cell-culture manufacture of a vaccine effective against a range of H5N1 strains, Hartmut J. Ehrlich et al., "A Clinical Trial of a Whole-Virus H5N1 Vaccine Manufactured from Cell Culture," *New England Journal of Medicine* 358 (2008): 2573–2584. The technique needs less lead time and is not dependent on egg culture—but does require enhanced biosafety protection. Swifter availability of larger supplies of vaccine would both ease the need for prioritization and require re-examination of prioritization categories.

administration depending on the severity of a pandemic. There are four categories: homeland and national security, health care and community support services, critical infrastructure, and the general population. Within each category, some groups have "level A" priority for vaccination—that is, highest priority for vaccination. In the level of homeland and national security, the level A group is "deployed and mission critical personnel"; in the category of health care and community support services, it is public health personnel, inpatient health-care providers, outpatient and home health providers, and health-care providers in long-term care facilities; in the category of critical infrastructure, it is emergency medical service personnel, law enforcement personnel, fire services personnel, manufacturers of pandemic vaccine and antivirals, and key government leaders; and in the category of the general population it is pregnant women and infants between 6 and 35 months. Within level A, there are tiered sub-rankings for administration depending on pandemic severity; for example, pregnant women and infants between 6 and 11 months are in the sixth tier, and other infants are in the final, seventh tier within level A.[12]

In reaching these priorities, the guidance attempts to strike a balance among several values: reciprocity and vaccinating those placed at risk in their jobs; maintaining essential services such as law enforcement and fire protection and vaccinating those who provide them; and protecting the vulnerable and vaccinating those who are likely to become sickest from infection. In the judgment of the draft guidance, this balance reflects values of reciprocity, fairness in the sense of treating everyone as equal, and flexibility.[13] The fairest observation to make about these priorities is that they attempt to strike a balance among these and other competing values. But it is not at all clear that this is the balance that would be struck from the PVV perspective—or that attempting to strike a balance that has something for each of these values is the best way to go about allocating vaccine in pandemic scarcity. To be sure, the emphasis on keeping public health, health care, and other essential services functioning would appear to be well placed, assuming these functions are carefully defined: without these services, efforts to prevent disease spread are more likely to collapse and victims are more likely to go unsupported. But from both the vector- and the victim-side of our PVV perspective, there are important questions to ask about the newest prioritization.

From the vector-side, a central problem is whether the most recent priorities have paid sufficient attention to targeted use of vaccination to prevent spread. An easy concern to raise is that, like the earlier recommended prioritization, this guidance will allocate vaccines to states on the basis of population—surely a strategy that is not the best way to think about prevention even though it may be politically expedient in a federalist system. A more complex question is whether the priorities pay sufficient attention to how pandemic

---

12. U.S. Federal Government, *Draft Guidance*, 5.
13. Ibid., 11.

disease might spread—and to the need to reassess this in the face of actual pandemic circumstances. To take one example: if people are still mobile during the onset of a pandemic, use of public transit is a likely means of disease spread, yet transit workers are not listed in top priority of "critical infrastructure" groups—they are only in level C of three levels within the critical infrastructure category.[14] To take another example: depending on the speed and distribution of pandemic spread (vaccines generally take two weeks to become effective), a plan to deploy vaccination quickly to areas of initial disease identification—and to couple it with a two-week course of antivirals—may be a more successful strategy than a plan to vaccinate people by occupational or disease-risk groups. And to take a final example: from the perspective of prevention, it is not at all clear that the way to protect the most vulnerable—say, infants—is through vaccination of them or whether it is through vaccination of those with whom they might come into contact—say, their parents who go out into the world.

From the victim-side, it might seem that the best strategy is to be in a group that is prioritized to receive vaccine. And so, it might seem, the desired policy is to protect those who are most likely to be vulnerable—that is, whose risks, should they be victims, are the greatest. But from the perspective of someone who does not know her actual circumstances of vulnerability, it is not at all clear that this would be the most justified policy. Obviously, one important goal would be to try to protect all potential victims; for example, by increasing vaccine manufacture capability or by developing prepandemic vaccines of likely efficacy. But if a pandemic is sufficiently severe and swift, these strategies might not be available. And there are other strategies to reduce the overall possibility of victimhood. One strategy is transparency: to make sure that people are fully aware of what the scarcities are and what the implications of those scarcities are for them so that they may take precautions to the extent that they are available; for example, by self-shielding until vaccine supplies increase. Another is the emphasis on prevention—that is, a shift back to the vector-side; the best strategy for possible victims who may not be prioritized for vaccine is to have vaccine deployed in such a way that it reduces and slows down disease spread. This is why emphasis on prevention in vaccine allocation, rather than on vulnerability, may be more justifiable *even to* the vulnerable. It is also why the border strategies that we discussed in Chapter 17 might remain important, even if they are only delaying tactics at best. It is also why attention to other aspects of victimhood, such as the delivery of essential supplies contemplated in the European planning process, might be so critical: if people know they have effective access to essential supplies, self-shielding is far more likely to be available as a protective strategy.

Finally, we note that the U.S. draft guidance does not discuss at all the question of how vaccine will actually be distributed. The United States has a

---

14. Ibid., 5.

history of difficulties over the respective roles of public and private health-care providers when vaccine supplies are scarce.[15] Allegations of favoritism and gaming the system surfaced, for example, when flu vaccine supplies were unexpectedly limited in the winter of 2004–2005.[16] Such favoritism with respect to essential supplies is both wrong and threatens to undermine trust just in the kind of emergency circumstances where trust is important to achieving prevention to the extent possible. Some states' plans, such as New Jersey's, recognize that current vaccine distribution occurs often through private providers and that there may be a need for public intervention in the distribution process.[17] Attending to this issue is thus also critical for pandemic planning in the United States.

In sum, the current U.S. draft guidance for vaccine prioritization is structured in a manner that attempts to reflect multiple values and political pressures, but that might be less effective in prevention than some other strategies. At the same time, it attends to victims in an incomplete way, continuing emphasis on those who might become worst off if they were to become ill but not fully considering other allocative strategies that might reduce their risks of illness overall.

Antivirals. As we have mentioned, antivirals interrupt the replication process of viruses. They may be given either as prophylaxis starting before infection occurs or as treatment that interrupts the course of the disease. As prophylaxis before infection, they must be given on an ongoing basis; thus prophylactic use may consume larger dose numbers and be less efficient overall when supplies are scarce, unless prophylaxis is carefully limited to those at known risk. Conversely, prophylaxis is effective in preventing infection, and such prophylaxis before infection may be the most efficient way to protect people at ongoing risk of exposure, such as health-care workers—at least, until vaccines can be administered and become effective. Because antivirals interrupt replication, once infection occurs they are more effective the earlier they are initiated. "Effective" here is a statistical term, meaning on average "more effective" than no intervention. One estimate of the magnitude of impact for antivirals administered within the first 24 hours of onset of symptoms is the reduction of

15. See, e.g., Monica Schoch-Spana, Joseph Fitzgerald, Bradley R. Kramer, and the UMPC Influenza Task Force, "Influenza Vaccine Scarcity 2004–05: Implications for Biosecurity and Public Health Preparedness," *Biosecurity and Bioterrorism: Biodefense Strategy, Practice, and Science* 3, no. 3 (2005): 211–234; Gardiner Harris, "U.S. Creates Ethics Panel for Priority on Flu Shots," *New York Times*, sec. A, October 28, 2004.
16. E.g., "Vaccine for Congress and the Bears," *New York Times*, sec. A, October 23, 2004, describing how some members of Congress and some players on the Chicago Bears football team had no qualms in lining up for scarce flu vaccine even though they were not in high priority groups.
17. New Jersey Department of Health and Senior Services, *Influenza Pandemic Plan* (draft February 1, 2006), http://www.state.nj.us/health/flu/documents/pandemic_draft_022006.pdf (accessed July 5, 2008), 32–41.

a degree of temperature and a day of illness—in healthy people with seasonal influenza. There is insufficient evidence to predict what the efficacy of antivirals might be in people who become ill with pandemic flu.[18]

An initial point to make about antivirals in pandemic planning, therefore, is that it may not be most sensible to consider the distribution of vaccines and antivirals as separate strategies. From the perspective of prevention, it may be most effective to deploy antivirals in tandem with vaccine, giving antivirals to people such as those care-providers who are at known exposure risk until vaccine becomes available and takes effect. It is also noteworthy that antivirals are quite expensive at least if taken for prolonged prophylaxis, although a treatment course would typically involve only four or five days. For example, one "discount" price advertised over the Internet in early 2008 for Roche's Tamiflu was $90 for a 10-tablet (75mg) package;[19] dosage is 2 tablets a day, so the effective cost per person of Tamiflu prophylaxis purchased in this way would be $18 per day. Another ongoing concern about antivirals is the possibility of resistance; there are recent, alarming reports about strains of seasonal influenza that are resistant to Tamiflu.[20] Strategies of stockpiling antivirals for treatment purposes thus consume scarce economic resources that might otherwise be devoted to developing faster techniques for vaccine manufacture, with gains that are at least somewhat uncertain.

Recommendations for the allocation of antivirals see treatment as the primary goal. The British plan, for example, comments that prophylactic use of antivirals is in general inefficient because it will consume large amounts of scarce dosage. Britain thus plans to use antivirals in initial containment efforts but primarily for treatment of symptomatic patients.[21] With treatment as one central goal in the allocation of antivirals, the U.S. federal plan recommendations allocate to priority groups in the following order: hospitalized patients, health-care

---

18. U.K Department of Health, *Pandemic Flu*, 75; N. Kawai et al., "A Comparison of the Effectiveness of Oseltamivir for the Treatment of Influenza A and Influenza B: A Japanese Multicenter Study of the 2003–2004 and 2004–2005 Influenza Seasons," *Clinical Infectious Diseases* 43, no. 4 (August 15, 2006)::439–444.

19. Mail-RX.com, http://www.mail-rx.com/shop/home.php?cat=255 (accessed February 9, 2008). It is also noteworthy that Roche, the manufacturer of the anti-viral Tamiflu, is now allowing businesses to pay an annual fee to stockpile Tamiflu reserves sufficient to protect their entire work force and hopefully available within 48 hours, http://www.pandemictoolkit.com/tamiflu-supplyordering/stockpiling-dilemma.aspx (accessed July 1, 2008).

20. European Center for Disease Prevention and Control, "Emergence of Seasonal Influenza Viruses Type A/H1N1 with Oseltamivir Resistance in Some European Countries at the Start of the 2007–8 Influenza Season" (January 27, 2008), http://ecdc.europa.eu/pdf/080127_os.pdf (accessed February 3, 2008); Lawrence K. Altman, "Mutant Flu Virus Is Found That Resists Popular Drugs," *New York Times*, January 31, 2008, A10. For mathematical modeling of the effects of population structure on the development of resistance with the use of treatment and prophylaxis during a pandemic, see Florence Debarre, Sebastian Bonhoeffer, and Roland R. Regoes, The Effect of Population Structure on the Emergence of Drug Resistance During Influenza Pandemics, *J. Royal Society Interface* 4 (2007): 893–906, argues that in fragmented populations, development of resistance is less.

21. U.K Department of Health, *Pandemic Flu*, 75–78.

workers and emergency service workers with direct patient contact, high-risk outpatients (e.g., people who are immune-compromised), pandemic health responders and government officials, increased risk outpatients, residents of nursing homes and residents in homes where there has been an outbreak).[22] The justifications for this priority list begin with protecting people at greatest risk of mortality and morbidity—hence the allocation to hospitalized patients for treatment even when they are outside the window in which administration of antivirals is most likely to be effective and at a point at which efficacy is unknown.[23] Protecting those who are most likely to suffer mortality and morbidity is also the rationale for prioritizing high and increased risk groups.[24] Maintaining health-care services, encouraging health-care workers to come to work, and reciprocal obligations to those who incur risks are all given as justifications for providing scarce antivirals to health-care workers—as is the observation that this allocation might be publicly acceptable because of the recognition that health-care workers incur risks in virtue of their jobs.[25]

As with vaccines, there are important questions from the PVV perspective about these allocations. From the vector-side, targeting prophylactics quickly to cases of known exposure will have the greatest impact in reducing viral replication and thus diminishing risks of transmission—but this is not an emphasis in U.S. prioritization. From the victim-side, giving highest priority to hospitalized patients—those whose disease has already become severe—also appears problematic. From the first level as an identified victim—someone who knows that she is already desperately ill—it might seem that any use of antivirals, no matter whether it has a low or unknown probability of success, would be desired. This allocation, however, runs the very real risk of benefiting no one at all. This result surely is not what would be justified from the perspective of our third level, someone who does not know his or her actual circumstances of vulnerability. From this perspective, the most justified policy is that which makes best use of antivirals in interrupting disease processes—that is, trying to target their use to cases of known exposure as well as early symptoms, when there is a very real chance of changing the course of disease. The prioritization of health-care workers reflects this concern to the extent that it is aimed at those who might have suffered exposures; it also responds to obligations to those who take risks in protecting others from disease.

---

22. U.S Department of Health and Human Services, *HHS Pandemic Influenza Plan*, app. D, 21. Like increased availability of vaccine, increased availability of Tamiflu would require rethinking these priorities; nonetheless, there remain questions of justice about proposals such as Roche's offer to stockpile supplies for employers willing to pay for the service, a quite different prioritization than that found in the federal plan.

23. Ibid., 22.

24. Ibid., 24.

25. Ibid., 23.

Priority level 6 in the U.S. recommendations—targeting antivirals as a response to outbreaks in care facilities and in residences—represents a clear effort to intervene where it might be most effective in interrupting the course of disease. However, it is noteworthy that this category groups together widely different cases: residents of long-term care facilities are in the same category as home caregivers for people who are ill and people who are subject to home quarantine because of known exposures. Long-term care residents may be highly likely to die from disease—but there are also questions about whether the administration of antivirals after symptoms have appeared is likely to be effective in altering their disease course and thus to be beneficial to them. Moreover, arguably there are far better ways to protect these residents—for example, by ensuring that during a time of pandemic they are cared for only by people who have been vaccinated or who are taking antiviral prophylaxis and who have followed proper hygienic practices such as hand washing.

By contrast, home caregivers are being relied on by victim-patients; indeed, in a pandemic of any degree of severity, it is likely that such care will be an integral part of efforts to attend to the circumstances of victims. We have already argued that pandemic plans should pay attention to protecting these caregivers through means such as the use of masks and careful instructions about hygiene; antiviral allocation is another aspect of this protection. Moreover, it is arguable that home caregivers are taking on some of the responsibilities of health-care providers, to the extent that they are filling in for health-care capacities that are insufficient to meet need, and therefore that obligations extend to them as well. Finally, people in home quarantine because of an exposure are being constrained as vectors; attention to them as victims requires allocation of antivirals to them as well.

Because of their mechanism of action, antivirals must be deployed rapidly to people who have become symptomatic, if they are to be effective at all. Many U.S. plans, at least in published versions to date, appear uninformative about how rapid distribution is to take place. Mechanisms for identifying exposure or illness in early stages—as by hotlines—are provided in some plans.[26] Methods of delivery need to be clear as well. In the United States, Alaska's plan is somewhat of an exception—it actually lists the planned locations and distribution amounts for Tamiflu.[27] The plan recommends as well that communities work out methods for delivering Tamiflu to homebound and vulnerable people. In comparison, Europe has recently made it an "acid test" for European Economic

26. State of Massachusetts, *Massachusetts Influenza Pandemic Preparedness Plan* (October 2006), http://www.mass.gov/dph/cdc/epii/flu/pandemic_plan_8.pdf (accessed February 9, 2008), 113; New Jersey Department of Health and Senior Services, *Influenza Pandemic Plan* (draft February 1, 2006), http://www.state.nj.us/health/flu/documents/pandemic_draft_022006.pdf (accessed July 5, 2008), 55.

27. State of Alaska, Division of Public Health, *Pandemic Influenza Response Plan* (February, 2008), http://www.pandemicflu.alaska.gov/panfluplan.pdf (accessed July 5, 2008), 35.

Area (EEA) countries in pandemic planning whether social services can deliver antivirals to all who need them within 48 hours of the onset of symptoms.[28] However, this comparison does not imply complete success in Europe: apparently an attempt to create a European stockpile of antivirals was unsuccessful, and different EEA nations have varying levels of supplies available.[29]

Surge Capacity and Palliative Care: Victims Without Care

A second, ethically critical issue in pandemic planning is allocation of treatment for the seriously ill. Pandemic planning models recognize that even in medium-bad case scenarios, some—perhaps even many—people will not receive optimal treatment, or very good treatment, or even any treatment at all. One plan—Idaho's—has chosen a remarkably honest epigram for its pandemic plan: the newspaper description of how Idaho hospitals were overwhelmed in the 1918 pandemic and had to turn to schools and churches as alternative facilities.[30] Many plans make quite clear that care facilities may be utterly inadequate should a pandemic become serious. The U.S. Department of Health and Human Services (HSS) in grim fashion advises health-care facilities that they should make provisions for security to deal with long lines and patients who "because [of] triage or treatment decisions [do] not receiv[e] the care they think they require."[31] Some plans contain milder messages about the need to communicate with the public about where to seek alternative care facilities. Yet many plans—at least the ones available on the Internet—are not fully transparent about the scenarios that may develop. Plans do not spell out where people should go, or where they will not be able to go, as rates of illness increase. Few plans are transparent about prioritization of hospital admission or intensive care services—a point to which we will return below. This is information that is critically important to people as potential victims—both so that they know what they might or might not be able to receive and so that they are aware of the nature of the choices being made.

Expanding "Surge Capacity." Beyond transparency, how should pandemic planning approach issues of scarcity in treatment? One possibility, of course,

---

28. European Centre for Disease Prevention and Control, *Technical Report: Pandemic Influenza Preparedness in the EU/EEA* (December 2007), 15.

29. European Centre for Disease Prevention and Control, "Report for Policymakers: Pandemic Preparedness in the European Union, Autumn 2007," http://ecdc.europa.eu/pdf/2007_12_05_Pand emic%20preparedness%20for%20policymakers.pdf (accessed February 4, 2008), 3.

30. *Idaho Pandemic Influenza Response* (March 2006), http://www.healthandwelfare.idaho.gov/ DesktopModules/Documents/DocumentsView.aspx?tabID=0&ItemID=4523&MId=11634&wversi on=Staging (accessed July 5, 2008), vi.

31. *HHS Pandemic Influenza Plan Supplement 3 Healthcare Planning*, http://www.hhs.gov/pandemicflu/plan/sup3.html#secur (accessed February 9, 2008).

is to attempt to expand capacities for treatment. The HHS high-end estimate is that nationwide 1.5 million people will need intensive care unit treatment in a predictable avian flu epidemic.[32] This will require extensive "surge capacity"—that is, the ability of facilities in a community to respond to a sudden patient load. California planning assumes that by the fifth week of a worst-case pandemic, demand for critical care beds will exceed surge capacity by 1,212% and for ventilators by 1,350%.[33] Other than relying on the Joint Commission on Accreditation of Healthcare Organizations (JCAHO) recommendation for "sufficient" care in emergencies, however, California had not yet laid out further recommendations for allocation of scarce treatment.[34] Massachusetts and Minnesota have quite fully developed plans, envisioning hospitals as critical-care facilities operating in tandem with intermediate care satellite facilities providing surge capacity.[35] New Jersey has innovative plans for mental health services, including telecounseling, as well as plans for outpatient rehydration stations to reduce the need for hospitalization in some cases.[36] As of this writing, none of these states have allocated funding for these or other resources.

In the United States as health-care costs have risen, hospitals and health-care systems have cut back on the numbers of available beds and occupancy rates of 100% or higher are now common.[37] Emergency room capacity has fallen as well. Despite some attention to coordinated disaster planning, estimates now are that the United States falls far short of reasonable levels of disaster preparedness. "Surge capacity" requires not only facilities, but also supplies and adequate staffing. Especially given current pressures on health-care financing in the United States, expanding surge capacity is a very difficult task. One problem is the acute shortage of personnel, especially nurses. Another problem is

32. *HHS Pandemic Influenza Plan* (2005), http://www.hhs.gov/pandemicflu/plan/pdf/HHSPandemicInfluenzaPlan.pdf (accessed May 2007).
33. California Department of Health Services, *Pandemic Influenza Preparedness and Response Plan* (September 8, 2006), http://www.cdph.ca.gov/HealthInfo/discond/Documents/pandemic_influenza_preparedness_response_plan_06.pdf (accessed July 7, 2008), 54.
34. California Department of Health Services, *Pandemic Influenza Preparedness and Response Plan*, 58. The JCAHO reference is JCAHO, *Surge Hospitals: Providing Safe Care During Emergencies* (2006), http://www.jointcommission.org/NR/rdonlyres/802E9DA4-AE80-4584-A205-48989C5BD684/0/surge_hospital.pdf (accessed February 12, 2008). Other illustrative plans clearly recognizing the problem of surge capacity but stopping short of making recommendations include the District of Columbia plan, *Pandemic Influenza Preparedness Plan* (March 2005), http://dchealth.dc.gov/doh/frames.asp?doc=/doh/lib/doh/information/influenza/pdf/dc_pandemic_influenza_plan.pdf (accessed July 4, 2008), 63.
35. State of Massachusetts, *Massachusetts Influenza Preparedness Plan*, 50; Minnesota Department of Health, *Pandemic Influenza Plan* (April 2006), http://www.health.state.mn.us/divs/idepc/diseases/flu/pandemic/plan/mdhpanfluplan.pdf (accessed July 5, 2008), 133–162.
36. New Jersey Department of Health and Senior Services, *Pandemic Preparedness Plan*, 59, 72.
37. The discussion in this paragraph is based on Amy H. Kaji, Kristi L. Koenig, and Roger J. Lewis, "Current Hospital Disaster Preparedness," *Journal of the American Medical Association* 298, no. 18: 2188–2190 (November 14, 2007).

the lack of adequate primary care networks as well as support for primary care that result in increased burdens on existing emergency departments. In other words, in the judgment of a recent analysis by Kaji, Koenig, and Lewis, the problem of surge capacity is deeply intertwined with other problems in the delivery of health care in the United States. Development of more adequate surge capacity may rest on attending to some of these more systemic problems—and not to a simpler solution such as purchasing additional ventilators or identifying alternatives to hospitals such as closed schools where very ill patients can be housed. In the United States, the Veterans' Administration medical system is attempting to implement a coordinated systemwide response, which includes improved primary care infrastructure (such as ensuring high rates of vaccination), attention to staffing needs, and the identification of alternative care facilities.[38] This need to embed surge capacity planning into issues of access to health care more generally is but one suggestion of how issues of justice within pandemic planning may raise larger questions of distributive justice in health care, a point to which we will return below.

Seeing the issue of surge capacity in the context of health infrastructure more generally is not just a practical matter of developing an effective strategy. It is also morally required. From the first level of our PVV perspective—this patient, now, confronted with a grave illness—it would seem that what is most desirable is immediate access to whatever form of intensive care has any possibility of proving effective. As we have argued throughout this volume, however, to view justification from this immediacy of victimhood is myopic. We are all in some respects potential victims or vectors; from that perspective, practices are most justifiable that reduce the possibility of vectorhood and thus reduce overall burdens of disease, as well as addressing the range of possible situations of victims. Efforts to develop primary care structures that identify disease early and that increase the likelihood that victims will be treated while disease is incipient and more easily addressed would be most important from our PVV justificatory perspective. Thus, attention to the infrastructure that can support surge capacity is both a useful strategy and a moral imperative.

Allocating Care. Unfortunately, it remains all too likely that the United States—and the world in general—will not have addressed issues of health infrastructure effectively before the advent of a pandemic. Moreover, even with improved infrastructure, it remains possible that natural—or bioterrorism-caused—pandemic conditions may obtain. In such circumstances, on what bases should

38. Department of Veterans Affairs, *VA Pandemic Influenza Plan* (March 2006), *http://www. publichealth.va.gov/Flu/documents/VAPandemicFluPlan_2006-03-31.pdf* (accessed July 2 2008), 12.

available care be allocated? These situations are what John Rawls called "partial compliance" contexts—situations in which ideal justice does not obtain. As we have noted, Rawls considers two importantly different kinds of partial compliance contexts, without discussion of the difference between the two: those that are infused by social injustice, in this case the injustice of failures to address issues of health infrastructure; and those that are in the main the result of disasters, either natural or manmade.[39] An important final question to address is the relevance of background injustice—whether social or natural—to pandemic allocation decisions.

Drawing from the Toronto Centre's *Stand on Guard for Thee*, several pandemic plans have begun to address quite directly prioritization of higher-level care on a principled ethical basis. In the United States, the Tennessee plan is an early example. Tennessee proposes to base allocation decisions on the values of "stewardship" and "reciprocity." Stewardship in the sense of careful use of scarce resources recommends giving lesser priority to people who are not expected to benefit from hospitalization, people with less than five years of expected survival, and people who are expected to need scarce resources for longer periods of time. The value of reciprocity leads Tennessee to give priority to health-care workers and others who have risked infection in pandemic control.[40]

A more recent example is a Canadian proposal,[41] also developed on the basis of *Stand on Guard for Thee* and later incorporated in a plan for Utah.[42] This proposal utilizes the values of equality of access and fairness of treatment. Equality of access is understood to mean that all have an equal claim to treatment evaluated in terms of inclusion and exclusion criteria. These criteria are developed through an assessment tool for survival and need for care. People will have low priority on the one hand if they have limited chances of survival even with treatment and on the other hand if they have very high chances of survival without treatment. Reassessment is on an ongoing basis; a patient who might have qualified for intensive care on one day may no longer qualify on the next.

From our victim/vector perspective, the decision of both Tennessee and the Canadian proposal to understand equal treatment in terms of stewardship of

39. John Rawls, *A Theory of Justice* (Cambridge: Harvard University Press, 1971), 244–245.
40. Tennessee Department of Health, *Pandemic Influenza Response Plan* (July 2006), http://health.state.tn.us/CEDS/PDFs/2006_PanFlu_Plan.pdf (accessed July 5, 2008), 129–130.
41. The proposal is Christian et al., Development of a Triage Protocol for Critical Care During an Influenza Pandemic," *Canadian Medical Association Journal* 175, no. 11 (November 21, 2006): 1377–1381. Although this protocol claims to be based on *Stand on Guard for Thee*, commentators have questioned whether the values in the latter are fully represented in the former. Ryan M. Melnychuk and Nuala P. Kenny, "Pandemic Triage: The Ethical Challenge," *Canadian Medical Association Journal* 175, no. 11 (November 21, 2006): 1393.
42. Utah Hospitals and Health Systems Association, *Utah Pandemic Influenza Hospital and ICU Triage Guidelines* (draft December 7, 2007), http://www.pandemicflu.utah.gov/plan/med_triage120707.pdf (accessed July 5 2008).

resources is a reasonable one. Such prioritization husbands resources to give people overall the best chance that effective treatment will be available for them. However, our PVV perspective also reminds us of several noteworthy aspects of these decisions. First, from the perspective of someone who might be a victim, it is especially important for the "deprioritization" that is contemplated not to mean "being ignored." The Canadian document, followed by Utah's proposal, mentions the importance of palliative care for those who are not prioritized. Yet while there is extensive attention in the proposals to assessment methods for triage, there is no further discussion of what palliative care might be required or how it might be provided. "Discharge to home" is the contemplated strategy when even ordinary hospital floors are full or patients do not meet triage criteria for hospital admission—but surely an adequate account of what discharge might involve includes pain management, methods to deal with distress from air hunger, and psychosocial support for both victims and their caregivers.

A second issue that is not attended to at all in pandemic advance care triage plans is raised by the possibility of partial compliance contexts that result from injustice in health care—and is especially noticeable from the population level of our PVV perspective. When care is triaged according to the proposed medical criteria of survivability and need, certain distributive patterns may emerge, as Tabery and Mackett have pointed out.[43] One pattern is that groups already disadvantaged in access to health care may be further disadvantaged in pandemic prioritization. For example, African-Americans for a variety of reasons may be over-represented among patients who are so severely ill when they come to medical attention that their probabilities of survival are lower than the survival probabilities of patients in other groups. African-Americans are less likely to have a source of primary care and so less likely to receive vaccine or to be seen early in the course of disease; they are more likely to live in crowded urban areas and to be dependent on modes of public transit where exposure might be more expected (especially if, as we have noted, prophylaxis is not prioritized to transportation workers); and they are more likely to be in poor health status and thus experience greater severity of disease. Depending on the type of pandemic, African-Americans thus might be over-represented among the sickest—and under-represented among those triaged to care. To be sure, the likelihood of any pattern such as this will depend on

---

43. James Tabery, Charles W. Mackett III, and the UPMC Pandemic Influenza Task Force's Triage Review Board, "The Ethics of Triage in the Event of an Influenza Pandemic," *Disaster Medicine and Public Health Preparedness* 2, no. 2 (June 2008): 114–118. These authors defend a hybrid ethical model of triage, emphasizing utility (who can most benefit), narrow social utility (who is most needed to maintain health care and social infrastructure during a pandemic), and egalitarianism (who is most needy; egalitarian considerations also temper utility when unintended patterns of racism or other forms of discrimination become apparent).

the nature and distribution of a pandemic. We are not arguing here for addition of a kind of "affirmative action" criterion to pandemic triage that disrupts attention to the effort to triage care where it will be most effective. What we do claim is that the possibility of a result such as this—although the subject of much attention in the aftermath of Hurricane Katrina—has gone largely unnoticed in pandemic triage discussions and that this is a matter of concern. At a minimum, we think, reducing the likelihood that pandemic triage will compound existing patterns of injustice is another argument for attention to basic health-care infrastructure: to the kind of primary care networks and trust in the health-care system that decrease existing injustice and thus the likelihood that pandemic planning would compound it.

Palliative Care. As we have already indicated, plans in the United States take quite different positions about responsibilities for home care. Some have attempted to identify agencies such as the Red Cross that may be available to help out. Others, however, view stockpiling essential supplies and home remedies as fundamentally an individual responsibility. By contrast, as we have also indicated, Britain's plan devotes far more attention to the development of the infrastructure that may be needed to deliver essential supplies to people in home isolation or quarantine. This question—whether home care is a social or an individual responsibility—looms with even greater urgency when people are triaged not to receive advanced care and sent home because there is insufficient surge capacity to include everyone who might otherwise receive treatment in hospitals or intensive care units.

These "deprioritized"—people who are sent home because treatment is not available for them—will include the sickest victims. Considering them as victims, therefore, requires significant attention to palliative care modalities that might be available for them in an out of hospital setting. For example, might it be possible to develop methods of dealing with respiratory distress that do not require the sophistication of hospital personnel and equipment? What kinds of pain medication might be appropriate to ease distress, and how can it be administered at home? Depending on the type of pandemic illness, what other forms of care might be needed to relieve distress: for example, is there likely to be vomiting or diarrhea, with the need for medication to relieve nausea or other forms of abdominal distress? Is there likely to be bleeding, with all the needs for care that might involve? These are questions that, as far as we know, have not been addressed extensively in pandemic planning to date—yet they are critical to the recognition of the deprioritized as victim. These questions are particularly challenging if a wider range of pandemics is contemplated: not only influenza, but hemorrhagic fevers, asphyxiating conditions, or any of the myriad designer diseases bioterrorists might concoct.

Compensation for the Deprioritized? A final question that has not been raised at all in pandemic planning discussions is compensation for those who are deprioritized for care. Although we do think there are significant differences between the social decisions that result in deprioritization and those that impose constraints, we also think some similarities warrant exploration. Like constraints, decisions to prioritize vaccines, antivirals, and intensive care represent social choices to treat individuals in specific ways and to provide scarce resources to some but not to others. Prioritization decisions are necessitated just in conditions of emergency and scarcity; that is, as explained above, "partial compliance" contexts in which ideal justice cannot be achieved. No matter how careful and well reasoned, prioritization may leave those who otherwise might have had access to supplies without them—or it may be yet another instance in which some are left without any access to care. Health-care facilities may be given over to treating infectious disease victims, thus displacing others who need ongoing care from the facilities, such as cancer patients in the midst of chemotherapy or dialysis patients who require ongoing treatment. Some state plans explicitly contemplate discharging patients who are less acutely ill, postponing elective procedures, and triaging patients more stringently.[44] This may be especially problematic for those who are dependent on public facilities (such as emergency rooms in public hospitals) for their health care and who thus may find themselves without access to care for other conditions such as diabetes or asthma.[45] Health-care workers who otherwise might have been available to treat the chronically ill also may be diverted to efforts to manage a pandemic.

The role of social choices in the imposition of constraints, we argued in Chapter 18, is part of what grounds obligations to compensate as a matter of response to constraints. As we have just considered, social choices are explicit in pandemic triage—or implicit in the background that generates at least some triage problems in the first place. Social choices are involved in whether government funding is directed toward production of vaccines or antivirals, or toward the purchase of additional therapeutic equipment such as respirators. For example, although in 2007, the Infectious Diseases Society of America (IDSA) recommended devoting $2.8 billion toward influenza vaccine development,[46] U.S. federal investment in vaccine technology in 2007 was far

---

44. See, e.g., Illinois Pandemic Response Plan, http://www.idph.state.il.us/pandemic_flu/Illinois%20Pandemic%20Flu%20Plan%20101006%20Final.pdf (accessed July 1, 2008), 19.
45. See, e.g., Mark Rothstein. "Are Traditional Public Health Strategies Consistent with Contemporary American Values?" *Temple Law Review* 77 (2004): 175–192 (179).
46. Infectious Diseases Society of America, *Pandemic and Seasonal Influenza*, http://www.idsociety.org/influenza.htm (accessed February 9, 2008).

below that amount.[47] Overall, the Bush administration's 2009 budget proposal for infectious disease contains cutbacks that will leave many infectious disease programs "in shock," in the judgment of the IDSA.[48] To take another example, the HHS influenza plan recommends stockpiling antivirals at a level necessary to treat only 25% of the U.S. population.[49]

Thus persons who are deprioritized in pandemic planning are treated by social choices in a manner that creates anticipated risks of harm to them. Furthermore, as we have argued, these choices may compound existing injustices. And the choices to prioritize are choices that are made to benefit everyone: sometimes by attempting to prevent the spread of disease, sometimes by maintaining health care and other services, sometimes as a response to the risks taken by health-care workers and others, and sometimes as a way to use scarce resources in a manner that has the greatest likelihood of proving benefit overall. These are all important similarities between the argument for compensating those who are harmed by constraints and the situation of those who are harmed by deprioritization.

But there are also differences between constraints and deprioritization that make extension of the argument problematic. As with constraints, a principal concern with this argument is that it proves too much. It may be difficult or impossible to trace causal chains from the deprioritization to the harm—would this person have survived if he or she had received antivirals in time, or been admitted to an intensive care unit? A reply is that it is the decision to deprioritize that is the basis of the claim for responsiveness, not a causal link between the prioritization and any harm. However, characterizing deprioritization as a "harm" assumes a baseline on which people ordinarily would have received the care in question. Arguably, it is more problematic to regard not reaching this baseline as "harm" than it is to judge the imposition of constraints as "harm." Moreover, if deprioritization during a pandemic is a "harm" warranting compensation, why does it not follow more generally that other deprioritization decisions in non-pandemic circumstances are also harms warranting compensation? If duties to compensate apply to those who are deprioritized during a pandemic, are there also duties to compensate people who are deprioritized in the delivery of health care in the United States today?

A simple response to this question is that the situations are different: in pandemic planning, it is the clear social decision about priority, made for the overall social good, that generates obligations in return. With respect to health

47. See, e.g., Maryn McKenna, "The Pandemic Vaccine Puzzle: Part 1," http://www.cidrap.umn.edu/cidrap/content/influenza/panflu/news/oct2507panvax1.html (accessed February 9, 2008).
48. Infectious Diseases Society of America, "President's FY 2009 Budget will Leave Many Infectious Disease Programs in Shock," (February 7, 2008), http://www.idsociety.org/Content.aspx?id=9772 (accessed February 11, 2008).
49. U.S Department of Health and Human Services, *HHS Pandemic Influenza Plan*, 6.

care in the United States, many different decisions or non-decisions lie behind
access to care and priorities are not established in a manner that limits access
for some specifically as a way to protect others in a situation of emergency.
This answer is too simple, however. The situations of deprioritization and lack
of access to health care are similar at least to the extent that some social decisions about health-care priorities disadvantage some to the benefit of others.
For example, decisions not to fund an expansion of the publicly funded S-CHIP
in the United States are tied to views about the desirability of reducing the role
of government and providing tax cuts to some who are reasonably well off—at
least, better off than the children who would have been insured. This is not
enough by itself to generate an obligation to compensate: after all, many social
decisions disadvantage some to the advantage of others. It would need to be
coupled with an argument that the prioritizations are unjust in such a way that
the benefits to some warrant compensating others for any resulting harms.[50]
We are not prepared to make that argument at this point; however, we do believe that our PVV perspective supports an argument that much of the failure
to provide for global health security in the world today is unjust, an argument
to which we now turn.

PVV, the Justice of Pandemic Planning, and Global Health Security

We have already noted a number of respects in which pandemic planning decisions require further attention to health infrastructure in order to be justified from our PVV perspective. Global surveillance—critically important to
the early identification of possible pandemic infection—depends both practically and ethically on structures that can offer treatment. Adequate health infrastructures are important in vaccine development, too: countries have been unwilling to share the viral samples needed for vaccine research and development
without assurance that they also will benefit.[51] Without access to primary care,

---

50. Thomas Pogge has argued that obligations to attempt to mitigate the health conditions of others
are dependent in part on relational factors: that is, on whether the conduct of some is related to
the health conditions of others. If the conduct of some impoverishes others, and impoverishment
is related to diminished health status, Pogge contends, the former have an obligation to attempt
to mitigate the health conditions of the latter. See Thomas W. Pogge, "Relational Conceptions of
Justice: Responsibilities for Health Outcomes," in *Public Health, Ethics, and Equity*, ed. Sudhir
Anand, Fabienne Peter, and Amartya Sen (Oxford: Oxford University Press, 2004), 131–161. An argument for compensation would take Pogge's reasoning a step further: that benefiting from practices that diminish the health status of others not only requires responsibility to attempt to ameliorate that ill health, but also requires compensation for the harm caused. Our argument in what
follows is that interconnection in a web of infectious disease—our PVV perspective—requires
provision for global health security, whether or not individuals or societies have benefited from
practices that adversely affect the health status of others.
51. USINFO.STATE.GOV, "Indonesia Agrees to Resume Sharing Avian Flu Samples," (March 27,
2007), http://www.america.gov/st/washfile-english/2007/March/200703271518131cnirellepo.7828638.

people are less likely to identify disease, receive vaccine or prophylaxis when needed, or identify symptoms early enough to permit antiviral treatment to be effective. Pandemic planners in Europe, for example, have judged that attention to the health infrastructure needed to provide ordinary care for people in the case of seasonal influenza is a critical strategy for preparation for pandemic influenza.[52] Arizona's effort in its pandemic plan to understand ways of communicating with special populations—the elderly, people with disabilities, and people who do not speak English—is an excellent example of how infrastructures might be developed to help build the trust that is essential for health-care delivery to be effective in crisis situations.[53] The development of surge capacity to improve health-care delivery in pandemics or in other emergencies likewise requires attention to health infrastructure. Allocation of scarce intensive care to patients who are most likely to benefit may compound patterns of disadvantage, if attention is not paid to these patterns in the first place.

Questions of justice within pandemic planning thus cannot be considered without attention to the justice *of* pandemic planning. By this claim, we do not mean that pandemic planning should be ignored. Rather, we mean that questions of justice within pandemic planning cannot be addressed in an ethically satisfactory manner without attention to health-care justice more generally—that is, that "pandemic myopia" is misguided. Thus we want to show how our PVV perspective can ground the claim that justice requires access to a decent minimum of primary care and treatment.

From the first level of our PVV analysis, individuals care about their individual health status and the health of their family and friends and thus about how health-care delivery structures are likely to affect them as actually likely victims or vectors of disease. From this perspective, people who have relatively secure access to health care may seem to have little interest in what happens to others and thus little interest in more robust systems of health security. As long as individuals are immunized, or otherwise unlikely to catch communicable diseases from others because of where they live or the health and living choices they make, it might seem that it does not matter to them how those others fare. But even at this first level, such insulated health security is unstable at best. The possibility of pandemic influenza is perhaps the most powerful illustration of this for people in the developed world today, but so are possibilities of measles, mumps, whooping cough, and other transmissible infectious diseases for which immunization rates remain less than optimal and have been declining.

---

html (accessed February 9, 2008).

52. European Centre for Disease Prevention and Control, *Technical Report: Pandemic Influenza*, 18.

53. Arizona Department of Health Services, *Demographics and Effective Risk Communication* (April 2005), http://www.azdhs.gov/phs/edc/edrp/es/pdf/adhsspecialpopstudy.pdf (accessed January 26, 2008).

What this analysis from our first level suggests is the importance of a robust public health infrastructure, where people are treated for diseases that they or others might catch, even in areas of the developed world where health security for some is relatively great. Critical here is funding for vaccination and vaccine development, as well as for inexpensive and widely available modes of treatment for infectious disease. Critical also is the presence of the kind of primary care system that encourages people to be vaccinated, as well as to seek treatment early for conditions that might prove contagious.

By contrast, from the actual circumstances of victims and vectors of infectious disease, health security for non-communicable conditions might at first glance seem less important. The intensive investment in the United States, for example, in treatment for diseases that are not communicable—heart disease, cancer, even diabetes—might at first glance seem unsupported from the first level of PVV, despite the use of the rhetoric of "epidemic" in referring to conditions such as diabetes, a rhetoric that appeals to the possibility of extensive victimhood.

Even at this first level, however, there are important arguments for the expansion of health security that this analysis overlooks. The more that public facilities or public funding are available for the treatment of common ailments such as diabetes for people who could not afford treatment, for example, the higher the likelihood that people will receive primary care in general. Robust health infrastructures such as this increase the likelihood of access to more general primary care and thus to routine immunization. Access to primary care also makes it more likely that people will have a source and the trust to seek care if they become ill with diseases that are communicable. Influenza surveillance is an example of the importance of such access to primary care. To take but one example, the current strategy for monitoring influenza infections in the United States involves identified sentinel providers submitting samples to state health department laboratories that in turn report infection sub-types to the CDC.[54] Unless patients access providers—whether for diabetes or for the flu—this system will not function to identify novel viral strains.

From this perspective, for many in the developed world, it might also seem that much of the untreated burden of diseases in the developing world is of little consequence. The diarrheal diseases that kill so many infants in areas of the world with unsanitary water, for example, seem unlikely to spread to the United States, even as air travel increases. Yet some of this sense of safety may be illusory. West Nile virus, unheard of in the United States 20 years ago, has now been reported in mosquito and avian populations in all states but Alaska,

54. The White House, *National Strategy for Pandemic Influenza Implementation Plan One Year Summary* (July 2007), http://www.whitehouse.gov/homeland/pandemic-influenza-oneyear.html (accessed January 26, 2008).

Hawaii, and Maine; in 2007, human cases were reported in every state but the above-mentioned three, as well as New Hampshire, Vermont, Washington, and West Virginia.[55] Dengue fever, hardly a disease familiar to most Americans, is now regarded as a potential threat to public health in the United States; the mosquito vectors of the disease have been multiplying and spreading at remarkable rates, perhaps owing to global climate change, and are now found in 36 states.[56] Gostin has recently argued that both narrow and enlightened self-interest support a moral interest of the developed world in the health status of people in the developing world.[57] The argument from narrow self-interest is the point we have just made about dengue fever: no one, anywhere in the world today, is safe from infectious diseases, both familiar and emerging ones. Gostin's argument from an enlightened self-interest perspective is that improving health status in impoverished countries benefits travel, world trade, and national security.

From our PVV perspective, Gostin's argument based on self-interest, even enlightened self-interest, is a "first-level" argument. That is, it is an argument based on how individuals from their real-life circumstances perceive themselves as victims or vectors, threats or the objects of threats. This perspective is inherently unstable, however, for it depends on current perceptions of apparent safety or apparent danger. These perceptions may be accurate—or they may be dangerously wrong. Moreover, they are not based on the deeper understanding of the way-station self that our PVV perspective reveals. From the third level of our PVV perspective, we see that we are enmeshed in a web of infectious disease such that we are all potential victims and vectors to each other. The interest we have in global health security is thus not a contingent interest: it is essential to who we are as human beings.

From the third level of our PVV perspective, the current failure to attend to global health security against the burden of infectious disease is unjustifiable. This conclusion is but a starting place for enormous questions about how such attention should ethically be achieved. Even establishing that global health security is a worldwide human responsibility is an important beginning, however. In the next chapter, we develop far more fully some of the ethical and political issues that might be involved in reducing the overall burden of infectious disease. Here, we merely sketch some issues that should come to the fore.

55. CDC, 2007 *West Nile Virus Activity in the United States* (reported as of January 8, 2008), http://www.cdc.gov/ncidod/dvbid/westnile/Mapsactivity/surv&contro107Maps.htm (accessed January 27, 2008).
56. David Morens and Anthony S. Fauci, "Dengue and Hemorrhagic Fever: A Potential Threat to Public Health in the United States," *Journal of the American Medical Association* 299, no.2 (2008): 214–216.
57. Lawrence O. Gostin, "Why Rich Countries Should Care About the World's Least Healthy People," *Journal of the American Medical Association* 298, no. 1 (2007): 89–92.

First, as vaccination is the best preventive—after all, someone who is vaccinated is unlikely to get sick and pass disease on to others, thus interrupting the chain of disease transmission—far more attention to vaccine development and vaccination is critical. Yet even in wealthy countries such as the United States, funding for vaccination and development of new vaccines has been lagging.[58] And elsewhere in the world, vaccination rates remain low for diseases such as measles[59] or even polio[60] in some areas. The WHO strategic plan of the Initiative for Vaccine Research emphasizes the need for development of vaccines against diseases that are major killers of people in poverty: especially HIV/AIDS, malaria, and tuberculosis.[61]

Second, investment in other forms of disease prevention remains problematic. Beyond poverty itself, poor sanitation and unclean water are major sources of infection, from infant diarrhea to cholera.[62] Bednets—the cheap and highly effective means for interrupting malaria transmission, especially for infants[63]—are still far from universally available.

Third, inexpensive forms of treatment are all-too-scarce, in the developing world but also in areas of the developed world. Treatment for HIV infection, as well as other essential medications, remains unaffordable in many areas of the developing world.[64] Over 45 million residents of the United States lack health insurance, many of them children. The problem of antimicrobial resistance also continues to grow, as we explained in Chapter 13, as does insufficient attention to the development of replacement drugs. In many areas of the world, simple primary care infrastructures—storefront clinics, mobile units, public clinics, and the like—are utterly unavailable; yet accessible care is, as we

---

58. See, e.g., Grace M. Lee et al., "Gaps in Vaccine Financing for Underinsured Children in the United States," *Journal of the American Medical Association* 298, no. 6 (August 2007): 638–643.

59. The WHO vaccine campaign against measles resulted in a 68% drop in the death rate from measles worldwide between 2000 and 2007; however, 600 children still die every day from this disease that is preventable with a vaccine that costs less than $1. Measles Initiative, http://www.measlesinitiative.org/index3.asp (accessed February 11, 2008).

60. Although progress continues to be made, in 2006 WHO estimated immunization rates of below 50% in some areas of sub-Saharan Africa and rates hovering between 50 and 75% in areas of Africa and Southeast Asia. WHO, "Immunization Coverage with 3rd Dose of Polio Vaccines in Infants, 2006," http://www.who.int/immunization_monitoring/diseases/Polio_coverage_map.jpg (accessed February 11, 2008).

61. WHO Initiative for Vaccine Research, *Strategic Plan* 2006–2009, http://www.who.int/vaccine_research/documents/Final_version.pdf (accessed February 11, 2008), 6.

62. WHO, "Cholera Prevention and Control," http://www.who.int/topics/cholera/control/en/index.html (accessed February 11, 2008).

63. See, e.g., CDC, "Malaria: Vector Control," http://www.cdc.gov/malaria/control_prevention/vector_control.htm (accessed February 11, 2008).

64. Robert Steinbrook, "Closing the Affordability Gap for Drugs in Low-Income Countries," *New England Journal of Medicine* 357, no. 20 (November 15, 2007): 1996–1999.

have suggested, critical to encouraging people to seek care and thus to the early identification of emerging disease.

Admittedly, identification of these priorities does not provide an argument from justice for advanced treatment of advanced cancer or of non-communicable or degenerative diseases such as Alzheimer's. In our PVV perspective, these priorities—so much the concern of health care in the United States—should take something of a back seat. But we should note that this back seat is not a vacant seat. For one thing, many of the infrastructural reforms that we are suggesting may reduce other disease risks. Moreover, better access to primary care may result in earlier diagnosis of non-infectious diseases. Arguably, access to at least a decent minimum of care overall—however this is to be defined in the wide variety of societies across the globe—is critical to the trust needed for the health-care infrastructure which, as we have argued, is ultimately critical to improving global health security against infectious disease. Therefore, even with respect to other conditions, we are all in this together—at least to some extent. Indeed, as we are learning more about the interplay between infectious disease and diseases once thought to be non-infectious—HPV and cervical cancer, for example—we may find that separating efforts to reduce the global burden of infectious disease from efforts to reduce global burdens of disease more generally may prove scientifically unfounded.

Nearly fifty years ago, in the context of racial discrimination, the Reverend Martin Luther King, Jr., wrote about social interconnectedness: "We are caught in an inescapable network of mutuality, tied in a single garment of destiny. Whatever affects one directly affects all indirectly."[65] Although King was writing about social interconnectedness, his language captures perfectly the biological interconnectedness that is the basis for our account of the way-station self and the implications for distributive justice of viewing human life in this way. In the final part of the book, we turn to a fuller account of what might be involved in reducing the global burden of infectious disease.

---

65. Rev. Martin Luther King, Jr., "Letter from Birmingham City Jail," http://www.crisispapers.org/liberty/king-letter.htm (accessed February 19, 2008).

PART V: MAKING USE OF THE *PATIENT AS VICTIM AND VECTOR* VIEW

THINKING BIG: EMERGING GLOBAL EFFORTS FOR THE CONTROL OF INFECTIOUS DISEASE

Despite the devastating pandemic of HIV/AIDS that erupted in the early 1980s, despite the failure to eradicate polio and the emergence of resistant forms of tuberculosis that came into focus in the 1990s, and despite newly emerging diseases like SARS in 2003 and the fearsome prospect of human-to-human avian flu, this is nevertheless a time of some excitement over prospects for effective control of much of infectious disease. Funded by national and international governmental and nongovernmental organizations (NGOs), private foundations, and even popular entertainers, large-scale new efforts are under way to address global killers like AIDS, tuberculosis, and malaria, among others. Legal standoffs over patent rights to antiretrovirals and other drugs have to some extent been resolved, and pressure is being exerted for the improvement of infrastructure issues, like clean water and improved sanitation. Research in the identification of pathogens, as well as in the prevention, diagnosis, and treatment of infectious diseases, has made very great progress in some areas, especially in vaccine development, the development of rapid tests, and in the establishment of globally coordinated disease outbreak surveillance networks. At last, attention is being focused on orphan infectious diseases and the so-called neglected tropical diseases. It is, we think, a moment of growing optimism. Finally, after what has seemed like a long hiatus—roughly since the late 1960s and early 1970s, when, as we saw at the outset of this book, the then Surgeon General apparently said that it was time to "close the book on infectious disease" and concern over infectious disease was slipping out of public view in the developed world—broad and publicly visible efforts at control are now again being made as a central part of the new concern for global health. Progress, it seems, is in the air.

This chapter is a modified and extended version of Margaret P. Battin, Charles B. Smith, Leslie P. Francis, and Jay A. Jacobson, "Toward the Control of Infectious Disease: Ethical Challenges for a Global Effort," in *International Public Health Policy and Ethics*, ed. Michael Boylan, Dordrecht, Netherlands: Springer, 2008, pp. 191-214. By kind permission of Springer Science and Business Media.

A "Marvelous Momentum" for the Control of Infectious Disease

It is important to understand how very recent the new optimism is—as of 2008 it is not quite a decade old. In 1999, the Gates Foundation announced that it would contribute $25 million to the International AIDS Vaccine Initiative (IAVI) to further the development of an AIDS vaccine, and the following year dedicated $90 million toward control of HIV/AIDS in Africa, especially to decrease the rates of new infections and maternal-child transmission and provide resources and training in palliative care to children orphaned by AIDS.[1] The impressive size of the Gates Foundation's contributions, together with the fact that they came from a private entity rather than a governmental organization, contributed to a new optimism that at last something could be done to try to bring under control one of the world's most devastating pandemics—one that echoes the plagues of the middle ages and the 1918 influenza.

In the perception of both the public and of many professionals, this infusion of money and energy served as the turning point after years in which many institutions and governments, including that of the United States, had done little or nothing to try to stop the AIDS pandemic as a global phenomenon—even after effective drugs had been developed.[2] The wealthy nations, especially the United States, had been attentive to issues of HIV treatment in their own populations and patent protections for their own pharmaceutical industries, but seemingly oblivious to the skyrocketing death rate in the developing world and the devastation of an entire continent. HIV control on a global scale seemed impossible. However, galvanized perhaps by the infusion of both optimism and cash from the Gates Foundation (its endowment nearly doubled by Warren Buffett's 2006 gift of most of his fortune), within the past decade governments, NGOs, public/private partnerships, multinational corporations, religious groups, and entertainers have rushed to contribute to a far more concerted effort to reduce the global burden of HIV and with it, other infectious diseases as well.

In fact, considerable progress toward the control of infectious disease had been made during the 1970s and 1980s in the development of vaccines, anti-infectives, and methods for disease prevention and treatment. With the emergence of HIV/AIDS on a global scale, the public awakened as well. The World Health Organization (WHO) had been making tireless efforts over the years, culminating in the ambitious 3 by 5 program to have 3 million HIV patients receiving antiretroviral therapy by 2005. In addition to Gates, other foundations had been concerned with global health, like the Rockefeller Foundation;

---

1. Bill and Melinda Gates Foundation, "The Bill & Melinda Gates Foundation Announces New HIV/AIDS Grants at World AIDS Conference," http://www.gatesfoundation.org/GlobalHealth/Pri_Diseases/HIVAIDS/Announcements/Announce-245.htm (accessed February 16, 2008).
2. Jon Cohen, "The New World of Global Health," *Science* 311, no. 5758 (January 13, 2006): 162–167.

so were many national and international governmental institutions. Evolving market forces and improved education also played some role. But the Gates Foundation's immense contribution of private funding to fight AIDS has served as a catalyst, giving focus to many other efforts, both those initiated beforehand and especially those introduced afterward. Governments of affluent countries have become major donors to efforts to improve global health: the United States, France, Italy, the United Kingdom, Canada, Germany, the Netherlands, Sweden, Spain, Norway Denmark, and Russia, ranked by size of contribution to the Global Fund as of early 2008;[3] but less affluent countries have also been donors: Romania, Brazil, Mexico, Slovenia, Poland and Hungary.[4] Funds have poured in from multiple sources—a total of some $35 billion, by one estimate, as of January 2006.[5] Laurie Garrett, seconded by Paul Farmer, calls this "a marvelous momentum" toward assistance in global health.[6]

This picture of progress and emerging comprehensive global efforts toward the improvement of global health and with it, the control of infectious disease, is hardly a fully coordinated or integrated one: efforts by one foundation or NGO sometimes reduplicate efforts by another, and related but not-quite-parallel research programs leave gaps where articulation of related efforts might be much closer. Competition between entities, international tensions, commercial agendas, and very different styles of research funding and priority-setting make the picture far from seamless. Political agendas sometimes undercut research; research sometimes violates local custom or understandings of fairness; popular misunderstandings sometimes block immunization drives and other efforts to control the transmission of disease. Officials at one organization complain of dominance by another.[7] There have been

---

3. The largest governmental donation to this international cause so far has come from the United States, with leadership from President George W. Bush and bipartisan support from Congress; over 19 billion U.S. dollars have been allocated to the President's Emergency Plan for AIDS Relief (PEPFAR) for prevention, treatment, and care in developing countries, Sheryl Gay Stolberg, "In Global Battle on AIDS, Bush Creates Legacy," *New York Times*, U.S. section, January 5, 2008. In his final State of the Union address on January 28, 2008 President Bush upped the ante by urging Congress to devote $30 billion over the next five years to combating the global AIDS epidemic, Sheryl Gay Stolberg, "Bush, Facing Troubles, Focuses on War and Taxes," *New York Times*, sec. A1, January 28, 2008.
4. The Global Fund, *Donors' Pledges and Contributions* (February 2008), www.theglobalfund.org (accessed February 14, 2008).
5. Jon Cohen, "The New World of Global Health," *Science* 311, no. 5758 (January 13, 2006): 162–167.
6. Laurie Garrett, "The Challenge of Global Health," *Foreign Affairs* 86, no. 1 (January/February 2007): 14–38; Paul Farmer and Laurie Garrett, "From 'Marvelous Momentum' to Health Care for All: Success Is Possible with the Right Programs," *Foreign Affairs* 86, no. 2 (March/April 2007), http://www.foreignaffairs.org/20070301faresponse86213/paul-farmer-laurie-garrett/from-marvelous-momentum-to-health-care-for-all-success-is-possible-with-the-right-programs.html (accessed February 16, 2008), 155.
7. For example, see Donald G. McNeil, Jr., "WHO Official Complains of Gates Foundation Dominance in Malaria Research," *New York Times*, February 16, 2008.

disappointments and failures: the 3 by 5 program for AIDS and Roll Back Malaria, for example, did not meet their ambitious initial goals. Only 1 million rather than 3 million people were receiving combination antiretroviral therapy for HIV/AIDS in developing countries by 2005, the target date[8]; by 2007 only 2 million were receiving treatment, representing just 28% of the 7.1 million people with advanced AIDS who need such therapy in poor and middle-income countries.[9] Roll Back Malaria's clear pledge in 1998 to cut deaths from malaria in half by 2010 was labeled a failure, its principal contributors admitting that it was "acting against a background of increasing malaria burden"—that is, that malaria deaths were going up, not down.[10]

Furthermore, attention to infectious disease has been patchwork in character, focusing on some high-profile diseases while ignoring others that cost far more lives. While AIDS, Ebola, and avian flu fuel widespread fear, some ongoing endemic killers, such as infantile diarrhea and childhood acute respiratory tract infections, receive little press and correspondingly little funding or policy attention. Indeed, Solomon Benatar laments the "siloed" character of approaches to infectious disease—one disease at a time.[11] Laurie Garrett despairs of "stovepipe" funding: aid that is piped down narrow channels relating to a particular program or disease, ignoring broader needs and concerns. She cites as an example the case in which a government receives considerable support for an antiretroviral distribution program for mothers and children in a specific area, but nothing else. The consequence: mothers who are HIV-positive receive drugs for their own infection and to prevent maternal/infant transmission at delivery, but they cannot obtain obstetric and gynecological care or infant immunizations.[12] Attention to specific diseases has seemed to be quite unequal: while massive research efforts have been directed toward development of a vaccine against HIV, with more than 30 candidates currently in the pipeline, no new tuberculosis vaccine has been developed since 1921, even though the TB bacillus is a technically easier target than the human immunodeficiency virus. In most developing countries TB is still diagnosed using a microscope and stain, the same type of method as that used in 1847.

---

8. The 3 by 5 Initiative, "Access to HIV Treatment Continues to Accelerate in Developing Countries, but Bottlenecks Persist, Says WHO/UNAIDS Report," (June 29, 2005), http://www.who.int/3by5/progressreportJune2005/en/ (accessed February 16, 2008).
9. Lawrence K. Altman, "AIDS Drugs Reach More People, U.N. Report Says, but Not Enough," *New York Times*, April 18, 2007.
10. Gavin Yamey, "Roll Back Malaria: A Failing Global Health Campaign," *British Medical Journal* 328, no. 7448 (May 8, 2004): 1086–1087.
11. Solomon R. Benatar, "Moral Imagination: The Missing Component in Global Health," *PLoS Medicine* 2, no. 12 (December 27, 2005): e400.
12. Laurie Garrett, "The Challenge of Global Health," *Foreign Affairs* 86, no. 1 (January/February 2007): 22–23.

Yet even if not fully coordinated and sometimes seeming to undercut each other, these disease-by-disease, program-by-program efforts all focus directly or indirectly on a common goal, the reduction of the global burden of infectious disease. Thus these varied efforts can all be seen as a sort of mosaic or kaleidoscope of specific efforts that form part of a broader global effort coming incrementally into being. The many programs of research in vaccines and antimicrobials, the various water purification and public sanitation projects, the various initiatives for the control of diseases from AIDS to HPV-caused cervical cancer to river blindness, and the multiple legal and social programs like model statutes and pandemic prioritization policies contribute to this emerging, newly coalescing global effort toward the ultimate goal of control of infectious disease, the details of which are being continuously filled in and modified as the various individual projects are developed and become more fully integrated. We can think of it as a projection forward of current efforts and an anticipation of future ones; an ongoing, overall project under continuous development. Call this still-emerging set of efforts by a unifying name: a *Comprehensive Global Effort for the Eradication, Elimination, or Control of Infectious Disease.*

A Vision for 2020–2030? A *Comprehensive Global Effort* for the Control of Infectious Disease

We want to take advantage of this forward-looking, unifying, optimistic picture of new progress and reenergized enthusiasm over the last seven or eight years to examine the ethical questions a genuinely global effort would raise. After all, practical success in the various components of this overall effort to move forward does not entail ethical success, either in their mosaic diversity or as a comprehensive whole.

One way to give the notion of an emerging *Comprehensive Global Effort* concreteness and urgency is to think about what would need to happen if we were to try to bring these various efforts to fruition within a given decade— for example, to imagine implementing it fully between, say, 2020 and 2030. A clearly defined *Comprehensive Global Effort* imagined as just far enough away to give some time for coordination and preparation would nevertheless be close enough to make a real difference to the world today. This is a somewhat visionary approach, but not just fantasy—rather, it is an approach that looks ahead to a future we can reasonably foresee.

To the degree that such an approach involves extrapolating into the future from current trends, we can hardly be sure what the conditions and events even in the future will be, or whether a *Comprehensive Global Effort* could or will succeed or even partly succeed. It might work; it might not; or it might be only a partial success. Yet using our PVV view, we can also reasonably foresee something about the ethical challenges that can be expected to arise along the way. It is these challenges we wish to explore here.

A more pessimistic version of the same projection of a *Comprehensive Global Effort* despairs of the possibility of ever achieving control of infectious disease or doing so within a specific period of time. It asks instead what are the crucial features in delay—what factors are operating now or might operate in the future to make such a goal unattainable? Could the fearsome prospect of virtually total collapse of public health portrayed so effectively by Laurie Garrett in *Betrayal of Trust* be inevitable?[13] Could the effects of climate change and global warming destroy advances in environmental preventives like vector control, or could the expansion of warfare and ethnic cleansing, especially that which employs deliberate tactics for spreading infectious disease, undercut any progress in disease-control programs? And what ethical failures in disease control are becoming increasingly evident, and what ethical objections might be so strong that they would be sufficient to warrant blocking any attempt to undertake comprehensive global efforts?

Leaving these concerns aside for the moment, the optimistic picture we explore here of an emerging *Comprehensive Global Effort for the Control of Infectious Disease* is in one sense an elaboration and expansion of the comparatively simple thought-experiment about airport surveillance presented in Chapter 15, a way of considering what constraints would be acceptable in the effort to eradicate, eliminate, or control the serious human infectious diseases. In another sense, it is a projection of the overall direction we discern in the many somewhat disparate enterprises already under way, a description of an overall project on which many organizations around the globe have already embarked. And in yet another sense, casting a *Comprehensive Global Effort* as highly time-focused, pursued within the specific decade of the 2020s, looks very much like a plan, something we have already embarked on and should continue pursuing.

This chapter's account of a *Comprehensive Global Effort* can thus be read in at least three not fully distinct ways. It lies somewhere between a sheer thought-experiment *("What if the serious human infectious diseases could be brought under control?")*, a factual account of events that are now taking place *("Look at all the remarkable progress that is going on!")*, and a practical proposal with a concrete, dated plan *("What would it take to bring the serious human infectious diseases under control, and to do so* [this is the visionary part] *by the end of the decade 2020–2030?")*. The power of a thought-experiment is to help identify moral fault lines, as in the airport thought-experiment, and the importance of a factual account of what is actually going on is to remind ourselves of the very substantial progress, as well as backsliding, that has been made so far. And the heuristic device of a time-pressured feature, of imagining the culmination of

---

13. Laurie Garrett, *Betrayal of Trust: The Collapse of Global Public Health* (New York: Hyperion, 2001).

this *Effort* in a fast-approaching, specific, and limited period of time—the decade 2020–2030—emphasizes the real-world challenges of global coordination and cooperation, if that is what would be necessary to bring the serious human communicable diseases under control. But most important for our concerns here, this chapter's broader and far more realistic exploration of what is afoot in the new "marvelous momentum" of efforts to reduce the global burden of disease also involves exploring concrete moral claims about what would be required to make this immense global effort go *ethically* well.

Some authors suggest that the moment for such a project is already past. Robert Baker, for instance, contends that humankind has "squandered" the opportunity to usher in a "Golden Age of protection from disease."[14] But that does not preclude a renewed, reinvigorated, and better-orchestrated effort as a revitalized attempt, something we see as again under way.

Other large-scale efforts are also beginning to attract at least some measure of global cooperation—for example, controlling global warming, rescuing endangered species, securing equitable access to water or establishing water justice, developing alternative energy sources, managing immigration, controlling drugs, and eliminating terrorism, ethnic cleansing, and war. But a common goal of the eradication, elimination, or full control of serious, human-affecting infectious disease may be, as we will consider later on, both more practicable and less controversial than the others, even though like them it may involve quite controversial policy initiatives.

In a *Comprehensive Global Effort,* coordination of effort or at least simultaneous effort on many different fronts is crucial, because the factors that need to be addressed are highly interrelated. Scientific advances accomplish little without infrastructure improvement, for example, or environmental control. Institutional cooperation and legal protections are inadequate in the face of cultural and religious attitudes that vilify carriers of infectious disease as sinful individuals, or characterize outbreaks of infectious disease as an appropriate scourge for sinful populations. To think about an emerging, coordinated, globe-wide effort is to "think big" about all the factors across the board that affect how we might address a challenge to human well-being that had almost disappeared from ethical dialogue in the late 1960s and early 1970s, before renewed ethical debate with the emergence of HIV, even though advances like the development of new antimicrobials and the eradication of smallpox were proceeding apace. It is an ongoing effort that has now come into view again with real force, re-energized and far more publicly visible in the last seven or eight years. That makes it imperative to "think big."

---

14. Robert Baker quoted in Tahla Khan Burki, "Review of Robert Baker, *Quiet Killers: The Fall and Rise of Deadly Diseases," New England Journal of Medicine* 357, no. 17 (October 25, 2007): 1784–1785.

"Thinking Big," Both Practically and Ethically

A number of "think big" efforts toward reducing the global burden of infectious disease are already under way, practical efforts of a variety of sorts focusing on social realities and scientific gains.[15] The UN Millennium Development Goals (MDG), for example, represent an effort to think globally about health and related problems. [16]

The Gates Foundation's Grand Challenges in Global Health Initiative is also global in scale: it seeks to achieve scientific breakthroughs against diseases that disproportionately affect the two billion poorest people on earth, though of course diseases like AIDS and tuberculosis can affect people everywhere. The Council of Science Editors has organized a global theme issue on poverty and human development involving more than 230 science and biomedical journals, focusing among other things on interventions to improve health among the poor.[17] These are all invaluable efforts involving many parts of the overall picture, and they all "think big."

At the same time that practical efforts are converging in the effort to control infectious disease, there is an efflorescence of efforts to consider the ethical issues involved. In Chapter 4, we have surveyed individual papers, journal issues, and collections of essays that are alert to ethics issues in infectious disease, though with the exception of those directed to HIV/AIDS, most date from 1999 or later. Think tanks like the American Enterprise Institute, the Brookings Institution, the CATO Institute, the Center for Strategic and International Studies, the Council on Foreign Relations, and the Harvard School of Public Health's AIDS Initiative Vaccine Think Tank, have begun to address issues in infectious disease in papers and conferences. Attention to the ethics issues in pandemic influenza planning, as we have seen in Section IV of this book, has been extensive, with reports, white papers, and articles exploring practical and ethical issues. Documents like that from WHO by Coleman, Reis, and Croisier[18] articulate policies; others, like the American Civil Liberties Union

---

15. We thank a number of people who helped us "think big" at a conference in July 2007, at the Uehiro Center for Ethics, Oxford University: Julian Savulescu, David Bradley, Nimalan Arinaminpathy, Angela McLean, Helen Fletcher, Paul Kelly, Anders Sandberg, Carl H. Coleman, Michael Parker, Harold Jaffe, Angus Dawson, Michael J. Selgelid, Marcel Verweij, Dan Brock, Soren Holm, Ray Zilinskas, and Matthew Liao.

16. United Nations, "UN Millennium Development Goals" (2008), http://www.un.org/millenniu mgoals (accessed February 16, 2008).

17. Annette Flanagin and Margaret A. Winker, "Global Theme Issue on Poverty and Human Development," *Journal of the American Medical Association* 298, no. 16 (October 24/31, 2007): 1942; Council of Science Editors, *Global Theme Issue on Poverty and Human Development* (October 22, 2007), http://www.councilscienceeditors.org/globalthemeissue.cfm (accessed February 16, 2008).

18. Carl Coleman, Andreas Reis, and Alice Croisier, "Ethical Considerations in Developing a Public Health Response to Pandemic Influenza" (2007), www.who.int/csr/resources/publications (accessed February 16, 2008).

(ACLU) document authored by Annas, Mariner, and Parmet,[19] vigorously critique already-developed policies on the basis of ethical inadequacies. And a major effort has been mounted by the Bill and Melinda Gates Foundation to look specifically at the ethical issues in the emerging concern with global health: this is the Ethical, Social and Cultural Program funded under the Grand Challenges in Global Health Initiative, designed to use bioethics considerations to assess the specific Grand Challenges projects that are planned or are currently under way.[20] In Chapter 4, we documented how infectious disease had been left out of bioethics during that new field's formative years; now it is moving back in, so to speak, with extraordinary rapidity, making up for lost time.

However, much of the burgeoning new work in the ethics of infectious disease employs the conceptual categories of traditional bioethics that, as we have documented in Chapter 4, were developed without specific attention to the moral issues in transmissibility. To be sure, this may be perfectly adequate in addressing issues like caged field trials of genetically modified mosquitoes, as is the subject of one of the current projects under the Gates Foundation's Grand Challenges program, but the traditional approaches of bioethics' usual ethical framework within which projects are assessed needs, as we argued there, to be augmented and expanded.

Of course, many writers and theorists already instinctively appeal to both victim-related and vector-related concerns, but as far as we are aware none have done this explicitly or systematically in a way that would *guarantee* that both concerns would be addressed on any given issue. This is what we have sought to do with our PVV view. Hence, we like to think of our objective here in exploring the notion of a comprehensive global project as in concert with and indeed admiring of the many efforts now afoot to explore the ethical issues in infectious disease, but pushing them a good step further—a step we believe necessary for morally adequate reflection on a very broad scale.

What, then, would be involved in a *Comprehensive Global Effort for the Eradication, Elimination, or Control of Infectious Disease for the Years 2020–2030*? We point to both practical and ethical issues and agendas for future research that would arise along five "tracks," different though interrelated directions:

1. What would be desirable in the spheres of national and international policy?
2. What would we need to bring about in terms of epidemiological and health-care infrastructure?
3. What are most crucial lines of pursuit in scientific development?

19. George J. Annas, Wendy K. Mariner, and Wendy E. Parmet, "Pandemic Preparedness: The Need for a Public Health—Not a Law Enforcement/National Security—Approach," *American Civil Liberties Union: Technology and Liberty Project* (2008), http://www.aclu.org/privacy/medical/33642pub20080114.html (accessed Jan 20, 2008).
20. Peter A. Singer et al., "Grand Challenges in Global Health: The Ethical, Social and Cultural Program" *PLoS Medicine* 4, no. 9 (September 11, 2007): 1440–1444.

418 Making Use of the Patient as Victim and Vector View

4. What would need to be thought about in light of religious, social, and cultural considerations?

5. What would need to be developed as ethical, legal and social protections for individuals?

These are all critical areas for research and policy development, most of them interdependent on each other, and all raising substantial ethical issues we will sketch here.

This *Global Effort* is not to be imagined as starting from zero. On the contrary, many of the critical areas in tracks 1–5 are already well known to participants in current efforts to address infectious disease across the globe, from researchers and clinical health-care providers to immense organizations concerned with global health. Indeed, everyone and every organization working in infectious disease participates in some part of the global effort explored here, whether aware of the emerging comprehensive effort or not. It is already in progress—indeed, in full swing.

Global Efforts: Results So Far

Can we even imagine a *Comprehensive Global Effort for the Eradication, Elimination, or Control of Infectious Disease?* In many respects the world is already halfway there, at least in developed countries. It is important to remember as we entertain the notion of a *Global Effort* the impressive list of infectious diseases affecting humans for which effective vaccines, treatments, and preventive measures have been developed. Some of these diseases have already been eradicated, eliminated, or brought under control, some globally, others in one hemisphere or various regions. For some diseases, however, immunization or other methods for prevention and treatment are known but not available in specific areas, including much of the developing world.

Here is a snapshot taken at the current moment in the history of our progress so far in bringing the serious human infectious diseases under control: here at the beginning of the 21st century, it is a shifting picture and highly variable from one area to another, but a picture of extraordinary achievement just the same. We provide, first, a list of vaccine-preventable diseases, presented in loosely chronological order to reflect the way in which the possibility of controlling these diseases has come into being. Of course, only some of this progress is due to the development of vaccines; much is due to sanitary reforms and infrastructure development, including swamp clearance (e.g. malaria in the U.S.), water purification (e.g. cholera), and milk pasteurization (e. g. brucellosis); effective preventive measures, including health education (some sexually transmitted diseases); the development of antibiotics and other drugs (e.g. rheumatic fever, syphilis); and the accidents of geography or environmental change, as with alterations in the ranges of animal or insect vectors. Some diseases are vaccine-preventable but pre-exposure prophylaxis is recommended only for high-risk individuals (e.g. rabies). Some vaccines are given in combination (e.g. DPT or MMRV), and some vaccines are given within specific age ranges. Some vaccines are more effective in children, less so in elderly adults (seasonal influenza, from which about 36,000 people in the U.S. die each year, almost all elderly; also the BCG tuberculosis vaccine). Some vaccines confer only partial immunity, or wane in effectiveness over time. Some vaccines are of limited use (e.g. Rift Valley fever); others have been widely used in the past but are now less common (for example, typhus, widely used in World War II but replaced by vector control with DDT). For many diseases, vaccine development has not been easy: particularly in the early days, efforts to provide protection from specific diseases often began with antiserums or antitoxins that were not true vaccines, and some initial vaccines were ineffective, dangerous, or both. There is no simple, straight-line story here, and yet this list of the major vaccine-preventable diseases does represent enormous progress in the effort to control serious human-affecting infectious disease—progress that is realized at least in the developed world.

Vaccine-preventable diseases[21]:

smallpox	*(vaccine, 1798; eradicated 1977)*
cholera	*(limited-effectiveness vaccines 1884, 1894; parenteral whole-cell vaccines 1920s; inactivated and live vaccines; sanitation, clean water)*
rabies	*(vaccine, 1885)*
plague	*(vaccine, 1895, 1896, 1897; antibiotics, vector control)*
dipththeria	*(antitoxin 1891; toxoid 1926; antibiotics)*
typhoid	*(antiserum/antitoxin, 1898; clean water, 1906–1942; vaccines, 1990, 1994)*
pertussis (whooping cough)	*(1914–1931, vaccines unsound; whole-cell vaccine 1930–40s; acellular vaccines licensed for routine immunization of children, 1996)*
tetanus (lockjaw)	*(antitoxin; toxoid vaccine, 1924)*
tuberculosis	*(BCG, bacille Calmette-Guérin vaccine, 1927; effective primarily in children)*
yellow fever	*(vaccine, 1931; vector control)*
influenza A, B (some seasonal strains)	*(vaccines 1936, 1945; antivirals; effective in children, less effective in elderly)*

21. This list, compiled together with Warren B.P. Pettey, Division of Clinical Epidemiology, University of Utah, and Amanda G. Pettey, draws from a number of varied (and sometimes inconsistent, hence the citation of differing dates) sources, including: Arthur Allen, *Vaccine* (New York: W. W. Norton, 2007); Barry R. Bloom and Paul-Henri Lambert, eds, *The Vaccine Book* (San Diego, CA: Elsevier Science, Academic Press, 2003); Centers for Disease Control and Prevention, Inactivated Japanese encephalitis virus vaccine. Recommendations of the advisory committee on immunization practices (ACIP),

Japanese encephalitis	*(vaccines in use by 1942; 1954; vector control)*
poliomyelitis	*(vaccines: IPV licensed 1955; OPV licensed, 1961)*
measles	*(vaccine licensed, 1963)*
mumps	*(vaccine licensed, 1967)*
rubella (German measles)	*(vaccine licensed, 1969)*
anthrax	*(vaccine, 1970)*
invasive pneumococcal disease	*(antiserum, 1930's; vaccines, 1976, 1977, age 2 and up; 2000, infants; antibiotics)*
meningococcal meningitis	*(vaccine, 1974, 1978)*
varicella (chickenpox)	*(vaccines, 1968;1974; vaccine licensed, 1995)*
hepatitis B	*(plasma-derived vaccine, 1981; recombinant vaccine 1986)*
Hib (Haemophilus influenzae type b)	*(vaccine licensed, 1987; conjugate vaccine licensed, 1990)*
hepatitis A	*(vaccine licensed, 1995)*
rotavirus	*(vaccine licensed, 1998, withdrawn 1999; vaccine 2006)*
Lyme Disease	*(antibiotics; vector avoidance; vaccine licensed 1998; discontinued in U.S., 2002)*
shingles (herpes zoster)	*(vaccine licensed, 2006)*
monkeypox	*(no vaccine for monkeypox; smallpox vaccine used)*
cervical cancer (HPV virus)	*(vaccine, 2008)*

Morbidity and Mortality Weekly Report, 42 (RR–01) (January 08, 1993); Centers for Disease Control and Prevention, *Epidemiology and Prevention of Vaccine-Preventable Diseases* (2nd Printing: 10th ed.) (Washington, D.C.: Public Health Foundation, 2008); Centers for Disease Control and Prevention, List of Vaccine-Preventable Diseases, http://www.cdc.gov/vaccines/vpd-vac.vpd-list.htm [accessed July 30, 2008]; Centers for Disease Control and Prevention, *Global Immunization Strategic Framework 2006–2010*, http://www.cdc.gov/vaccines/programs/global/downloads/gisf-2006–2010.pdf [accessed July 29, 2008); J. Cohen & W.G Powderly, *Infectious diseases* (2nd ed.) (St. Louis, Mo. and London: Mosby, 2003); A.S. Evans & P.S. Brachman, *Bacterial infections of humans: epidemiology and control* (3rd ed.) (New York: Plenum Medical Book Co., 1998); G.L. Mandell, R.G. Douglas, J. E. Bennett & R. Dolin, Mandell, Douglas, and Bennett's principles and practice of infectious diseases, *MDConsult* 6th. from http://atoz.ebsco.com/link.asp?id=7227&sid=128189840&rid=400072&urlSource =AtoZ&lang=en; K. Nicholson, R.G. Webster & A.J. Hay, Eds., *Textbook of influenza* (Oxford and Malden, MA, USA: Blackwell Science, 1998); S.A. Plotkin, W.A. Orenstein, and P.A. Offit, *Vaccines* (5th ed.) (New York: Saunders, 2008); A. Sauerbrei, E. Rubtcova, P. Wutzler, D.S. Schmid & V.N. Loparev, Genetic profile of an Oka varicella vaccine virus variant isolated from an infant with zoster, *J Clin Microbiol*, 42(12), 5604–5608 (2004); R. Titball, *Plague Vaccines and Assessment of Immune Responses*, Paper presented at the Public Workshop on Animal Models and Correlates of Protection for Plague Vaccines, Gaithersburg, Maryland (October 13, 2004); University of Pennsylvania, Center for Bioethics, Ethics of Vaccines Project, "Vaccines: A Timeline," http://www.bioethics.upenn.edu/vaccines/?pageId=3&subpage=196 [accessed May 9, 2008]; M. Vazquez, P.S. LaRussa, A.A. Gershon, L.M. Niccolai, C.E. Muehlenbein, S.P. Steinberg, et al., Effectiveness over time of varicella vaccine. *JAMA*, 291(7), 851–855 (2004).

Diseases controllable or partly controllable by antimicrobials include:

Most bacterial infections (including pneumonias), parasites, and fungi.
leprosy (Hansen's Disease)
syphilis
group A streptococcal complications:
  scarlet fever
  rheumatic fever
Cytomegalovirus
Respiratory syncytial virus
Legionnaire's Disease (legionellosis)

Other infectious diseases, particularly those common in developing countries, have effective or largely effective vaccines, antimicrobial therapies, vector reduction strategies, or other methods for treatment or control, but in many regions—especially the developing world—these controls have not been adequately implemented. These include many of the above, especially:

tuberculosis, including MDR-TB, XDR-TB
malaria
AIDS (human immunodeficiency virus)
cholera
trypanosomiasis (sleeping sickness, Chagas disease)
Leishmaniasis (sandfly fever)
hemolytic uremic syndrome (diarrhea due to toxigenic *E. coli*)

"Neglected tropical diseases" including: (for this group, effective oral treatments are known):[22]

  roundworm
  whipworm
  hookworm
  schistosomiasis (snail fever or bilharziasis)
  elephantiasis
  trachoma
  river blindness

Diseases for which there is currently no effective vaccine or antimicrobial therapy include:

Ebola
Marburg

---

22. Madhuri Reddy et al., "Oral Drug Therapy for Multiple Neglected Tropical Diseases: A Systematic Review," *Journal of the American Medical Association* 298, no. 16 (October 24/31, 2007): 1911–1924, table 1.

dengue fever and dengue hemorrhagic fever
West Nile encephalitis
hantavirus pneumonia
SARS
Creutzfeldt-Jakob Disease and variant Creutzfeldt-Jakob Disease

So far, successes in reducing the burden of disease in the developed world have been remarkable. In the United States, the death rates for smallpox, diphtheria, and polio have declined by 100% since vaccines were approved; for another nine diseases, they have declined by 90%.[23] Despite that, there have been major setbacks (like the reemergence of tuberculosis, polio, yellow fever, even plague[24]), but in general progress toward the full control of infectious disease is astonishing—at least where it is fully implemented, as in the wealthier parts of the world. There is progress in the developing parts of the world: some 78% of the world's infants receive diptheria-tetanus-pertussis vaccine, and an estimated 20 million deaths from vaccine-preventable diseases have been prevented by immunization during the past two decades. In contemplating the possibility of eradication, elimination, or control of the serious human infectious diseases, it might be said, we are halfway there, at least in the developed world.

"Halfway there," it might be said, but this must be understood in a loose and metaphorical way. One serious difficulty with any general claim about the proportion of human-affecting infectious diseases that are now in principle eradicated, eliminable, or can in principle be brought under control is how to individuate diseases. Different classificatory systems have very different understandings of how diseases should be categorized: by symptoms, by causative organism, etc.; various Committees on Taxonomy attempt to address such problems. The role of genetics in interaction with infectious conditions is part of the picture. A second difficulty involves identifying what diseases "count": is it just the widespread, serious or fatal diseases, those with high estimated mortality? What about those with the capacity to disrupt normal life, but that are not serious or life-threatening, like the common cold, or those that are neither but have considerable nuisance value, like athlete's foot? A third barrier to

23. Donald G McNeil. Jr., "Sharp Drop Seen in Deaths from Ills Fought by Vaccine," *New York Times*, Health Section, November 14, 2007.
24. Michael Kahn, "Plague a Growing but Overlooked Threat: Study," *Reuters* (January 15, 2008). http://www.reuters.com/article/scienceNews/idUSL1446129320080115?pageNumber=2&virtualBrand Channel=o&sp=true. "Plague, the disease that devastated medieval Europe, is re-emerging worldwide and poses a growing but overlooked threat, researchers warned on Tuesday. While it has only killed some 100 to 200 people annually over the past 20 years, plague has appeared in new countries in recent decades and is now shifting in to Africa," Michael Begon, an ecologist at the University of Liverpool and colleagues said (Nils Chr. Stenseth et al., "Plague: Past, Present, and Future," *PLoS Medicine* 5, no. 1 [January 15, 2008]: 9–13).

ascertaining whether we are "halfway there" in any precise sense is that it is not possible to predict what new, emerging zoonotic or other natural diseases or designer bioweapons will come to exist in the future; thus it is in principle impossible to compare the proportion of diseases already controllable to those not yet conquered. Attempting to quantify an exact count of diseases subject to control versus those still to go would require agreement on the underlying categorical structure, a deeply fraught metaphysical question as well as an enormously complex practical challenge.

Nevertheless, as we consider the progress so far and imagine the thought experiment of a *Comprehensive Global Effort for the Control of Infectious Disease in the Decade 2020-2030*, we wish to convey the sense that "we're halfway there" still does have intuitive meaning—thanks to among other things dedicated work in vaccine research and in public health, much of it in very recent decades. This optimism is reflected for example in the CDC *Global Immunization Strategic Framework 2006–2010*, a vision statement imagining "a world without vaccine preventable disease, disability, and death." We've made enormous progress, and at the same time still have a very long way to go. Recognizing this is central in motivating a *Global Effort*.

Human Health in Epidemiological Perspective

The already impressive successes of an emerging *Comprehensive Global Effort*, if we can think of them as part of a long-term effort, are after all evident in the history of demographic shifts in causes of human mortality. Up through the middle of the nineteenth century, everywhere in the world, parasitic and infectious diseases were the principal cause of human mortality.[25] With the development of clean water, public sanitation, immunization, the germ theory of disease, hand washing by physicians, antibiotics, and many other factors, infectious disease, with the single exception of pneumonia, is not even on the standard list of the top ten causes of death in the developed world. At the same time, infectious diseases remain a major factor in the developing world, where death rates—particularly for children—remain high. Just a century ago, infectious and parasitic diseases were the way most people everywhere in the world died; in the developed world, they are a much reduced threat, and where they do kill, kill mainly the old. Infectious disease mortality in the United States has declined remarkably in the twentieth century, and now represents a small

---

25. S. Jay Olshansky and A. Brian Ault, "The Fourth Stage of the Epidemiologic Transition: The Age of Delayed Degenerative Disease," in *Should Medical Care Be Rationed by Age?* ed. Timothy M. Smeeding et al. (Totowa, NJ: Rowman & Littlefield, 1987), 11–43; and S. J. Olshansky et al., "Emerging Infectious Diseases: The Fifth Stage of the Epidemiologic Transition?" *World Health Statistics Quarterly* 51, nos. 2–4 (1998): 207–217.

percentage (<5%) of disability-adjusted life-years lost.[26] The stark differences in life expectancy around the world, ranging roughly from a high of between 75 and 85.5 for women in Japan, Australia, Iceland, Canada, the Netherlands, Cuba, and the UK downward to between 40 and 60 in the poorer, developing nations, and in some countries, like Malawi, Mozambique, Zimbabwe, Zambia, still lower, to Sierra Leone, with a low for men between 37.3 and 40, is not just a matter of disparate human development indices but differential death rates from infectious disease.[27] Efforts to reduce the burden of infectious disease, it is painfully obvious, have already been remarkably successful in the developed world—this may be part of what has allowed the developed world to become developed—but have a long, long way to go in those countries left behind.

Is a *Comprehensive Global Effort* Realistic? On Eradication, Elimination, and Control

It is crucial in understanding any *Global Effort* to recognize the differences between eradication, elimination, and control. Complete eradication by eliminating entirely the pathogen that causes disease is realistic in only a small proportion of cases, those that involve human vectors only and no intermediate stages: for example, smallpox, polio, measles, and tuberculosis. The eradication of all human infectious disease—that is, completely ridding the world of all disease-causing pathogens in the wild—is not a realistic goal, because many human-affecting infectious diseases also have nonhuman vectors or reservoirs. Tetanus, for example, lives in the soil; so do the spores of coccidioidomycosis, a fungal infection responsible for Valley Fever.[28] Malaria involves a transmission stage in mosquitoes; so do yellow fever, dengue fever, and many other arthropod-borne infectious diseases. Other common infections—such as staphylococcal skin infections, or peritonitis due to ruptured bowel—are due to organisms that we normally carry on our skin or in our gastrointestinal tracts, and attempts to eliminate one pathogen would be foiled by the rapid appearance of other potential pathogens to refill the microbial niche in the skin or GI tract.

---

26. Gregory L. Armstrong, Laura A. Conn, and Robert W. Pinner, "Trends in Infectious Disease Mortality in the United States During the 20th Century," *Journal of the American Medical Association* 281, no. 1 (January 6, 1999): 61–66. The study shows a flattening of the curve of decline in ID mortality beginning in 1960, and a rise in ID mortality of 58% from 1980 to 1992 (presumably due to AIDS).

27. Life expectancy data are for 2005; World Health Organization, http://www.who.int/countries/en/ (accessed February 16, 2008).

28. Jesse McKinley, "Infection Hits a California Prison Hard, and Experts Ask Why," *New York Times*, (December 30, 2007), http://query.nytimes.com/gst/fullpage.html?res=9A06E6D81130F933 A05751C1A9619C8B63&scp=2&sq=Valley±Fever&st=nyt (accessed January 21, 2008).

Furthermore, many pathogenic organisms do not require humans for their perpetuation and are not acquired from other humans. Elimination of these organisms in humans, for instance by means of universal immunization or effective treatment, would still not eliminate these organisms, and the diseases they cause will remain a continuing threat. Some human-affecting diseases also affect animals and are carried by animals—Rift Valley Fever, for example—and unless contact between these animals and humans were completely interrupted, control of these diseases in humans could not be complete without achieving control in the animal population as well. Some pathogens affect both people and plants, like the bacterium *Burkholderia cepacia* (people and onions), which can be lethal for people with cystic fibrosis, or *Serratia marcescens* (people and squash plants), which reaches immunocompromised hospital patients through floral arrangements, salads, and intravenous tubes;[29] it is hard to see how these pathogens could be entirely eradicated. And some infectious diseases, such as influenza and HIV, reappear in modified form and potentially require ongoing prevention or treatment in generation after generation.

At this point in the human history of infectious disease, there is just one extant example of complete eradication: smallpox. But there are many examples of elimination, that is, reduction to a very low level, like leprosy, plague, and polio, the latter on the verge of eradication despite recent outbreaks.[30] And there are many examples of full or nearly full control, at least in the developed world, where disease is preventable, treatable, or curable by means of immunization, antimicrobials, sanitation measures (e.g., clean water) or other effective prevention or treatment.

Of course, there is an immense gap between diseases that can be eliminated and diseases that are in fact eliminated. Leprosy, for example, falls in this category, as do many of the so-called neglected tropical diseases for which effective treatment is known but not widely available: here the gulf between the developed world and the developing world is at its greatest. It is already possible in principle, despite enormous practical obstacles, to reduce dramatically much of the huge burden of disease suffered by those in poorest parts of the globe, and as new diagnostic technologies, vaccines, and treatment modalities are developed, so is the likelihood of elimination or full control for many additional diseases.

Obviously, even in the developed world control of infectious disease will never be complete. There will always be newly emerging diseases: in recent years, some 39 new communicable diseases with the potential to become pandemic have jumped species, including SARS, monkeypox, and bird flu.[31] The prospect

29. Susan Milius, "Not Just Hitchhikers: Human Pathogens Make Homes on Plants," *Science News*, October 20, 2007, 251.

30. Elimination is defined as the level at which a disease no longer constitutes a public health problem. See http://www.cdc.gov/mmwr/preview/mmwrhtml/su48a9.htm.

31. Harriet Rubin, "Google's Searches Now Include Ways to Make a Better World," *New York Times*, sec. C1, January 18, 2008.

of newly designed or already known pathogens used as bioweapons cannot be ruled out.[32] Climate change, settlement of newly cleared land, and warfare and its dislocations can also play a role in the emergence or evolution of disease.

Some theorists might argue that certain serious diseases should not be eliminated because they are useful in other respects, as when pneumonia serves as the "old man's friend"—a bringer of death more easeful than that from other human maladies. Others might point to research suggesting that exposure to infectious disease has played a major role in mammalian evolution, resulting among other things in the development of the amniotic sac and other adaptive advantages, and thus argue that continuing exposure should not be eliminated, lest further evolutionary gains be lost.[33] Still others claim that the overuse of antibacterial soaps and other "germ-proofing" methods results in higher rates of asthma and allergies. A *Comprehensive Global Effort* certainly would not seek to exterminate all parasites, fungi, bacteria, viruses, and prions—the microorganisms that affect human beings—because many are essential for human health, but only the pathogenic ones that do not also have beneficial functions and are responsible for extensive human morbidity and mortality. It is this process of overcoming *disease* that we see as already well under way in any long-term *Comprehensive Global Effort*.

If we see a *Comprehensive Global Effort* in three ways—as a thought-experiment, as a report of current activity, or as a plan—we may ask: what would it be like if, what is happening that, or what do we need to do to try to achieve the eradication, elimination, or full control of serious human-affecting infectious disease, say within the decade 2020–2030, around the globe? The question, in each of these forms, is not just about what practical projects of research, policy development, or implementation would be most urgent, but also about what ethical issues most urgently require attention as a *Global Effort* proceeds. As we have said, these issues arise in five, often overlapping, tracks of inquiry.

Track 1: National and International Organizations and the Development of Global Will

If a *Comprehensive Global Effort* is to succeed fully, it would be important to foster the cooperation of institutions and players of all sorts. Many are already committed—but not all. Thus the first step is to consider what sorts of institutions are critical to infectious disease control, which are helpful, which are

---

32. Michael J. Selgelid, "Dual Use Discoveries: Censorship Policy Making," lecture at Oxford University, July 4, 2007; Ray Zilinskas, "Assessing the Bioterrorism Threat: Problems and Possibilities," lecture at Oxford University, July 4, 2007.
33. Marlene Zuk, *Riddled with Life: Friendly Worms, Ladybug Sex, and the Parasites That Make Us Who We Are* (Orlando, FL: Harcourt, 2007).

problematic—and how the support of such institutions could be enlisted and maintained, or modified where it has been counterproductive. This is to seek to establish and maintain the global will to try to reduce the burden of infectious disease to as low a level as possible. Many institutions and individuals are relevant to infectious disease control, and of these, many have already been playing a substantial role, whether in developing health policy, in supplying goods or services, in conducting research, or in raising and contributing money. Institutions involved include international organizations, like the World Health Organization, the World Bank, United Nations Children's Fund (UNICEF), Joint United Nations Programme on HIV/AIDS (UNAIDS), the Global Alliance for Vaccines and Immunization (GAVI), the Millennium Fund, the International AIDS Vaccine Initiative (IAVI), the Global Fund to Fight AIDS, Tuberculosis and Malaria, and the World Organization for Animal Health, among many others. They also include both affluent and poorer governments. Moreover, governmental organizations play a major role: for example, the Centers for Disease Control and its counterparts in other nations, the Institute of Medicine, the National Institutes of Health's Fogarty International Center, the U.S. Agency for International Development, the Walter Reed Army Research Institute, the Food and Agriculture Organization, the National Institute of Allergy and Infectious Disease, and the President's Emergency Plan for AIDS Relief (PEPFAR). They include private philanthropic foundations, like the Bill and Melinda Gates Foundation, the Rockefeller Foundation, Rotary International, Save the Children, and many more. Catholic, Protestant, Islamic, and many other religious groups are very much involved in providing care, including funding relief societies and maintaining mission clinics and hospitals in developing countries. Private enterprise contributes too: for example, donors to the Global Fund include (Product) RED and Partners, American Express, Apple, Converse, Dell + Windows, GAP, Giorgio Armani, Hallmark, Motorola, and Media Partners.[34] Pharmaceutical firms like Pfizer ($12 million to the Uganda HIV program in collaboration with the U.S. Infectious Disease Society) and Lilly contribute funds and free or discounted drugs. Google.org has joined the ranks of major contributors. Public figures have had a major voice: Jimmy Carter, Bill Clinton, Tony Blair, Kofi Annan, Paul Farmer, Jeffrey Sachs, to name only a few. And entertainers and impresarios have also played a major role in raising funds and focusing public attention on global health needs: Bono, Richard Gere, and Angelina Jolie, among many others. The complete roster of members of the Global Health Council lists some 526 organizations,

---

34. The Global Fund, *Donors' Pledges and Contributions* (February 2008), www.theglobalfund.org (accessed February 14, 2008).

many but not all focused on infectious disease, including many public–private partnerships.[35]

Impressive as this list of organizations and individuals already participating in effect in a *Comprehensive Global Effort* is, however, they are to varying degrees independent actors. Many smaller agencies address one piece of the puzzle or another. But some are entities with vast expertise and resources, committed to making a global difference, and are already "thinking big" in a global way. Part of the question here about how to generate and perpetuate sufficient collective will to achieve global control of infectious disease is whether a more extensively coordinated effort of the globe's major institutions is required, as well as how to respond to differing political and social circumstances, successes and setbacks, and competing priorities. Some specific entities might emphasize local cooperation and grassroots involvement; others might serve to secure major funding or provide extensive scientific, technological, or social research. That major institutions like governments, multinational corporations, private sponsors, or religious organizations cooperate need not dictate what specific projects they undertake or methods they use, or for that matter whether cooperation is enshrined in treaties, cross-border agreements, contracts, good-faith promises, or other ways. But a *Comprehensive Global Effort* clearly requires far fuller and quite substantial cooperation on at least some institutional levels. The practical challenge is to develop the global political will to try to work together to bring infectious disease under control in the first place, and it is substantial: if the many sorts of institutions listed are all to cooperate, it would require laying aside infighting, reducing political competition, avoiding distraction by shifting from one to another "short-term numerical target,"[36] avoiding turf wars, and other friction that could derail progress.[37] Could all these institutions contribute cooperatively in their myriad ways to a common project, even for just a decade? And what ethical as well as practical challenges would the effort to generate a cooperative global effort raise? Here are four.

The Question of Global Architecture. A number of authors have pointed to the disease-by-disease character of many efforts at controlling infectious disease, and the way they sometimes undercut each others' success. Laurie Garrett warns that because the extraordinary generosity of public and private giving is paying for efforts that are largely uncoordinated and directed mostly at specific high-profile diseases like AIDS, tuberculosis, and malaria, there is danger

---

35. Global Health Council, *Member Organizations* (2008), http://globalhealth.org/view_top.php3?id=232 (accessed February 16, 2008).

36. Farmer and Laurie Garrett, "Marvelous Momentum."

37. Jon Cohen, "The New World of Global Health," *Science* 311, no. 5758 (January 13, 2006): 162–167.

of making things worse on the ground.[38] There is no central, fully effective co-ordinating authority for integrating global health efforts around the world. The WHO has clearly been extraordinarily successful in generating cooperation among countries, but even it is sometimes constrained by political disagreements. Furthermore, there is no central mechanism for prioritizing efforts at disease control in comparison to many other global concerns, for example, environmental protection, international and intranational hostility reduction, elimination of human trafficking, global drug control, and much more. Global disease-control efforts may be well under way, but often in a piecemeal fashion. Writing from a collaboration between the CDC and WHO, McNabb et al. argue that many developing countries have poor performance in both infectious disease surveillance and action due to duplicative, independent, vertical disease-oriented public health systems, focusing for example on tuberculosis control versus HIV control. These lead to redundant use of personnel, excessive costs, and in general inefficient, ineffective systems; part of the problem here is that control priorities are set by distant foreign countries or NGOs.[39] As Barry Bloom puts it, there is no "global architecture" to deal with health threats that cross national boundaries, which is what would be necessary for the full global control of infectious disease.[40] This is not to say there is no global cooperation: the WHO, for example, has been conducting worldwide influenza surveillance since 1947[41] and is currently coordinating pandemic flu control efforts, but this is still to concentrate on a specific threat rather than on the full range of infectious diseases.

As any *Global Effort* emerges in full, then, will it be necessary or even desirable to identify a central coordinating entity? Must the various organizations work together? Coordination is clearly essential for matters like surveillance, for example in reporting disease outbreaks, or managing border controls. However, coordination of any enterprise where a central authority has the ability to manage all the resources raises the risk of crushing creative and unique approaches to solving problems, and it is sometimes said that the more structured and principled a program gets, the harder it is for truly original ideas to be put forward. It may well be that heavy-handed centralization both undermines trust and is

---

38. Laurie Garrett, "The Challenge of Global Health," *Foreign Affairs* 86, no. 1 (January/February 2007), 14.

39. Cohen, "The New World," 165; Barry R. Bloom, "Public Health in Transition," *Scientific American* 293, no. 3 (September 2005): 92–99.

40. Scott, J.N. McNabb, Stella Chungong, Mike Ryan, Tadesse Wuhib, Peter Nsubuga, Wondi Alemu, Vilma Carande-Kulis, Guenael Rodier, "Conceptual framework of public health surveillance and action and its application in health sector reform," *BMC Public Health* 2(2) (2002), Epub January 29, p. 2 of 9.

41. Laurie Garrett, "The Next Pandemic? Probable Cause," *Foreign Affairs* 84, no 4. (July/August 2005): 22.

disruptive of local values and cultures, and thus would undermine the prospects for a *Global Effort* overall. In any case, issues of institutional design and international coordination are immensely complex—witness the tensions in the formation of the European Union—and a highly coordinated, focused *Comprehensive Global Effort* slated to culminate within a specific decade would no doubt exhibit many of the same stresses.

Funding for a Comprehensive Global Effort. Funding for a *Global Effort* of the scale we are envisioning would require very substantial financial support, perhaps in the form of taxes to be levied on or contributions expected from the major institutions, not only governments but public–private partnerships, philanthropic organizations, multinational corporations, NGOs, religious groups, private sponsors, and others committed to the *Global Effort;* equitably shared contributions would be especially important as an alternative to taxes in locales where governments are unstable or abjectly poor. Contributions to funding might be in financial form or in kind, depending on the institution. Yet either way, the issue of financial support raises enormous questions of distributive justice. One possibility would be to fund a *Global Effort* relative to the capacity of each entity involved, whether it be a government, international organization, corporation, private sponsor, or religious group: the idea is that if all such entities could be signed on for a decade, presumably in rough proportion to their capacities, the financial burden for each might be manageable.

In Chapter 19, we used our PVV perspective to show how there are shared interests in global health security. To be sure, any given individual cares about his own fate—but, we argued, in caring about his own fate, he needs to care more broadly about society in general. So he has reason to care about how groups of which he is a member fare, too—and this will probably include his country as well as his clan, state, ethnic group, or tribe, especially given the role of national borders. But borders are porous—so there is reason to care about what happens everywhere, all the time——and thus there is reason for everyone to contribute, too. But these are all parts of the overall perspective of what it means to be victim and vector. Translating this individual point of view to a perspective about funding raises the possibility of mutual requests or claims that could be directed by institutional entities to each other about the importance of their participation in such a burden-sharing arrangement. Because infectious disease can travel as rapidly as a single intercontinental airplane flight, no country or institution is safe, and hence it might be argued, every institution around the globe should be held accountable for sharing in this global task.

However, not all countries or institutions are equally at risk for specific diseases or even for an equal overall burden of disease: some are at high risk of the rapid spread of dangerous diseases—cholera, for example, in poor countries with inadequate sanitation and water systems—while others are not. These differences raise the possibility that burden-sharing should be tagged somehow to the disease burden a country actually suffers, though it is not clear whether this should be directly or inversely. Is it just the countries where dengue flourishes or the *Aedes aegypti* mosquito is enlarging its range that ought to be held responsible for dengue control?[42] Ought the United States be held responsible for contributions to the global spread of HIV because its own burden of HIV infection has been so great, and is further increasing? Should Russia be assessed for heavy contributions to tuberculosis management, given its role in allowing drug-resistant TB to develop in its prisons? In contrast, it is by and large the poorest countries that are at highest risk but least able to contribute to a burden-sharing arrangement. Global fairness might dictate that burden-sharing should be the other way around, because these countries are already victims of these diseases, not just vectors of them.

Utilizing the PVV view not just at the individual level, but with respect to countries as well, helps to argue that an account of fair burden-sharing would need to recognize that while actual, currently poor countries have the greatest burden of disease but the least capacity for financial burden-sharing (partly because the burden of disease is so high), it could be quite different. For example, there is always the possibility of a new pathogen (or for that matter a designer bioweapon) that strikes (or is aimed at) primarily the richer countries and leaves the poor ones unscathed. This is to view the issue of fair burden-sharing from the third as well as first and second perspectives within the PVV view—the Rawlsian-influenced perspective of deep uncertainty. From this perspective, policies for financing disease control would need to take most seriously the underlying notion of people's and indeed countries' mutual embeddedness in a web of disease, the idea that "we're all in this together." Indeed, it is this that underwrites the very notion of a global *Comprehensive Effort*.

Alterations in Economic Structures and Incentives for Contribution. Alterations in economic structures and incentives for contribution to a comprehensive global effort are a central concern. The existence of differing legal and economic systems in various regions of the world may raise issues about the development, testing, and production of vaccines and treatment drugs, especially where property rights and patent issues conflict with the need for low cost to ensure broad distribution. As well, the training and deployment of health professionals and international "brain drains" depleting the number of physicians and health-care workers, particularly in countries or regions where infectious

42. David M. Morens and Anthony S. Fauci, "Dengue and Hemorrhagic Fever: A Potential Threat to Public Health in the United States," *Journal of the American Medical Association* 299, no. 2 (January 9/16, 2008): 214–216.

disease is least well controlled, not only disastrously affect those health-care systems but undercut the interests of us all, residents of the developed as well as developing world. To think about brain drain issues just from the point of view of the personal choices of health-care professionals about where they want to practice, or for that matter from humanitarian motives alone, overlooks these broader concerns. If everyone has an interest in reducing the burden of disease, then there is an argument against taking physicians or other health-care providers away from where disease is most severe and problems of control are greatest—yet that is what the rich countries may be permitting to occur to poor countries right now. Instead, arguably, wealthier countries have an interest in making up for those who leave, whether by means of financial contributions or exchange of personnel. Finally, wealthier countries also have an interest in supporting health infrastructure everywhere, not just within their own borders, to the extent that better health infrastructure discourages health-care providers from moving away from their home countries of need in the first place.

Other questions about economic structures challenge underlying assumptions about the financial status and economic incentives of entire industries, especially the pharmaceutical industry, which is most involved with the development and marketing of vaccines and treatment drugs for infectious disease. In exploring the tensions between the profit motive in private industry and the needs of populations where poverty rates are high and the prevalence of preventable disease great, Thomas Pogge, for instance, argues that new drug development for vaccines and certain treatment measures should be rewarded as a function of the number of lives saved, not as a function of the units of drug purchased.[43] Even if they do not favor his solution to the problem, many theorists agree with the claim that current drug pricing schemes yield perverse drug development incentives and that this problem must eventually be addressed. A proposal like Pogge's or other similar ones would have bigger impact in the area of infectious disease than perhaps any other area of human health, because, as we have pointed out in Chapter 3, infectious disease can often be prevented with a single immunization or treated effectively with a one-time administration of an antibiotic. Unlike the continuing medical attention and drug treatment required to protect function or preserve life in chronic illnesses like heart disease, diabetes, emphysema, or cancer, in many infectious diseases serious illness or death can be prevented easily and cheaply. Thus economic incentives in the pharmaceutical industry favor research and development of drugs for chronic illnesses, where far more money is to be made, but

---

43. Thomas Pogge, "Human Rights and Global Health: A Research Program," in *Ethics and Infectious Disease,* ed. Michael J. Selgelid, Margaret P. Battin, and Charles B. Smith (Oxford: Blackwell, 2006), 285–306.

not for easy-to-treat infectious ones, yielding the perverse outcome that simple, cheap solutions to many infectious diseases are ignored.

Major changes could thus be in store if economic incentives are changed, particularly for the so-called neglected tropical diseases. As mentioned earlier, research finally now in progress suggests that immunization or full control would be possible with a single oral drug treatment for as many as seven of these diseases: roundworm, whipworm, hookworm, snail fever, elephantiasis, trachoma, and river blindness.[44] There are various other proposals for revising the economic incentives in the pharmaceutical industry; virtually all observers agree that the current incentives do not work in favor of the most efficient, effective infectious-disease control. A *Global Effort*, both in the period before the 2020–2030 decade of full implementation and during it, would need to address such issues in the varying contexts of international trade and patent protection, industry supports, and other economic differences around the globe.

Constraints or Sanctions for Non-Cooperation. Another substantial institutional issue concerns the appropriateness of constraints or sanctions for non-cooperation in a *Global Effort*. Some entities are unlikely to volunteer their resources, and some are not only unwilling to volunteer resources, but adopt policies or continue practices that undercut coordinated, cooperative global efforts. Specific recent and current governments, institutions, religious groups, and others have, for example, at times refused to recognize that AIDS is a virus-caused, human-to-human transmissible infectious disease; refused to cooperate in containing the spread of polio; refused to acknowledge the condom as a method of preventing the transmission of HIV and other sexually transmitted infectious diseases; refused to provide the WHO with information about the spread of SARS; refused to acknowledge the reality of sex trafficking and prostitution and so made control of HIV transmission in these contexts far more difficult;[45] insisted on ideologically driven practices like the "social marketing" of bednets by selling them for a price rather than giving them away;[46] refused to provide prisoners with effective tuberculosis medication that would not engender resistance; or refused to share H5N1 avian flu virus samples. Worse still, these specific actions that interfere with efforts to control infectious disease happen against a background in which some governments initiate or prolong war, sectarian strife, ethnic cleansing, and other hostilities that worsen a population's vulnerability to infectious disease, or in some cases deliberately encourage disease spread.

---

44. Madhuri Reddy et al., "Oral Drug Therapy for Multiple Neglected Tropical Diseases," table 1.

45. Louise Brown, *Sex Slaves: The Trafficking of Women in Asia* (London: Virago Press, 2000).

46. M. J. Friedrich, "Jeffrey Sachs, PhD," *Journal of the American Medical Association* 298, no. 16 (2007): 1850.

One ethical argument worthy of further exploration is that if institutions expect others to contribute, they are obligated in turn not to undermine the efforts of those who are involved in contributory practices from which they benefit.[47] There are examples in the world today of such contributory expectations: for example, the disease reporting requirements implemented by the WHO in the summer of 2007. Countries that benefit from such surveillance arguably have an obligation not to undermine its efficacy—as, for example, they might be in fostering intellectual property regimes that apparently work to the disadvantage of nations where diseases are endemic and thus potentially discourage cooperation in surveillance. How such matters should be addressed is a crucial issue for reflection in the development of this track of a *Global Effort to Close the Book on Infectious Disease*. After all, the *Effort* cannot succeed, or succeed quickly, if some institutions undercut the efforts of the whole.

Track 2: Epidemiologic and Health-Care Infrastructure

Track 2, epidemiologic and health-care infrastructure, is widely recognized as indispensable in the control of infectious disease. The absence of adequate health-care infrastructure, including the absence of adequate diagnostic and surveillance measures as well as adequate immunization and treatment measures, can contribute dramatically to the unchecked spread of infectious disease. An outbreak unnoticed (or ignored) can have an immense amplification effect down the road; the "stitch in time" approach to infectious disease is key to prevention, in that it is almost always easier to stop one case now than ten cases—or a hundred, or a hundred thousand—later on. Poverty and war have crucial amplifying effects: diseases that might be mild or resisted altogether by individuals who are healthy and well-nourished may spread rapidly in disrupted conditions where people endure malnourishment, parasites, and chronic illness. Natural disasters can also produce similar effects, if populations are cut off from care, and if the conditions of the disaster—standing water after a flood, for instance—create risks of disease. Economic practices can also affect disease transmission: for example, the practice common in many developing countries that physicians see private patients rather than poor, charity ones, exacerbates disease transmission, because it is poor, charity patients who are most likely to be afflicted because of their crowded living conditions and lack of access to clean water and adequate sanitation. And as was pointed out in Chapter 2, it is essential to keep in mind the mutual relationship of poverty and infectious disease: the socially destructive effects of uncontrolled AIDS, malaria, tuberculosis, and

---

47. Leslie Francis, "Global Systemic Problems and Interconnected Duties," *Environmental Ethics* 25 (2003): 115–128.

other plagues on the developing world are major causative factors in suppressing the economies of many developing nations.

Poverty, war, and natural disaster are also typically associated with inadequate infrastructure: for those who do become ill, health care is hardly available: clinics, if there are any, are overcrowded, personnel are inadequately trained and hopelessly stressed, medications are outmoded or unavailable. Poverty and war are often hopelessly intertwined: northeast Kenya, for example, has a million refugees from Somalia, people for whom the risks of infectious disease are compounded over the already difficult lives they had previously led. Kenya also saw another 300,000 people internally displaced following the post-election violence in early 2008, and chief among the many health risks these refugees face is cholera.[48] Life in refugee camps or urban slums, often without adequate sanitation facilities, is, as our PVV view might describe it, life most fully "enmeshed in the web of disease," life in which people are most obviously way-station selves as microorganisms travel unchecked among them. Thus, in seeking greater control of infectious disease, attention to infrastructure issues is crucial:

- enhancement of social and sanitary infrastructure:
  - clean water
  - sanitation
  - waste disposal
  - control of insect and animal vectors (mosquitoes, fleas, rats, etc.)
  - control of environmental toxins
  - health-related transportation, including roads or airlifts and other ways bringing health care to people in remote or disrupted communities
- enhancement of health-care delivery systems, especially vaccine delivery systems, treatment facilities, and easy-access clinics
- encouragement of use of low-tech, low-cost modalities for infectious-disease prevention: bednets,[49] water filters and "drinking straws," pond attendants, etc.
- development of novel health-care delivery modalities, e.g., "accompagnateurs"[50] as *Partners in Health* has utilized in HIV/TB treatment in Haiti
- attention to the causes of poverty associated with infectious disease, particularly those associated with the neglected tropical diseases and with disease outbreaks among dislocated populations like refugees

---

48. Harvard World Health News, "Kenya: Homeless Face Myriad Risks," January 17, 2008, quoting *The Standard, Nairobi.*
49. David Bradley, discussion of insecticide-treated mosquito nets, "Ethical Barriers to Malaria Control," lecture at Oxford University, July 4, 2007.
50. Paul Farmer and Laurie Garrett, "From 'Marvelous Momentum' to Health Care for All: Success Is Possible with the Right Programs," *Foreign Affairs* 86, no. 2 (March/April 2007), http://www.foreignaffairs.org/20070301faresponse86213/paul-farmer-laurie-garrett/from-marvelous-momentum-to-health-care-for-all-success-is-possible-with-the-right-programs.html.

- attention to the causes of war, civil conflict, guerilla actions, and related hostilities that exacerbate the risks of infectious disease
- rapid response to natural disasters, with particular attention to special characteristics of a disaster that might encourage the spread of disease

To be sure, there are compelling reasons for attempting to reduce poverty, war, and the impact of natural diseases beyond that related to the control of infectious disease; our point here, obviously, is that these factors compound the difficulties of disease control to an enormous degree. Of course, to insist that infrastructure issues are essential is not to insist that they are more fundamental or more pressing than access to vaccines[51]; in a *Global Effort*, both are essential.

Attention to surveillance mechanisms, balanced against considerations of privacy and confidentiality, is also essential in tracking infectious disease; we have discussed these issues in Chapter 19. Projects such as these, many already well developed, are essential:

- enhanced local surveillance and communication systems
- enhanced global surveillance mechanisms for monitoring disease outbreaks
- improved methods of global communication and systems for increasing speed of reporting, etc.
- improved methods of developing the technical infrastructure for protecting data security and privacy

It is also crucial to use population-wide epidemiological approaches as well as clinical approaches for tracking disease spread and control. Here, advanced modeling and other methods come into play:

- enhanced modeling methods for determining the interaction of poverty, war, natural disaster, and other reasons for the lack of health-care resources with factors associated with infectious disease
- improved modeling methods for determining how to use prophylaxis and postexposure treatments effectively, for example stockpiles of antivirals[52]
- improved historical and modeling methods for determining the effect of social distancing—and whether this is an effective method of controlling spread.[53]

Ethical questions associated with this enormous variety of concerns might range from consideration of who should receive how many bednets and what they may or may not do with them, to requiring financial contributions or

---

51. Nim Pathy (Nimalan Arinamipathy), "Using Antiviral Stockpiles Effectively," lecture at Oxford University, July 4, 2007.

52. Dave A. Chokshi, Aaron S. Kesselheim. 2008. "Rethinking global access to vaccines," *British Medical Journal* 336 (April 5, 2008): 750-753.

53. Angela McLean, "Impact of Social Distancing on Influenza Transmission" lecture at Oxford University, Oxford, England, July 4, 2007.

labor for the installation of sanitary systems, to the very substantial privacy and confidentiality issues that arise with local and global surveillance systems.[54] Modeling methods used in planning, whether for endemic disease in poverty and war or for outbreaks associated with pandemics of newly emerging diseases or in natural disasters, are of particular ethical significance under the PVV view, because they often incorporate assumptions about what levels of disease can be tolerated; the PVV view warns against cavalier acceptance of leaving a significant proportion—indeed, any proportion—of a population still subject to preventable or treatable disease, because that is to ignore the fact that those who suffer disease are indeed victims.

Infrastructure improvement and, more broadly, societal development raise immense issues of global distributive justice. Although such issues are already extensively pursued by many philosophers, social policy experts, political theorists, and global health thinkers, our PVV view invites the re-examination of these views with specific attention to the ways in which they regard people in every part of the world as both (potential) victims and (potential) vectors, either as individuals or as population groups. We will take a more sustained look at Amartya Sen and especially Martha Nussbaum's capabilities approach in the next chapter, recognizing that the background philosophical issues are of enormous complexity, but will simply note here that the PVV demands that, among other things:

- attempts to alter infrastructure do not exacerbate poverty
- attempts to relieve poverty do not destroy social fabrics
- attempts to alter infrastructure or alter economic conditions do not incite war that might worsen the health conditions of populations
- diagnostic and surveillance methods are not abused, particularly by violations of privacy or confidentiality
- modeling methods do not write off portions of a population—that is, that they do not make victims of some people in the effort to protect others from vectors

These demands may be so immense as to seem implausible. But there is another way of thinking about the immense issue of epidemiologic and health-care infrastructure, in all its varied social and political settings: this is to recognize the role of what is often called the "know–do gap" in infectious disease—the fact that we know how to control many infectious diseases, among them malaria, TB, and AIDS; we just do not do it.[55] What kind of self-regarding

---

54. In some areas, fishermen are reported to use bednets as fishing nets rather than to protect children from mosquitoes. David Bradley, "Ethical Barriers to Malaria Control," lecture at Oxford University, July 4, 2007.
55. Jessika van Kammen, Don de Savigny, and Nelson Sewankambo, "Using Knowledge Brokering to Promote Evidence-Based Policy-Making: The Need for Support Structures," *Bulletin of the World Health Organization* 84, no. 8 (October 3, 2006): 608–612.

discipline, and what moral obligations must we assume, in order to break the know–do barrier? This is an enormous area for ethical reflection, one we can only have sketched most briefly here.

Particularly important under the PVV view, especially at its second, population-wide level, is attention to how large-scale programs are formulated. Classic epidemiology tracks disease movement through populations. Research agendas focus on issues of particular salience in specific populations but leave aside others. Treatment programs often target just those populations or population subgroups at highest risk of contracting and transmitting disease. There are obvious advantages of design and efficiency here, but at some moral cost. Our PVV view insists that those left outside these categories—people not in high-risk groups who nevertheless contract disease, people whose groups are not the focus of research efforts, and sufferers from "orphan diseases"—be recognized too, both in their roles as vectors but especially as victims.

Track 3: Scientific Development

Effective control of human infectious disease cannot be possible without continuing scientific development. Examples of scientific efforts—many already well under way—that would be essential to achieving any measure of success involve better diagnosis; better treatment; better mechanisms for prevention; and better background science in the understanding of microbial pathogenesis, defense mechanisms in humans, and evolutionary, genetic and other factors relevant to human vulnerability to infectious disease. The Gates Foundation's handsomely funded Grand Challenges in Global Health program already includes some 14 research incentives, which serve seven long-term goals in global health: improving childhood vaccines, creating new vaccines, controlling insects that transmit agents of disease, improving nutrition to promote health, improving drug treatment of infectious diseases, curing latent and chronic infection, and measuring health status accurately and economically in developing countries.[56]

These are immensely important goals; many others are in progress or remain to be developed. A group of comparatively realistic research goals would include:

- improvement or development of rapid, reliable tests for all infectious diseases, based on polymerase chain reaction, proteomic, or nanotechnology methods:
  - Goal: 100% specificity, 100% sensitivity: no false positives, no false negatives, including field-usable tests available at point-of-care
  - Goal: rapid speed of identification, in minutes or seconds
  - Goal: low cost, easy use

---

56. Singer et al., "Grand Challenges in Global Health: The Ethical, Social and Cultural Program."

- improvement of genetic identification methods for pathogens and other means for transmission tracking
  - in humans
  - in animal vectors
- development of improved methods of rapid identification of emerging diseases

Pathogen identification and disease diagnosis are crucial in prevention, and central to a *Global Effort* already under way. Particularly challenging scientific goals include treatment as well, especially because treatment possibilities change with the rapid replication rate of many infectious organisms, with the development of drug resistance, and other factors. A drug that may have worked in one region may not work in others; for instance chloroquin resistance on the part of the falciparum malaria parasite is widespread in some areas endemic for the parasite.[57] Developing effective prevention and treatment is an ongoing challenge.

Among the particular scientific research projects that constitute further components of an overall PVV research agenda for a *Global Effort* are:

- development of improved vaccines and vaccine production methods
  - cell culture based vaccines
  - toll-Like receptor ligand vaccines, coupled to antigen-presenting cells, for activating innate immune response
  - transcutaneous immunization, including adjuvant patches for pandemic influenza
  - muscosal vaccines, e.g., for HIV
  - reverse vaccinology approaches[58]
  - a current dream: one vaccine for HIV, TB, and malaria[59]
  - a future dream: one vaccine, administered once, for all serious human infectious diseases
- development of improved antimicrobials and other forms of treatment for all infectious diseases, including
  - orphan diseases
  - the so-called neglected tropical diseases
  - animal and plant diseases that contribute to human diseases
- dedicated effort to develop strategies for drug design to evade resistance, including combating resistance that may develop when control or elimination efforts are incomplete and disease rebounds

---

57. Bradley, "Ethical Barriers to Malaria Control."
58. "5th Annual Vaccines: All Things Considered," GTC Bio Conference, Washington DC., November 7–9, 2007.
59. Helen Fletcher, "TB Research in Developing Countries," lecture at Oxford University, July 4, 2007; Paul Kelly, "Public Health and Ethical Challenges in Tuberculosis Treatment and Control," lecture at Oxford University, July 4, 2007.

- development of safer insecticides and other vector controls
- development of novel, noninvasive diagnostic and surveillance mechanisms, for example:
  - ○ cell phones that take a person's temperature, or test for disease[60]
  - ○ temperature-sensing fabrics made into clothing[61]
  - ○ noninvasive temperature-monitoring devices[62]
- preparation for further research even after control or eradication: secure storage of organism samples, tissue samples, etc.

Furthermore, a particularly crucial direction of scientific development and research, if a genuinely *global* project were undertaken with the aim of reducing the burden of infectious disease to as low a point as possible, would involve enhancing our understanding of how infectious disease actually works, and whether elimination of disease is always a benefit.

- development of better understanding of atypical individuals, for example
  - ○ people who are contagious but asymptomatic
  - ○ people with chronic high temperature who might inappropriately trigger diagnostic mechanisms
  - ○ people with genetic protection against or vulnerabilities to specific diseases
- pursuit of careful research on whether any infectious diseases or processes confer evolutionary or survival advantage, either to individuals or groups

The latter is particularly important. Many diseases, including smallpox, diphtheria, malaria, yellow fever, and polio, are already under control, eliminated, or eradicated at least in some areas of the world: is there any downside to this other than risk of retransmission from areas where the disease is not eradicated? What, indeed, is the relationship between specific infectious diseases and other conditions afflicting human beings, for example, asthma or sickle cell disease? After all, at our current stage of scientific development, we may not know whether by eradicating or eliminating one disease we are increasing our susceptibility to other, perhaps related conditions, or disrupting human evolutionary development. Eradication or elimination might also create naive populations that are more likely to become severely ill when or if an infectious agent re-emerges or is developed as a bioweapon; this too is a serious risk.

Popular conflation over diseases with similar symptoms might also regard some as too minor to be the focus of control efforts. Noroviruses, including Norwalk virus, are the most common cause of focal outbreaks of vomiting and

---

60. Anders Sandberg, personal communication to M. Battin, July 4, 2007.
61. Gemma O'Doherty, "Power Dressing," *Irish Independent*, August 28, 2007, 31, reporting on the Siggraph 2007 exhibition in San Diego.
62. Sumita Roy, Keith Powell, and Lowell W. Gerson, "Temporal Artery Temperature Measurements in Healthy Infants, Children, and Adolescents," *Clinical Pediatrics* 42 (2003): 433–437.

diarrhea in the United States, but without serious aftereffects—unlike *E. coli*,[63] salmonella, shigella, or campylobacter, which are also the causes of acute food-borne illness that are sometimes fatal or followed by serious later problems.[64]

Scientists have also raised questions about whether some bacteria, viruses, or other human-affecting microorganisms are not just beneficial—they clearly are—but whether at least some infectious *diseases* are functional. On this worry, a thoroughgoing control program might risk higher rates of asthma, autoimmune disorders, or other unforeseen hazards that outweigh the benefits of eliminating at least some infectious diseases. A *Global Effort* must of course anticipate such questions, and this third track thus includes provision for extensive scientific research into these questions. A *Comprehensive Global Effort* seeks only human extrication from those conditions among the web of disease we would be better off without. It is already clear, however, that there are many diseases we are better off without, and nobody mourns the passing of smallpox or the imminent passing of polio.

The scientific track of the *Global Effort* also involves a number of ethical conditions and constraints, not as a function of the science itself but of the way it is pursued, funded, and administered. Under our PVV view, the scientific component of the *Global Effort* should meet certain moral criteria, a function of the overall ethical concern that all parties who are affected be treated as (potentially) both victims and vectors. Thus the science involved in the *Global Effort* should aim to achieve:

- the lowest possible false-negative and false-positive rates for diagnostic and surveillance measures consonant with effective disease control
- the lowest possible vaccine risks consonant with effective immunization
- the lowest side effect and failure rates for antibiotics and other treatments consonant with effective disease control
- progress in prevention or control of *all* serious human diseases, including orphan diseases and the so-called neglected tropical diseases, not just diseases of the rich or of rich countries
- pursuit of basic science as well as medical applications, sufficient to understand the long-range implications of control of infectious disease

---

63. There are an estimated 17 million cases of diarrhea each year attributed to bacteria that contaminate food and water in developing countries; a strain of *Escherichia coli* is responsible for a large fraction of these. A vaccine now under development by the Iomai Corporation, Gaithersburg, Md., involves a skin patch that contains a toxin made by the bacterium; the toxin induces an immune response without causing disease. Nathan Seppa, "Patch Guards Against Montezuma's Revenge," *Science News* 172, no. 22 (December 1, 2007): 350.

64. Paul S. Mead et al., "Food-Related Illness and Death in the United States," *Emerging Infectious Diseases* 5, no. 5 (September/October 1999): 607–617.

The way science is pursued is not value-free, moreover. The *Global Effort* would need to be attentive to how values affect the conduct of science, including such questions as the role of economic incentives in the reporting of research data or the selection of research problems.

A related kind of tension that might interfere with a *Comprehensive Global Effort for the Control of Infectious Disease* is competition for funding. Whether competitive enterprise is more or less productive in yielding new and effective scientific development is, of course, a familiar question in political theory, but here our PVV view insists that whatever system is in force, it takes the interests of *all* parties into account both as victims and vectors. There are many ways of violating PVV in doing science. For example, competition can be destructive: there is clearly a sense in Africa that there is now a very competitive environment for researchers competing for big donor money, and arguments over "turf" abound. Nongovernmental organizations and their expatriate technical experts have sometimes undermined local control of health programs, contributed to social inequality in the locations in which they work, and fragmented the local health systems.[65]

The PVV view also urges that governments and entities recognize the hypothetical as well as actual reasons for support of scientific research and cooperation in a *Comprehensive Global Effort*: although epidemics may at the current historical moment seem particularly likely to afflict some countries or continents rather than others, when it comes to globally transmissible disease, it could be otherwise. After all, dengue may be spreading to areas that, it is claimed, are warming with global climate change, but influenza flourishes in colder weather, and we may be unable to predict the ranges of future, not-as-yet emerging diseases.

Track 4: Religious, Social, and Cultural Considerations

Track 1's concern with developing cooperation among the various major institutions of the world—governmental, corporate, private, intergovernmental, and so on—also included religious institutions. Inasmuch as religious traditions and their institutions influence much of what people in every part of the globe think about disease and also govern their disease-transmission behavior, from hand washing before meals to sexual contact, the participation of religious institutions is crucial to the success of a *Global Effort*. However, some religious traditions preserve scriptural or traditional characterizations of infectious disease as "scourge," as "punishment" that is divinely ordained, or as the product of wrong behavior in this or previous lives. Addressing archaic

---

65. James Pfeifer, "International NGOs and Primary Health Care in Mozambique: The Need for a New Model of Collaboration," *Social Science & Medicine* 56, no. 4 (2003): 725–738.

characterizations of infectious disease is of consummate importance in securing the cooperation of people and their religious institutions, often enormously powerful, around the globe.

Consider the various portrayals of leprosy or plague or other infectious diseases in the scriptures of religious traditions. In the Hebrew/Christian Bible, for example, God allows Satan to test the loyal Job with any hardship that is short of fatal, and Satan begins with infectious disease (perhaps leprosy or a staph infection): Satan "smote Job with running sores from head to foot, so that he took a piece of broken pot to scratch himself as he sat among the ashes."[66] In the al-Bukhari *Hadith*, plague is described as "a means of torture which Allah used to send upon whom-so-ever He wished, but He made it a source of mercy for the believers, for anyone who is residing in a town in which this disease is present, and remains there and does not leave that town, but has patience and hopes for Allah's reward, and knows that nothing will befall him except what Allah has written for him, then he will get such reward as that of a martyr"—in other words, plague is a punishment, though it can also become a blessing for those who believe.[67] The Xhosa people of Lusikisiki, a district in the Eastern Cape Province of South Africa, an area in which many people dying of AIDS do not get tested or do not take antiretroviral drugs even if they are available, are said to see sickness as "a kind of bewitchment, something sent to you by ancestors you have offended or by those who wish you ill."[68] In many religious and cultural traditions, the implication is that people or groups afflicted by disease in some way deserve it, and that such illnesses are a product of divine wrath visited upon them or perhaps an opportunity for spiritual growth.

Attitudes about HIV/AIDS or other STDs expressed in some contemporary religious groups sometimes construe contracting the disease as punishment for homosexuality, infidelity, promiscuity, or other sinful behavior, either of individuals or of groups. Fatalism may also be associated with religious views, as when it is held that the visitation of infectious disease is God's will and hence that nothing can be done about it. Both religious and cultural attitudes may be involved in ancient practices like belling lepers or shunning victims with pocks, boils, open sores, or other visible evidence of disease. In some traditions, such attitudes may include views that the afflicted not only deserve it but are "not our problem," that justice is being done and others have either no obligation to intervene, or no intervention is appropriate. Some religious

---

66. Job 2:7–9.
67. Al-Bukhari, Sahih, *Hadith*, vol. 8, book 77, no. 616, tr. Muhammad Mushin Khan,"The translation of the meanings of Sahih Al-Bukhari," in *Fath Al-Bari*, Egyptian Press of Mustafa Al-Babi Al-Halabi, 1959.
68. Adam Hochschild, "'Death March,' review of Johnny Steinberg, *Siswe's Test: A Young Man's Journey Through Africa's AIDS Epidemic* (New York: Simon and Schuster, 2008)," *New York Times Book Review* (February 10): 28–29.

groups appear to fear that attempts to reduce infectious disease transmission, especially of sexually transmitted diseases like HIV or HPV, might interfere with teachings prohibiting homosexuality or encouraging chastity. And some religious traditions value the contingency of human life per se, appearing to hold that efforts to forestall illness or delay death are contrary to divine plan.

Some religious groups or religious authorities also hold specific views about infectious disease or its preventives or treatment that might play a major role in contributing to or undercutting the success of the *Global Effort*. The imams of Kano, northern Nigeria, were reported to believe and encourage their parishioners to believe that polio vaccine was part of a U.S. plot to spread HIV and make Muslim girls sterile; this resulted in a year-long boycott of polio vaccine, and thus contributed to the outbreak of polio emanating from that state in 2003. The Catholic Church does not officially permit the use of condoms for disease prevention as distinct from contraception, though it has been considering changing the condom ban for married couples in which one partner is already infected.[69] And whether or not such views are rooted in religious differences or are largely cultural or political, some individuals, groups, and countries may be hostile to a *Global Effort*, in ways ranging from non-cooperation to sabotage, if it is seen as a "western" project imposed as yet another legacy of colonialism on the non-white peoples of the world.

Religious beliefs and attitudes can of course play a strongly positive role in encouraging cooperation with a societal project to protect the life and health of human beings. Religious commandments like "do not kill" and "respect life" speak in favor of bringing potentially lethal infectious diseases under control. Traditions that stress compassion and the relief of suffering would presumably also support the underlying concern of a *Global Effort* to extricate humankind from the web of disease within which it is enmeshed. Some religious traditions stress the unity of human beings in divine creation; some stress stewardship of the environment and, with it, concern for human health; some emphasize attitudes of caring, concern, compassion for those who are ill. And many stress the value of sacrifice and dedicated work for the good of the community, a commitment believed to be viewed favorably by the divine or rewarded well in the next life. These are all attitudes that suggest that religious institutions might play a powerful role in engendering cooperation with a *Global Effort* by the world's faithful who subscribe to these views. Specific examples can be cited such as cooperation among Islamic officials in requiring polio immunization for children on the hajj in the wake of the 2003 outbreak. Even a religious group that rejects conventional medicine, like Christian Science, recognizes

---

69. Alfonso Cardinal Lopez Trujillo, "Family Values Verses Safe Sex" (December 1, 2003), http://www.vatican.va/roman_curia/pontifical_councils/family/documents/rc_pc_family_doc_20031201_family-values-safe-sex-trujillo_en.html (accessed February 16, 2008).

the importance of reducing transmission: a Church of Christ, Scientist, practitioner and teacher in Chicago writes of using spiritual means of healing for "Making Colds Uncommon—For the Common Good";[70] Christian Science also permits its members to accept immunization where it is legally required, for example for travel or school entry. But a larger *Comprehensive Global Effort* might involve enlisting the cooperation of both major and minor religious groups, for instance by holding ongoing all-faiths councils on infectious disease: here the aim might usefully be not only to cooperate in practical projects like operating medical missions in severely affected areas, but to think through together how traditional beliefs might undercut or support a *Global Effort*.

Social and cultural attitudes may also dramatically affect capacities to control infectious disease, from beliefs about science and research, to views about desert in allocation of resources, to views about the intrinsic nature or purposes of humankind. Such attitudes cover a vast range, but several quite different examples might suggest the variety of attitudes and the role they can play. Some are comparatively easy to address: for example, white-colored bednets have been viewed as culturally inappropriate in some communities in which they were used. Carl Coleman describes the social attitudes that fuel the over-prescribing of antibiotics in the medical cultures of the developed world.[71] Paul Farmer describes attitudes about poverty that allow HIV and tuberculosis to decimate a country like Haiti.[72] Social and cultural attitudes affect virtually all the issues discussed in this volume, but it is important to think through the degree to which they serve, or disserve, a *Global Effort*, and in particular whether they succeed in enacting the PVV view, managing to view every party affected as both (potential) victim and (potential) vector. Many social attitudes are either victim-blaming or demand draconian control over vectors; religious, social, and cultural attitudes should be explored, under the PVV view, for ways they might avoid both. Doing so would also be an essential component of a *Global Effort*'s task, an immense undertaking we can only sketch here.

In a *Global Effort*'s attention to religious, social, and cultural contexts, a primary concern must involve respect for people's cultural, religious, and social structures, intervening or attempting to modify them only to the least extent necessary to achieve elimination or control of infectious disease. Very small accommodations can sometimes make a considerable difference in disease

---

70. Bea Roegge, "Making Colds Uncommon—For the Common Good," *Christian Science Sentinel* (February 6, 2006), http://www.spirituality.com/tte/article_display.jhtml?ElementId=/repositories/shcomarticle/Jan2006/1138043707.xml&ElementName=Making%20colds%20uncommon%14for%20the%20common%20good (accessed February 16, 2008).

71. Carl Coleman, "The Role of Law in Limiting the Over-Prescription of Antibiotics," lecture at Oxford University, July 4, 2007.

72. Paul Farmer, *Pathologies of Power: Health, Human Rights, and the New War on the Poor* (Berkeley: University of California Press, 2004).

control without disrupting religious practice. For example, the Roman Catholic practice of Communion involves having many people drink the sacramental wine one after another from a common cup, but this ritual practice is adapted in the effort to diminish health concerns by having the priest wipe the lip of the cup with a cloth after one communicant has drunk, before offering it to the next.[73] Somewhat larger accommodations can also sometimes be approached in different ways: for example, after outbreaks of polio among Orthodox Reformed groups in the Netherlands that do not accept immunizations, Dutch health authorities went to meet with the leaders and members of the community, letting them know that it would be about 10 years before another outbreak could be expected. The authorities agreed that there was insufficient political and social basis for mandatory vaccination, and concluded that global eradication would be the only way to protect these groups.[74] Sometimes, however, a religious or cultural practice cannot be sustained at all if the risks of disease are to be controlled—for example, the Fore language group in Papua New Guinea practice of eating human brains as part of a funeral ritual, a ritual that led to the transmission of the prion disease, Kuru. After elimination of this practice, Kuru has nearly disappeared.[75] But other programs to control infectious disease have sometimes been quite heavy-handed, in effect attempting to eliminate certain social, religious, or cultural practices associated with infectious disease rather than attempting to eliminate just the disease.

To challenge entrenched social or religious beliefs is never easy, and rarely fully successful. But this is the issue our PVV view expects us to put on the table: that entrenched beliefs and practices may fail to regard people, as individuals and in groups or populations, in light of both their victimhood and their vectorhood.

Track 5: Legal, Social, and Ethical Protections for Individuals and Groups

Our PVV view here also recognizes that a *Global Effort* for the control of infectious disease cannot satisfy the conditions of this view unless it attends to legal, social, and ethical protections for individuals and groups, to ensure that neither individuals nor groups are victimized by institutional measures, scientific research programs, infrastructure changes, or other matters that are part

---

73. Archdiocesan Liturgy Office, *Suggestions for the Administration of Holy Communion and the Sharing of the Sign of Peace During the Cold and Flu Season* (June 19, 2007), www.liturgy.sydney.catholic.org.au/documents/pdf/20070719_CommunionPaxColdFluSeason.pdf (accessed February 16, 2008).

74. Marina A.E. Conyn-van Spaendonck et al., "Immunity to Poliomyelitis in the Netherlands," *American Journal of Epidemiology* 153 no. 3 (February 1, 2001): 207–214.

75. James Chin, *Control of Communicable Diseases Manual* (Washington, DC: American Public Health Association, 2000), 186.

of the *Global Effort*. This is to recognize that, under our PVV view, "victim-hood" can have a dual sense: a person or group, or entire population, may be the victim of a disease—this is the primary sense of "victim" in the PVV view—but may also be the victim, so to speak, of policies, programs, prejudices, and other matters associated with disease, or both.

Protections for individuals, groups, and populations, under our PVV view, should include, as we have been arguing throughout this book, at least:

- development of rigorous local, national, and international protections for privacy and confidentiality of individual information in surveillance systems
  - in reporting of data
  - in contact tracing and transmission tracking
  - in follow up for health care
- development of policies concerning rights to privacy and/or confidentiality for information that poses a risk to other people, or a right to privacy in a public place
- development of protections and systems for maximum communication among families and social groups during isolation, quarantine, home quarantine, or other restrictions in epidemics
- development of protections for things that matter to people, e.g., pets, property.
  - attention to animal-rights, animal-welfare issues
- erection of special protections for the least well off (and most likely to be
  - affected by infectious disease):
  - refugees
  - prisoners
  - the institutionalized, including those in mental institutions
  - the homeless
  - the elderly
  - infants and children
  - people with disabilities, in poor health, or with compromised immune systems

As Michael Parker puts it, echoing the British pandemic plan, "Everyone matters."[76] This notion is essential to our PVV view: while it recognizes that tradeoffs between concerns like privacy and surveillance or confidentiality and interruption of transmission must sometimes be made, it still insists that policies must always consider everyone as both victim and vector—so that attention to vectorhood is tempered by the circumstances of victims, and solicitation for victims by the risks of vectorhood, at one and the same time.

As with issues concerning infrastructure development, this track too involves not merely practical measures, but continuing philosophical attention to background issues in constraints. In preceding chapters, we have discussed constraints

76. Michael Parker, "Methods of Pandemic Planning—the UK Task Force," lecture at Oxford University, July 4, 2007.

in general and in the specific context of pandemic planning, particularly for avian flu, but we imagine here that under a *Comprehensive Global Effort* and in the years leading up to it there would be extensive academic, professional, and public reflection on which constraints are legitimate and which are not. These discussions will require open dialogue; they will require sensitivity to cultural difference; they will require political finesse; but they will be a crucial element of a *Global Effort.*

After all, effective constraints on individuals, groups, institutions, and even countries may play a central role in achieving control of infectious disease, both as it spreads from one person to another and from one global region to another, and will require at least basic global agreement, though not necessarily identical practices, if parties are to work together, even for a single decade. When and under what conditions is the imposition of such measures as quarantine, isolation, required immunization, and other transmission-control measures legitimate? As we have seen in earlier chapters, these are not easy questions. Nor are questions about infractions of constraints, and whether responses to non-cooperation and evasion of constraints should be non-punitive and non-blaming, or be modeled on elements of civil or criminal law where one party's actions constitute a harm to another or another's interests. Here is where questions about contemporary versions of Typhoid Mary need to be addressed: for example, Andrew Speaker's evasion of no-fly constraints; superspreaders who remain sexually active, like Patient Zero; or deliberate "bug-chasers" who either seek to contract HIV or volunteer to transmit it to someone else. What about countries that are said to have disguised the occurrence of cases of SARS during the 2003 epidemic, or to have allowed drug-resistant tuberculosis to develop in their prison populations, or to have ignored scientific evidence about disease transmission, like the United States, where then-President Ronald Reagan refused to mention AIDS in public for several years after the epidemic began, and South Africa, where then-President Thabo Mbeki refused to acknowledge the viral etiology of AIDS, in both cases contributing to unchecked spread. Such specific issues as whether opt out as distinct from opt in testing is appropriate[77] or what is meant by the "least restrictive alternative" in constraints of any kind[78] will be crucial here, among many others. The kind of theoretical and policy work that would need to be done in preparation for a *Global Effort* would need to address all these issues, so that appropriate policies could be in place but also so that the public affected by them could know them in advance.

We have not tried to take a stand on every specific question, focusing instead on the moral conditions that any constraint must meet. For this reason,

77. Harold Jaffe, "Opt-out HIV Testing," lecture at Oxford University, July 4, 2007.
78. Angus Dawson, "Tuberculosis and the Ethical Justification of the 'Least Restrictive Alternative'," lecture at Oxford University, July 4, 2007.

we have avoided taking sides in vivid current controversies, like that for example between policy theorists Larry Gostin and George Annas. But we do note
that Gostin's *Model Plan*[79] for pandemic mitigation is exquisitely sensitive to
issues of vector control, while Annas, Mariner, and Parmet's attack on it, prepared for the American Civil Liberties Union,[80] is equally sensitive to the situations of victims, both of such policies and of disease. (Indeed we think Gostin
and Annas are both right in considerable measure, but each is one-sided at the
same time.)

There are also a number of specific additional issues that fall within Track 5's
concern with legal, ethical, and social protections for individuals and groups.

Press and Public Information Issues. In a genuine global cooperative effort to
bring infectious disease under control, there would be (as there already are)
issues about how to respond to popular information, involving clashes of freedom of the press and freedom of religion with the need for a sound scientific
basis for public disease-control policy. What about popular but erroneous beliefs concerning the dangers of vaccines—for example, that vaccines cause autism or inflammatory bowel disease, or that they sterilize girls? Currently, as
we have seen in Chapter 14 on HPV, this issue is to some degree ignored by relying on herd immunity: if some parents refuse to immunize their children
because of these unfounded beliefs, their children and others are still in the
main protected—provided vaccine uptake in the surrounding population remains at adequate levels. Even in developed countries, however, immunization
rates have slipped low enough in recent years that herd immunity sometimes
fails. For example, a 2005 outbreak of measles occurred in Indiana among people
who declined vaccination,[81] and in August 2007 Britain's National Health Protection Agency warned of the worst outbreak of measles in 20 years, occurring in
geographic areas with the lowest uptake of the MMR vaccine; by then there
had already been 480 confirmed cases and one death, a 14-year-old boy.[82]

Many other examples of popular misinformation can have broad consequences as well—for example, that HIV has been unleashed in Africa by foreign governments, either as part of bio-warfare or due to contamination of

79. Lawrence Gostin, *Model Plan*.
80. Annas, Mariner, and Parmet, "Pandemic Preparedness."
81. Amy A. Parker et al., "Implications of a 2005 Measles Outbreak in Indiana for Sustained Elimination of Measles in the United States," *New England Journal of Medicine* 355, no. 5 (August 3,
2006): 447–455.
82. Donald G McNeil, Jr., "Sharp Drop Seen in Deaths From Ills Fought by Vaccine," *New York
Times*, Health Section, November 14, 2007; Polly Curtis, "Vaccination of Children in UK Urged as
Measles Cases Soar," *Irish Times*, August 31, 2007, 12.

vaccines made in wealthy countries.[83] The press may sometimes also contribute to popular misunderstanding, for example when it reports isolated incidents of abuses or excesses, when it generalizes from isolated anecdotes, when it fans exaggerated fear-mongering (especially of pandemic outbreaks), or when it labels subgroup populations as foci of infection but fails to make clear that others are infected too (for instance, that it is Haitians or gay men or blacks who have HIV, or that it is women who have HPV). In January 2008, the Infectious Diseases Society of America implored the Disney-ABC television network not to release an episode of "Eli Stone," featuring a legal case in which a child becomes autistic as the result of having been vaccinated, warning that it was not based on fact and had the potential to undercut immunization rates.[84] While the press could in general be a tremendously effective force in galvanizing support for a *Global Effort* to rid the world of the major human-affecting infectious diseases, it could also undercut such an effort. There are ample areas for further focused ethical attention here, weighing freedom of the press against accuracy in conveying the facts of infectious disease distribution and how it spreads.

Variations in Policy. Policies about legal and social issues of all sorts may vary considerably among democratic, authoritarian, tribal, religion-based, and other communities. A *Global Effort* need not be committed to changing governmental or cultural structures; it is concerned rather with how entities within all these environments could cooperate in pursuing a single common interest, namely reducing the burden of infectious disease in all parts of the world, from urban metropolis to tribal homeland. Local policies may differ greatly, yet still permit cooperation or at least progress in tandem toward the elimination or control of disease. In the United States, for example, protections for privacy and confidentiality for people who are HIV-positive are extensive, while in contrast, a policy now being introduced among the Enga of Papua New Guinea stresses traditional cultural values about community knowledge of illness, and reinforces open, public announcement of HIV status.[85]

83. Brooke Grundfest Schoepf, "AIDS, History, and Struggles over Meaning," in *HIV and AIDS in Africa: Beyond Epidemiology*, ed. Ezekiel Kalipeni et al. (Malden, MA: Blackwell, 2004), 20.

84. Benjamin Kruskal and Carole Allen, "Perpetrating the Autism Myth," *Boston Globe* (January 31, 2008), http://www.boston.com/news/health/articles/2008/01/31/perpetrating_the_autism_myth/ (accessed January 8, 2008). Letter from Donald Poretz, M.D., IDSA President, to Anne Sweeney, President, Disney-ABC Television Group, January 28, 2008.

85. See Enga Provincial HIV/AIDS Committee, the Tradition and Transition Centre, and the Tambukini, Aipos and Tetemanda Communities, "Community Initiative to Curb the HIV/AIDS Epidemic: A Pilot Project in Enga Province [Papua New Guinea] [2007]," manuscript. For more information contact: Dr. Polly Wiessner, Department of Anthropology, University of Utah.

Among the Enga, current HIV/AIDS awareness programs are rejected as centered on the individual as the sole responsible actor, a posture which is seen as having little impact; instead, the Enga seek a project that, according to the policy proposal, "treats health as a public good to be fostered by collective action."[86] The Enga are described as having had

> ... numerous traditions of openness in the past. One was the *yanda aiputi miningi* held to unite fighters when tribal wars took a turn for the worse. Men assembled, confessed the most atrocious past thoughts and deeds towards one another, went through rituals of cleansing, and emerged united.
>
> Health status was public knowledge because it was the community who cared for the sick at home. Relatives and sub-clan members provided pigs for healing rituals. Disfigured lepers were cared for and included in social events, although housed in separate dwellings near the family house to avoid intimate daily contact. Today family members accompany their relatives to medical consultations; diagnoses and papers bearing test results are circulated by the patient. . . . Only with HIV/AIDS has confidentiality of individual health status been emphasized, leading to rumor, suspicion, and stigma. Secrets are regarded as lies.[87]

In the United States, control of the HIV/ADIS epidemic is usually (but not always) regarded as best served by rigorous protection for privacy and confidentiality; among the Enga, in contrast, openness about diagnoses is seen as the best way to stem the epidemic before it worsens. Tensions of this sort, which we have explored in other contexts throughout this volume, may be great if viewed through the lens of clinical bioethics, which has been particularly concerned with privacy and confidentiality as well as other traditional issues in the doctor–patient relationship, or the lens of public health, which has been in contrast particularly concerned with transmission control. Our PVV view insists on the need to accommodate both; the more creative the solutions to this tension, no doubt the better. Part of the route to a satisfactory solution is to recognize that while HIV confidentiality policies in the United States and among the Enga are different, they share two common goals: protecting affected individuals from becoming victims of either their illness or of social condemnation, and reducing transmission of a devastating human disease.

Legal and social protections for individuals and groups will also need to be adapted to specific circumstances of infectious disease, from endemic and often inconsequential, self-resolving infections like that in HPV to pandemic and highly dangerous infection like that of the most lethal and rapidly transmissible influenzas. Those engaged in devising legal and social protections will

---

86. Ibid., 1.
87. Ibid., 2.

need to do at much more extensive length what we have considered in the previous chapters: engage in open dialogue and careful policy construction about priority-setting both in endemic and especially pandemic emergency conditions, where scarcity of resources,[88] personnel, vaccines, treatment facilities, and aftercare may be extreme.[89] In the previous chapters on constraints we have provided a sketch of what we think this dialogue ought to include and some problems we see as currently overlooked. In preparation for and during a *Comprehensive Global Effort*, especially as imagined for the decade 2020–2030, attention to these issues will be of paramount importance—especially should a major epidemic of serious or lethal disease occur during that time.

Also relevant to legal and social protections (as well as to scientific development and other tracks), are issues of aftermath, both of a *Global Effort* and in the wake of any specific outbreaks or pandemics that might occur. Attention to aftermath issues is essential in achieving full control of infectious disease, because it will influence the willingness of people to participate in global efforts. Thus, it will be necessary to engage in open dialogue and policy construction concerning compensation,[90] as we have discussed in Chapter 18, for such matters as:

- losses to those constrained, deprioritized, harmed, or otherwise made worse off under policies for control or eradication of infectious disease
  - those placed in quarantine or isolation
  - those injured by vaccines or treatments
  - those who suffer losses from livestock culling, lost work days, etc.
  - those who become ill as a result of doing necessary jobs that may involve exposure (e.g., health-care workers, transport workers, morgue and cemetery workers)
  - those who are last on the list for treatment

A further area of concern about legal and social protections for individuals and groups involves attention to micro- and macroeconomic issues. What will be the impact of a *Global Effort* on all parties? Some concerns might involve those whose current income depends on treatment of infectious disease. After all, if a *Global Effort* were to succeed and the global burden of infectious disease dramatically reduced, this income would be eliminated. Who will be out of a job? Larger economic concerns might focus for instance on the impact of higher rates of infant and child survival on domestic and social situations where poverty is severe, or on changed patterns of survival—reflecting the

---

88. Marcel Verweij, "Hard Choices: Allocation of Scarce Medical Resources in an Influenza Pandemic," lecture at Oxford University, July 4, 2007.

89. Dan Brock, "Pandemic Flu: Scenarios for Planning and Teaching," lecture at Oxford University, July 4, 2007.

90. Søren Holm, "Justifiable Detention and the Question of Compensation," lecture at Oxford University, July 4, 2007.

success of a *Global Effort* in reducing death rates—on economies around the world. There would presumably be relatively little effect on economies in the advanced industrial nations where infectious disease is already largely under control, but there could be dramatic effect in the worst-off nations of the world. Like everything else associated with it, a *Comprehensive Global Effort* should be subjected to adequate scrutiny in the decades prior to and during the culminating phase itself, with of course an eye to mitigating economic damage where it threatens to occur and but reaping the economic benefits of effective disease control as well.

Follow Up for the Five Practice and Policy Tracks of a Global Effort

Crucial to the success of all five of the practical and policy tracks that a *Comprehensive Global Effort* would pursue are issues of follow up, both the short and long term after the end of the decade in which a *Global Effort* is pursued. Adequate follow up would need to involve:

- continuing inquiry into what followup is appropriate:
    - ongoing information about risks averted
    - registry of diseases under control or eradicated
- maintenance of continuing global coordination, cooperation; keep sign-ons from all parties in place
- adaptation of practical and ethical concerns in conditions of political instability and background injustice
- addressing questions about how to calculate and distribute costs fairly, including costs after the fact. These include the costs of initial surveillance, intervention, treatment and the costs of endemic and pandemic control
- addressing questions of how to calculate savings from diseases brought under control, eliminated, or eradicated
    - How to calculate savings for developed countries, where much ID is already under control, but risks may still be large?
    - How to calculate savings for less developed countries, where economic impact is great but human costs even greater?
    - how to calculate savings to future generations? (try calculating the savings over the last 200 years from smallpox eradication)
- addressing questions of failure and success:
    If complete success doesn't occur within a decade, remember why:
    - some pathogens have nonhuman vectors that cannot be controlled[91]
    - some pathogens are not yet identified

---

91. Angela McLean, "Impact of Social Distancing on Influenza Transmission," lecture at Oxford University, July 4, 2007.

- some pathogens are not yet treatable
- some pathogens evolve, re-emerge, emerge anew, become resistant
- preparation for temporary resurgences, new emergence of disease; prevention of breakdowns in infrastructure and surveillance systems
- pursuit of ongoing conceptual analysis of the distinctions between success and failure:
    - delays and disappointments are not necessarily failures
    - new emergences are not failures
    - but there are real failures: e.g., reemergence of malaria in Peru, TB in Russia and America, trypanosomiasis in Angola, Congo, and Sudan, yellow fever in Paraguay, and more
- also attending to the risks of success:
    - the likelihood of distraction, diversion, and other demands on funds as success increases and infectious disease is no longer seen as a threat
    - how to announce, celebrate (even partial) success without letting up on being on guard?

Responding to a review of current global approaches to neglected tropical diseases, two Australian researchers stress the importance of vigilant ongoing post-intervention surveillance programs that should continue well after the use of a "rapid-impact package of drugs" to control or eliminate these diseases.[92] They recognize that surveillance poses not just a resource challenge, but also a statistical challenge as diseases become less common. As the perceived benefits of incidence reduction decrease and the costs of going after the last few cases increase, priorities may seem to change; there is extensive discussion of whether these are false economies or appropriate changes in the use of resources. In any case, the Australian researchers' concern here, voiced with respect to parasitic diseases in the developing world, would in fact be a concern for a *Comprehensive Global Effort* as a whole: not letting attention be diverted by other priorities for funding, and not assuming a problem is solved just because incidence declines, in a premature way that actually serves to court resurgence.

A Comprehensive Global Effort: From Thought Experiment to Plan

Attempts to control infectious disease are already going on in many areas— indeed, in all five practical and policy tracks considered above—and they all raise important ethical issues. A *Comprehensive Global Effort for the Control of Infectious Disease*, incompletely developed as it is, is already well under way,

---

92. Clare Huppatz and David N. Durrheim, "Letter to the Editor: Control of Neglected Tropical Diseases," *New England Journal of Medicine* 357, no. 23 (December 6): 2407.

whether we see it as a thought experiment, a description of current events, or a plan. Whichever way we interpret it, it requires us to consider the importance of not only of global coordination and cooperation, but also the importance of coordinated, across-the-board *ethical* reflection. This reflection must include comparatively focused issues considered earlier in this book, like how to balance considerations of confidentiality versus public interest, how to weigh the impact of mandated treatment, or how to prioritize access to prevention and care in epidemics. It also extends to deeper but at the moment more diffuse sorts of philosophical issues, such as whether attempts to control infectious disease should be given priority over attempts to control cancer[93] or

---

93. Michael Selgelid trenchantly asks, what if we had a way of curing or preventing cancer—shouldn't we put our efforts here instead? (Personal communication with L. Francis and M. Battin, July 2007). Two responses are important. First, the question of whether we should put our efforts into curing cancer or preventing infectious disease is in part a question about efficiency: infectious disease strikes from outside, so to speak, transmitted from one human or other host to the person who becomes victim, while most (though not all) forms of cancer, as far as we know at the moment, result from or in concert with deteriorative processes within the body itself. Of course, if it is possible to completely eradicate a particular infectious pathogen—smallpox is our best and so far only example—that is the maximally efficient form of protection, since once eradication has been achieved (leaving aside deliberate reintroduction, as in biowarfare), no measures need be taken ever again to protect anyone from that disease. It is "cured" once and for all. Even immunization is no longer necessary, though it was essential in achieving eradication in the first place, and ongoing "protection" from then on involves no further risks, burdens, or costs. Even if the costs of eradication are huge, they will not equal the cumulative savings from eradication over time.

In contrast, deteriorative and degenerative diseases like many forms of cancer that are associated with or are the result of the normal aging processes of the human body and hence need to be addressed over and over again for each new aging individual, always balancing issues of risks, burdens, and costs. Even a "cure" for such forms of cancer would need to be deployed for each individual now and in the future who contracts cancer; as far as we currently know, there can be no analogue to eradication of these cancers once and for all, so that they never strike anyone ever again. Thus the eradication of a given infectious disease, assuming roughly similar morbidity and mortality, is at least in terms of cost-effectiveness far more appropriate than attempting to prevent or cure deteriorative diseases like cancer. It is well to remember, however, that most human-affecting infectious diseases are not eradicable, only eliminable or controllable.

Second, the question of controlling cancer versus infectious disease raises age-related intergenerational issues of justice. Cancer is typically (though not always) a disease of late middle age, a function in part of degenerative physical conditions in the human body. In contrast, infectious diseases, attacking so to speak from the outside, occur at any age, often unpredictably. To be sure, some age ranges are more susceptible to certain kinds of infectious diseases—babies and young children are particularly susceptible to infantile diarrhea (a major killer in the Third World), women of childbearing age who are delivering babies are the ones susceptible to puerperal sepsis, and young adults with active immune systems were particularly vulnerable to the 1918 flu. But many infectious diseases, like cholera or yellow fever can strike at any time during the normal human lifespan, thus potentially cutting life short at earlier and less predictable points than late-life diseases like most cancer. Thus, it is possible to save more quality life-years by preventing the infectious diseases at the beginning or mid-years of life than later-life diseases such as certain forms of cancer—especially infectious diseases that strike children in the developing world, since treatment is generally cheap and these diseases easy to prevent. To save a child from cancer is a sustained, complex, resource-intensive

whether bioweaponry is intrinsically worse than conventional arms.[94] In part because attention to the full control of infectious disease on a global scale has not so far been unified, the ethical issues each distinct effort raises have not been unified either, and have to a considerable extent been treated in comparatively isolated, discrete, "siloed" ways, even now that they are finally coming to be discussed in bioethics and other fields. This is not to say that ethical issues are to be viewed in a monolithic way, but that reflection on them must include understanding them in the larger context of a world in which we are "all in this together," all potentially victims and vectors of transmissible infectious disease.

---

project; to save a child from tetanus or polio or infantile diarrhea takes just an injection or a bit of oral rehydration solution. These are issues of intercontinental justice as well: in the United States, as in other developed countries, not only are there many fewer deaths from infectious disease but the vast proportion of them occur in older people; in Africa, it is the other way around, many deaths and an enormous proportion of them in children. In developed countries, thus, comparatively little life is to be saved: fewer years toward the end of the lifespan, for fewer people; in Africa, the amount of life to be saved with the effective control of infectious disease is huge.

To be sure, the questions of efficiency and justice are muddied when infection control is just that—ongoing control, rather than permanent eradication or elimination—and hence repeated, ongoing measures like immunization (or repeated immunization) or antibiotic treatment are required for each new individual. Questions of efficiency and justice also become more complex as we begin to discover viral associations with some forms of cancer—HIV-related lymphomas and Kaposi's sarcoma, EBV-related Burkett's lymphoma, and others; as scientific knowledge improves, it is increasingly difficult to separate out cancer (and also heart disease) from infectious diseases. And the questions are muddied still further as we keep in mind the ever present possibilities of new emergences—new "attacks from outside"—as new zoonotic diseases affect human populations or designer pathogens are unleashed in warfare or terrorism. Nevertheless, such issues of efficiency and justice in tradeoffs between dedicating resources to the control of infectious disease versus addressing other causes of human mortality must also be an important part of the continued ethical reflection the *Global Project* demands. The general issue is whether it is ethically defensible to try to achieve permanent, for-all-time control of the serious human infectious diseases through eradication, elimination, or reliable forms of control in contrast with non-eliminable, recurring causes of death. The best answer, of course, is to try to do both, but where the resources and political will are not sufficient and a choice of focus must be made, part of the *Global Effort's* underlying philosophical charge will be to explore the case in favor of either one.

94. It is widely assumed that the weaponization of infectious disease, from aerosolized smallpox and anthrax to designer pathogens based on the most lethal human plagues, is somehow worse than the use of conventional military and terrorist weaponry like guns and bombs. The issue is whether a bioweapon that killed, say, about 90,000 people within two to four months of its release would be intrinsically better or worse, or neither, other things being equal, than say the atomic bomb at Hiroshima, which killed an estimated 90,000 people within two to four months after it was dropped. Is the prospect of designing temporarily disabling but not lethal bioweapons (for example, the salmonella that the Rajneeshee religious sect sprinkled on salad bars in the Dalles and Wasco Counties, Oregon, in 1984 to sicken people long enough to prevent them from voting in the local election), a point against or in favor of the use of bioweapons in contrast to conventional weapons, if weapons are to be used at all, somewhat analogous to the development of stun guns and other sublethal weaponry that does not involve killing people? What about the fact that contemporary infectious-disease surveillance and reporting systems serve dual-use functions with biowarfare prevention; is there something problematic about technological development in this dual-use way?

In Chapter 15, which introduced the section on constraints in this volume, we entertained a comparatively simple thought experiment designed to test our conceptions of the appropriate limits of constraints in the effort to control the spread of infectious disease. At airports, we imagined, and at other places of public contact, people might be routinely screened by means of PCR, antibody, proteomic, nanotechnology, or other rapid tests that can detect infectious disease with virtually perfect accuracy, within a matter of minutes or seconds. When a person tests positive for any disease that he or she could transmit to others—whether in an airplane, after the plane lands, or in any other context—they would be detained, given treatment, if available, and either sent on their way or isolated until the contagious stage had passed. Surveillance and treatment need not be confined to airports, we assumed, but if tests were rapid, cheap, easy, and reliable, could be used in any areas of public contact—hospitals, shopping markets and malls, churches, and stadiums. Though this might work less well for some conditions like emerging pandemics where a virus had not yet been identified but very well for others like syphilis, easily detectable and treatable, we conjectured that if careful surveillance-and-treatment were done routinely in all areas of the world, it might take a decade or so to eradicate, eliminate, or bring under control the principal known infectious diseases in which human-to-human transmission is central, and surveillance could be relaxed except when new outbreaks occurred. In this thought experiment, a decade of universal surveillance and treatment would usher in the "Golden Age of protection from disease" that Robert Baker thinks we have already squandered. Universal surveillance and treatment would not of course rid the world of all infectious disease, but it would come close, a truly major achievement for humankind. Indeed, we suggested that this universal surveillance-and-treatment thought-experiment might be thought of as a way of starting to "close the book" on infectious disease.

But that was just an initial step, a mere thought-experiment, and indeed one that might seem impossibly demanding especially in the developing world. In this chapter we have pushed beyond the realm of intellectual fantasy to a consideration of what it might take to make desirable levels of control of infectious disease actual, both by continuing measures already in progress and developing new ones, and to do this within a relatively short time frame—envisioned in this broader account as the decade 2020–2030. What, we have been asking, might the moral costs as well as gains be? This is a much more serious and practical reflection on what forms of global cooperative effort and mutual constraint might be underwritten by a genuine attempt to extricate humankind from our embeddedness in a global web of transmissible infectious disease—and the very real burdens the everpresent reality of transmissible infectious disease constitutes.

No writer, as far as we are aware, is currently advocating the kind of universal surveillance or mandated treatment imagined in our airport thought-experiment, and no writer is advocating a decade of single-minded dedication to infectious disease control. The point of a thought-experiment like this is to test the ethical challenges to be faced in the real world, not just in a fictional one, and hence the challenges that would and do arise in what we see as an already emerging *Comprehensive Global Effort.* This thought experiment demonstrates that ethical reflection in the context of infectious disease, we have been arguing all along, must be far broader than it has been, even during the efflorescence of the last seven or eight years. That is why we appeal not only to a limited thought-experiment about airport surveillance but to the much broader constellation of developments we have called an emerging *Comprehensive Global Effort for the Control of Infectious Disease.* Indeed, we imagine it as culminating in the decade 2020–2030—that is the visionary part, as we said. But we also see it in a much more factual way, not just as a thought-experiment but also as an extrapolation from trends already under way, a projection from the astonishing variety of work toward this goal already in progress around the world. It is thus descriptive, we think, of the current decade's "marvelous momentum," a global effort at the moment not yet fully coordinated but yet entirely plausible and increasingly actual. This *Comprehensive Global Effort* encompasses all efforts to eradicate, eliminate, or control infectious disease.

It is this broader view that the notion of a *Comprehensive Global Effort* requires us to see. We cannot treat ethical issues in the same focused, siloed way that some efforts to combat disease have been, as concrete but little connected with other efforts toward the same goal. Ethical questions about specific projects like the Grand Challenges projects or pandemic influenza plans as well as every other effort to control infectious disease must also be viewed through a still broader theoretical lens that sees the "individual" not just as the tall-standing, health-enjoying, competent, rational, individually discrete figure envisioned in many accounts in liberal normative theory, so central in bioethics, but as a way-station self, as a person-in-disease-relationships, as enmeshed in a web of disease, as part of humanity whose biological nature as an organism inhabited by literally trillions of microorganisms, some beneficial or neutral but some seriously harmful or lethal, is central in human reality.

The notion of a *Global Effort* culminating in a specific time-limited period is thus not only partly thought-experiment and partly projection from practical efforts already well underway, but also partly a device for pressing the most serious ethical meta-issue: how can we attain a sufficiently comprehensive view of the distinctive ethics issues that infectious disease raises to be useful not only now but also in the future, in order to make sure that our global efforts to control infectious disease go *ethically* well? We cannot do ethics piecemeal, considering for example issues about infectious disease research in children, or mandated testing during pregnancy, or mandatory immunization for adolescents, or broad-scale surveillance measures, without an adequate conceptual underpinning. We have considered all these issues in previous chapters, but always in the light of our complex but unitary theoretical view that is sensitive to issues of communicability, which we call the *patient as victim and vector* view.

If a *Global Effort* as imagined here seems too grand—an overly far-fetched thought-experiment, a misdescription of current reality, or an unworkable concrete plan—imagine what is involved in trying to extricate the globe from any *one* of the particularly devastating diseases that are currently widespread—say, HIV/AIDS, or tuberculosis, or malaria. These are all recognized as devastating. AIDS has already killed 19 million people and, as of 2007, another 33.2 million are infected with the HIV virus. Tuberculosis infects or has infected an estimated 30% of the global population and kills about 2 million people a year. Worldwide, malaria infects between 350 and 500 million people every year, and between 2 to 3 million die from it—90% of them in Africa, where it is estimated that one child dies from malaria every 30 seconds.[95] The new movement for global health, building on the steady work of the WHO and others over many years and galvanized less than a decade ago by the remarkable private contribution of the Gates Foundation, is already committed to the elimination of these diseases; it has become a top global priority. Yet—here is the key to our project in this "think big" chapter—eliminating any one of these diseases will raise virtually *all* the issues we have posed in the five tracks outlined above. So would eliminating all three diseases. Indeed, for any disease or group of diseases for which we might consider trying to achieve global or even local eradication, elimination, or control, issues about institutional cooperation, infrastructure improvement, scientific development, religious and cultural attitudes, and social and legal protections are all relevant. Comprehensive ethical reflection is crucial in such an enterprise as well: although it is important to be sensitive to the specific, factual features of any given case, we cannot do ethics, as we have said, piecemeal, as an iterated effort one disease after another for the indefinite future, or in response to one new technology, or one political challenge, or one scientific development at a time, without a larger picture of human "thrownness," human embeddedness in webs of mutual disease transmission, within which they occur.

"Think big" thought-experiments are unlimited in scope, in this case fueled by an elective optimism and bounded only by the limits of plausibility in assembling the resources of the world to confront one of its most pervasive problems. We can imagine, as we have said, other *Global Efforts* directed toward other global problems—climate change and global warming, endangered species rescue,

---

95. Randall M. Packard, *The Making of a Tropical Disease: A Short History of Malaria* (Baltimore: Johns Hopkins University Press, 2007), xvi.

water justice, immigration management, global drug control, and so on. But the vision of a *Comprehensive Global Effort for the Eradication, Elimination, or Control of Infectious Disease for the Years 2020–2030* may be, in contrast, simpler: its overall purpose of reducing the burden of infectious disease may be less controversial; its methods are not technically impossible; its science is reasonably well understood; and it does not require the change of institutions, only coordination and cooperation. Imagining such an effort is of course to "think big," but we can certainly imagine what this project would take, as the culmination of the efforts of several centuries, to achieve within a single decade a goal with which the fate of humankind might be dramatically improved. There is no way to guarantee that it would succeed. But it is an effort already well under way, since the time of Jenner and with the best efforts of dedicated researchers, clinicians, and workers in public health. There is no practical or moral reason not to undertake this project, though plenty of reason to be cautious about how to do so—that is what we have tried to explore.

There is another, darker reason for exploring the practical and ethical issues in the *Global Effort* in this comprehensive way. A *Global Effort*, or even just continuing ordinary efforts to control infectious disease, might contain repressive, biased, insensitive, or otherwise morally indefensible elements, particularly if it were pursued under a tight time schedule by zealous institutions or highly competitive players. That there is a current efflorescence of ethical reflection does not entail that the various components of the overall global effort will go ethically well, and ethical reflection by itself will not prevent abuse. It is important to understand how even an admirable effort with a highly desirable goal—extricating humankind from the web of infectious disease—could go wrong, that is, how it could be done, but not done well. In the final chapter, then, we will look at a variety of policies of the sort that might be involved in a *Global Effort* to see what can go wrong with them as well as right, using our PVV view as a tool for examining actual, real-world policies as a way of thinking about larger aims.

THE *PATIENT AS VICTIM AND VECTOR* VIEW AS CRITICAL AND DIAGNOSTIC TOOL

This book began with gaps, lapses, and failures to see the ethical inconsistencies in medical and public health management of infectious diseases. There were a number of explanations of these gaps, as we have detailed in our previous chapters. First, bioethics was developing during the same decade when it was said to be "time to close the book on infectious disease," and consequently gave virtually no attention to issues of transmissibility, even when examining cases involving conditions like hepatitis at Willowbrook or the syphilis study at Tuskegee. Second, when AIDS emerged at the beginning of the 1980s, it was cast as an exception, a condition that because of the sensitive social issues surrounding it, at least in the United States, could not be addressed with the same surveillance and containment measures as other communicable disease epidemics. Even as international bodies call for universal testing of pregnant women for HIV, current global programs designed to reduce maternal/infant transmission of HIV still fail to appreciate fully the situation of these women not only as vectors but also as victims themselves. And political tensions currently erupting over proposals like requiring immunization for 11-and 12-year-old girls for HPV provide still further evidence, we believe, of the complexity of ethical dilemmas concerning infectious disease. Lacunae like these are at the root of the serious ethical issues that we have hoped to expose in this book.

Along the way, this book has also touched on a variety of historical examples, both distant and more recent: the shunning and belling of lepers in ancient times, efforts at *cordon sanitaire* containment of the plague, offshore quarantine of ships for cholera and holding of passengers on islands like Grosse Île, the pursuit and banishment of lepers in Hawaii, the forced quarantine of Chinese (but not whites) for plague in San Francisco's Chinatown in 1900, the global catastrophe (despite efforts at containment) of the 1918–1919 flu, Cuban isolation policy for HIV/AIDS, quarantine and isolation in Hong Kong and Toronto during the SARS outbreak in 2003, and, in quite recent dispute, mandatory treatment for drug-resistant TB and required school-entry immunization for HPV.

In most (but not all) of these infamous or controversial cases, it is easy to see that gross violations of ethical principles have occurred—particularly in the vivid, long-past historical cases. Of course, these are often cases in which hindsight is clear but ethically acceptable decision making was not easy at the time, especially where etiology was unknown or where immunization or treatment that is available now was not even imagined at the time—for instance in leprosy, plague, cholera, and tuberculosis. Just the same, these cases are still important; seeing that there were gross violations of ethical principles is not the same as explaining exactly what would have been more ethical social policies, even in those cases now regarded as most problematic. In this book, we hope to have brought assessing these lapses, gaps, and failures to see ethical inconsistencies into better focus, by clarifying just what went wrong in them, but also in some respects what went at least partially right. We have also pointed to a number of challenges for ethical theory and specific ethical questions along the way. In this final chapter, we will address both of these concerns.

The PVV View

Our effort throughout has been to develop a theoretical account of both philosophical and practical problems associated with communicable infectious disease. This account began, in Chapter 6, on "embedded autonomy," with a re-understanding of the individual as "embedded" in a web of disease, a "way-station self" that serves as a launching pad and breeding ground for trillions of organisms that move from one human being to another, either directly or by way of intermediate vectors. It is this human "individual" whom we see in a moral framework involving three essential perspectives, developed in Chapter 7. First is the perspective of the "individual" himself or herself, in a real-world, actual situation, as either ill or not ill, and hence as vulnerable or not so vulnerable to certain kinds of infectious disease. Second is the population perspective that is concerned with how groups and populations fare, including the entire global population. Third is the hypothetical, naturalized-Rawlsian perspective that recognizes the deep uncertainty of infectious disease, given that we do not and cannot know what new diseases may emerge, either naturally from zoonoses or evolutionary processes or as a product of deliberate engineering, or how great our capacities will be to outrun the development of antibiotic resistance, or how we can contain disease in other ways. Even if a *Comprehensive Global Effort* like the one we explored in Chapter 20 were to be virtually completely successful in bringing the known human-affecting serious infectious diseases under control, our infectious-disease future still remains deeply uncertain and deeply serious. "Control" of infectious disease is, after all, far from "eradication." This perspective forces us to recognize that in structuring policies, we cannot take our own current situation as primary or our beliefs about our relative safety or risk as assured. Nor can we take the current state of infectious-disease reality as permanent; with respect to vulnerability to disease, we must recognize that things could be quite different, and that this is true for all human beings.

This view, we acknowledged, is elaborate, drawing on three perspectives that, although intuitively clear, might be difficult to hold in view in all respects in practice. Each of the three perspectives is inadequate by itself, and each must modify and reform the others. But we have also offered a shortcut: the view we call *the patient as victim and vector* or, even shorter, *the PVV view*, which incorporates all these components but need not articulate them explicitly at every moment. We have been using this shortcut all along. It is intuitively easy to grasp but powerful in practice, and its utility and power in practice are what we want to conclude by exploring here. We put it this way in Chapter 1 and again in Chapter 7:

> *Ethical problems in infectious disease should be analyzed, and clinical practices, research agendas, and public policies developed, that always take into account the possibility that a person with communicable infectious disease is both victim* and *vector.*

In this concluding chapter, we want to show how we can use this PVV view as a tool, in two different ways: first, more briefly, as a critical theoretical tool for examining philosophical argumentation in a variety of contexts, and second, more extensively, as a practical diagnostic tool for examining public policy concerning medical and public health practice.

The PVV View as a Philosophical Tool

The enormous range of philosophic argumentation over the centuries about issues having to do with human existence and well-being, we think, exhibits a curious characteristic: very little of it refers explicitly to the basic human situation of life and health as enmeshed in a web of communicable infectious diseases. Philosophers and other thinkers have of course been aware of the vulnerability of human life and its limits—all human beings die, and this awareness of mortality has been central in many religious and philosophical systems. But few philosophers or others have concerned themselves with the specific fact that humans are vulnerable to, and die from, communicable infectious disease; that is, that human beings sicken and die from illnesses that are brought to them by other human beings, and that they in turn transmit diseases that cause others to sicken or die. This "embeddedness" has been so central in the history of human experience that failure to attend to it might seem astonishing. Indeed, it is only since about the mid-nineteenth century and particularly in the twentieth century that some parts of the world, the developed ones, have achieved enough distance from this embeddedness in the web of disease that it is possible to comprehend what it would be like for human experience to be otherwise—that is, to live a life relatively free from serious infectious disease. Although it would be impossible here to rewrite all of philosophy with this concern in mind, we would like to explore three examples of philosophic reflection with different sorts of focus as a way of seeing how the PVV view might make a difference. First, we take a brief look at an account of principles that has become central in bioethics teaching and clinical practice. Second, we look—again, briefly—at the capabilities view of human functioning developed by Amartya Sen and Martha Nussbaum; this is a view not developed within the field of bioethics, but with wider implications for it. Finally, we look—once again, briefly—at what the PVV might mean for classical liberal theory, originally expounded by John Stuart Mill and a central tradition in contemporary Anglo-American philosophic reflection—this is to take the broadest of views. These are just three examples among many that we could explore, but they illustrate ways in which the PVV view can augment, enrich, and enhance philosophic theory at varying ranges of focus.

A First Example: The Implications of the PVV View for Principlist Bioethics

Four principles make up the basis of what has been called "principlist" bioethics. Originally put forth by Tom Beauchamp and James Childress, these four principles—autonomy, beneficence, non-maleficence, and justice—have become a staple of bioethics analysis in the United States, used over and over again by hospital ethics committees, health-care providers, and social commentators.[1] These principles are so ubiquitous that they are sometimes (affectionately) characterized as the "Georgetown Mantra," acknowledging the fact that Beauchamp and Childress were at Georgetown University when they were developed. Yet, as we detailed in Chapter 6, the fundamental conceptualization of human life underlying these principles requires re-examination in light of the biological interconnectedness of the way-station self.

Take respect for autonomy, for example. The standard view requires that if "patients" have necessary mental capacity and offer voluntary informed consent or refusal for a recommended intervention, this choice should be honored.

---

1. Tom L. Beauchamp and James F. Childress, *Principles of Biomedical Ethics* (New York: Oxford University Press, 1983).

Yet it is not at all clear, on this view, whether the risks and benefits presented to patients should include the risks and benefits to others. Instead, attention is directed to whether the patient is competent—for incompetence presents the most compelling reason for overriding a patient's choice. From our PVV view, however, this picture is critically incomplete: the consequences to others of possible contagious disease are part of the patient's *own* interests, when the patient is understood in a web of infectious disease relationships.

Or consider the second and third principles, beneficence and non-maleficence. Here, the focus is on benefits to the patient—or preventing harms to him or her. Once again, however, the physician's focus is unidirectional, considering only harms or benefits for *this* patient. This is the message of the Hippocratic Oath's classical statement, "I will follow that system or regimen which, according to my ability and judgment, I consider for the benefit of my patients, and will abstain from whatever is deleterious or mischievous."[2] Understanding the patient through the lens of PVV, however, requires considering how doing what is best for this patient may harm others—and thus in a sense also harms the patient himself or herself as well. The need to further educate, inform, or even coerce or constrain the patient, which could be understood as harm to him, is also something that the patient has an interest in because the patient has an interest in reducing the overall burden of disease that can affect himself or herself. There remain difficult tradeoffs—between, say, the harms of failure to protect and the harms of constraint—but it is too simple to regard these tradeoffs as one person against others. Instead, they are tradeoffs for everyone enmeshed in a web of disease.

The final of the four original principles proposed by Beauchamp and Childress was justice—in the sense of distributive justice. Unfortunately, it has too often remained an afterthought in the uses to which principlist bioethics have been put. In the United States, the question of distributive justice in health care has remained a vexed one, with the defense of individual responsibility for health and health care remaining a powerful political argument. This individualism is less apparent in Europe and in many other countries of the world, where shared social responsibilities for health care have been recognized for decades. Yet as costs of care continue to mount, pressures on the social fabric of health care have been increasing. As we have explained in Chapter 19, we think that the PVV view provides a theoretical basis for regarding justice in health care as a shared issue for all. *Everyone* has an interest in the access to care and development of health infrastructure that is needed as a bulwark against the ever present reality of transmissible disease. Pandemic disease is only one threat of this kind—but it is at present the greatest reminder of the

---

2. The Oath of Hippocrates, http://classics.mit.edu/Hippocrates/hippooath.html (accessed February 19, 2008).

need for global health security as a matter of doing justice to "way station" selves.

A Second Example: The Implications of the PVV View for Theorizing About Capabilities

As a second example of how the PVV approach can augment analysis, consider the ways in which it can challenge and enrich theoretical positions in philosophy that are not specifically addressed to bioethics or medical topics. While we certainly cannot consider all of the various theoretical positions advanced by philosophers on topics of social justice relevant to human existence, we take as one example the influential account known as the *capabilities approach*, developed (in somewhat different ways) by Amartya Sen and Martha Nussbaum. Sen and Nussbaum have been concerned with such issues as poverty, famine, gender inequality, and other circumstances that undermine human well-being—that is, with the political and social situations of many societies in which people live around the globe. They have developed the view that people's well-being is not best measured by the amount of material resources or income a person has, and that a society's well-being is not best measured by indices of production, spending, consumer goods, or the like; on such a view, rich people and rich societies would always be better off than poor ones. Instead, though Sen and Nussbaum develop these views in somewhat different ways, they hold that the important measures are what people are able to experience and do within the society in which they live, what range of choices they are able to exercise effectively. What is necessary for a person to live at least a minimally decent life? Can this person form important social bonds? Does this person have enough to eat to sustain herself in whatever activities she undertakes? Does this person have a sufficient measure of security, including physical and economic security, to be able to engage in recreation and play? As Sen observed, one might have many resources but lack well-being, if one has certain kinds of needs; well-being is associated not with what one has, but what one can choose and do.

Nussbaum identifies ten "central human functional capabilities":[3]

1. the capability for physical survival;
2. the capability for bodily health;
3. the capability for bodily integrity;
4. the capability for the exercise of imagination;

---

3. Martha Nussbaum, *Sex and Social Justice* (New York: Oxford University Press, 1999), 41. Nussbaum's descriptions for these capabilities are more extensive, and the parsing of them here is taken from Stuart White's account in *Stanford Encyclopedia of Philosophy*, ed. Edward N. Zalta, s.v. "Social Minimum," http://plato.stanford.edu/entries/social-minimum/ (accessed December 1, 2007).

5. the capability for emotional response and exploration;
6. the capability for practical reason;
7. the capability for love and friendship;
8. the capability for connection with nature and other species;
9. the capability for play;
10. the capability for the exercise of control over environment, including political control.

This list and the more extensive descriptions Nussbaum supplies of these capabilities have of course engendered extensive critical discussion among philosophers, but it is fair to say that hers is an impressive attempt to try to characterize what is essential for a decent human life in a way that does not fall prey to cultural relativism or entail that the rich automatically have better lives than the poor.[4] Whether one subscribes to the capabilities approach in the first place or not, it is nevertheless an influential view in contemporary ethics, and it is thus informative to see how our PVV view might enhance it. In brief, whatever route one takes toward enriching the understanding of capabilities, whether by exploring what is needed for people to exercise freedom as does Sen,[5] by expanding the characterization of one or more of the capabilities listed by Nussbaum, or by adding a new capability to the list, what is clear is that sensitivity to the way in which human beings are enmeshed in a web of communicable infectious disease dramatically influences whether they are able to lead decent human lives.

Consider initially, whether the capabilities set Nussbaum articulates is as sensitive as it might be to the realities of communicable infectious disease, especially in the situations of poverty and inequality with which she and Sen are particularly concerned. These situations are, after all, the situations in which a majority of human beings actually do live. Her list of capabilities, those matters that a society has a positive obligation to try to protect and ensure, explicitly includes #1,—the capability for physical survival and #2—the capability for bodily health: these would preclude malnutrition, injury, congenital, acute, and chronic illness, and fatal disease; with #6—the capability for practical reason, they would include some degree of mental health as well. These capabilities—for survival, bodily health, and reason—jointly require freedom from serious or life-threatening infectious as well as other disease. Thus far, the capabilities list Nussbaum has articulated appears to cover what is involved in being a victim of infectious disease.

However, as PVV requires us to see, there is more to infectious disease than not being made ill or killed by it oneself. The other part of the role in which

---

4. The most extensive statement of her capability view is found in Martha Nussbaum, *Frontiers of Justice: disability, nationality, species membership* (Cambridge: Harvard University Press, 2006).
5. Amartya Sen, *Development as Freedom* (New York: Alfred A. Knopf, 1999).

communicable infectious disease casts a given person is that of transmitter of disease to others. The transmission of disease to others can occur in many of the circumstances involved in other capabilities on Nussbaum's list: #7—love and friendship, #9—play, and even perhaps #4—the exercise of imagination as well as #5—emotional response and exploration, where it involves emotional response to others or projects involving working or playing together with others. Consider for instance, how the capability for love, especially in sexual expression, is affected by embeddedness in a web of sexually transmitted disease: traditionally feared conditions like gonorrhea and syphilis, newly emerged conditions like HIV/AIDS; and endemic pathogens like HPV and herpes. Protective measures like condom use may reduce the likelihood of becoming infected or transmitting infection, but are ineffective for some pathogens (like HPV) and 100% effective for none. Love expressed in sexual intimacy is everywhere limited by the possibility of disease transmission; intimacy might be rather different, and much more fully expressed, without this risk. Similarly, other human activities on Nussbaum's list of capabilities are also affected by the possibility of disease transmission: working together, playing together, exploring together, and so on, are always subject to the transmission of aerosolized diseases, vectorborne diseases, diseases harbored in water contaminated by human bacteria or parasites, and so on. Part of the challenge to capabilities theorists, then, would be to spell out more fully what would be involved in extending the relevant capabilities to articulate explicitly what is essential for a decent life, in being free as far as possible from a role in which one not only is not made ill or killed by diseases transmitted by others, but does not make ill or kill others oneself. This is part of the victim *and* vector insight that is essential to the PVV view.

An alternative, supplementarist approach in enhancing or enriching the capabilities approach would be to recommend the addition of a further capability to the list, a capability that captures the victim/vector duality we have described as obtaining at all three levels of the PVV view: the interest in 1) both not being a victim of disease oneself and in not transmitting it to others, in 2) not being a member of a population in which infectious disease circulates, and 3) not being even potentially either victim or vector of infectious disease that has not yet and may or may not occur. This would be to address directly the notion that to be able to live a decent human life, it is essential to extricate oneself and indeed one's society from its current condition of being enmeshed, as we have put it, in the web of infectious disease in which we all live.

It is important to see that this eleventh capability, if it is indeed that—what we could dub the "capability for transmission-immunity"—is something that many inhabitants of the developed world already have to a large extent in their daily lives. Inhabitants of the developed world, where immunization is virtually universal, work together without transmitting whooping cough, play together without transmitting measles, make love without transmitting syphilis, and if they are by some chance unprotected, find treatment readily available. But many, many other inhabitants of the world do not have this capability, or have it for only some but not many other diseases: work, play, and love are all occasions for the transmission of infection.

Extrication from (much of) the web of communicable infectious disease tracks in general the economic development of societies and in particular their health care and public health systems: inhabitants of rich countries do in general have this capability, at least as far as the diseases on the long list in chapter 20 of diseases that have been eradicated, eliminated, or brought under control (among them smallpox, leprosy, plague, diphtheria, typhoid, yellow fever, cholera, and polio) are concerned. Thanks to prevention, immunization, and effective treatment, the inhabitants of rich countries are able to live largely protected against these—although always with the cautionary reminder that spread of many serious infectious diseases may be just a plane ride away, including reintroduction of diseases that have been eliminated in the developed world. This protection is essential, we believe, to a decent human life: both not to become a victim and also not to become a vector of such diseases, and to live in a society in which serious infectious disease does not circulate. Of course it has not always been possible (especially not before Jenner and before the enormous gains in immunizations and antimicrobials of recent decades), and it still is not possible for some diseases. But it is possible for a very long list of diseases—and already actualized for some of these in the developed world.

Nussbaum's list of capabilities constitutes a list of what decent societies should assure their members. We admire the scope and sensitivity of this list. As we've shown, we think this list can be enriched either by exploring a number of the capabilities already on the list of ten, or by augmenting it with this eleventh capability: either route, we think, would enhance the richness of their already influential view. Other writers exploring issues in global justice direct attention to health-related issues such as poverty, gender inequality, inadequate health-care infrastructure, and the heavy and inequitable burden of disease, as well as to specific practical issues like pharmaceutical patenting or drug testing in the developing world. There has been, however, little focus on the moral implications of the fact that much of the burden of disease involves diseases that are transmissible. This is an astonishing omission: after all, mutual contagion has always been among the most basic realities of human existence—especially for those who are poor.

A Third Example: Liberal Individualism

As we discussed in Chapter 6, a hallmark of liberal theory developed originally by John Stuart Mill is the "harm principle," that the sole reason for which coercion is permissible is to prevent the person coerced from harming others.

As we also explained, in the PVV view the contrast between "harm to self" and "harm to others" on which this harm principle is based is inadequate. From the perspective of the way-station self, there simply is no clear distinction between harm to self and harm to another. For example, in deciding whether or not to be immunized, it may seem that an individual is only risking harm to herself: she may contract disease that she would not have, had she accepted the protection that immunization might bring. But she is also risking harm to others, if she becomes a vector. From the perspective of deep uncertainty about victimhood and vectorhood, moreover, she may be presenting unknown possibilities of harm to herself by risking contribution to the overall burden of infectious disease.

A second hallmark of Millian liberalism, related to the harm principle, is the distinction between the public and the private. Core to liberal theory has been the idea that there is a "private sphere": homes, bodies, minds, into which the state has no business penetrating. As we have discussed in considering the relative importance of privacy and confidentiality, however, this distinction between the public and the private is challenged by contagious disease. Sex may take place within the confines of a home, but the organisms exchanged in the sexual act may spread far and wide. Someone may feel ill and go home to crawl into bed—but having touched doorknobs, coughed, and breathed in the vicinity of others, spreading disease-causing microbes all along the way. No person, that is, is an island, or even an archipelago,[6] in a world of transmissible infectious disease.

This is not to say that liberal theory got it wrong in trying to figure out how to respect persons as individuals. The idea of individual human dignity remains the enduring insight of theoreticians in the liberal tradition. It is to say, rather, that what it means to respect human dignity must be understood in an enriched way, in terms of their situation as both victims and vectors. If social policies aim to respect individuals by protecting privacy or individual choice, but end up creating the circumstances in which deadly diseases such as HIV/AIDS proliferate into epidemics, they have respected dignity in a sense that is far too narrow. Instead, we believe, efforts to protect freedom and liberty must come to terms with the balance between choice and constraint that is presented over and over again, to every way-station self.

The Implications of the PVV View for Policy Analysis

In addition to these implications for philosophy, which we have just sketched in the barest outline, the *"patient as victim and vector"* view also has implications for public policy. The philosophical and public policy questions are both

---

6. The archipelago image is from Chandran Kukathas, *The Liberal Archipelago: A Theory of Diversity and Freedom* (New York: Oxford University Press, 2003).

illuminated by the PVV view, but their thrust is quite different. Philosophical exploration typically makes things harder—assumptions that had not been questioned are exposed to the light of day; arguments that had seemed sound are dismembered; issues that had seemed far-fetched, if they had been raised at all, are brought to the center of concern, like the seemingly obvious question, what is wrong with disease? In contrast, policy analysis can make things easier: our effort here is to see clearly what is wrong and also what is right about a variety of policies that have been erected both in the past and the present to control infectious disease.

The PVV View as a Practical Diagnostic Tool for Examining Public Policy

Although it might be cumbersome to employ in its fully elaborated form, the PVV view can be used in a simple, shortcut form as an effective diagnostic and assessment tool for examining many practices and policies. It can be used retrospectively, to assess past practices as well as the critiques of them. It can be used to assess contemporary clinical practice, including both immediate physician–patient relationships and the policies of health-care organizations that influence physician practice. It can be used to assess research, including research priorities and the conduct of research studies. It can be used to scrutinize prevention and infection-control measures, including public health programs and policies and the rationales for them, as well as international infectious-disease control programs, including both containment and eradication programs. It can be used to evaluate public presentations of infectious-disease issues, including advertising campaigns for public health measures and public service announcements, as well as the attitudes about choice and responsibility they convey. And, as we have seen in Chapters 16 through 19, it can be used to assess pandemic planning for outbreaks that have not yet occurred. Indeed, it can be used to examine virtually everything that has to do with infectious disease, retrospectively, currently, or prospectively, to critique or shape the design of past, current, and future practices, research agendas, plans, and policies. It asks an exquisitely simple question even when the answer may be hard to supply: does it—the practice, agenda, program, policy, plan—*always consider any person it affects as (potentially) both victim AND vector?*

The PVV view has already been serving as a tool in developing and critiquing both past and existing policies and practices as well as hypothetical ones. It has been at work in both expanded and shortcut forms in the applied chapters of Part III of this book, and it has been the basis for our discussion of constraints in Part IV. That the patient—the individual person, including all persons affected—should be treated to the fullest extent possible as both victim and vector has been the basis for our account of constraints, including violations of autonomy and bodily integrity, even by the use of force, violations of privacy and confidentiality, subjection to increased risks, and violations of justice. We do not hold that constraints, whether modest constrictions of liberty or sheer force, should never be used, but rather that constraints of whatever degree must be countered by specific protections and guarantees, as we have outlined, if attention to the people affected is to recognize that they are to be regarded also as victims, not wholly as vectors. This is true even in particularly problematic or difficult situations, like surveillance that includes many false positives, decision making that occurs under extreme uncertainty, or eradication programs where complete elimination of a disease can be sought only at the expense of other goals and where cooperation with transmission-control public health measures is not voluntary. Our procedural protections and substantive guarantees developed in Chapter 16, indispensable in morally defensible constraints, are designed to serve this function: to not let us overlook the fact that in constraints involving communicable infectious disease, it is people who are, may become, or could become victims who are affected. This is especially relevant in questions about what is owed those who have been constrained and about those who have been deprioritized for access to health care in situations of pandemic crisis, as we have seen.

But the PVV view as diagnostic and assessment tool also requires that infectious-disease practices and policies respond to the fact that, as way-station individuals embedded in a web of disease, *all* of us—all human beings, not to mention other animals and organisms—are actually or potentially vectors as well. Transmissible infectious disease is not always about *other* people; it is always also about *each one* him or herself. It is easy to miss this fact in developed, privileged countries, where many of the most serious infectious agents are already under control. Yet a large proportion of the human population is still vulnerable to an enormous range of infectious diseases, including all those just mentioned as well as HIV, tuberculosis, malaria, dengue, cholera, and the so-called neglected tropical diseases. Just the same, that ought not delude the affluent parts of the world where infectious disease is under greater control into thinking they are safe. Situations can change—witness the eruption of HIV, the emergence of diseases like hantavirus and SARS, the reemergence of tuberculosis on a global scale, and the possibility of person-to-person avian flu or another lethal global outbreak.

It is also easy to miss this fact if history is forgotten. Human "individuals" have always been embedded in a web of mutually transmissible disease, but as global travel and commerce become more interconnected, issues of transmission grow and come increasingly into view. Historical antecedents about intercontinental transmission are sobering: the transmission of the plague from Asia to Europe, killing an estimated one-quarter to one-third of Europe's population; the transmission of smallpox and measles from Europe to North America, resulting in the virtual annihilation of Native American populations, when as many as 90% to 100% of people in some areas died[7]; the transmission of the most serious form of syphilis from the New World to Europe[8]; the decimation of the native population of Hawaii and other islands by introduced disease[9]; and the intercontinental transmission of the so-called Spanish flu from American soldiers to Europe in 1918, where it evolved into its deadly form and killed some 40–100 million people worldwide. Disease travels in many directions, both predictably and unpredictably, and it is part of the concern of this book to guard against complacency about vectorhood, just as much as it is the concern of this book to guard against insensitivity to victimhood. The idea is to see both at once, the individual person and indeed groups and populations comprised of individual persons as both victim *and* vector.

Using the PVV View as a Tool: Lopsided, Controversial, and Well-Balanced Policies and Practices

Using the PVV view as a diagnostic tool, it becomes possible to group morally problematic historical and recent infectious-disease practices and policies into two initial basic groups: those that err by overemphasizing vectorhood to the relative exclusion of victimhood, and those that err the other way around. This can be done with any of the cases already discussed here, or new cases as well.

Practices and Policies That Overemphasize Vectorhood, Underemphasize Victimhood. Consider, first, several historical cases in which practices, policies, and social responses have generally overemphasized vectorhood to the exclusion of victimhood. For example, traditional practices of belling and isolating people with leprosy have meant banishing these people from society without means of support, disrupting their social ties, denying any form of compensation, and refusing them any measure of respect: the very term "leper" has come to mean *complete social outcast.* These practices regard persons with what is now known as Hansen's Disease wholly as vectors, while ignoring their plight as victims. To be sure, some slightly more humane practices have involved setting up residential areas with at least some maintenance and treatment facilities—"leper colonies"—but issues about exclusion from society were rarely fully addressed.

For example, literally millennia after the earliest recorded exclusions of people with leprosy, lepers were still being rounded up and banished. In nine-

---

7. Noble David Cook, *Born to Die: Disease and New World Conquest, 1492–1650* (New York: Cambridge University Press, 1998).
8. K.N. Harper, P.S. Ocampo, B.M. Steiner, R.W. George, M.S. Silverman et al., "On the Origin of the Treponematoses: A Phylogenetic Approach," *PLoS Neglected Tropical Diseases* 2(1): e148.
9. John Tayman, The Colony: The Harrowing True Story of the Exiles of Molokai (New York: Scribner, 2006).

teenth-century Hawaii, in one of the most notorious and largest-scale quarantine programs in U.S. history, people with leprosy were isolated for the rest of their lives on an inaccessible stretch of land on Molokai, Kaluapapa. Deceived by government promises of treatment, summarily diagnosed by health inspectors on sometimes the flimsiest of grounds (those quarantined often included people with skin rashes merely suspected of leprosy), and sometimes hunted down as if they were criminals, these people were shipped to a makeshift colony where they were dumped (sometimes literally by being pushed off a boat into the surf) to spend the rest of their lives in virtually complete isolation from their spouses, families, communities, and the rest of the world, in a community controlled by often brutal thugs. They were categorized as legally dead. Those policies were infected with racism—native Hawaiians were far more frequently identified as lepers than colonizing whites (although to some extent this may have been a function of differential susceptibility to disease)—and were often brutal in their execution; they provided virtually no assistance in living, no health care, and no compensation either to the victims or their families for the loss of freedom.[10]

Yet despite the callousness of this policy, it cannot simply be dismissed. Our PVV view as a tool insists that we see both what was morally wrong, but also in part right about a case like this—the effort to control transmission, when no known treatment was available (though there were experiments with a vaccine) and the disease was believed both lethal and highly contagious. The history of infectious disease in Hawaii is relevant here. Hawaii, with a native population that had no natural immunities to European or Asian diseases, had been swept by waves of introduced disease. Syphilis and gonorrhea had been brought in 1778 by Will Bradley, a sailor aboard one of Captain Cook's ships. With other sailors and other voyages came measles, mumps, chickenpox, typhoid fever (which killed nearly every child born in 1848), dysentery, and whooping cough. Finally smallpox arrived, and between the day the *Charles Mallory,* sailing from San Francisco, landed in Honolulu harbor, February 10, 1853, and January 1854, it produced a raging epidemic that killed as much as a fifth of the Hawaiian population and almost half the population of Oahu.[11] What was in part right about the isolation policy for leprosy was its alertness to the prospect of transmission of yet another devastating disease, but was among the many things that were wrong was the failure to confirm whether the evidence then available really indicated that leprosy constituted another

---

10. Tayman, *The Colony.* See also W.S. Merwin, *The Folding Cliffs* (New York: Knopf, 1998) for a vivid poetic account of this policy in practice; Zachary Gussow, *Leprosy, Racism, and the Public Health* (Boulder, CO: Westview Press, 1989) for an historical account; Penne Moblo, "Blessed Damien of Moloka'i: The Critical Analysis of Contemporary Myth," *Ethnohistory* 44, no. 4 (1997): 691–726.

11. Tayman, *The Colony,* 25–26.

rapidly spreading threat and especially the failure to treat people thus afflicted as victims, the failure to care for them or about them in any significant way.

The older, historical cases typically provide the more vivid examples of lopsided practices (that is why we mention them again here), while newer, more contemporary practices and policies are often still out of balance but in ways that are sometimes more difficult to discern. We think it is important to attend not only to current dilemmas but to see clearly what is—and is not—ethically troubling about even the most egregious past cases. In virtually all of the vivid historical cases, an initial reaction is that this "parade of horrors" of past abuses is too dreadful to remember and too dreadful to repeat. But this is to miss the point of the PVV view as a tool, which reminds us that there is of-ten *also* something in some respects morally legitimate even in the most distressing of past cases, and that it is imperative that we succeed in identifying what it was if we are to think clearly about practice and policy in the present and the future. This is not to say that there is anything at all right about the horrific aspects of such policies—force, violence, official lies, and the like—but that the policies themselves may have reflected legitimate concerns, albeit in morally troubling ways. The PVV tool brings important moral considerations to the fore, recognizing that policies may have both horrific aspects (both as a matter of policy and as a matter of application of the policy) but reveal moral insights in other respects. This point is often overlooked in the rush to condemn policies viewed as unconscionable, especially those that were indeed unconscionable overall.

There have been many other examples of similarly lopsided emphasis on vectorhood but overlooking of victimhood. We have already mentioned the quarantine of Chinese (but not white) residents of San Francisco's Chinatown in 1900 for bubonic plague—another vivid case in the painful annals of public health that involved abusive policies, inattention to the needs of those affected as victims, unwarranted aggression in constraining the afflicted as vectors, and other abuses like preventing residents from going to work, burning their pos-sessions, or beating those who were uncooperative with the Health Depart-ment's quarantine.

Using our PVV view as a tool, we can now see how out of balance this pub-lic health effort was. This attempt to prevent an outbreak of plague was ad-dressed virtually entirely toward potential vectorhood; this, our PVV view lets us see, was supported by an important moral reason, given what was known about plague at the time, even if the attempt was extraordinarily heavy-handed and on balance deeply morally problematic. But our PVV view also lets us see how no attempt was made to address the quarantined Chinese as victims, when it was only Levi Strauss who succeeded in organizing a group of busi-nessmen that began to provide food for the quarantined Chinese; in this respect, the public policy put in place was wholly wrong. Except for the four individuals who did actually have plague, the Chinese were victims of the Health Department policy rather than of the disease itself, but it is still the case under our PVV view that this form of victimhood must be attended to as well. To pass full ethical muster, the policy would have had to take both concerns, victimhood (both of disease and of policy) and vectorhood, into account.

There are many other egregious historical examples. Mary Mallon, the Irish cook in New York City who came to be known as Typhoid Mary, was clearly treated in lopsided ways, with public opprobrium focused almost exclusively on her irresponsibility as a vector. The public reviled her for returning to cooking even though she knew she carried (and transmitted) typhoid, but did nothing to attend to her plight as victim—in her case, victim both of her carriage of the disease and of public hostility toward her because of it. She was hounded, reviled, and quarantined on North Brother Island. But Mary Mallon was also a victim, both of the heavy-handed efforts to control her and of the way in which her disease, although asymptomatic and not a cause of physical distress to her, nevertheless put her in an unconscionable position vis-à-vis others: she became a cook in a *hospital*, spreading typhoid to the most vulnerable of others. In a sympathetic contemporary documentary, Judith Walzer Leavitt describes Mary's plight:

> Consider her circumstances. She had been abruptly, even violently, wrenched from her life, a life in which she found various satisfactions and from which she earned a decent living. She was physically separated from all that was familiar to her and isolated on an island. She was labeled a monster and a freak. . . . She was not permitted to work at a job that had sustained her, but she was not retrained for any comparable work. . . . The health department, for all of [New York City Health Commissioner] Lederle's words of obligation to help her in 1910, did not provide her with long-term gainful employment. . . . There was no viable "safety net," practical or intellectual, for an unemployed middle-aged Irish immigrant single woman.[12]

It was only when she was eventually removed from the kitchen and given a job in the hospital laboratory, where her disease would no longer be transmitted, that a more defensible balance of attention to both her vectorhood and victimhood was achieved.

Many other cases likewise display a shift in time from lopsidedness to better balance between concerns about the person as victim and the person as vector. In the case of the homeless man dying of drug-resistant tuberculosis who wanted to go home to be with his dog, recounted in Chapter 9—a multiple-year history of both misattention to his situation as victim and overly strong

---

12. Judith Walzer Leavitt, "Typhoid Mary: Villain or Victim?" *PBS NOVA Special*. http//www.pbs.org/wgbh/nova/typhoid/mary.html (accessed October 27, 2007).

constraint as vector—was finally resolved in a way that allowed attention to both: he would remain hospitalized to prevent transmission, but his dog was brought in to be with him. Public opinion about Andrew Speaker, the Atlanta lawyer who evaded no-fly restrictions in 2007 in returning from his wedding in Greece, initially reviled him as an irresponsible vector, likely to have infected other passengers on the plane with XDR-TB. Only as further details of his diagnosis and illness became available—in particular, that he did not after all have XDR-TB but a less contagious and more treatable form, and that thousands of other travelers with minimal transmission risks are routinely allowed travel or immigration into the United States[13]—did public opinion soften enough to begin to see him as a victim, too, a man with a serious illness who needed treatment for what might otherwise become a fatal disease. "Typhoid Mary," who passed on her infection to many, and "Patient Zero," the airline steward widely although perhaps erroneously singled out for blame for unleashing the AIDS epidemic in the United States—two of the most thoroughly demonized transmitters of infectious disease of all—are now also recognized as victims as well.

Neither the procedural nor the substantive principles we have defended in Chapter 16 would permit any of these historical cases as they occurred—herding Hawaiians with leprosy into permanent quarantine on an isolated coast, blockading San Francisco's Chinatown by establishing a race-based *cordon sanitaire* and imposing forcible but inadequately tested inoculation for plague, jailing Mary Mallon, or reviling Gaetan Dugas for his sexual life or Andrew Speaker for his wedding trip. This is not just because some containment measures were unwarranted, though given the comparatively primitive science of the time especially in the early cases, some may have been unnecessary or ineffective. The containment measures were unjust because there was inadequate, if any, effort in these cases to consider the strength of the justification, to use the least restrictive alternative, to make the rationale transparent to the community, or to consider redress. Nor, it appears, were there any efforts to respond in an ethically sensitive and appropriate way to the people constrained, whether by providing them with basic health needs (including food), personal security, communication, or recognition of their very substantial losses of liberty, privacy, property, bodily integrity, rights to travel and associate freely, and other important matters. They were treated as vectors only, at least

13. Timothy Brewer, "Extensively Drug-Resistant Tuberculosis and Public Health," *Journal of the American Medical Association* 298, no.16 (2007): 1861. Speaker's signs and symptoms, however, would classify him as active and infectious, and were he not a U.S. citizen, he would be inadmissible to the United States until rendered noninfectious. See Howard Markel, Lawrence O. Gostin, and David P. Fidler, "Extensively Drug-Resistant Tuberculosis and Public Health—Reply," *Journal of the American Medical Association* 298, no. 16 (2007): 1861–1862.

initially, not also as victims. Indeed, many of the early public health measures, including social exclusion, public labeling (like belling), the *cordon sanitaire* method of containing an outbreak area, and other traditional public health measures may be called into question, if it means ejecting, humiliating, or walling off people infected, exposed, or uninfected, and failing to provide further attention to their serious needs.

Some of what is required by these considerations is quite simple and, as medical science improves, increasingly easy to satisfy. Leprosy, plague, typhoid, and cholera are now easily preventable or treatable. Just the same, some of what is required by a PVV-informed principle of legitimate constraint could have been satisfied in any of these cases, even then, without advances in medical science. For example, relief of suffering and promotion of recovery both require adequate nutrition—and yet, in many cases, including the quarantine of Hawaiians with leprosy and the blockade of San Francisco's Chinatown, people suspected of disease or who might contract disease were allowed to starve—in the latter case, until Levi Strauss intervened. Relief of suffering can also be promoted by all the usual comforts in medical and nursing care for those who are ill: not only adequate nutrition, but adequate warmth, shelter, clothing, and so on. Promotion of recovery or cure, where possible, is also required; thus, victims of infectious disease, even though potentially dangerous to others as vectors, are entitled to whatever medication or other treatment is possible to try to release them from the grip of the disease. Half a century after the blockade of Chinatown, the Tuskegee syphilis study involved the egregious violation of the PVV requirement of attending to victimhood as well as to vectorhood—though unremarked at the time—in failing to provide penicillin, a treatment that was known to be effective, to the syphilis victims under study.

Under the PVV view, the prevention of recurrence, as with, say, malaria, and the prevention of a person's illness from exacerbating other health conditions from which that person also suffers are, where possible, also required as a matter of attentiveness to both victimhood and vectorhood. If a society imposes constraints on a person to protect others from the disease he or she harbors, it must also attempt to do what it can to prevent the disease from worsening for that person or for making their other health conditions worse, as for example HIV and tuberculosis may exacerbate each other.

Finally, it is important to remember that not all the egregious cases of treating people as vectors only without regard to their victimhood occurred in the distant historical past. Early in the HIV epidemic, for example, the United States imposed isolation policies on HIV positive Haitians, most of whom were refugees who had arrived by boat and who refused to return to Haiti for fear of persecution after the coup d'état that had deposed the elected president

Jean-Bertrand Aristide. Several hundred refuges were sent to Guantanamo "detention camps" for up to two years. Paul Farmer relays one internee's account:

> We were in a space cordoned off with barbed wire. Wherever they put you, you were meant to stay right there; there was no place to move. The latrines were brimming over. There was never any cool water to drink, to wet our lips. There was only water in a cistern, boiling in the hot sun. When you drank it, it gave you diarrhea .. . Rats crawled over us at night ... When we saw all these things, we thought, it's not possible, it can't go on like this. We're humans, just like everyone else.[14]

Practices and Policies That Overemphasize Victimhood, Underemphasize Vectorhood. Lopsided cases overemphasizing vectorhood and underemphasizing victimhood are, however, not the only ways practices and policies can err. Policies and practices can also err in the other, equally unbalanced direction as well. Another early parade of horrors viewed retrospectively here also requires closer inspection, to see not only exactly what was wrong with them but also what was partially right.

The notorious Tuskegee syphilis study violated a central requirement of concern for infectious-disease patients as victims in failing to provide the syphilis carriers under study with treatment already known to be effective. This study also failed to attend to issues of vectorhood: in keeping these men untreated, it failed to consider the consequences for their wives or sexual partners or for any future children. Although transmission is most likely in the early phase of syphilis and less likely during the many years of second-stage latency, suffering untreated syphilis over a 40-year period meant that these men may have remained potential, if less likely, vectors for 40 years. Indeed, given the state of knowledge of syphilis at the time, there was no reason for complacency about such risks of vectorhood. This fact, as we have seen, went unattended to in study protocols, public critique, or popular literature. To be sure, there is *nothing* to be said in favor of the continuation of the Tuskegee study after the development of penicillin. Intense moral critique has been appropriately aimed at this study, and it is recognized as perhaps the most appalling violation of research ethics in the history of medical research in the United States. Just the same, it remains important to diagnose precisely what is wrong with the Tuskegee picture.

Under our PVV view, the later critique of the Tuskegee study has only partially hit the mark. The critique itself, as distinct from the study, has erred by failing to achieve an adequate balance of attention to the victimhood and

---

14. Paul Farmer, *Pathologies of Power: Health, Human Rights, and the New War on the Poor* (Berkeley: University of California Press, 2003), 52, relaying the account of Yolande Jean, interned at Guantanamo for 11 months, based on interviews conducted by Farmer in 1993.

vectorhood of the men in the study. The Tuskegee study itself erred in both ways, failing in attending to victimhood—it violated the interests of the study subjects in an appalling way—and failing in attending to vectorhood—it ignored this aspect altogether. Yet the critique of the Tuskegee experiment has been lopsided, alert to the study's failings in one direction only. As we have seen in Chapter 4, when documenting bioethics' initial inattention to problems of transmissibility, critique of the Tuskegee experiment was itself lopsided, noticing the unconscionable and racist mistreatment of these men insofar as they were victims of the disease, but failing to notice the equally unconscionable way in which they were also made to remain carriers of the disease that could have potentially infected others around them. It is not known whether there were any actual cases of transmission to wives or sexual partners during the 40-year period of the study or cases of babies with congenital syphilis, but what is not excusable is the apparent failure to consider this possibility either in the study itself or in the critique of it.

A second, more recent case in which practices and policies have underweighted vectorhood is to be found in responses to the 2003 polio outbreak that originated in Kano, northern Nigeria, involving religious issues and suspicion of foreign meddling that led to an interruption of the polio immunization program. Imams in the area believed that immunization was a U.S. plot to make girls sterile. The case is not precisely apposite, because it did not involve overweighting the Nigerian girls' situation as victims *of polio* and underweighting their role as vectors, though it quickly became the case that even clear evidence that polio was being spread as a result of the imams' policy was rejected or ignored by those who imposed the policy. The global response to it, at least at first, also erred in underweighting vectorhood, deploring but not taking action to stop the situation, apparently out of concern for national sovereignty or perhaps religious liberty.

Our PVV view can diagnose not only practices and policies, but also attitudes and ways of framing matters. A third case in which victimhood has been very strongly emphasized to the diminishment of issues about vectorhood is the selling of HPV vaccine in the United States. As we have seen in Chapter 14, the new HPV vaccine has been very heavily advertised as protecting girls from future cervical cancer, but comparatively little is said about reducing the burden of HPV infection in the population as a whole, or, more specifically, reducing the burden of HPV infection in boys and men, who are both carriers and also (though less frequently) themselves victims of HPV-related disease, including cancer of the anus, cancer of the penis, and neck and throat cancer. Here, one of the principal rationales for mandating or encouraging widespread use of the vaccine in girls and boys should be to reduce transmission—that would be to base the campaign for its use on controlling vectorhood—but immunization is actually publicly promoted by emphasizing victimhood instead—and, indeed, the victimhood just of women.

Similarly, immunization campaigns often stress victimhood to the virtual exclusion of vectorhood. Why have a flu shot? Do it to protect yourself, say the ads and the public service announcements, but they rarely mention doing it to protect others to whom you might transmit the flu. At least in the United States (unlike Canada), virtually none of the annual public-service flu immunization campaigns approach potential acceptors by encouraging them to think of themselves as vectors; all the emphasis is on the individual's own risk of becoming victim.

Failing to distinguish between reasoning that is primarily alert to victimhood and reasoning that is primarily alert to vectorhood is at work in many other contexts. Even some seemingly simple practices like respect for patients' refusals of immunization look more problematic under the scrutiny of our PVV tool. For example, as we have seen in Chapter 8, allowing a competent patient to refuse immunization is often understood as a variety of the more general principle that a competent patient must be allowed to refuse any treatment at all. But refusing treatment and refusing immunization cannot be equated. They may look the same if one is considering the patient as victim only—the potential victim, for instance, of side effects like bruising at an injection site, an overwhelming fear of needles, or a serious reaction to the injection medium, but this is to view the patient as victim only and fail to keep in mind that the unimmunized patient is a potential vector. Vectorhood is not at issue when the patient is refusing other forms of medical treatment, and perhaps for this reason it is often overlooked in refusals of infectious-disease treatment or prevention as well.

Practices and Policies in Which the Relative Emphasis of Victimhood and Vectorhood Is Controversial. Of course, PVV analysis reveals not just two forms of lopsided policy, but also others where the balance is unclear, erratic, or controversial. For example, as we have explored at length in Chapters 16–19, pandemic planning may appear to be unclear, inconsistent, erratic, or fluctuating, especially while plans are still in development. Some pandemic plans appear to overemphasize vectorhood and fail to focus on the care of victims, especially people who are or become ill but are deprioritized for care, as we have argued. Some plans, we thus might like to say, are in effect plans for controlling vectorhood but not really plans for attending to victimhood. Such plans are best viewed as "half-plans," good in part but missing an essential complement if they are to be fully morally satisfactory. Similarly, any plan that overemphasizes victimhood—for example, a plan that failed to attend sufficiently to how social distancing measures might affect disease transmission—would demonstrate the opposite flaw.

Perhaps no recent infectious-disease control policy has been a greater focus of controversy than Cuba's treatment of HIV-positive patients, especially in the early days after the outbreak of the AIDS epidemic. Cuba's initial HIV quarantine policy involved quite severe constraints: isolation of infected individuals from the rest of the population was mandatory and, for those who were unwilling, sometimes involved the use of force. This policy did not merely prohibit people who were HIV-positive from entering the country (as U.S. policy did and still does), but removed Cuban citizens from their everyday lives. People who tested positive were taken away from their homes and sent to a sanatorium located in a suburb of Havana, Santiago de las Vegas.[15] Cuba's HIV policy might seem to involve as severe a violation of liberty as did the forcible relocation of lepers and suspected lepers in Hawaii to an isolated location. It might also seem to treat people who were HIV-positive primarily as vectors. But Cuba's policy had a real difference, and arguably met some of the basic requirements we have defended here at least to some extent: it attempted to do what it could to improve the conditions of people with HIV even while isolating them in sequestered facilities. The housing at Santiago de las Vegas to which they were moved, at first an "ugly medicalized army barracks," was transformed after the Ministry of Public Health took over from the military into a "community" of homes typically far better than those from which the residents had come, and they were paid their full, regular salaries, whether they worked or not.[16] This was a far cry from being dumped on a remote spit of land without any resources, as were the Hawaiian lepers exiled to Molokai. The Cuban detainees, it is claimed, were given housing equipped with air conditioning and television, and provided with education about HIV disease and how to protect their partners—as well as up-to-date health care.[17] We do not wish to argue that Cuba's policy was ideal, or even to claim that it was actually motivated by concerns for the victimhood of those in isolation. There remains considerable dispute (no doubt influenced by ideological concerns) about the actual conditions for patients and the strategies of containment that were put in place. Nevertheless, we do recognize that Cuba's HIV policy went further toward satisfying most of the procedural and substantive principles we identify as essential in putting our PVV view into practice than those of constraining infectious-disease control programs in many other countries.

This is for two reasons, one about victims, the other about vectors. Cuba's policy worked to treat HIV victims as precisely that, as victims—victims of a feared, life-threatening disease as well as victims of social prejudice—and in that victim-role provided health care and protection for them. But it also recognized

15. Ronald Bayer and Cheryl Healton, "Controlling AIDS in Cuba: The Logic of Quarantine," *New England Journal of Medicine* 320, no. 15 (1989): 1022-1024 (1023).
16. Nancy Scheper-Hughes, "Aids, Public Health and Human Rights in Cuba," *Lancet* 342, no. 8877 (October 16, 1993): 965-967.
17. Ibid.

that these same individuals could be vectors and pose a risk to others, hence the use of isolation to prevent transmission by them. Cuba's policy, it thus can be argued, at least to some extent took both victimhood and vectorhood considerations into account, without giving exaggerated weight to one over the other.

In contrast, many other countries have failed to achieve a defensible balance between responsibility to people with HIV disease as victims and as vectors. Countries with imbalanced, overly weak policies have allowed the HIV epidemic to spread unconscionably; examples might include many countries in Africa as well as those, arguably, in the developed world, especially the United States. The AIDS epidemic in the United States, for example, had by 2007 already claimed about half a million lives. Some observers pointed to an over-emphasis on victimhood as problematic. For example, writing in 1996, only a dozen years after the beginning of the AIDS epidemic in the United States, Bernard Rabinowitz denounced U.S. policies protecting confidentiality and permitting anonymous testing for HIV infectious as a "great hijack" by special interests, where, in his view, "the rights to secrecy of a tiny minority were deemed ethically more important than the rights of the huge uninfected majority," thus producing the "first legally protected epidemic in medical history."[18] Indeed, had the AIDS epidemic been controlled in the United States as effectively as in Cuba so that the rate of spread was the same, literally hundreds of thousands might not have died. At the same time, to focus only on prevention, as Rabinowitz's critique appeared to do, would tip the balance once again too far in the other direction.

Other areas have treated victims far too harshly. The unconfirmed report from an anthropologist working in Papua New Guinea, mentioned above, that when villagers are known (or suspected) of having AIDS, they are often summarily shot and their bodies dumped in the river, suggests a community that fails egregiously in satisfying the basic principles essential in constraint, based in recognition of these people's situations as victims. Killing someone is not the least restrictive alternative for curtailing the spread of disease; it does not protect personal security; it does not allow communication from the one constrained to those he or she cares about; and it permits no redress. In every respect, it violates this full set of principles.

It is also not the case that a country's policy necessarily succeeds in satisfying all of the basic procedural and substantive principles even if it satisfies many of them. For example while Cuba's policy, especially as it evolved, clearly met requirements for important interest, transparency, treatment of basic health needs, personal security, and communication, it may not have met the basic procedural requirement of reconsideration and redress: were Cubans

---

18. Bernard Rabinowitz, "The Great Hijack," *British Medical Journal* 313, no. 7060 (1996): 826.

484 *Making Use of the* Patient as Victim and Vector *View*

sent to the HIV facilities able to protest their detention or seek adequate redress afterward? Cuba's policy has clearly been regarded as controversial by
many outside observers, and it will require a far more sustained analysis (no
doubt not fully available until the HIV pandemic subsides), to assess whether
Cuba's policy succeeded or failed to weigh considerations of victimhood and
considerations of vectorhood in appropriate proportion. But it was clearly
more successful in doing so than the policies of many other countries on both
sides of the victim-protecting, vector-constraining divide.

Not all practices where the appropriate balance between attention to victimhood and vectorhood is unclear need involve massive quarantine programs
or other clear invasions of liberties. Some occur in familiar clinical settings.
For example, modern hospitals routinely isolate patients who are identified as
carriers of Vancomycin resistant enterococci or of methicillin resistant *Staphylococcus aureus.* The patient might be a person who has been hospitalized for a
fractured hip, but whose carriage has been identified by a nasal culture. The
hospital's response may be an isolation room, with signs proclaiming "special
pathogen precautions" and "gowns, masks required for entry" posted on the
door. These are burdens: it is known, for example, that fewer people go into that
room—the signs themselves are a symbolic barrier. A patient in isolation gets
fewer visits, and perhaps less good care—at least, less attentive care. Such patients
in isolation do get physical therapy and other needed treatment—including antibiotics that hopefully will still prove effective against their infection. But they
are victims as well—not just of a bad hip, not just of a staph infection, but
perhaps of less caring and less humane treatment.

Of course, policies may be well-crafted with adequate attention to both
victimhood and vectorhood, but simply not observed in practice. Particularly
egregious have been low rates of vaccination of health-care workers in the
United States, and health-care workers who report to work even when they
are not feeling well: they can easily serve, in the words of a physician writing
in the *New England Journal of Medicine,* as "vehicles of doom" for their patients.[19] The PVV tool is useful in assessing compliance with policy as well as
policy itself, and clearly recognizes in such cases that these health-care workers
egregiously underemphasize their own roles as vectors.

To be sure, there are some very hard cases: for example, those in which the
disease in question is both potentially lethal and easily communicable, but effective treatment is not available in the circumstances, whether because it is
not available in the region or because it is instituted too late. We have discussed one such case in detail in Chapter 9, in the case of the homeless man
dying of drug-resistant tuberculosis who wanted to be at home with his dog.

---

19. John D. Treanor, "Influenza—The Goal of Control," *New England Journal of Medicine* 357, no.
14 (2007): 1440.

The tension in this difficult case—though, we think, ultimately resolved in a satisfactory way—was how to recognize Mr. K's dangerousness as a vector and at the same time his vulnerability as a victim. In allowing Mr. K to have the dog with him in the hospital at the end of his life, a reasonable and humane balance of these concerns was finally—albeit after a long and distressing time—achieved. This is what PVV tells us to do: always look for new solutions, but at the end of the day recognize the ineluctable tensions between victimhood and vectorhood and attempt to reason through what anyone would want from the perspective of deep uncertainty about whether at any given time they are victim or vector, or, of course, potentially both.

Practices and Policies in Which Relative Emphasis of Victimhood and Vectorhood Is Well-Balanced. Compare these lopsided and controversial examples with a contemporary example of a better-balanced and hence, in our view, more ethically acceptable policy. This is Canada's *Guidelines Regarding Departure from Canada of Persons with Suspected Respiratory Tuberculosis (TB), Untreated Active Respiratory TB or Partially Treated Active Respiratory TB*, issued July 18, 2006, by the Public Health Agency of Canada.[20] This document sets out exit guidelines for people with active TB or suspected active TB leaving Canada. It applies to everyone, including ordinary citizens and visitors, deportees, and prisoners being transferred to a correctional system in another country. It provides a list of quarantine stations at the major airports, contact information for the Tuberculosis Prevention and Control official at the Public Health Agency of Canada, and various emergency provisions, like the possibility of convening a teleconference to determine the best course of action in given circumstances. But what is central to these guidelines is their recognition that patients who do not have access to adequate therapy meeting WHO standards are at risk, in dual ways, both to themselves and to others. They are both vectors *and* victims at the same time.

This policy's emphasis is on transfer of *care* as well as on prevention of transmission. Its strategy is to insist that when TB-infected persons leave Canada, continuity of care with a provider in the destination country must be arranged in advance. For areas of the world where TB treatment meets WHO standards (normally, at least 6 months of treatment), the policy requires only that information about the patient's case be sent to the new provider, and if the patient cannot identify one, the Public Health Agency of Canada or another Canadian

---

20. Public Health Agency of Canada, "Guidelines Regarding Departure from Canada of Persons with Suspected Respiratory Tuberculosis (TB), Untreated Active Respiratory TB or Partially Treated Active Respiratory TB," (2006), http://www.phac-aspc.gc.ca/tbpc-latb/tb_guide-ld_depart_e.html, 1–5 (accessed April 27, 2008).

agency will do so. Furthermore, it directs that the patient be given a supply (usually one month) of medication by the Canadian TB care provider to last until the first visit to the new provider in the destination country: this is intended to ensure continuity of care. But for the many countries where adequate TB treatment is not available, the policy also recognizes that the person receiving only erratic or substandard treatment may well develop chronic illness and drug-resistant disease, which—as the policy succinctly puts it, "can have serious consequences for those with TB disease as well as for society at large."[21] It therefore prohibits patients with active TB from leaving Canada for such countries. These patients may travel to another suitable country until their TB treatment is complete, or they will be required to remain in Canada until that time. Quarantine may be invoked if necessary, and the introduction to the policy points out that every jurisdiction in Canada has a legal mechanism that allows provincial or territorial public health authorities to maintain patients with active, contagious TB in respiratory isolation, usually about two to three weeks with appropriate drug treatment, until they are no longer deemed contagious.[22] If the patient has XDR-TB, the time for treatment will be longer. If the patient wants to travel against medical advice, the policy holds, the provincial or territorial public health acts should be used when possible to prevent travel.[23]

Canada's policy thus serves to protect the person with active TB from becoming a more serious victim of his disease, because if treatment is discontinuous or erratic he may develop drug-resistant disease and thus become far more difficult to treat. This may have substantial social costs for him, for instance, if he is prevented from traveling to his home country for important business, political, or family reasons, or if he is detained in respiratory isolation for a substantial period of time. Family members who are non-infectious may travel and the public health authority will sometimes provide letters for family members certifying that they have been examined and are non-infectious, lest they too be subject to the border service's exit controls. What typically happens is that people who refuse treatment and are therefore placed in respiratory isolation decide, after a couple of days, to accept treatment after all.[24] Nevertheless, under Canadian law, exit travel without treatment is non-negotiable for persons with active TB.

At the same time, Canada's policy also recognizes a *global* obligation to try to prevent transmission, even when the person is actually leaving Canada permanently and presumably will not further affect Canadians directly. The Canadian

21. Ibid., 2.
22. Ibid., 3.
23. Ibid.
24. Edward Ellis, M.D., Tuberculosis Prevention and Control, Public Health Agency of Canada, personal communication to M. Battin, February 15, 2008.

policy's alertness to the possibilities of global vectorhood is explicit, in that it insists that the policy is intended in part to prevent a situation in which "Canada will be contributing to the global burden of TB in countries that can least afford it."[25] The policy does not merely oblige commercial transportation carriers (like airlines) to refuse passage to someone for communicable disease reasons or require infection control measures if non-commercial transport is used (say, in deportation or in the transfer of prisoners), but concerns itself with that person's health, as both victim and vector, even after he or she is outside Canada. It is not an expensive policy, and not one that requires new legal powers. But in contrast to U.S. federal law, which, as Larry Gostin observes, focuses on preventing disease importation and does not mention preventing disease exportation,[26] the Canadian policy takes a much wider, global view. Indeed, the Canadian plan is much closer to ideal from a PVV point of view: it sees the patient as both victim and vector at the same time. This short document is thus a prime example of how practical policy can concern itself both with the well-being of the patient as victim and with that person's threat to others as vector, within one workable and coherent policy.

Furthermore, it satisfies the demands of the PVV view with respect to all three of the perspectives of which our shortcut tool is a composite: the real-life individual perspective, the population perspective, and the naturalized Rawlsian perspective. This policy is alert to the patient's immediate, personal circumstances and his current victim/vector status. It is at the same time concerned with the impact of disease transmission on populations, especially in the developing world where spread is more likely. And, although because it is written as a policy specifically concerning tuberculosis this is not explicit, the principles the policy develops governing who may be permitted to travel to what other countries under what conditions are readily applicable to other diseases with similar transmission and treatment profiles, and could of course be adapted to relevant emerging diseases should they appear. In this way, Canada's TB exit policy can include responsiveness to the deep uncertainty that is also part of the complex PVV view: things could be otherwise, and something else equally (or more) contagious and equally (or more) dangerous could emerge at any time. With a simple modification in the disease focus, this policy would be ready for it. Thus, while we have considered the PVV view in this chapter as a "simple" tool, it in fact incorporates a set of considerations that is quite complex.

---

25. Public Health Agency of Canada, 2.
26. Howard Markel, Lawrence O. Gostin, and David P. Fidler, "Extensively Drug-Resistant Tuberculosis: An Isolation Order, Public Health Powers, and a Global Crisis," *Journal of the American Medical Association* 298, no. 1 (2007): 85.

The Goal: Enhancing Philosophy and Policies

The lens of PVV is useful as a diagnostic and assessment tool both for philosophical reflection in ethics and for examining distant past, recent, and current practices and policies. But it is of particular importance in future philosophical reflection or designing new policies. Its demands are simple: incorporate an understanding of human reality in philosophical reflection that captures human vulnerability to serious communicable disease, and design the policy or implement the practice in ways that take both the victimhood and vectorhood of individuals into account; if not, the philosophy or the policy must be adjudged seriously deficient. Accounts of bioethics principles and theories of social justice, for example, may need to be augmented; policies like that involving pandemic planning require attention to what may be serious gaps (as for example the gap concerning the deprioritized)—matters that may not be evident without the dual sensitivities of the PVV view.

From our PVV view, we can work to see how deficiencies in philosophical theory and gaps in practical planning need correction. Once this is recognized, the directions further reflection and policy development should pursue are, if not easy, at least clearer. Indeed, rightly used, this PVV view would be brought to bear on all new philosophy and policy construction, to diagnose confusion, conflation, gaps, and other deficiencies. These may be more easily remedied once it is evident that *any* philosophical account of human circumstances, and *any* policy development that affects the health of human beings, should attend to the human beings in light of their embeddedness in a web of infectious disease, where the person, the patient, is both victim and vector at the same time. And thus, we hope, the book on infectious disease can be reopened in increasingly constructive ways.

REFERENCES

8 U.S.C. § 1182(1)(A)(1) (2007).

42 U.S.C § 1396a (2007).

42 U.S.C. § 300aa-10 (2007).

42 U.S.C. § 300aa-11(c) (2007).

42 U.S.C. § 300aa-13(1)(B) (2007).

42 U.S.C. § 300aa-14(c) (2007).

42 C.F.R § 100.3 (2007).

45 C.F.R. § 164.514(e) (2007).

45 C.F.R. § 46.102(f) (2007).

45 C.F.R. § 46.111(a)(1)(i) (2007).

45 C.F.R. § 46.111(a)(2) (2007).

45 C.F.R. §§ 46.116(a)(2), (3) (2007).

45 C.F.R Parts 160 and 164 (2007) (HIPAA Privacy Rule).

AAEM/SAEM Smallpox Vaccination Working Group. 2003. Smallpox vaccination for emergency physicians. *Academic Emergency Medicine* 10, no. 6 (June): 681–683.

Acuff, K.L., and R.R. Faden. 1991. A history of prenatal and newborn screening programs: Lessons for the future. In *AIDS, women and the next generation*, ed. R.R. Faden, G. Geller, and M. Powers. New York: Oxford University Press.

Aglionby, John. 2004. Farmers count flu's bitter cost. *The Observer*, news, January 25, 26.

Agosti, Jan M., and Sue J. Goldie. 2007. Introducing HPV vaccine in developing countries—Key challenges and issues. *New England Journal of Medicine* 356, no. 19 (May 10): 1908–1910.

Ahronheim, Judith C., Jonathan D. Moreno, and Connie Zuckerman. 2000. *Ethics in clinical practice.* 2nd ed. Gaithersburg, MD: Aspen Publishers.

Albert, Michael, Kristen Ostheimer, and Joel Breman. 2001. The last smallpox epidemic in Boston and the vaccination controversy, 1901–1903. *New England Journal of Medicine* 344, no. 5 (February 1): 375–379. Al-Bukhari, Sahih. 1959. *Hadith*, vol. 8, book 77, no. 616, tr. Muhammad Mushin Khan. Egyptian Press of Mustafa Al-Babi Al-Halabi.

Alford, Peter. 2006. Bird flu financial help for Jakarta. *The Australian*, local, June 26, 2.

Allen, Arthur. 2007. *Vaccine: The Controversial Story of Medicine's Greatest Lifesaver.* New York: W.W. Norton.

Almanac of Policy Issues. Unemployment compensation. Available at http://www.policyalmanac.org/social_welfare/archive/unemployment_compensation.shtml (accessed February 9, 2008).

Altman, Lawrence K. 1998. *Who goes first? The story of self-experimentation in medicine.* 2nd ed. Berkeley: University of California Press.

Altman, Lawrence K. 2007. AIDS Drugs Reach More People, U.N. Report Says, but Not Enough. *New York Times,* sec. A, April 18, 7.

Altman, Lawrence K. 2008. Mutant flu virus is found that resists popular drugs. *New York Times,* sec. A, January 31, 10.

American Academy of Family Physicians. AFFP policy statement regarding consideration of the mandated use of HPV for school attendance. Approved February 7, 2007, available at http://www.aafp.org/online/en/home/clinical/immunizationres/mandatedhpv.html (accessed January 5, 2008).

American Academy of Pediatrics and American Academy of Family Physicians, Subcommittee on Management of Acute Otitis Media. 2004. Diagnosis and management of acute otitis media. *Pediatrics* 113, no. 5 (May): 1451–1465.

American Academy of Pediatrics Committee on Infectious Diseases. 2007. Recommended immunization schedules for children and adolescents—United States, 2007. *Pediatrics* 119, no. 1 (January): 207–208.

American Academy of Pediatrics. 2002. *Guidelines for perinatal care.* 5th ed. Elk Grove Village, IL: American Academy of Pediatrics.

American College of Obstetricians and Gynecologists. 2001. *Cystic fibrosis carrier testing: The decision is yours.* Washington, DC: The American College of Obstetricians and Gynecologists, available at http://www.acog.org/publications/patient_education/cf001.cfm (accessed December 31, 2007).

American College of Obstetricians and Gynecologists. 2003. *Special procedures: The PAP test.* Washington, DC: American College of Obstetricians and Gynecologists, available at http://www.acog.org/publications/patient_education/bp085.cfm (accessed January 5, 2008).

American College of Obstetricians and Gynecologists and American College of Medical Genetics. 2001. *Preconception and prenatal carrier screening for cystic fibrosis: Clinical and laboratory guidelines.* Washington, DC: American College of Obstetricians and Gynecologists.

American College of Physicians. 2002. Medical professionalism in the new millennium: A physician charter. *Annals of Internal Medicine* 136, no. 3 (February 5): 243–246.

American Medical Association. Report of the council on ethical and judicial affairs. CEJA Report 1-I-05, available at http://www.ama–assn.org/ama1/pub/upload/mm/31/quarantine15726.pdf (accessed February 1, 2008).

Andrews, Lori. 2001. A conceptual framework for genetic policy: Comparing the medical, public health, and fundamental rights models. *Washington University Law Quarterly* 79: 221–285.

Angell, Marcia. 1997. The ethics of clinical research in the third world. *New England Journal of Medicine* 337, no. 12 (September 18): 847–849.

Annas, George J. 1993. Control of tuberculosis—The law and the public's health. *New England Journal of Medicine* 328, no. 8 (February 25): 585–588.

Annas, George. 2003. Puppy love: Bioterrorism, civil rights, and the public's health. *University of Florida Law Review* 55: 1171–1190.

Annas, George, Wendy K. Mariner, and Wendy E. Parmet. 2008. Pandemic preparedness: The need for a public health—Not a law enforcement/national security—Approach. *American Civil Liberties Union: Technology and Liberty Project* (January), available at http://www.aclu.org/privacy/medical/33642pub-20080114.html (accessed January 10, 2008).

Archdiocesan Liturgy Office. 2007. *Suggestions for the administration of holy communion and the sharing of the sign of peace during the cold and flu season.* Available at www.liturgy.sydney.catholic.org.au/documents/pdf/20070719_CommunionPaxColdFluSeason.pdf (accessed January 10, 2008).

Arinaminpathy, Nimalan. 2007. Using antiviral stockpiles effectively. Lecture, Uehiro Center, Oxford University, Oxford, England, July 4.

Arizona Department of Health Services. 2005. *Demographics and effective risk communication.* April, available at http://www.azdhs.gov/phs/edc/edrp/es/pdf/adhsspecialpopstudy.pdf (accessed January 26, 2008).

Arkansas Department of Health and Human Services. 2006. *Arkansas influenza pandemic response plan.* August, available at http://www.healthyarkansas.com/pandemic_influenza/pandemic_influenza_plan.pdf (accessed February 9, 2008; link no longer valid).

Armstrong, Conn, and Robert W. Pinner. 1999. Trends in infectious disease mortality in the United States during the 20th century. *Journal of the American Medical Association* 281, no. 1 (January 6): 61–66.

Arnold, Wayne. 2003. In Singapore, 1970's law becomes weapon against SARS. *New York Times*, sec. F, June 10, 5.

ASEAN Secretariat. 2007. ASEAN cooperation in combating avian influenza. November, available at http://www.cafte.gov.cn/include/linshiwenjian/download/6ASEAN.ppt#256 (accessed January 24, 2008).

Asser, S.M., and R. Swan. 1998. Child fatalities from religion-motivated medical neglect. *Pediatrics* 101: 625–629.

Associated Press. 2005. Rare drug-resistant HIV hits NYC. CBS News.com, February 12, available at http://www.cbsnews.com/stories/2005/02/12/health/main 673667.shtml (accessed January 2007).

Associated Press. 2006. New Hampshire to offer free HPV vaccine. *The Olympian*, November 30, available at http://www.theolympian.com/news/story/53188.html (accessed January 6, 2008).

Associated Press. 2007. Drugmaker stops lobbying efforts for STD shots: Merck criticized by parents and doctors for pushing cervical cancer vaccine. February 20, available at http://www.msnbc.msn.com/id/17246920/ (accessed January 6, 2008).

Associated Press. 2008. Passengers flew with infected woman. *New York Times*, sec. A, January 4, 12.

Association of Southeast Asian Nations. 2005 East Asia summit declaration on avian influenza prevention, control and response. December, available at http://www.aseansec.org/18101.htm (accessed January 24, 2008).

Ault, K. 2006. Vaccines for the prevention of human papillomavirus-related diseases: A review. *Obstetrical & Gynecological Survey* 61, no. 6, supplement 1 (June): S26–S31.

Baker, M.G., and D.P. Fidler. 2006. Global public health surveillance under new international health regulations. *Emerging Infectious Diseases* 12, no. 7 (July): 1058–1065.

Bale, J.F. 2002. Congenital infections. *Neurological Clinics of North America* 20, no. 4: 1039–1060.

Banta, D. 2002. Economic development Key to healthier world. *Journal of the American Medical Association* 287, no. 24 (June 26): 3195–3197.

Barnett, Daniel J. et al. 2005. A systematic analytic approach to pandemic influenza preparedness planning. *PLoS Med* 12, no. 2 (December): e359.

Baron, Dicker, and K.E. Bussell et al. 1988. Assessing trends in mortality in 121 US cities, 1970–79, from all causes and from pneumonia and influenza. *Public Health Report* 103: 120.

Barrett, R, and P.J Brown. 2008. Stigma in the Time of Influenza: Social and Institutional Responses to Pandemic Influenza. *Journal of Infectious Diseases* 197 (Suppl 1): S34-37.

Barry, Carolyn. 2007. The breast solution. *Science News* 172, no. 12 (September 22): 187.

Barry, John M. 2004. *The great influenza.* London: Penguin.

Bates, Betsy. 2003. Prenatal screening halves CF births: Data from large screening program. *OB. Gyn. News* 38, no. 24 (December 15): 1–2.

Bayer, Ronald. 1994. Ethical challenges posed by Zidovudine treatment to reduce vertical transmission of HIV. *New England Journal of Medicine* 331, no. 18 (November 3): 1223–1225.

Bayer, Ronald, and D. Wilkinson. 1995. Directly observed therapy for tuberculosis: History of an idea. *Lancet* 345: 545–1548.

Bayer, Ronald, and A.L. Fairchild. 2006. Changing the paradigm for HIV testing—The end of exceptionalism. *New England Journal of Medicine* 355, no. 7 (August 17): 647–649.

Bayer, Ronald, and Cheryl Healton. 1989. Controlling AIDS in Cuba: The Logic of Quarantine. *New England Journal of Medicine* 320, no. 15:1022-1024.

Bayer, Ronald. 1989. *Private acts, social consequences.* New York: Free Press.

Bayer, Ronald. 1991. Public health policy and the AIDS epidemic: An end to HIV exceptionalism? *New England Journal of Medicine* 324, no. 21 (May 23): 1500–1504.

Bayer, Ronald. 1999. Clinical progress and the future of HIV exceptionalism. *Archives of Internal Medicine* 159: 1042–1048.

Beauchamp, Dan E. 1975. Public health: Alien ethic in a strange land. *American Journal of Public Health* 65: 1338–1339.

Beauchamp, Dan E., and Bonnie Steinbock, eds. 1999. *New ethics for the public's health.* Oxford: Oxford University Press.

Beauchamp, Tom L., and James F. Childress. 2001 [1978]. *Principles of biomedical ethics.* 5th ed. New York: Oxford University Press.

Beauchamp, Tom L., and Leroy Walters, eds. 1978. *Contemporary issues in bioethics.* Encino, CA: Dickenson.

Beecher, Henry K. 1966. Ethics and clinical research. *New England Journal of Medicine* 274, no. 24: 1354–1360.

Beliefnet. Christian science basics: Main tenets. Available at http://www.beliefnet.com/index/index_10123.html (accessed January 6, 2008).

Benatar, Solomon R. 1998. Global disparities in health and human rights: A critical commentary. *American Journal of Public Health* 88 (2): 295–300.

Benatar, Solomon R. 2001. Commentary: Justice and medical research: A global perspective. *Bioethics* 15, no. 4: 333–340. Benatar, Solomon R. 2003. Bioethics: Power and Injustice: IAB Presidential Address, *Bioethics* 17, nos. 5/6 (October): 387–400.

Benatar, Solomon R. 2005. Moral imagination: The missing component in global health. *PLoS Medicine* 2, no. 12 (December 27), available at http://medicine. plosjournals.org/perlserv?request=get-document&doi=10.1371/journal.pmed .0020400 (accessed February 16, 2008).

Benitez, Mary Ann. 2004. One fifth of live poultry stalls agree to close in flu buy-back. *South China Morning Post*, news, August 26, 1.

Bensimon, Cecile, and Ross Upshur. 2007. Evidence and effectiveness in decision-making for quarantine. *American Journal of Public Health* 97: S44–S48.

Berk, Ariel. 2004. Handwashing lessens MRSA risk. *Johns Hopkins Newsletter*. November 15, available at http://media.www.jhunewsletter.com/media/storage /paper932/news/2004/11/05/Science/Hand-Washing.Lessens.Mrsa.Risk–2244064 .shtml (accessed December 29, 2007).

Bhattacharya, Shaoni. 2005. Multi-drug-resistant HIV strain raises alarm. *New Scientist* 16 (February 14): 15. Available at http://www.newscientist.com/article .ns?id=dn7007 (accessed January 2007).

Bill and Melinda Gates Foundation. 2000. *The Bill & Melinda Gates Foundation announces new HIV/AIDS grants at World AIDS Conference.* July, available at http://www.gatesfoundation.org/GlobalHealth/Pri_Diseases/HIVAIDS/Announcements/Announce–245.htm (accessed February 1, 2008).

Bill and Melinda Gates Foundation. 2005. Grand challenges in global health selects 43 groundbreaking research projects for more than $436 million in funding. June 27, available at http://www.gatesfoundation.org/GlobalHealth /BreakthroughScience/GrandChallenges/Announcements/Announce-050627 .htm (accessed January 22, 2008).

Bisno, A.L. 2001. Acute pharyngitis. *New England Journal of Medicine* 344, no. 3 (January 18): 205–211.

Bisno, A.L., M.A. Gerber, J.M. Gwaltney, Jr., E.L. Kaplan, R.H. Schwartz, and Infectious Diseases Society of America. 2002. Practice guidelines for the diagnosis and management of group A streptococcal pharyngitis. *Clinical Infectious Diseases* 35, no. 2 (July 15): 113–125.

Blendon, Robert J., Catherine M. DesRoches, Martin S. Cetron, John M. Benson, Theodore Meinhart, and William Pollard. 2006. Attitudes toward the use of quarantine in a public health emergency in four countries. *Health Affairs* 25, no. 2 (March–April): w15–w25.

Bloom, Barry R. 2005. Public health in transition. *Scientific American* 293, no. 3 (September): 92–99.

Bloom, Barry R., and Paul-Henri Lambert, eds. 2003. *The Vaccine Book.* San Diego, CA: Elsevier Science, Academic Press.

Bluestone, Naomi R. 1976. The teaching of ethics in schools of public health. *American Journal of Public Health* 66 (5): 478–479.

Bootsma, M.C.J., and N.M. Ferguson. 2007. The effect of public health measures on the 1918 influenza pandemic in U.S. Cities. *Proceedings of the National Academy of Sciences of the United States* 104, no. 18 (May 1): 7588–7593.

Bosch, F.X., X. Castellsagué, N. Muñoz, S. de Sanjosé, A.M. Ghaffari, L.C. González, M. Gili et al. 1996. Male sexual behaviors and human papillomavirus DNA: Key risk factors for cervical cancer in Spain. *Journal of the National Cancer Institute* 88, no. 15 (August 7): 1060–1067.

Bostick, N.A., R. Sade, J.W. McMahon, and R. Benjamin. 2006. Report of the American medical association council on ethical and judicial affairs: Withholding information from patients, rethinking the propriety of "therapeutic privilege." *Journal of Clinical Ethics* 17, no. 4: 302–306.

Boston Globe. 1901. Virus squad out. *Boston Globe*, November 18, 7. In Albert, Ostheimer, and Breman 2001, 375–379.

Boston University School of Public Health. Health law, bioethics and human rights: Research. Available at http://sph.bu.edu/index.php?option=com_content&task=view&id=66&Itemid=94 (accessed December 29, 2007).

Botkin, Jeffrey R. 2001. Protecting the privacy of family members in survey and pedigree research. *Journal of the American Medical Association* 285, no. 2 (January 10): 207–211.

Boylan, Michael, ed. 2004. *Public health policy and ethics.* Dordrecht, the Netherlands: Kluwer Academic.

Bozzette, S.A. 2005. Routine screening for HIV infection—Timely and cost-effective. *New England Journal of Medicine* 352, no. 6 (February 10): 620–621.

Bozzette S.A., R. Boer, V. Bhatnagar, J.L. Brower, E.B. Keeler, S.C. Morton, and M. A. Stoto. 2003. A model for a smallpox vaccination policy. *New England Journal of Medicine* 348, no. 5 (January 30): 416–425.

Bradley, David. 2007. Ethical barriers to malaria control. Lecture, Uehiro Center, Oxford University, Oxford, England, July 4.

Bradely, J. 2006. Delivering, safe, effective and acceptable cervical cancer prevention services in low resource settings. Presentation at 2006 XVIII FIGO World Congress of Gynecology and Obstetrics, available at http://www.alliance-cxca.org (accessed January 5, 2008).

Bradsher, Keith, and Lawrence K Altman. 2004. A war and a mystery: Confronting avian flu. *New York Times*, sec. 4, October 12, 1.

Bradsher, Keith. 2005. The front lines in the battle against avian flu are running short of money. *New York Times*, sec. 1, October 9, 10.

Brandt, Allan M. 1979. Polio, politics, publicity, and duplicity: Ethical aspects in the development of the Salk vaccine. *Connecticut Medicine* 43, no. 9: 581–590.

Branson, B.M. 2000. Rapid tests for HIV antibody. *AIDS Reviews* 2: 76–83.

Branson, B.M. 2005. Rapid HIV Testing: 2005 Update, Routine HIV Screening for Emergency Department Patients. Slide no. 34, available at www.cdc.gov/hiv/topics/testing/resources/slidesets/pdf/USCA_Branson.pdf (accessed January 3, 2008). Brewer, Timothy F. 2007. Extensively drug-resistant tuberculosis and public health. *Journal of the American Medical Association* 298, no. 16: 1861.

Brewer, Timothy F., and S. Jody Heymann. 2004. The long journey to health equity. *Journal of the American Medical Association* 292, no. 2 (July 14): 269–271.

Bridges, C.B., M.J. Kuehnert, and C.B. Hall. 2003. Transmission of influenza: Implications for control in health care settings. *Clinical Infectious Diseases* 37: 1094–1101.

Brock, Dan. 2007. Pandemic flu: Scenarios for planning and teaching. Lecture, Uehiro Center, Oxford University, Oxford, England, July 4.

Brouqui, P., B. Lascola, V. Roux, and D. Raoult. 1999. Chronic *Bartonella quintana* bacteremia in homeless patients. *New England Journal of Medicine* 340, no. 3 (January 21): 184–189.

Brown, Louise. 2000. *Sex slaves: The trafficking of women in Asia*. London: Virago Press.

Brown, Theodore M., Marcus Cueto, and Elizabeth Fee. 2006. The World Health Organization and the transition from "international" to "global" public health. *American Journal of Public Health* 96: 62–72.

Buchanan, Allen, and Dan Brock. 1989. *Deciding for others*. Cambridge: Cambridge University Press.

Bulterys, M., D.J. Jamieson, M.J. O'Sullivan, M.H. Cohen, R. Maupin, S. Nesheim, M.P. Webber et al. 2004. Rapid HIV-1 testing during labor: A multicenter study. *Journal of the American Medical Association* 292, no. 2 (July 14): 219–223

Burki, Talha Khan. 2007. Review of Robert Baker, Quiet killers: The fall and rise of deadly diseases. *New England Journal of Medicine* 357, no. 17 (October 25): 1784–1785.

Calabresi, Guido, and Philip Bobbitt. 1978. *Tragic choices*. New York: Norton.

California Department of Health Services. 2006. *Pandemic influenza preparedness and response plan* (September 8). Available at http://www.dhs.ca.gov/ps/dcdc/izgroup/pdf/pandemic.pdf (accessed July 7, 2008).

Callahan, Daniel and Bruce Jennings. 2002. Ethics and public health: Forging a strong relationship. *American Journal of Public Health* 92: 169–176.

Campion, E.W. 1999. Liberty and the control of tuberculosis. *New England Journal of Medicine* 340, no. 5 (February 4): 385–386.

Carson, Rachel. 1962. *Silent spring*. Boston: Houghton-Mifflin.

Castellsagué, X. et al. 2002. Male circumcision, penile human papillomavirus infection, and cervical cancer in female partners. *New England Journal of Medicine* 346, no. 15 (April 11): 1105–1112.

Centers for Law and the Public's Health. 2008. Model state public health laws. Available at http://www.publichealthlaw.net/Resources/Modellaws.htm#MSEHPA (accessed July 4, 2008).

Centers for Law and the Public's Health. 2008. The turning point model state public health act state legislative matrix table. Available at http://www.publichealth-law.net/Resources/ResourcesPDFs/MSPHA%20Matrix%20Table.pdf (accessed July 4, 2008).

Centers for Law and the Public's Health. 2001. The model state emergency health powers act. December 21, sec. 604(b)(2), available at http://www.publichealthlaw.net/MSEHPA/MSEHPA2.pdf (accessed January 24, 2008).

Centers for Law and the Public's Health. 2001. The model state emergency health powers act. December 21, sec. 506, available at http://www.publichealthlaw.net/MSEHPA/MSEHPA2.pdf (accessed January 24, 2008).

Center on the Evaluation of Value and Risk in Health. *The Cost-Effectiveness Analysis Registry: Cost-Utility Analyses Published in 2002 and 2003.* Boston: Tufts-New England Medical Center, ICRHPS, available at http://160.109.101.132/cearegistry/data/docs/PhaseIIIACompleteLeagueTable.pdf (accessed January 5, 2008).

Centers for Disease Control and Prevention. 1993. Inactivated Japanese encephalitis virus vaccine. Recommendations of the advisory committee on immunization practices (ACIP). *Morbidity and Mortality Weekly Report,* 42, no. RR-01 (January 8).

Centers for Disease Control and Prevention. 1994. Outbreak of measles among Christian Science students—Missouri and Indiana, 1994. *Mortality and Morbidity Weekly Report* 43, no. 25 (July 1): 463–465.

Centers for Disease Control and Prevention. 1995. Essential components of a tuberculosis control program: Recommendations of the advisory council for the elimination of tuberculosis. *Mortality and Morbidity Weekly Report* 44, no. RR–11 (September 8): 1–16.

Centers for Disease Control and Prevention. 1997. Immunization of health-care workers: Recommendations of the advisory committee on immunization practices (ACIP) and the hospital infection control practices advisory committee (HICPAC). *Mortality and Morbidity Weekly Report* 46, no. RR-18 (December 26): 1–42.

Centers for Disease Control and Prevention. 1997. Poliomyelitis prevention in the United States: Introduction of a sequential vaccination schedule of inactivated poliovirus vaccine followed by oral poliovirus vaccine; Recommendations of the Advisory Committee on Immunization Practices (ACIP). *Mortality and Morbidity Weekly Report* 46, no. RR-3 (January 24): 1–25.

Centers for Disease Control and Prevention. 2002. Discontinuation of Cefixime tablets—United States. *Mortality and Morbidity Weekly Report* 51, no. 46 (November 22): 1052.

Centers for Disease Control and Prevention. 2002. Notice to readers: Approval of a new rapid test for HIV antibody. *Morbidity and Mortality Weekly Report* 51, no. 46 (November 22): 1051–1052.

Centers for Disease Control and Prevention. 2002. Probable variant Creutzfeldt-Jakob disease in a US resident – Florida, 2002. *Mortality and Morbidity Weekly Report* 51, no. 41 (October 18): 927–929.

Centers for Disease Control and Prevention. 2003. 2002 national STD surveillance report: STDs in women and infants. Available at http://www.cdc.gov/std/stats02/women&inf.htm (accessed January 1, 2008).

Centers for Disease Control and Prevention. 2003. Guidance for the healthcare community concerning section 304 of the Homeland Security Act. Available at http://www.bt.cdc.gov/agent/smallpox/vaccination/healthcare-304-guidance.asp (accessed February 9, 2008).

Centers for Disease Control and Prevention. 2003. Use of quarantine to prevent transmission of severe acute respiratory syndrome—Taiwan, 2003. *Mortality and Morbidity Weekly Report* 52, no. 29 (July 23): 680–683.

Centers for Disease Control and Prevention. 2004. Congenital syphilis—United States 2002. *Morbidity and Mortality Weekly Report* 53, no. 31 (August 13): 716–719.

Centers for Disease Control and Prevention. 2004. Introduction of routine HIV testing in prenatal care—Botswana, 2004. *Morbidity and Mortality Weekly Report* 53, no. 46 (November 26): 1083–1086.

Centers for Disease Control and Prevention. 2004. Oral alternatives to Cefixime for the treatment of uncomplicated Neisseria gonorrhoeae urogenital infections. Available at http://www.cdc.gov/std/treatment/cefixime.htm (accessed December 29, 2007).

Centers for Disease Control and Prevention. 2004. *Rapid HIV–1 antibody testing during labor and delivery for women of unknown HIV status: A practical guide and model protocol.* January 30. Available at http://www.cdc.gov/hiv/topics /testing/resources/guidelines/rt--labor&delivery.htm (accessed January 1, 2008).

Centers for Disease Control and Prevention. 2006. *ACIP meeting minutes October 25–26, 2006: Update on the quadrivalent HPV vaccine.* Available at http://www.cdc .gov/vaccines/recs/acip/downloads/min–oct06.pdf (accessed January 5, 2008).

Centers for Disease Control and Prevention. 2006. Emergence of mycobacterium tuberculosis with extensive resistance to second-line drugs—Worldwide, 2000–2004. *Mortality and Morbidity Weekly Report* 55, no. 11 (March 24): 301–305.

Centers for Disease Control and Prevention. 2006. *The national plan to eliminate syphilis from the United States* (May). Available at http://www.cdc.gov/ stopsyphilis/SEE Plan2006.pdf (accessed December 31, 2007).

Centers for Disease Control and Prevention. 2006. Revised recommendations for HIV testing of adults, adolescents, and pregnant women in health-care settings. *Morbidity and Mortality Weekly Report* 55, no. RR-14 (September 22): 1–17.

Centers for Disease Control and Prevention. 2006–2007. Influenza season summary. Available at http://www.cdc.gov/flu/weekly/weeklyarchives2006-2007 /06-07summary.htm (accessed February 6, 2008).

Centers for Disease Control and Prevention. 2007. HPV vaccine—Questions & answers for the public (June 28). Available at http://www.cdc.gov/vaccines /vpd-vac/hpv/hpv-vacsafe-effic.htm (accessed January 6, 2008).

Centers for Disease Control and Prevention. 2007. National vaccination coverage among adolescents aged 13-17 years—United States, 2006. *Mortality and Morbidity Weekly Report* 56, no. 34 (August 1): 885–888.

Centers for Disease Control and Prevention. 2007. Progress toward interruption of wild poliovirus transmission—worldwide, January 2006–May 2007. *Mortality and Morbidity Weekly Report* 56, no. 27 (July 13): 682–685.

Centers for Disease Control and Prevention. 2007. Quadrivalent human papillomavirus vaccine: Recommendations of the Advisory Committee on Immunization Practices (ACIP). *Mortality and Morbidity Weekly Report* 56, no. RR-02 (March 23): 1–24.

Centers for Disease Control and Prevention. 2007. *Vaccine information statement (interim): Varicella vaccine.* January 10, available at http://www.cdc.gov/vaccines/pubs/vis/downloads/vis-varicella.pdf (accessed January 4, 2008).

Centers for Disease Control and Prevention. CDC vaccine price list. Available at http://www.cdc.gov/vaccines/programs/vfc/cdc–vac–price–list.htm (accessed February 9, 2008).

Centers for Disease Control and Prevention. FluAid 2.0. Available at http://www2 .cdc.gov/od/fluaid/default.htm (accessed February 6, 2008).

Centers for Disease Control and Prevention. Get smart: Know when antibiotics work. available at http://www.cdc.gov/drugresistance/community/faqs.htm#1 (accessed January 3, 2008).

Centers for Disease Control and Prevention. HIV/AIDS Surveillance Supplemental Report: Deaths among Persons with AIDS through December 2000. Available at www.cdc.gov/hiv/topics/surveillance/resources/reports/2002supp_vol8no1/table2.htm (accessed January 22, 2008).

Centers for Disease Control and Prevention. *Public health action plan to combat antibiotic resistance: Antimicrobial resistance interagency task force* 2001 *annual report.* Available at http://www.cdc.gov/drugresistance/actionplan /index.htm (accessed January 3, 2008).

Centers for Disease Control and Prevention. Sexually transmitted diseases: Surveillance 2006. Available at www.cdc.gov/std/stats/syphilis.htm (accessed November 2007).

Centers for Disease Control and Prevention. 2008. 2007 *West Nile Virus Activity in the United States.* Reported as of January 8. Available at http://www.cdc.gov /ncidod/dvbid/westnile/Mapsactivity/surv&control07Maps.htm (accessed January 27, 2008).

Centers for Disease Control and Prevention. 2008. U.S. public health service syphilis study at Tuskegee. Available at http://www.cdc.gov/tuskegee/timeline. htm (accessed July 4, 2008).

Centers for Disease Control. 2007. History of quarantine. Available at http://www.cdc .gov/ncidod/dq/history.htm (accessed July 4, 2008).

Centers for Disease Control and Prevention. 2008. Availability of Cefixime 400 mg. Tablets. United States, April 2008. *Morbidity and Mortality Weekly Report* 57, no. 16 (April 25): 435.

Centers for Disease Control and Prevention. 2008. *Epidemiology and Prevention of Vaccine-Preventable Diseases* (2nd Printing: 10th ed.). Washington, D.C.: Public Health Foundation.

Centers for Disease Control and Prevention. 2008. *CDC Global Immunization Strategic Framework 2006–2010.* Available at http://www.cdc.gov/vaccines/ programs/global/downloads/gisf-2006–2010.pdf (accessed July 29, 2008).

Chakraborti, Chaanda. 2006. Ethics of care and HIV: A case for rural women in India. *Developing World Bioethics* 6: 89–94.

Chakraborti, Chaanda. Forthcoming. "Pandemic Management and Developing World Bioethics: Bird Flu in West Bengal," *Developing World Bioethics.*

Chang, Howard F. 2002. Migration regulation goes local: The role of states in U.S. immigration policy. *New York University Annual Survey of American Law* 58: 357–370.

Charo, R. Alta. 2007. Politics, parents, and prophylaxis—Mandating HPV vaccination in the United States. *New England Journal of Medicine* 356, no. 19 (May 10): 1905–1908.

Chen, R.T. 1999. Vaccine risks: real, perceived and unknown. *Vaccine* 17, supplement 3 (October 29): S41–S46.

Childress, James F., and Ruth Gaare Bernheim. 2003. Beyond the liberal and communitarian impasse: A framework and vision for public health, *Florida Law Review* 55: 1191–1219.

Chin, James. 2000. *Control of communicable diseases manual*. Washington, DC: American Public Health Association.

Chio, A., D. Cocito, and M. Leone. 2003. Guillain-Barré syndrome: A prospective, population-based incidence and outcome survey. *Neurology* 60: 1146–1150.

Chokshi, Dave A., and Aaron S. Kesselheim. 2008. "Rethinking global access to vaccines," *British Medical Journal* 336:750-753 (April 5).

Chou, Roger, et al. 2005. Prenatal screening for HIV: A review of the evidence for the US Preventive Services Task Force. *Annals of Internal Medicine* 143, no. 1 (July 5): 38–54.

Christian, M.D., et al. 2006. Development of a Triage Protocol for Critical Care During an Influenza Pandemic. *Canadian Medical Association Journal* 175, no. 11 (November 21): 1377–1381.

Christian Medical & Dental Associations. 2007. *Position statement: Human papilloma virus vaccine.* (January 26). Available at http://www.cmda.org/AM/Template.cfm?Section= Ethics_and_Position_Statements&Template=/CM/ContentDisplay.cfm&ContentID=4293 (accessed January 5, 2008).

Clark, Margaret A. 1999. This little piggy went to market: The xenotranplantation and xenozoonose debate. *Journal of Law, Medicine & Ethics* 27, no. 1: 137–152.

Clark, Richard A. 1999. Finding the right balance against bioterrorism. *Emerging Infectious Diseases Special Issue* 5, no. 4 (July/August): 502.

Cochrane Collaboration. 2007. Interventions for the interruption or reduction of the spread of respiratory viruses (Review). Available at http://www.thecochranelibrary.com (accessed January 30, 2008).

Cohen, Jon. 2006. The new world of global health. *Science* 311, no. 5758 (January 13): 162–167.

Cohen, J., & W.G. Powderly. 2003. *Infectious diseases* (2nd ed.). St. Louis, Mo. London: Mosby.

Coker, R. 2001. Just coercion? Detention of nonadherent tuberculosis patients. *Annals of the New York Academies of Sciences* 953 (December): 216–222.

Coleman, Carl. 2007. The role of law in limiting the over—prescription of antibiotics. Lecture, Uehiro Center, Oxford Univeristy, Oxford, England, July 4.

Coleman, Carl, Andreas Reis, and Alice Croisier. 2007. Ethical considerations in developing a public health response to pandemic influenza. World Health Organization, available at www.who.int/csr/resources/publications (accessed February 16, 2008).

Collignon, P., and F.J. Angulo. 2006. Fluoroquinolone-resistant *Escherichia coli*: Food for thought. *Journal of Infectious Diseases* 194, no. 1 (July 1, 2006): 8–10.

Colorado Department of Public Health. 2006. *CDPHE internal emergency response implementation plan, annex U: Disease outbreak, appendix 1: pandemic influenza attachment* (December 14). Available at http://www.cdphe.state.co.us/epr/Public/InternalResponsePlan/Attachment7.pdf (accessed January 26, 2008).

Combs, O'Brien, and L.J. Geiter. 1990. USPHS tuberculosis short-course chemotherapy trial 21: Effectiveness, toxicity, and acceptability. *Annals of Internal Medicine* 112: 397–406.

Commission of the European Communities. 2004. *Commission Working Document on Community Influenza Preparedness and Response Planning.* COM(2004)201 final, Brussels, March 26. Available at http://europa.eu/eur-lex/en/com/wdc/2004/com2004_0201en01.pdf (accessed January 24, 2008).

Commission of the European Communities. 2005. *Communication from the Commission to The Council, the European Parliament, the European Economic and Social Committee and the Committee of the Regions on pandemic influenza preparedness and response planning in the European community.* COM(2005) 607 final, Brussels, November 28. Available at http://eur-lex.europa.eu/LexUriServ/site/en/com/2005/com2005_0607en01.pdf (accessed February 7, 2008).

Connor, Edward M., et al. 1994. Reduction of maternal-infant transmission of human immunodeficiency virus type 1 with Zidovudine treatment. *New England Journal of Medicine* 331, no. 18 (November 3): 1173–1180.

Conyers, Boomer, and Brian T. McMahon. 2005. Workplace discrimination and HIV/AIDS: The national EEOC ADA research project. *Work* 25, no. 1: 37–48.

Conyn-van Spaendonck, Marina A. E. et al. 2001. Immunity to poliomyelitis in the Netherlands. *American Journal of Epidemiology* 153, no. 3 (February 1): 207–214.

Cook, Noble David. 1998. *Born to Die: Disease and New World Conquest, 1492–1650.* New York: Cambridge University Press.

Coughlin, Steven S., Wendy H. Katz, and Donald R. Mattison. 1999. Ethics instruction at schools of public health in the United States. *American Journal of Public Health* 89, no. 5: 768–770.

Council of Science Editors. 2007. *Global theme issue on poverty and human development.* October 22. Available at http://www.councilscienceeditors.org/globalthemeissue.cfm (accessed February 16, 2008).

Cranford, Ron E. 1991. Helga Wanglie's ventilator. *Hastings Center Report* 21, no. 4: 23–24.

Curtis, Polly. 2007. Vaccination of Children in UK Urged as Measles Cases Soar. *Irish Times* (August 31) 12.

Cystic Fibrosis Foundation. 2007. Newborn screening. Available at http://www.cff.org/AboutCF/Testing/NewbornScreening/#What_states_do_newborn_screening_for_CF (accessed December 31, 2007).

Da Silva, Carlos, and Henrique Martins. 2004. Not telling the truth in the patient–physician relationship. *Bioethics* 17, nos. 5–6: 417–424.

Dabis, F., and E.R. Ekpini. 2002. HIV-1/AIDS and maternal and child health in Africa. *Lancet* 359: 2097–2104.

Dales, L.G. et al. 1993. Measles epidemic from failure to immunize. *Western Journal of Medicine* 159, no. 4: 455–464.

Dalton, Larry R. 2007. Theory-Guided Nano-Engineering: A Technology Revolution! Lecture at the University of Utah (October 24).

Daniels, Norman. 1985. *Just Health Care.* Cambridge: Cambridge University Press.

Daniels, Norman. 2008. *Just health: Meeting health needs fairly.* Cambridge: Cambridge University Press.

Daniels, Norman, and James Sabin. 2002. *Setting limits fairly: Can we learn to share medical resources?* New York: Oxford University Press.

Daubert, Michelle A. 2007. Comment: Pandemic fears and contemporary quarantine: Protecting liberty through a continuum of due process rights. *Buffalo Law Review.* 54: 1299–1353.

Davenport, F.M. 1977. Influenza viruses. In *Viral infections of humans,* ed. A.S. Evans, 273–296. New York: Plenum.

Davis, John. W., Barry Hoffmaster, and Sarah Shorten, eds. 1978. *Contemporary issues in biomedical ethics.* Clifton, NJ: Humana Press.

Dawson, Angus. 2007. Tuberculosis and the ethical justification of the "least restrictive alternative." Lecture, Uehiro Center, Oxford University, Oxford, England, July 4.

de Melo–Martín, Inmaculada. 2006. The promise of human papillomavirus vaccine does not confer immunity against ethical reflection. *Oncologist* 11, no. 4 (April): 393–396.

De Zulueta, Paquita. 2001. Randomised placebo-controlled trials and HIV-infected pregnant women in developing countries: Ethical imperialism or unethical exploitation. *Bioethics* 1, no. 4: 289–311.

Debarre, Florence, Sebastian, Bonhoeffer, and Roland R. Regoes. 2007. The effect of population structure on the emergence of drug resistance during influenza pandemics. *Journal of the Royal Society Interface* 4, no. 16 (October 22): 893–906.

Deber, Raisa B., and Goel Vivek. 1990. Using explicit decision rules to manage issues of justice, risk, and ethics in decision analysis: When is it not rational to maximize expected utility. *Medical Decision Making* 10, no. 3: 181–194.

Deem, David S., and W. Burke. 2006. Ethical issues arising from the participation of children in genetic research. *Journal of Pediatrics* 149, supplement 1 (July): S34–S38.

Del Rio, C., and J. Sepulveda. 2002. AIDS in Mexico: Lessons learned and implications for developing countries. *AIDS* 16: 1445–1457.

Delaware Department of Health and Social Services Division of Public Health. 2007. *Delaware pandemic influenza plan.* April. Available at http://www.dhss.delaware.gov/dhss/dph/files/depanfluplan.pdf (accessed July 4, 2008).

Department of Health. 2007. *Responding to pandemic influenza: The ethical framework for policy and planning.* November 22, available at http://www.dh.gov.uk/en/Publicationsandstatistics/Publications/PublicationsPolicyAndGuidance/DH_080751 (accessed January 21, 2008).

Department of Health and Human Services. 2006. *Pandemic planning update.* March 13, available at http://www.pandemicflu.gov/plan/pdf/panflu20060313.pdf (accessed February 6, 2008).

Department of Veterans Affairs. 2006. *VA Pandemic Influenza Plan.* Available at http://www.publichealth.va.gov/Flu/documents/VAPandemicFluPlan_2006-03-31.pdf (accessed July 2, 2008).

Department of Health and Human Services. 2006. *Pandemic planning update III.* November, available at http://www.pandemicflu.gov/plan/pdf/panflure port3. pdf (accessed February 6, 2008).

DeVille, K.A. 1994. Nothing to fear but fear itself: HIV-infected physicians and the law of informed consent. *Journal of Law, Medicine, and Ethics* 22: 163–175.

Diamond, Jared. 1999. *Guns, germs and steel.* New York: W.W. Norton.

Dib, Jacobo, Jr. 2007. Letter: Nonpharmaceutical Interventions implemented during the 1918–1919 influenza pandemic. *Journal of the American Medical Association* 298, no. 19 (November 21): 2260.

Diekema, D.S., and the Committee on Bioethics. 2005. Responding to parental refusals of immunization of children. *Pediatrics* 115: 1428–1431.

District of Columbia Department of Health. 2005. *Pandemic influenza preparedness plan.* March. Available at http://dchealth.dc.gov/doh/frames.asp?doc=/doh/lib/doh/information/influenza/pdf/dc_pandemic_influenza_plan.pdf (accessed July 4, 2008).

Dixon, Lloyd, and Rachel Kaganoff Stern. 2004. *Compensation for losses from the 9/11 attacks.* Rand Corporation, available at http://www.rand.org/pubs/monographs/2004/RAND_MG264.pdf (accessed February 9, 2008).

Dobkin, Jay F. 2006. HIV management: Time for a public health approach? *Infections in Medicine* 23: 48–49.

Domingo, P., and N. Barquet. 1994. The first epidemic of cerebrospinal meningitis. *Gesnerus* 51, nos. 3–4: 280–282.

Dondero, T.J. Jr., M. Pappaioanou, and J.W. Curran. 1988. Monitoring the levels and trends of HIV infection: The Public Health Service's HIV surveillance program. *Public Health Reports* 103, no. 3 (May–June): 213–220.

Doughty, Roger. 1994. The confidentiality of HIV related information: Responding to the resurgence of aggressive public health interventions in the AIDS epidemic. *California Law Review* 82: 113–184.

Dove, Alan W., and Vincent R. Racaniello. 1997. The polio eradication effort: Should vaccine eradication be next? *Science* 277 (5372): 779–780.

Doyal, L. 2001. Moral problems in the use of coercion in dealing with nonadherence in the diagnosis and treatment of tuberculosis. *Annals of the New York Academies of Sciences* 953 (December): 208–215.

Drake, John M., Suok Kai Chew, and Stefan Ma. 2006. Societal learning in epidemics: Intervention effectiveness during the 2003 SARS outbreak in Singapore. *PLoS One* 1 (December 20): e20.

Drane, James. 1985. The many faces of competency. *Hastings Center Report* 15, no. 4: 17–21.

Drexler, M. 2002. *Secret agents: The menace of emerging infections.* Washington, DC: Joseph Henry Press.

D'Souza G., A.R. Kreimer, R. Viscidi, M. Pawlita, C. Fakhry, W.M. Koch, W.H. Westra, and M.L. Gillison. 2007. Case-control study of human papillomavirus and oropharyngeal cancer. *New England Journal of Medicine* 356, no. 19 (May 10): 1944–1956.

Dubler, N.N., R. Bayer, S. Landesman, and A. White. 1992. *The tuberculosis revival: Individual rights and societal obligations in a time of AIDS.* New York: United Hospital Fund of New York.

Dubler, Nancy, Jeffrey Blustein, Rohit Bhalla, and David Bernard. 2007. Informed participation: An alternative ethical process for including patients in quality improvement projects. In *Health care quality improvement: Ethical and regulatory issues*, ed. Bruce Jennings, Mary Ann Baily, Melissa Bottrell, and Joanne Lynn, 69–87. Garrison, NY: Hastings Center.

Dubos, R., and J. Dubos. 1952. *The White Plague: Tuberculosis, Man and Society*. Boston: Little, Brown.

Dugger, Celia W. 2005. U.N. proposes doubling of aid to cut poverty. *New York Times*, sec. A, January 18, 1.

Dunne, E.F., E.R. Unger, M. Sternberg, G. McQuillan, D.C. Swan, S.S. Patel, and L. E. Markowitz. 2007. Prevalence of HPV infection among females in the United States. *Journal of the American Medical Association* 297, no. 8 (February 28): 813–819.

Dye, C., et al, and the WHO Global Surveillance and Monitoring Project. 1999. Global burden of tuberculosis: Estimated incidence, prevalence, and mortality by country. *Journal of the American Medical Association* 282, no. 7 (August 18): 677–686.

Dyer, Claire. 1999. BMA's patient confidentiality rules are deemed unlawful. *British Medical Journal* 319: 1221. Available at -dyn/articles/A34467-2004Mar29.html (accessed December 29, 2007).

Edmunds, Vincent, and C. Gordon Scorer, eds. 1967. *Ethical responsibility in medicine: A Christian approach*. London: E. & S. Livingstone.

H.J. Ehrlich, et al. 2008. A clinical trial of a whole-virus H5N1 vaccine derived from cell culture. *New England Journal of Medicine* 358, no. 24 (June 12): 2573–84.

Elbasha, E.H., E.J. Dasbach, and R.P. Insinga. 2007. Model for assessing human papillomavirus vaccination strategies. *Emerging Infectious Diseases* 13, no. 1 (January): 28–41.

Ellickson, Robert C. 1991. *Order without law: How neighbors settle disputes*. Cambridge: Harvard University Press.

Enarson, D.A. 1994. Why not the elimination of tuberculosis? *Mayo Clinic Proceedings* 69: 85–86.

Engemann, J.J., Y. Carmeli, S.E. Cosgrove, V.G. Fowler, M.Z. Bronstein, S.L. Trivette, J.P. Briggs, D.J. Sexton, and K.S. Kaye. 2003. Adverse clinical and economic outcomes attributable to methicillin resistance among patients with Staphylococcus aureus surgical site infection. *Clinical Infectious Diseases* 36, no. 5 (March 1): 592–598.

Epstein, Richard A. 2004. In defense of the "old" public health: The legal framework for the regulation of public health. *Brooklyn Law Review* 69: 1421–1470.

European Center for Disease Prevention and Control. 2007. Report for policymakers: Pandemic preparedness in the European Union. Autumn. Available at http://ecdc.europa.eu/pdf/2007_12_05_Pandemic%20preparedness%20for %20policymakers.pdf (accessed February 4, 2008).

European Center for Disease Prevention and Control. 2007. *Technical report: Pandemic influenza preparedness in the EU/EEA*. December. Available at http:// ecdc.europa.eu/Health_topics/Pandemic_Influenza/pdf/Pandemic%20prep are%20web%201.pdf (accessed February 4, 2008).

European Center for Disease Prevention and Control. 2008. Emergence of seasonal influenza viruses type A/H1N1 with oseltamivir resistance in some European Countries at the start of the 2007–8 influenza season. January 27. Available at http://ecdc.europa.eu/pdf/080127_os.pdf (accessed February 3, 2008)

Evans, A. S., & Brachman, P. S. 1998. *Bacterial infections of humans: epidemiology and control* (3rd ed.). New York: Plenum Medical Book Co.

Evans, G. 1999. Vaccine injury compensation programs worldwide. *Vaccine* 17, supplement 3 (October 29): S25–S35.

Ewing, Charles Patrick. 2005. Tarasoff reconsidered. *APA Monitor on Psychology* 36, no. 7: 112. Available at http://www.apa.org/monitor/julaug05/jn.html.

Faden, Ruth R., Patrick S. Duggan, and Ruth Karron. 2007. Who pays to stop a pandemic. *New York Times*, sec. A, February 9, 19.

Farmer, Paul. 2001. *Infections and inequalities: The modern plagues.* Berkeley: University of California Press.

Farmer, P. 2001. The major infectious diseases in the world—To treat or not to treat? *New England Journal of Medicine* 345, no. 3 (July 19): 208–210.

Farmer, Paul. 2003. *Pathologies of power: Health, human rights, and the new war on the poor.* Berkeley: University of California Press.

Farmer, P., and N.G. Campos. 2004. Rethinking medical ethics: A view from below. *Developing World Bioethics* 4, no. 1 (May): 17–41.

Farmer, Paul, and Laurie Garrett. 2007. From "marvelous momentum" to health care for all. *Foreign Affairs* 86, no. 2, available at http://www.foreignaffairs.org/20070301faresponse86213/paul-farmer-laurie-garrett/from-marvelous-momentum-to-health-care-for-all-success-is-possible-with-the-right-programs.html (accessed February 16, 2008).

Farmer P.E., J.Y. Kim, C. Mitnick, and R.Timperi. 2000. Responding to outbreaks of MDRTB: Introducing "DOTS–Plus." In *Tuberculosis: A comprehensive international approach*, ed. L.B. Reichman and E.S. Hershfield, 447–469. 2nd ed. New York: Marcel Dekker.

Fed News. 2005. *World summit examines progress in meeting development financing commitments made five years ago in Monterrey.* September 14.

Fenner, F. et al., eds. 1988. Early efforts at control: Variolation, vaccination, and isolation and quarantine. In *Smallpox and its eradication*, 245–276. Geneva: World Health Organization.

Fidler, David P. 1999. *International law and infectious diseases.* Oxford: Oxford University Press.

Finucane, Thomas. 2001. Thinking about life-sustaining treatment late in the life of a demented patient. *Georgia Law Review* 35: 691–705.

Firth, Roderick. 1952. Ethical absolutism and the ideal observer. *Philosophy & Phenomenological Research* 12: 317–345.

Flanagin, and Margaret A. Winker. 2007. Global Theme Issue on Poverty and Human Development. *Journal of the American Medical Association* 298, no. 16 (October 24): 1942.

Fletcher, Faith, and Paul Ndebele. 2006. The infant-feeding dilemma of an HIV-infected mother in Southern Africa. Paper presented at the annual meeting of the American Society for Bioethics and Humanities.

Fletcher, F., P. Ndebele, and M. Kelley. "To Nourish Her Young: Ethical Dilemmas Associated With HIV-infected Mothers and Infant–Feeding," manuscript in progress.

Fletcher, Helen. 2007. TB research in developing countries. Lecture, Uehiro Center, Oxford University, Oxford, England, July 4.

Fletcher, Joseph F. 1954; 1979. Morals and medicine: The moral problems of the patient's right to know the truth, contraception, artificial insemination, sterilization, euthanasia. Princeton, N.J.: Princeton University Press.

Florida Department of Health. 2006. *Pandemic influenza annex* (October). Available at http://www.doh.state.fl.us/rw_Bulletins/flpanfluv104final.pdf (accessed July 7, 2008).

Flume, Patrick A. et al. 2007. Cystic fibrosis pulmonary guidelines. *American Journal of Respiratory and Critical Care Medicine* 176 (November 15): 957–969.

Forget, E.J., and D. Menzies. 2006. Adverse reactions to first-line antituberculosis drugs. *Expert Opinion on Drug Safety* 5, no. 2 (March): 231–249.

Foster, Kevin R., and Hajo Grundmann. 2006. Do we need to put society first? The potential for tragedy in antimicrobial resistance. *PLoS Medicine* 3, no. 2 (January 10): e29.

Francis, Leslie. 2003. Global systemic problems and interconnected duties. *Environmental Ethics* 25: 115–128.

Francis, Leslie. 2008. Privacy and confidentiality; the importance of context. *Monist* 91, no. 1 (January): 53–68.

Fraser, C., S. Riley, R.M. Anderson, and N.M. Ferguson. 2004. Factors that make an infectious disease outbreak controllable. *Proceedings of the National Academy of Sciences* 101:6146–6151.

Fraser, M.R., and D.L. Brown. 2000. Bioterrorism preparedness and local public health agencies: Building response capacity. *Public Health Reports* 115: 326–330.

Freeman, Gregory A. 2007. Bugchasers: The men who long to be HIV+. *Rolling Stone* (February 6), Available at http://www.solargeneral.com/library/Bug Chasers.pdf (accessed December 29, 2007).

Frieden, T.R., T. Sterling, A. Pablos–Mendez, J.O. Kilburn, G.M. Cauthen, and S.W. Dooley. The emergence of drug-resistant tuberculosis in New York City. *New England Journal of Medicine* 328, no. 8 (February 25): 521–526.

Frieden, Thomas R., et al. 2005. Applying public health principles to the HIV epidemic. *New England Journal of Medicine* 353, no. 22 (December 1): 2397–2402.

Friedrich, M.J. 2007. Jeffrey Sachs, PhD. *Journal of the American Medical Association* 298, no. 16 (October 24): 1850.

Fritsch, P., M. Pottinger, and L. Chang. 2003. Divergent Asian responses show difficulties in dealing with SARS. *Wall Street Journal*, sec. A, April 7, 1.

Frosch, Dan. 2007. Texas house rejects order by governor on vaccines. *New York Times*, sec. A, March 14, 14.

Fugh-Berman, Adriane. 2007. Cervical cancer vaccines and industry influence. *Bioethics Forum*, March 15, available at http://www.bioethicsforum.org/Merck-Gardasil-pharmaceutical-marketing.asp (accessed January 5, 2008).

Fumento, M.A. 2007. A Merck-y business. The case against mandatory HPV vaccinations. *Weekly Standard* 12, no. 25 (March 12).

Furin, J. 2007. The clinical management of drug-resistant tuberculosis. *Current Opinion in Pulmonary Medicine* 13, no. 3 (May): 212–217.

Future II Study Group. 2007. Quadrivalent HPV vaccine against human papillomavirus to prevent high-grade cervical lesions. *New England Journal of Medicine* 356, no. 19 (May 10): 1915–1927.

Fylkesnes, K., A. Haworth, C. Rosensvard, and P.M. Kwapa. 1999. HIV counseling and testing: Overemphasizing high acceptance rates a threat to confidentiality and the right not to know. *AIDS* 13: 2469–2474.

Gandhi, N.R., A. Moll, A.W. Sturm, R. Pawinski, T. Govender, U. Lalloo, K. Zeller, J. Andrews, and G. Friedland. 2006. Extensively drug-resistant tuberculosis as a cause of death in patients co-infected with tuberculosis and HIV in a rural area of South Africa. *Lancet* 368, no. 9547 (November 4): 1575–1580.

Gangarosa, E.J., A.M. Galazka, C.R. Wolfe, L.M. Phillips, R.E. Gangarosa, E. Miller, and R.T. Chen. 1998. Impact of anti-vaccine movements on pertussis control: The untold story. *Lancet* 351, no. 9099 (January 31): 356–361.

Gao, Zhan, Chi-hong Tseng, Zhiheng Pei, and Martin J. Blaser. 2007. Molecular analysis of human forearm superficial skin bacterial biota. *Proceedings of the National Academy of Sciences* 104 (February): 2927–2932.

Gardiner, Stephen. 2001. The real tragedy of the commons. *Philosophy & Public Affairs* 30: 387–416.

Gardiner, Stephen. 2006. A core precautionary principle. *Journal of Political Philosophy* 14, no. 1: 33–60.

Garnett, G.P. 2005. Role of herd immunity in determining the effect of vaccines against sexually transmitted disease. *Journal of Infectious Diseases* 191, supplement 1: S97–S106.

Garrett, Laurie. 1994. *The coming plague: Newly emerging diseases in a world out of balance.* New York: Penguin Books.

Garrett, Laurie. 2001. *Betray of trust: The collapse of global public health.* New York: Hyperion.

Garrett, Laurie. 2005. The next pandemic? Probable cause. *Foreign Affairs* 84, no. 4 (July/August): 22.

Garrett, Laurie. 2007. The challenge of global health. *Foreign Affairs* 86, no. 1 (January/February).

Gasner, M.R., K.L. Maw, G.E. Feldman et al. 1999. The use of legal action in New York City to ensure treatment of tuberculosis. *New England Journal of Medicine* 340, no. 5 (February 4): 359–366.

Gellin, B.G., E.W. Maibach, and E.K. Marcuse. 2000. Do parents understand immunizations? A national telephone survey. *Pediatrics* 106: 1097–1102.

Gilbert, M. Thomas P., Andrew Rambaut, Gabriela Wlasiuk, Thomas J. Spira, Arthur E. Pitchenik, and Michael Worobey. 2007. The emergence of HIV/AIDS in the Americas and beyond. *Proceedings of the National Academy of Sciences* 104, no. 47 (November 20): 18566–18570.

Gilchrist, Mary J., Christiana Greko, David B. Wallinga, George W. Beran, David G. Riley, and Peter S. Thorne. 2007. The potential role of concentrated animal feeding operations in infectious disease epidemics and antibiotic resistance. *Environmental Health Perspectives* 115, no. 2 (February): 313–316.

Global Health Council. *Member organization* Available at http://global health.org /view_top.php3?id=232 (accessed February 16, 2008).

Global Security.org. *Pandemic flu mitigation—Social distancing.* Available at http:// www.globalsecurity.org/security/ops/hsc-scen-3_flu-pandemic-distancing. htm (accessed January 28, 2008).

Goldby, Stephen. 1971. Letter: Experiments at the Willowbrook state school. *Lancet* (April 10): 749.

Goldie, Sue J., Michele Kohli, Daniel Grima et al. 2004. "Projected Clinical Benefits and Cost-effectiveness of the Human Papillomavirus 16/18 Vaccine," *Journal of the National Cancer Institute* 96, no. 3: 604–615.

Gorovitz, Samuel. 1982. *Doctors' dilemmas: Moral conflict and medical care.* New York: Oxford University Press.

Gorovitz, Samuel, Ruth Macklin, Andrew L. Jameton, John M. O'Connor, and Susan Sherwin, eds. 1976; 1983. *Moral problems in medicine.* 1st ed., 2nd ed. Englewood Cliffs, N.J.: Prentice–Hall.

Gostin, Lawrence O. 1993. Controlling the resurgent tuberculosis epidemic: A 50-state survey of statutes and proposals for reform. *Journal of the American Medical Association* 269, no. 2 (January 13): 255–261.

Gostin, Lawrence O. 2000. *Public health law: power, duty, restraint.* Berkeley: University of California Press.

Gostin, Lawrence O. 2003. The model state emergency health powers act: Public health and civil liberties in a time of terrorism. *Health Matrix* 13: 3–32.

Gostin, Lawrence O. 2006. Public health strategies for pandemic influenza. *Journal of the American Medical Association* 295, no. 14 (April 12): 1700–1704.

Gostin, Lawrence O. 2007. Why Rich Countries Should Care About the World's Least Healthy People. *Journal of the American Medical Association* 298, no. 1: 89–92.

Gostin, Lawrence O., and Catherine D. DeAngelis. 2007. Mandatory HPV vaccination: Public health vs. private wealth. *Journal of the American Medical Association* 297, no. 17 (May 2): 1921–1923.

Gostin, Lawrence O., and Zita Lazzarini. 1997. *Human rights and public health in the AIDS pandemic.* New York: Oxford University Press.

Gostin, Lawrence O., Ronald Bayer, and Amy L. Fairchild. 2003. Ethical and legal challenges posed by SARS: Implications for the control of serious infectious disease threats. *Journal of the American Medical Association* 290, no. 24 (December 24/31): 3229–3237.

Grady, Denise. 2007. A vital discussion, clouded. *New York Times*, sec. F, March 6, 5.

Green, Michael J., and Jeffery R. Botkin. 2003. "Genetic exceptionalism" in medicine: Clarifying the differences between genetic and nongenetic tests. *Annals of Internal Medicine* 138, no. 7 (April 1): 571–575.

Groginsky, E., N. Bowdler, and J. Yankowitz. 1998. Update on vertical HIV transmission. *Journal of Reproductive Medicine* 43, no. 8 (August): 637–646.

Gruen, Russell L., Steven D. Pearson, and Troyen A. Brennan. 2004. Physician-citizens—Public roles and professional obligations. *Journal of the American Medical Association* 291, no. 1 (January 7): 94–98.

Gruskin, Sofia, and Daniel Tarantola. 2002. Health and human rights. In *Oxford Textbook of Public Health*, ed. Roger Detels, James McEwen, Robert Beaglehole, and Heizo Tanada. Vol. 1. 4th ed. Oxford: Oxford University Press.

GTC Bio Conference. 2007. 5th annual vaccines: All things considered. Washington, DC, November 7–9.

Guam Department of Public Health and Social Services. 2006. *Guam pandemic influenza plan: draft*. January 25, available at http://www.guamhs.org/pdf/2006/Guam_Pandemic_Influenza_Plan_1-25-2006_DRAFT_.pdf?PHPSESSID=6241a277611dee8a84a88f721f7b2f7d (accessed July 5, 2008).

Gupta, S., D. Berg; F. de Lott, P. Kellner, and C. Driver. 2004. Directly observed therapy for tuberculosis in New York City: Factors associated with refusal. *International Journal of Tuberculosis and Lung Disease* 8, no. 4: 480–485.

Gussow, Zachary. 1989. *Leprosy, Racism, and the Public Health*. Boulder, Colo.: Westview Press.

Haas, D.W., and R.M. Des Pres. 1995. Mycobacterium Tuberculosis. In *Principles and practice of infectious diseases*, ed. G.L. Mandell, J.E. Bennett, and R. Dolin. 4th ed. New York: Churchill Livingstone.

Hall, Mark A. and Stephen S. Rich. 2000. Genetic privacy laws and patients' fear of discrimination by health insurers: The view from genetic counselors. *Journal of Law, Medicine & Ethics* 28: 245–255.

Halloran, M.E., et al. 2008. Modeling targeted layered containment of an influenza pandemic in the United States, *Proceedings of the National Academy of Science* 105(12): 4639–4644 (March 25).

Halpern, SD, PA Ubel, DA Asch, 2007. Harnessing the Power of Default Options to Improve Health Care. *New England Journal of Medicine* 357(13) (September 27):1340-1344.

Hamilton, Carey. 2007. Cervical cancer battle gets a $1 million jolt. *Salt Lake Tribune*, local, April 5.

Hanlon, John J. 1974. *Public health administration and practice*. 6th ed. St. Louis: C.V. Mosby.

Hanna, Donald, and Yiping Huang. 2004. The impact of SARS on Asian economies. *Asian Economic Papers* 3, no. 1: 102–112.

Hansell, D.A. 1993. The TB and HIV epidemics: History learned and unlearned. *Journal of Law, Medicine & Ethics* 21, nos. 3–4 (Fall–Winter): 376–381.

Hanson, Norwood Russell. 1958. *Patterns of discovery: An inquiry into the conceptual foundations of science*. Cambridge: Cambridge University Press.

Hardin, Garrett. 1968. The tragedy of the commons. *Science* 162: 1243–1244.

Hardwig, John. 1996. Is there a duty to die? *Hastings Center Report* 27, no. 2: 34–42.

Harper, K.N., P.S. Ocampo, B.M. Steiner, R.W. George, M.S. Silverman et al. 2008. On the Origin of the Treponematoses: A Phylogenetic Approach. *PLoS Neglected Tropical Diseases* 2(1): e148.

Harris, Gardiner. 2004. U.S. Creates Ethics Panel for Priority on Flu Shots. *New York Times*, sec. A, October 28.

Harris, John, and Soren Holm. 1995. Is there a moral obligation not to infect others? *British Medical Journal* 311, no. 7014 (November 4): 1215–1217.

Harris, John, and Kirsty Keywood. 2001. Ignorance, information, and autonomy. *Theoretical Medicine* 22: 415–436.

Harris, Paul. 2002. The plague upon our village. *Observer*, news, January 20, 13.

Harsanyi, John. 1953. Cardinal utility in welfare economics and in the theory of risk taking. *Journal of Political Economy* 61: 434–435.

Harsanyi, John. 1955. Cardinal welfare, individualistic ethics, and interpersonal comparisons of utility. *Journal of Political Economy* 63: 309–321.

Hart, H.L.A., and Tony Honore. 1962. *Causation in the law*. Oxford: Clarendon.

Hatchett, R.J., C.E. Mecher, and M. Lipsitch. 2007. Public health interventions and epidemic intensity during the 1918 influenza pandemic. *Proceedings of the National Academy of Sciences of the United States* 104, no. 18 (May 1): 7582–7587.

Hawaii State Department of Health. 2008. *Hawaii pandemic influenza preparedness & response plan*. Version 08.1. January. Available at http://hawaii.gov/health/family-child-health/contagious-disease/pandemic-flu/fluplan.pdf (accessed July 5, 2008).

Healy, Edwin F. 1956. *Medical ethics*. Chicago: Loyola University Press.

Heise, L. 2006. HIV disclosure holds no added risk. Presented at Microbicides Conference, Cape Town, Africa, April. *AIDS Reader* (June): 289–290.

Hellman, Deborah. 2003. What makes genetic discrimination exceptional? *American Journal of Law & Medicine* 29: 77–116.

Hendley, J. Owen. 2006. Hotel rooms have unseen guests. Study presented at the Interscience Conference on Antimicrobial Agents and Chemotherapy, San Francisco, CA, (September).

Hersh, Adam S. 1994. Go home, stranger: An analysis of unequal workers' compensation death benefits to nonresident alien beneficiaries. *Florida State University Law Review* 22, no. 1 (Summer): 217–241.

Highberg, Nels P. 2007. Lecture at American Society for Bioethics and Humanities (October).

Hildesheim, A., R. Herrero, S. Wacholder, et al. 2007. Effect of Human Papillomavirus 16/18 L1 Viruslike Particle Vaccination Among Young Women With Preexisting Infection. *Journal of the American Medical Association* 298, no. 7 (August 15): 743–753.

Hinman, Alan R., Jeffrey P. Koplan, Walter A. Orenstein, and Edward W. Brink. 1988. Decision analysis and polio immunization policy. *American Journal of Public Health* 78, no. 3: 301–303.

Hochschild, Adam. 2008. "Death March," review of Johnny Steinberg, *Siswe's Test: A Young Man's Journey Through Africa's AIDS Epidemic* (New York: Simon and Schuster, 2008), *New York Times Book Review* (February 10):28–29.

Hodge, James G., and Lawrence O. Gostin. 2001–2002. School vaccination requirements: Historical, social, and legal perspectives. *Kentucky Law Journal* 90:
831–890.

Hollier, LM, J. Hill, J.S. Sheffield, and G.D. Wendel. 2003. State laws regarding prenatal syphilis screening in the United States. *American Journal of Obstetrics
and Gynecology* 184: 1178–1183.

Holm, Søren. 2007. Justifiable detention and the question of compensation. Lecture, Uehiro Center, Oxford University, Oxford, England, July 4.

Homeland Security Council. 2005. *National strategy for pandemic influenza.* Available at http://www.whitehouse.gov/homeland/pandemic-influenza.html# sec-
tion6 (accessed February 1, 2008).

Homeland Security Council. 2007. *National strategy for pandemic influenza implementation plan one year summary.* July, available at http://www.whitehouse.
gov/homeland/pandemic-influenza-oneyear.html (accessed January 26, 2008).

Hopewell, P.C., M. Pai, D. Maher, M. Uplekar, and M.C. Raviglione. 2006. International standards for tuberculosis care. *Lancet Infectious Diseases* 6, no. 11
(November): 710–725.

Horn, Peter. 2003. *Clinical ethics casebook.* Belmont, CA: Wadsworth.

Horsburgh, C.R. 2004. Priorities for the treatment of latent tuberculosis infection
in the United States. *New England Journal of Medicine* 350, no. 20 (May 13):
2060–2067.

Horton, R. 2004. Vioxx, the implosion of Merck, and aftershocks at the FDA. *Lancet* 364, no. 9450 (December 4–10): 1995–1996.

HPV Today. 2007. Approaches to the use of HPV vaccines: Interview with Ian Fraser. *HPV Today* 10 (February), available at www.hpvtoday.com (accessed
January 6, 2008).

HPV Today. 2007. Evaluation of the quadrivalent HPV vaccine by the regulatory
agencies in 2006. *HPV Today* 10 (February), available at www.hpvtoday.com
(accessed January 6, 2008).

Humphreys, Margaret. 1992. *Yellow fever and the South.* New Brunswick, NJ:
Rutgers University Press. In Peter Patton, "Quarantine: Historical Lessons
Learned," Center for Policing Terrorism, Chemical, Biological, radiological,
and Nuclear Working Group (CPT/CBRN), 2004.

Hunt, Robert, and John Arras. 1977. *Ethical issues in modern medicine.* Palo Alto,
CA: Mayfield.

Huppatz, Clare, and David N. Durrheim. 2007. Letter to the editor: Control of neglected tropical diseases. *New England Journal of Medicine* 357, no. 23 (December 6): 2407.

Idaho Department of Health and Welfare. 2006. *Idaho pandemic influenza response.*
March. Available at http://www.healthandwelfare.idaho.gov/DesktopModules/
Docu ments/DocumentsView.aspx?tabID=0&ItemID=4523&MId=11634&wv
ersion=Staging (accessed July 5, 2008).

Indiana State Department of Health. 2006. *Pandemic influenza plan.* October.
Available at http://www.in.gov/isdh/files/PandemicInfluenzaPlan.pdf (accessed
July 5, 2008).

Infectious Diseases Society of America. 1993. Guidelines for ethical conduct by members and fellows. *Journal of Infectious Diseases* 16, no. 1: 257–258.

Infectious Diseases Society of America. Statement on the human papillomavirus (HPV) vaccine. Available at http://www.idsociety.org/Content.aspx?id=6532 (accessed January 5, 2008).

Institute of Medicine. 1988. *The future of public health.* Washington, DC: National Academy Press.

Institute of Medicine. 2000. *Ending neglect: The elimination of tuberculosis in the United States.* Ed. Lawrence Geiter. Washington DC: National Academy Press.

Institute of Medicine. 2000. *To err is human: Building a safer health system.* Ed. Linda T. Kohn, Janet M. Corrigan, and Molla S. Donaldson. Washington, DC: National Academy Press.

Institute of Medicine. 2003. Board on health promotion and disease prevention: letter report #3, May 27.

Ippolito, G., V. Puro, J. Heptonstal, et al. 1999. Occupational human immunodeficiency virus infection in health care workers: Worldwide cases through September 1997. *Clinical Infectious Diseases* 28, no. 2 (February): 365–383.

Iseman, M.D., D.L. Cohn, and J.A. Sbarbaro. 1993. Directly observed treatment for tuberculosis—We can't afford not to try it. *New England Journal of Medicine* 328, no. 8 (February 25): 576–578.

Issenberg, Sasha. 2007. House fails to override veto of SCHIP—Democrats vow to continue pushing a bill. *Boston Globe,* sec. A, October 19, 2.

Jacobs, M.R. 1999. Emergence of antibiotic resistance in upper and lower respiratory tract infections. *American Journal of Managed Care* 5: S651–S661.

Jaffe, Harold. 2007. Opt-out HIV testing. Lecture, Uehiro Center, Oxford University, Oxford, England, July 4.

JCAHO. 2006. *Surge hospitals: Providing safe care during emergencies.* Available at http://www.jointcommission.org/NR/rdonlyres/802E9DA4-AE80-4584-A205-48989C5BD684/0/surge_hospital.pdf (accessed February 9, 2008).

Jefferson, T., R. Foxlee, C. Del Mar, L. Dooley, E. Ferroni, B. Hewak, A. Prabhala, S Nair, and A. Rivetti. 2007. Interventions for the interruption or reduction of the spread of respiratory viruses. *Cochrane Database of Systemic Reviews* 4 (October 17): CD006207.

Jennings, Bruce. 2003. The liberalism of life: Bioethics in the face of biopower. *Raritan Review* 23, no. 4 (Spring): 132–146.

John, T.J., and R. Samuel. 2000. Herd immunity and herd effect: new insights and definitions. *European Journal of Epidemiology* 16, no. 7: 601–606.

Johns Hopkins Berman Institute of Bioethics. About the institute. Available at http://www.bioethicsinstitute.org/web/page/387/sectionid/387/pagelevel/1/interior.asp (accessed December 29, 2007).

Joint United Nations Programme on HIV/AIDS. 2005. *Call to action: Towards an HIV-free and AIDS-free generation.* Prevention of mother to child transmission (PMTCT) High Level Global Partners Forum, Abuja, Nigeria, available at http://www.unfpa.org/upload/lib_pub_file/523_filename_abuja_call-to-action.pdf (accessed January 3, 2008).

Joint United Nations Programme on HIV/AIDS. 2006. 2006 *report on the global AIDS epidemic.* Available at http://www.unaids.org/en/KnowledgeCentre/HIV Data / GlobalReport/default.asp (accessed January 1, 2008).

Joint United Nations Programme on HIV/AIDS. 2007. *AIDS epidemic update: December* 2007. Available at http://data.unaids.org/pub/EPISlides/2007/2007_ epiup date_ en.pdf (accessed January 1, 2008).

Jones, James. 1993. *Bad blood.* New York: Free Press.

Jonsen, Albert R. 1998. *The birth of bioethics.* Oxford: Oxford University Press.

Jonsen, Albert R. 2000. *A short history of medical ethics.* Oxford: Oxford University Press.

Jonsen, Albert R., Mark Siegler, and William J. Winslade. 1982. *Clinical ethics: A practical approach to ethical decisions in clinical medicine.* New York: Macmillan.

Jourdain, Gonzague, Nicole Ngo-Giang-Huong, Sophie Le Coeur, Chureeratana Bowonwatanuwong, Pacharee Kantipong, Pranee Leechanachai, Surabhon Ariyadej, Prattana Leenasirimakul, Scott Hammer, and Marc Lallemant. 2004. Intrapartum exposure to Nevirapine and subsequent maternal responses to Nevirapine-based antiretroviral therapy. *New England Journal of Medicine* 351, no. 3 (July 15): 229–240.

Kahn, C. 2007. Man with drug-resistant TB locked up. *USA Today,* April 2, 2007. In P. Sampathkumar. Dealing with threat of drug—resistant tuberculosis: Background information for interpreting the Andrew Speaker and related cases. *Mayo Clinic Proceedings* 82, no. 7 (July 2007): 799–802.

Kahn, Michael. 2008. Plague a growing but overlooked threat: Study. *Reuters.* January 15, available at http://www.reuters.com/article/scienceNews/idUSL1446 12932008015?pageNumber=2&virtualBrandChannel=0&sp=true (accessed February 16, 2008).

Kaiser Family Foundation. 2007. *The uninsured: A primer.* October, available at http://www.kff.org/uninsured/upload/7451-03.pdf (accessed January 26, 2008).

Kammen, Savigny, and Nelsom Sewankambo. 2006. Using knowledge brokering to promote evidence-based policy-making: The need for support structures. *Bulletin of the World Health Organization* 84, no. 8: 608–612.

Karon, J.M., P.L. Fleming, R.W. Steketee, and K.M. De Cock. 2001. HIV in the United States at the turn of the century: An epidemic in transition. *American Journal of Public Health* 92, no. 7: 1060–1068.

Kass, Nancy E. 2001. An ethics framework for public health. *American Journal of Public Health* 91, no. 11: 1776–1782.

Kass, Nancy. 2004. Public health ethics: From foundations and frameworks to justice and global public health. *The Journal of Law, Medicine & Ethics* 32, no. 2: 232–242.

Katz-Wise, Sabra L. 2006. Rapid strep test for strep throat. WebMD Medical Reference from Healthwise. August 29, available at http://www.webmd.com/a-to-z-guides/rapid-strep-test-for-strep-throat (accessed January 8, 2008).

Kawai, N., et al. 2006. A Comparison of the Effectiveness of Oseltamivir for the Treatment of Influenza A and Influenza B: A Japanese Multicenter Study of the 2003–2004 and 2004–2005 Influenza Seasons. *Clinical Infectious Diseases* 43, no. 4 (August 15): 439–444.

Kelly, Paul. 2007. Public health and ethical challenges in tuberculosis treatment and control. Lecture, Uehiro Center, Oxford University, Oxford, England, July 4.

Kennedy, D. 2006. News on women's health—Editorial. *Science* 313: 273.

Kentucky Cabinet for Health and Family Services. 2007. *Kentucky pandemic influenza preparedness plan.* April, available at http://chfs.ky.gov/NR/rdonlyres/6CD366D2-6726-4AD0-85BB-E83CF769560E/0/KyPandemicInfluenzaPrepared ness Plan.pdf (accessed July 5, 2008).

Kidder, Tracy. 2003. *Mountains beyond mountains: The quest of Dr. Paul Farmer, a man who would cure the world.* New York: Random House.

Kim, Jim Yong. and Arthur Ammann. 2004. Is the "3 by 5" initiative the best approach to tackling the HIV pandemic? *PLoS Medicine* 1, no. 2 (November 30): e37.

Kimball, Ann Marie. 2006. *Risky trade: Infectious disease in the era of global trade.* Aldershot, UK: Ashgate.

King, Nancy J., Sukanya Pillay, and Gail A. Lasprogata. 2006. Workplace privacy and discrimination issues related to genetic data: A comparative law study of the European Union and the United States. *American Business Law Journal* 43: 79–171.

Kipnis, Kenneth. 2006. Medical confidentiality. In *Blackwell Guide to Medical Ethics*, ed. Rosamond Rhodes, Leslie Francis, and Anita Silvers, 104–127. Oxford: Basil Blackwell.

Kittay, Eva Feder. 1998. *Love's Labor. Essays on Women, Equality, and Dependency.* New York: Routledge.

Klevens, R. Monina, et al. 2007. Invasive methicillin-resistant *staphylococcus aureus* infections in the United States. *Journal of the American Medical Association* 298, no. 15 (October 17): 1763–1771.

Koenig, Linda J., Daniel J. Whitaker, Rachel A. Royce, Tracey E. Wilson, Kathleen Ethier, and M. Isabel Fernandez. 2006. Physical and sexual violence during pregnancy and after delivery: A prospective multistate study of women with or at risk of HIV infection. *American Journal of Public Health* 96, no. 6 (June): 1052–1059.

Kotalik, Jaro. 2005. Preparing for an influenza pandemic: Ethical Issues. *Bioethics* 19, no. 4 (August): 422–431.

Kraut, Alan M. 1988. Germs, genes, and American efficiency, 1890–1924. *Social Science History*, 12, no. 4 (Winter): 377–394.

Krugman, Saul. 1986. The Willowbrook hepatitis studies revisited: Ethical aspects. *Reviews of Infectious Diseases* 8, no. 1: 157–162.

Krugman, Saul, Joan P. Giles, and Jack Hammond. 1967. Infectious hepatitis: Evidence for two distinctive clinical, epidemiological, and immunological types of infection. *Journal of the American Medical Association* 200, no. 5 (May 1): 365–373. Republished in 1984 as "Landmark Article," *Journal of the American Medical Association* 252, no. 3 (July 20): 393–401.

Kruskal, Benjamin and Carole Allen. 2008. Perpetrating the autism myth. *Boston Globe*, January 31, available at http://www.boston.com/news/health/articles/2008/01/31/perpetrating_the_autism_myth/. (accessed January 8, 2008).

Kuehn, B.M. Benefits of newer vaccines lauded. *Journal of the American Medical Association* 298, no. 18 (November 14): 2123–2125.

Kuhn, Thomas. 1970. *The structure of scientific revolutions.* Chicago: University of Chicago Press.

Kukathas, Chandran. 2003. *The Liberal Archipelago: A Theory of Diversity and Freedom.* New York: Oxford University Press.

Kunduru, Vindhya, and Shalini Prasad. 2007. Electrokinetic Formation of 'Microbridges' for Detection of Proteins. *Journal of the Association for Laboratory Automation* 12, no. 5 (October): 311–317.

Lab Tests Online. 2005. New DNA test approved for cystic fibrosis carrier screening and diagnosis. June 24, available at http://www.labtestsonline.org/news /cfo50624.html (accessed December 31, 2007).

Lacey, Marc. 2007. Mexican immigrants carry HIV home to unready rural areas. *New York Times,* sec. A, July 17, 1.

Lamunu, M., J.J. Lutwama, J. Kamugisha, A. Opio, J. Nambooze, N. Ndayimirije, and S. Okware. 2004. Containing a haemorrhagic fever epidemic: the Ebola experience in Uganda (October 2000–January 2001). *International Journal of Infectious Diseases* 8, no. 1 (January): 27–37.

Lancet. 1904. The spread of small-pox by tramps. *Lancet* 1: 446–447. In Albert, Ostheimer, and Breman, 2001, 375–379.

Lancet. 2000. Measles, MMR, and autism: The confusion continues. *Lancet* 355, no. 9213 (April 22): 1379.

Lancet. 2006. Rolling out HPV vaccines worldwide. *Lancet* 367, no. 9528 (June 24): 2034.

Lane, J.M., F.L. Ruben, J.M. Neff, and J.D. Millar. 1969. Complications of smallpox vaccination: 1968 national surveillance in the United States. *New England Journal of Medicine* 281: 1201–1208.

Lappe, M. 1995. *Breakout: The evolving threat of drug-resistant disease.* San Francisco: Sierra Club Books.

Last, John. 1992. Ethics and public health policy. In *Maxcy-Rosenau-Last public health and preventive medicine,* ed. John M. Last and Robert B. Wallace, 1187–1196. 13th ed. Norwalk, CT: Appleton and Lange.

Lazzarini, Zita. 2001. What lessons can we learn from the exceptionalism debate (finally)? *Journal of Law, Medicine & Ethics* 29: 149–151.

Leavitt, Judith Walzer. 1996. Typhoid Mary: Captive to the public's health. Boston: Beacon Press.

Leavitt, Judity Walzer. Typhoid Mary: Villain or victim? PBS NOVA Special. Available at http://www.pbs.org/wgbh/nova/typhoid/mary.html (accessed October 27, 2007).

Lee, Grace M. et al. 2007. Gaps in vaccine financing for underinsured children in the United States. *Journal of the American Medical Association* 298, no. 6 (August 8): 638–643.

LeFever, Linda L. 2006. Religious exemptions from school immunization: A sincere belief or a legal loophole? *Penn State Law Review* 110: 1047–1067.

Leland, J. 2005. U.S. weighs whether to open an era of rapid H.I.V. detection in the home. *New York Times*, sec. A, November 5, 11.

Lepage, Kenneth R. 1995. Lead-based paint litigation and the problem of causation: Toward a unified theory of market share liability. *Boston College Law Review* 37: 155–182.

Lerner, B.H. 1998. *Contagion and confinement: Controlling tuberculosis along the skid road*. Baltimore: John Hopkins University Press.

Levin, Betty Wolder, and Alan R. Fleishman. 2002. Public health and bioethics: The benefits of collaboration. *American Journal of Public Health* 92: 165–167.

Levine, Carol, ed. 1989. *Cases in bioethics: Selections from the Hastings Center Report*. New York: St. Martin's Press.

Levine, Carol, and Robert M. Veatch, eds. 1982. *Cases in bioethics from the Hastings Center Report*. New York: Hastings Center.

Levy, S.B. 2002. *The antibiotic paradox: How the misuse of antibiotics destroys their curative powers*. 2nd ed. Cambridge, MA: Perseus.

Lewis, Charles E., Mary Ann Lewis, and Muriel Ifekwunigue. 1978. Informed consent by children and participation in an influenza vaccine trial. *American Journal of Public Health* 68, no. 11: 1079–1083.

Lipkin, Mack. 1979. On telling patients the truth. *Newsweek*, June 4, 13. Reprinted in Ronald Munson, *Intervention and Reflection: Basic Issues in Medical Ethics*, 152–154. 8th ed. Belmont, CA: Thomson/Wadsworth, 2008.

Lipton, Eric, and Kirk Johnson. 2001. A nation challenged: The anthrax trail. *New York Times*, sec. A, December 26, 1.

Lo, B. 2006. HPV vaccine and adolescents' sexual activity. *British Medical Journal* 332, no. 7550 (May 13): 1106–1107.

Lockman, Shahin, Roger L. Shapiro, Laura M. Smeaton, Carolyn Wester, Ibou Thior, Lisa Stevens, and Fatima Chand. 2007. Response to antiretroviral therapy after a single, peripartum dose of Nevirapine. *New England Journal of Medicine* 356, no. 2 (January 11): 135–147.

Lockwood, Michael, ed. 1985. *Moral dilemmas in modern medicine*. Oxford: Oxford University Press.

Loewenstein, George, Troyen Brennan, and Kevin G. Volpp. 2007. Asymmetric paternalism to improve health behaviors. *Journal of the American Medical Association* 298(20)(November 28):2415-2417.

London, Alex John. 2001. Equipoise and international human-subjects research. *Bioethics* 15, no 4: 312–332.

Lopez, Marissa C. 2007. Society debated HPV vaccine. *Harvard Crimson, Online Edition*, March 7, available at http://www.thecrimson.com/article.aspx? ref= 517523 (accessed January 6, 2008).

MacKenzie, Catriona, and Natalie Stoljar. 2000. *Relational autonomy: Feminist perspectives on autonomy, agency, and the social self*. New York: Oxford University Press.

Maheux, B., N. Haley, M. Rivard, and A. Gervais. 1999. Do physicians assess lifestyle health risks during general medical examinations? A survey of general practitioners and obstetrician–gynecologists in Quebec. *Canadian Medical Association Journal* 160, no. 13 (June 29):1830–1834.

Maine Department of Health and Human Services. 2005. *Pandemic influenza plan,* July. Available at www.maine.gov/dhhs/boh/DRAFT%20Pan%20Flu%20Plan%20071205_revised_rb.pdf (accessed July 5, 2008).

Mandell, Gerald L., John E. Bennett, and Raphael Dolin, eds. 2005. *Principles and Practice of Infectious Diseases.* 2 vols. 6th ed. Philadelphia: Elsevier.

Mandell, G. L., R.G. Douglas, J.E. Bennett, & R. Dolin, 2005. Mandell, Douglas, and Bennett's principles and practice of infectious diseases. *MDConsult* 6th. from http://atoz.ebsco.com/link.asp?id=7227&sid=128189840&rid=400072 &urlSource=AtoZ&lang=en

Manhart, L.E., and L.A. Koutsky. 2002. Do condoms prevent genital HPV infection, external genital warts, or cervical neoplasia? A meta-analysis. *Sexually Transmitted Diseases* 29, no. 11: 725–735.

Mann, Jonathan M. 1997. Medicine and public health, ethics and human rights. *Hastings Center Report* 27: 6–13.

Mann, Thomas. 1929. *The magic mountain.* Trans. H.T. Lowe-Porter. London: M. Secker.

Manno, Catherine S., Amy J. Chew, Sylvia Hutchison, Peter J. Larson, Roland W. Herzog, Valder R. Arruda, Shing Jen Tai, et al. 2003. AAV-mediated factor IX gene transfer to skeletal muscle in patients with severe hemophilia B. *Blood* 101, no. 8 (April 15): 2963–2972.

Mappes, Thomas A., and Jane S. Zembaty. 1981. *Biomedical ethics.* New York: McGraw-Hill.

Marcus, Esther-Lee, A. Mark Clarfield, and Allon E. Moses. 2001. Ethical issues relating to the use of antimicrobial therapy in older adults. *Clinical Infectious Diseases* 33: 1697–1705.

Mariner, Wendy K. 2005. Law and public health: Beyond emergency preparedness. *Journal of Health Law* 38: 247–285.

Mariner, Wendy K. 2007. Mission creep: Public health surveillance and medical privacy. *Boston University Law Review* 87: 347–395.

Markel, Howard. 2004. *When germs travel: Six major epidemics that have invaded America and the fears they have unleashed.* New York: Random House.

Markel, Howard, Lawrence O. Gostin, and David P. Fidler. 2007. Extensively drug-resistant tuberculosis and public health—reply. *Journal of the American Medical Association* 298, no. 16: 1861–1862.

Markel, Howard, Lawrence O. Gostin, and David P. Fidler. 2007. Extensively drug-resistant tuberculosis: An isolation order, public health powers, and a global crisis. *Journal of the American Medical Association* 298, no. 1: 85.

Markel, Howard, Harvey B. Lipman, J. Alexander Navarro, Alexandra Sloan, Joseph R. Michalsen, Alexandra Minna Stern, and Martin S. Cetron. 2007. Non-pharmaceutical Interventions Implemented by US Cities During the 1918–1919 Influenza Pandemic. *Journal of the American Medical Association* 298, no. 6 (August 8): 644–654.

Markovits, Daniel. 2005. Quarantines and distributive justice. *Journal of Law, Medicine, & Ethics* 33: 323–338.

Marrazzo, J.M., K. Stine, and L.A. Koufsky. 2000. Genital human papillomavirus infection in women who have sex with women: A review. *American Journal of Obstetrics and Gynecology* 183, no. 3 (September): 770–774.

Martin, Margaret E. 1977. Statisticians, confidentiality, and privacy. *American Journal of Public Health* 67, no. 2: 165–167.

Maryland Department of Health and Mental Hygiene. 2006. *Draft pandemic influenza plan for Maryland*. Version 6.0, December. Available at http://bioterrorism.dhmh.state.md.us/docs_and_pdfs/DRAFTFluPlanDec2006Part2.pdf (accessed July 5, 2008).

Massachusetts Department of Public Health. 2006. *Community disease control and prevention: Draft*. October 9, available at http://www.mass.gov/dph/cdc/epii/flu/pandemic_plan_public_comments.pdf (accessed February 8, 2008).

Massachusetts Department of Public Health. 2006. *Massachusetts influenza pandemic preparedness plan*. October, available at http://www.mass.gov/dph/cdc/epii/flu/pandemic_plan_2.pdf (accessed July 5, 2008).

Maxcy, Kenneth, ed. 1956. *Rosenau preventive medicine and public health*. 8th ed. New York: Appleton Century Crofts.

May, Thomas. 2005. The concept of autonomy in bioethics: An unwarranted fall from grace. In *Personal Autonomy: New Essays on Personal Autonomy and Its Role in Contemporary Moral Philosophy*, ed. James Stacey Taylor, 299–309. Cambridge: Cambridge University Press.

McCallum and Barbara Ann Hocking. 2006. Reflecting on ethical and legal issues in wildlife disease. In *Ethics and Infectious Disease*, ed. Michael J. Selgelid, Margaret P. Battin, and Charles B. Smith, 83–94. Oxford: Blackwell.

McFadden, Charles J. 1956. *Medical ethics*. 4th ed. Philadelphia: F.A. Davis.

McIntyre, J. 2005. Preventing mother-to-child transmission of HIV: Successes and failures. *BJOG: An International Journal of Obstetrics and Gynecology* 112, no. 9 (September): 1196–1203.

McKenna, J.J. 1996. Where ignorance is not bliss: A proposal for mandatory HIV testing of pregnant women. *Stanford Law and Policy Review* 7: 133–157.

McKinley, Jesse. 2007. Infection hits a California prison hard, and experts ask why. *New York Times*, December 30, available at http://query.nytimes.com/gst/fullpage.html?res=9A06E6D81130F933A05751C1A9619C8B63&scp=2&sq=Valley±Fever&st=nyt (accessed January 21, 2008).

McKusick, L., J.A. Wiley, T.J. Coates, R. Stall, G. Saika, S. Morin, K. Charles, W. Horstman, M.A. Conant. 1985. Reported changes in the sexual behavior of men at risk for AIDS, San Francisco, 1982–84—The AIDS behavioral research project. *Public Health Reports* 100, no. 6: 622–629.

McLean, Angela. 2007. Impact of social distancing on influenza transmission. Lecture, Uehiro Center, Oxford University, Oxford, England, July 4.

McMahan, Jeff. 2002. *The ethics of killing*. New York: Oxford University Press.

McNabb, Scott J.N., Stella Chungong, Mike Ryan, Tadesse Wuhib, Peter Nsubuga, Wondi Alemu, Vilma Carande-Kulis, and Guenael Rodier. 2002. Conceptual framework of public health surveillance and action and its application in health sector reform. *BMC Public Health* 2(2), Epub January 29, p. 2 of 9.

McNeil, Donald G. Jr., 2007. Sharp drop seen in deaths from ills fought by vaccine. *New York Times*, sec. A, November 14, 18.

McPartland, T.S., B.A. Weaver, S. Lee, and L.A. Koutsky. 2005. Men's perceptions and knowledge of human papillomavirus (HPV) infection and cervical cancer. *Journal of American College Health* 53, no. 5 (March–April): 225–230.

Mead, Paul S., Laurence Slutsker, Vance Dietz, Linda F. McCaig, Joseph S. Bresee, Craig Shapiro, Patricia M. Griffin, and Robert V. Tauxe. 1999. Food–related illness and death in the United States. *Emerging Infectious Diseases* 5, no. 5 (September/October): 607–617.

Medical Institute for Sexual Health. 2007. The Medical Institute's statement on mandatory HPV vaccination. February. Available at http://www.medinstitute.org/content.php?name=HPVVaccineStatement (accessed January 6, 2008).

Melnychuk, Ryan M., and Nuala P. Kenny. 2006. Pandemic Triage: The Ethical Challenge," *Canadian Medical Association Journal* 175, no. 11 (November 21): 1393.

Meltzer, Martin I., Nancy J. Cox, and Keiji Fukuda. 1999. The economic impact of pandemic influenza in the United States: Priorities for intervention. *Emerging Infectious Diseases* 5, no. 5 (September–October): 659–671.

Merritt, Deborah Jones. 1986. Communicable disease and constitutional law: Controlling AIDS. *New York University Law Review* 61: 739–799.

Merwin, W.S. 1998. *The Folding Cliffs*. New York: Knopf.

Michigan Department of Community Health. 2007. *Pandemic influenza plan.* Version 3.1. May. Available at http://www.michigan.gov/documents/mdch/MDCH_Pandemic_Influenza_v_3.1_final_draft_060107_2_198392_7.pdf (accessed July 5, 2008).

Milius, Susan. 2007. Not just hitchhikers: Human pathogens make homes on plants. *Science News* (October 20): 251.

Mill, John Stuart. 1859. *On liberty.* London: Oxford University. Available at http://books.google.com/books?id=qCQCAAAAQAAJ&printsec=titlepage (accessed December 29, 2007).

Ministry of Health, Labour and Welfare. 2005. *Pandemic influenza preparedness action plan of the Japanese government.* November, available at http://www.mhlw.go.jp/english/topics/influenza/pandemic01.html (accessed July 5, 2008).

Minnesota Department of Health. 2006. *Pandemic influenza plan.* Draft version 2.5. April, available at http://www.health.state.mn.us/divs/idepc/diseases/flu/pandemic/plan/mdhpanfluplan.pdf (accessed July 5, 2008).

Minnesota Department of Health. 2007. *Mitigation strategies: Use of non-pharmaceutical interventions.* April, available at http://www.health.state.mn.us/divs/idepc/diseases/flu/pandemic/plan/npioverview.pdf (accessed January 30, 2008).

Missouri Department of Health and Senior Services. 2006. *Pandemic influenza plan.* Working document version 2.0 (February 9), available at http://www.dhss.mo.gov/PandemicInfluenza/PandemicPlan.pdf (accessed July 1, 2008).

Moblo, Penne. 1997. Blessed Damien of Moloka'i: The critical analysis of contemporary myth. *Ethnohistory* 44, no. 4: 691–726.

Moodley, Keymanthri. 2002. Vaccine trial participation in South Africa—An ethical assessment. *Journal of Medicine and Philosophy* 27, no. 2: 197–215.

Moore, A., and M. Richer. 2001. Re–emergence of epidemic sleeping sickness in southern Sudan. *Tropical Medicine & International Health* 6, no. 5: 342–347.

Morabia, A., and F.F. Zhang. 2004. History of medical screening: From concepts to action. *Postgrad Medical Journal.* 80: 463–469.

Moran, N.E., D. Shickle, C. Munthe, et al. 2006. Are compulsory immunization and incentives to immunize effective ways to achieve herd immunity in Europe? In *Ethics and Infectious Disease,* ed. Selgelid, Battin, and Smith, 215–231.

Morens, David M., and Anthony S. Fauci. 2008. Dengue and hemorrhagic fever: A potential threat to public health in the United States. *Journal of the American Medical Association* 299, no. 2 (January 9): 214–216.

Moser, M.R., T.R. Bender, H.S. Margolis, et al. 1979. An outbreak of influenza aboard a commercial airliner. *American Journal of Epidemiology* 110: 1–6.

Motomura, Hiroshi. 1993. Haitian asylum seekers: Interdiction and immigrants' rights. *Cornell International Law Journal* 26: 695–717.

Mount Sinai Hospital. PandemicWatch.ca. Available at http://microbiology.mtsinai.on.ca/avian/all-pandemic-plans.asp (accessed July 1, 2008).

Muñoz, Nubia, F. Xavier Bosch, Silvia de Sanjosé et al. 2003. "Epidemiological Classification of Human Papillomavirus Types Associated with Cervical Cancer," *New England Journal of Medicine* 348, no. 6: 518–527.

Nagel, Thomas. 1979. Moral luck. In *Mortal questions,*. New York: Cambridge University Press.

Nakchbandi, Inaam A., J. Craig Longenecker, Ann Ricksecker, Richard A. Latta, Cheryl Healton, and David G. Smith. 1998. A decision analysis of mandatory compared with voluntary HIV testing in pregnant women. *Annals of Internal Medicine* 128, no. 9 (May 1): 760–767.

National Conference of State Legislatures. HPV vaccine legislation 2007. Available at http://ncsl.org/programs/health/hpvvaccine.htm (accessed January 6, 2008).

National Ethics Advisory Committee. 2007. *Getting through together: Ethical values for a pandemic.* Wellington: Ministry of Health. Available at http://www .neac.health.govt.nz/moh.nsf/pagescm/1090/$File/getting-through-to-gether-jul07.pdf (accessed January 26, 2008).

National Institutes of Health. 1997. Genetic testing for cystic fibrosis. *NIH Consensus Statement Online* 15, no. 4 (April 14–16): 1–37, available at http://consensus.nih.gov/1997/1997GeneticTestCysticFibrosis106html.htm (accessed January 1, 2008).

National Network for Immunization Information. Vaccine information. Available at http://www.immunizationinfo.org/VaccineInfo/index.cfm (accessed January 6, 2008).

National Park Service. Ellis Island: History and culture. Available at http://www .nps.gov/elis/historyculture/index.htm (accessed December 29, 2007).

National Vaccine Information Center. 2007. NVIC letter to ACIP chairman regarding HPV VAERS reports. August 14, available at http://www.909shot.com/ Diseases/HPV/D.Morse_in_PDF_2%5B1%5D.pdf (accessed January 6, 2008).

Neff, J.M, J.M. Lane, V.A. Fulginiti, and D.A. Henderson. 2002. Contact vaccinia—Transmission of vaccinia from smallpox vaccination. *Journal of the American Medical Association* 288, no. 15 (October 16): 1901–1905.

Nelson, Roxanne. 2004. Tougher bugs, few new drugs: Dearth of new antibiotics threatens public health. *Washington Post* March 31. Available at http://www.washingtonpost.com/wp.

New Jersey Department of Health and Senior Services. 2006. *Influenza pandemic plan: Draft.* February 1, available at http://www.state.nj.us/health/flu/documents/pandemic_draft_022006.pdf (accessed July 5, 2008).

New Mexico Department of Health. 2007. *Pandemic Influenza Plan* (April 16), Suppl. 10. Available at http://www.health.state.nm.us/ohem/documents/supplement10publicinfo.pdf (accessed July 5, 2008).

New York Times. 1911. How we guard against the introduction of cholera: Where the scourge originated and how the government copes with it when it gets to these shores. Dr. Doty explodes some erroneous beliefs on the subject of the dread disease. *New York Times Sunday Magazine*, July 23.

New York Times. 2006. Editorial, extreme tuberculosis. *New York Times*, sec. A, September 14, 26.

New York Times. 2007. A vaccine to save women's lives. *New York Times*, sec. A, February 6, 20.

Nicholson, K.G., and J.M. Wood. 2003. Influenza. *Lancet* 362: 1733–1745.

Nicholson, K., R.G. Webster, & A.J. Hay, eds. 1998. *Textbook of influenza.* Oxford; Malden, MA, USA: Blackwell Science.

Nightingale, Elena O. 1977. Recommendations for a national policy on poliomyelitis vaccination. *New England Journal of Medicine* 297, no. 5 (August 4): 249–253.

Nordell, E.A., and W.F. Piessens. 2000. Transmission of tuberculosis. In *Tuberculosis: A comprehensive international approach*, ed. Reichman, L.B. and E.S. Hershfield, 224. 2nd ed. New York: Marcel Dekker.

North Carolina State Laboratory of Public Health. 2007. *N.C. Pandemic Influenza Plan.* January. Available at http://www.epi.state.nc.us/epi/gcdc/pandemic.html (accessed July 1, 2008).

NOVA. The most dangerous woman in America: History of quarantine. Available at http://www.pbs.org/wgbh/nova/typhoid/quarantine.html (accessed January 24, 2008).

Nussbaum, Martha. 1999. *Sex and social justice.* New York: Oxford.

Nussbaum, Martha. 2006. *Frontiers of Justice: disability, nationality, species membership.* Cambridge: Harvard University Press.

Oath of Hippocrates. Available at http://classics.mit.edu/Hippocrates/hippooath.html (accessed February 19, 2008).

O'Doherty, Gemma. 2007. Power Dressing. *Irish Independent* (August 28), 31.

Ohio Department of Health Bureau of Infectious Disease Control Immunization Program. 2005. *Influenza pandemic response plan.* Version 2.0, September. Available at http://www.odh.ohio.gov/ASSETS/399540667CF446508D5E663610B7396A/ODHFluPlan.pdf (accessed July 5, 2008).

Ojikutu, B.O., and V.E. Stone. 2005. Women, inequality, and the burden of HIV. *New England Journal of Medicine* 352, no. 7 (February 17): 649–652.

Okie, Susan. 2006. Fighting HIV—Lessons from Brazil. *New England Journal of Medicine* 354, no. 19 (May 11): 1977–1981.

Olshansky, S. Jay. and A. Brian Ault. 1987. The fourth stage of the epidemiological transition: The age of delayed degenerative disease. In *Should Medical Care be Rationed by Age?* ed. Timothy M. Smeeding et al. Totowa, N.J.: Rowman & Littlefield, 11–43.

Olshansky, S. Jay, et al. 1998. Emerging infectious diseases: The fifth stage of the epidemiological transition? *World Health Statistics Quarterly* 51, nos. 2–4: 207–217.

Olson, Elizabeth. 2003. Panel urges shift of focus in preparing for smallpox. *New York Times*, sec. A, August 12, 22.

Oregon Death with Dignity Act, Ore. Rev. Stat. §§ 127.800 *et seq.* (2007).

Orenstein, W.A., and A.R. Hinman. 1999. The immunization system in the United States—The role of school immunization laws. *Vaccine* 17, supplement 3 (October 29): S19–S24.

Osler, William. 1909. *The principles and practice of medicine: Designed for the use of practitioners and students of medicine.* 7th ed. New York: Appleton.

Ostrom, Elinor. 1990. *Governing the commons: The evolution of institutions for collective action.* Cambridge: Cambridge University Press.

Ostrow, D.E., K.J. Fox, J.S. Chmiel, A. Silvestre, B.R. Visscher, P.A. Vanable, L.P. Jacobson, and S.A. Strathdee. 2002. Attitudes towards highly active antiretroviral therapy are associated with sexual risk taking among HIV-infected and uninfected homosexual men. *AIDS* 16, no. 5: 775–780.

Packard, Randall M. 2007. *The making of a tropical disease: A short history of malaria.* Baltimore: Johns Hopkins University Press.

Palmer, Carol J., Jose M. Dubon, Ellen Koenig, Eddy Perez, Arba Ager, Dushyantha Jayaweera, Raul R. Cuadrado, Ada Rivera, Alex Rubido, and Dennis A. Palmer. 1999. Field evaluation of the determine rapid human immunodeficiency virus diagnostic test in Honduras and the Dominican Republic. *Journal of Clinical Microbiology* 37, no. 11 (November): 3698–3700.

Paolo, William F., Jr., and Joshua D. Nosanchuk. 2004. Tuberculosis in New York City: Recent lessons and a look ahead. *Lancet Infectious Diseases* 4, no. 5: 287–293.

Parent, W.A. 1983. Privacy, morality, and the law. *Philosophy and Public Affairs* 12, no. 4: 269–288.

Parker, Amy A., W. Staggs, G.H. Dayan, et al. 2006. Implications of a 2005 measles outbreak in Indiana for sustained elimination of measles in the United States. *New England Journal of Medicine* 355, no. 5 (August 3): 447–5045.

Parker, Michael. 2007. Methods of pandemic planning—The UK task force. Lecture, Uehiro Center, Oxford University, Oxford, England, July 4.

Parker-Pope, Tara. 2007. Germ fighters may lead to hardier germs. *New York Times*, sec. F, October 30, 5.

Parkin, D.M. 2006. The global health burden of infection–associated cancers in the year 2002. *International Journal of Cancer* 118: 3030–3044.

Parks Canada. Grosse Île and the Irish memorial national historic site of Canada: Management plan, a terrible toll. Available at www.pc.gc.ca/lhn-nhs/qc/grosseile/docs/plan1/sec3/page2biii_E.asp (accessed January 22, 2008).

Parmet, Wendy E. 2006. Unprepared: Why health law fails to prepare us for a pandemic. *Journal of Health & Biomedical Law* 2: 157–193.

Parmet, Wendy E. 2007. Legal power and legal rights—Isolation and quarantine in the case of drug–resistant tuberculosis. *New England Journal of Medicine* 357, no. 5 (August 2): 433–435.

Parmet, Wendy E. 2007. Public health and constitutional law: Recognizing the relationship. *Journal of Health Care Law & Policy* 10: 13–24.

Parmet, Wendy E., R.A. Goodman, and A. Farber. 2005. Individual rights versus the public's health—100 years after Jacobson v. Massachusetts. *New England Journal of Medicine* 352, no. 7 (February 17): 652–654.

Parran, Thomas. 1938. Syphilis: A public health problem. *Science* 87, no. 2251: 147–152.

Partridge, J.M., and L.A. Koutsky. 2006. Genital human papillomavirus infection in men. *Lancet Infectious Diseases* 6, no. 1 (January): 21–31.

Paul, Y., and A. Dawson. 2006. Some ethical issues arising from polio eradication programmes in India. In *Ethics and Infectious Disease*, ed. Selgelid, Battin, and Smith, 246–258.

Pence, Gregory. 1990–2008. *Classic cases in medical ethics.* Boston: McGraw-Hill.

Peng, Philip W.H., David T. Wong, David Bevan, and Michael Gardam. 2003. Infectious control and anaesthesia: Lessons learned from the Toronto SARS outbreak. *Canadian Journal of Anesthesia* 50: 989–997.

Pfeifer, James. 2003. International NGOs and primary health care in Mozambique: the need for a new model of collaboration. *Social Science & Medicine* 56, no. 4: 725–738.

Pichichero, Michael E., and Janet R. Casey. 2007. Emergence of a Multiresistant Serotype 19A Pneumococcal Strain Not Included in the 7-Valent Conjugate Vaccine as an Otopathogen in Children, *Journal of the American Medical Association* 298, no. 5 (October 17): 1772–1778.

Pincock, Stephen. 2004. Poliovirus spreads beyond Nigeria after vaccine uptake drops. *British Medical Journal* 328: 310.

Plotkin, S. A., W.A. Orenstein, & P.A. Offit. 2008. *Vaccines* (5th ed.). New York: Saunders.

Pogge, Thomas. 2005. World poverty and human rights. *Ethics & International Affairs* 19, no. 1: 1–7.

Pogge, Thomas. 2006. Human rights and global health. In *Ethics and Infectious Disease*, ed. Selgelid, Battin, and Smith, 285–306.

Powers, Madison, and Ruth Faden. 2006. *Social justice: The moral foundations of public health and health policy.* New York: Oxford University Press.

Program for Appropriate Technology in Health (PATH). 2006. PATH to pave the way for cervical cancer vaccines in the developing world. News release (June 5), available at http://path.org/news/pr060606-cervical_cancer_vaccine.php (accessed January 5, 2008).

Program for Appropriate Technology in Health (PATH). Rapid tests for HIV: Commercially available rapid tests for HIV. Available at http://www.rapid-diagnostics.org/rti-hiv-com.htm (accessed January 3, 2008).

Psaty, Bruce M., and R. Alta Charo. 2007. FDA responds to Institute of Medicine drug safety recommendations—in part. *Journal of the American Medical Association* 297, no. 17 (May 2): 1917–1920.

Public Health Agency of Canada. 2006. Guidelines Regarding Departure from Canada of Persons with Suspected Respiratory Tuberculosis (TB), Untreated Active Respiratory TB or Partially Treated Active Respiratory TB. Available at http://www.phac-aspc.gc.ca/tbpc-Iatb/tb_guide-Id_depart_e.html, 1–5 (accessed April 27, 2008).

Public Health Leadership Society. 2002. *Principles of the ethical practice of public health.* Version 2.2, available at http://www.apha.org/NR/rdonlyres/1CED3 CEA-287E-4185-9CBD-BD405FC60856/0/ethicsbrochure.pdf (accessed December 29, 2007).

Purdy, Laura. 1999. Genetics and reproductive risk: Can having children be immoral? In *Bioethics,* ed. Helga Kuhse and Peter Singer, 123–129. Oxford: Blackwell.

Quetel, C., and J. Braddoch. 1992. *The History of Syphilis.* Baltimore, MD: Johns Hopkins University Press.

Quinn, Thomas C., Maria J. Wawer, Nelson Sewankambo, David Serwadda, Chuanjun Li, Fred Wabwire–Mangen, Mary O. Meehan, Thomas Lutalo, and Ronald H. Gray. 2000. Viral load and heterosexual transmission of human immunodeficiency virus type 1. *New England Journal of Medicine* 342, no. 13 (March 30): 921–929.

Rabinowitz, Bernard. 1996. The Great Hijack. *British Medical Journal* 313, no. 7060: 826.

Radiation Effects Research Foundation. 2007. *Frequently asked questions.* Available at http://www.rerf.or.jp/general/qa_e/qa1.html. (accessed February 8, 2008).

Ramsey, Paul. 1970; 1973. *The patient as person: Explorations in medical ethics.* 1st ed.; 3rd ed. New Haven: Yale University Press.

Raviglione, M.C., and I.M. Smith. 2007. XDR tuberculosis—implications for global public health. *New England Journal of Medicine* 356, no. 7 (February 15): 656–659.

Rawls, John. 1971. *A theory of justice.* Cambridge: Harvard University Press.

Reddy, Madhuri et al. 2007. Oral Drug Therapy for Multiple Neglected Tropical Diseases: A Systematic Review. *Journal of the American Medical Association* 298, no. 16 (October 24): 1911–1924.

Reddy, R.K.K. et al. 2008. Electrical immunoassays toward clinical diagnostics: Identification of vulnerable cardiovascular plaque. *Journal of the Association of Laboratory Automation* 13, no. 1 (February).

Reid, Lynette. 2005. Diminishing returns? Risk and the duty to care in the SARS epidemic. *Bioethics* 19, no. 4: 348–361.

Reiser, Stanley Joel, Arthur J. Dyck, and William J. Curran, eds. 1977. *Ethics in medicine: Historical perspectives and contemporary concerns.* Cambridge: MIT Press.

Rennie, S., and F. Behets. 2006. AIDS care and treatment in Sub-Saharan Africa: Implementation ethics. *Hastings Center Report* 36, no. 3 (May–June): 23–31.

Reverby, Susan, ed. 2000. *Tuskegee's truths: Rethinking the Tuskegee syphilis study.* Chapel Hill: University of North Carolina Press.

Reynolds, Gretchen. 2004. Why were doctors afraid to treat Rebecca McLester? *New York Times,* sec. 6, April 18, 32.

Rhodes, Rosamond 1998. Genetic links, family ties, and social bonds: Rights and responsibilities in the face of genetic knowledge. *Journal of Medicine & Philosophy* 23: 18.

Rhodes, Rosamond. 2005. Justice in medicine and public health. *Cambridge Quarterly of Health Care Ethics* 14, no. 1: 13–26.

Roberts, Leslie. 2004. The exit strategy. *Science* 303 (March): 1969–1971.

Roberts, Leslie. 2004. Fighting polio block by block, shack by shack. *Science* 303 (March): 1965–1966.

Roberts, Leslie. 2004. Health workers scramble to contain African epidemic. *Science* 305 (July): 24–25.

Roberts, Leslie. 2004. Two steps forward, one step back in polio fight. *Science* 304 (May): 1096.

Robison, Wade, and Michael Pritchard. 1979. *Medical responsibility.* Clifton, NJ: Humana Press.

Roegge, Bea. 2006. Making colds uncommon—for the common good. *Christian Science Sentinel.* February 6, available at http://www.spirituality.com/tte/article_display.jhtml?ElementId=/repositories/shcomarticle/Jan2006/1138043707.xml&ElementName=Making%20colds%20uncommon%14for%20the%20common%20good (accessed February 16, 2008).

Roemer, Milton and Ruth Roemer. 1990. Global health, national development, and the role of government., *American Journal of Public Health* 80, no. 10: 88–92.

Rogers, Wendy, and Dan Brock, eds. 2004. Ethics and public health. *Bioethics Special Issue* 18, no. 6 (November).

Roisman, Florence Wagman. 2005. National ingratitude: The egregious deficiencies of the United States' housing programs for veterans and the "public scandal" of veterans' homelessness. *Indiana Law Review* 38: 103–176.

Ropper, A.H., and M. Victor. 1998. Influenza vaccination and the Guillain–Barré syndrome. *New England Journal of Medicine* 339, no. 25 (December 17): 1845–1846.

Rose, Carol. 1986. The comedy of the commons: Custom, commerce, and inherently public property. *University of Chicago Law Review* 53: 711–781.

Rosenbaum, David E., and Sheryl Gay Stolberg. 2001. A nation challenged: The vaccine. *New York Times*, sec. B, December 20, 1.

Rosenbaum, J.E. 2006. Reborn a virgin: Adolescents retracting of virginity pledges and sexual histories. *American Journal of Public Health* 96, no. 61: 1098-1103.

Rosenbaum, Julie, and Ken Sepkowitz. 2002. Infectious disease experimentation involving human volunteers. *Clinical Infectious Diseases* 34 (April 1): 963–971.

Rosenfeld, R.M. 2003. Clinical efficacy of medical therapy. In *Evidence-based otitis media,* ed. Rosenfeld and C.D. Bluestone, 199–226.

Rosenfeld, R.M., and C.D. Bluestone, eds. 2003. *Evidence-based otitis media.* 2nd ed. Hamilton, Ontario: BC Decker.

Rosenstein, N.E., B.A. Perkins, D.S. Stephens et al. 2001. Meningococcal disease. *New England Journal of Medicine* 344, no. 18 (May 3): 1378–1388.

Ross, Lainie Friedman. 2001. Genetic exceptionalism vs. paradigm shift: Lessons from HIV. *Journal of Law, Medicine & Ethics* 29: 141–146.

Ross, Lainie Friedman, and T. Aspinwell. 1997. Religious exemptions to the immunization statutes: Balancing public health and religious freedom. *Journal of Law, Medicine & Ethics* 25: 202–209.

Rothman, David J. 1991. *Strangers at the bedside: A history of how law and bioethics transformed medical decision making.* New York: Basic Books.

Rothman, S.M. 1992. The sanitorium experience: Myths and realities. In *The tuberculosis revival: Individual rights and societal obligations in a time of aids,* ed. Dubler, Nancy N., Ronald Bayer, Sheldon Landesman, and Amanda White, 67–73. New York: United Hospital Fund of New York.

Rothstein, Mark. 2004. Are traditional public health strategies consistent with contemporary American values? *Temple Law Review* 77: 175–192.

Rothstein, Mark, and Meghan Talbott. 2007. Encouraging compliance with quarantine: A proposal to provide job security and income replacement. *American Journal of Public Health* 97 (April): S49–S56.

Rothstein, Mark, and Meghan Talbott. 2007. Job security and income replacement for individuals in quarantine: The need for legislation. *Journal of Health Care Law & Policy* 10, no. 2: 239–257.

Roush S.W., T.V. Murphy, and the Vaccine-Preventable Disease Table Working Group. 2007. Historical comparisons of morbidity and mortality for vaccine-preventable diseases in the United States. *Journal of the American Medical Association* 298, no. 18 (November 14): 2155–2163.

Roy, Powell, and Lowell W. Gerson. 2003. Temporal artery temperature measurements in healthy infants, children, and adolescents. *Clinical Pediatrics* 42: 433–437.

Ruben, R.J. 2003. Sequelae of antibiotic therapy. In *Evidence-based otitis media,* ed. Rosenfeld and Bluestone, 303–314.

Rubin, Harriet. 2008. Google's searches now include ways to make a better world. *New York Times,* sec. C1, January 18, 1.

Ruddick, Sara. 1989. *Maternal thinking: Toward a politics of peace.* Boston: Beacon Press.

Runowicz, Carolyn D. 2008. "Molecular Screening for Cervical Cancer—Time to Give up Pap Tests?" *New England Journal of Medicine* 357, no. 16: 1650–1652.

Rutkow, Lainie, Brad Maggy, Joanna Zablotsky, and Thomas R. Oliver, et al. 2007. Balancing consumer and industry interests in public health: The national vaccine injury compensation program and its influence during the last two decades. *Penn State Law Review* 111: 681–735.

Saah, A. 1996. The epidemiology of HIV and AIDS in women. In *HIV, AIDS, and childbearing,* ed. R.R. Faden and N.E. Kass, 9–11. New York: Oxford University Press.

Sage, William M., Kathleen E. Hastings, and Robert A. Berenson. 1994. Enterprise liability for medical malpractice and health care quality improvement. *American Journal of Law & Medicine* 20: 1–28.

Sagoff, Mark. 1984. Animal liberation and environmental ethics: Bad marriage, quick divorce. *Osgoode Hall Law Journal* 22: 297–307.

Salk, Jonas. 1979. Immunization against poliomyelitis: Risk/benefit/cost in a changing context. *Developments in Biological Standardization* 43: 151–157.

Samore, M.H., M.K. Magill, S.C. Alder, E. Severina, L. Morrison-De Boer, J.L. Lyon, K. Carroll, et al. 2001. High rates of multiple antibiotic resistance in Streptococcus pneumoniae from healthy children living in isolated rural communities: Association with cephalosporin use and intrafamilial transmission. *Pediatrics* 108, no. 4 (October 2001): 856–860.

Sartwell, Philip E., ed. 1973. *Maxcy-Rosenau preventive medicine and public health*. 10th ed. New York: Appleton Century Crofts.

Saslow, D., P.E. Castle, J.T. Cox, D.D. Davey, M.H. Einstein, D.G. Ferris, S.J. Goldie, et al. American Cancer Society guideline for human papillomavirus (HPV) vaccine use to prevent cervical cancer and its precursors. *CA: A Cancer Journal for Clinicans* 57, no. 1 (January–February): 7–28.

Sauerbrei, A., E. Rubtcova, P. Wutzler, D.S. Schmid, & V.N. Loparev. 2004. Genetic profile of an Oka varicella vaccine virus variant isolated from an infant with zoster. *Journal of Clinical Microbiology* 42, no. 12: 5604–5608.

Sbarbaro, J.A. 1979. Compliance: Inducements and enforcements. *Chest* 76, no. 6 (December): 750–756.

Scanlon, Thomas. 1975. Thomson on privacy. *Philosophy & Public Affairs* 4, no. 4: 315–322.

Scheper-Hughes, Nancy. 1993. AIDS, Public Health, and Human Rights in Cuba. *Lancet* 342, no. 8877 (October 16).

Schiffman M., and P.E. Castle. 2005. The promise of global cervical cancer prevention. *New England Journal of Medicine* 353, no. 20 (November 17): 2101–2104.

Schoch-Spana, Monica, Joseph Fitzgerald, Bradley R. Kramer, and the UMPC Influenza Task Force. 2005. Influenza Vaccine Scarcity 2004–05: Implications for Biosecurity and Public Health Preparedness. *Biosecurity and Bioterrorism: Biodefense Strategy, Practice, and Science* 3, no. 3: 211–234.

Schoenbaum, S.C. 1987. Economic impact of influenza. *American Journal of Medicine* 82, supp. 6A: 26.

Schoepf, Brooke Grundfest. 2004. AIDS, history, and struggles over meaning. In *HIV and AIDS in Africa: Beyond epidemiology*, ed. Ezekiel Kalipeni et al. Malden, MA: Blackwell.

Schuklenk, Udo, and Anita Kleinsmidt. 2007. Rethinking mandatory HIV testing during pregnancy in areas with high HIV prevalence rates: Ethical and policy issues. *American Journal of Public Health* 97, no. 7 (July): 1179–1183.

Schwartz, Jason L. 2007. Gardasil: CDC response on safety/efficacy; survey on parental support for mandates. University of Pennsylvania, Center for Bioethics, June 15, available at http://www.vaccineethics.org/2007_06_01_archive.html (accessed January 5, 2008).

Schwartz, Jason L. 2007. Gardasil: Profile of Merck vaccines president; feature on early HPV–Cancer link proponent. University of Pennsylvania, Center for Bioethics, January 3. http://www.vaccineethics.org/2007/01/gardasil-profile-of-merck-vaccines.html (accessed January 5, 2008).

Schwartz, J.L., A.L. Caplan, R.R. Faden, and J. Sugarman. 2007. Lessons from the failure of human papillomavirus vaccine state requirements. *Clinical Pharmacology and Therapeutics* 82, no. 6 (December): 760–763.

Schwartz, John. 2007. Tangle of conflicting accounts in TB patient's 12–day odyssey. *New York Times*, sec. A, June 2, 1.

Scott, J.N. McNabb, Stella Chungong, Mike Ryan, Tadesse Wuhib, Peter Nsubuga, Wondi Alemu, Vilma Carande-Kulis, Guenael Rodier. 2002. Conceptual framework of public health surveillance and action and its application in health sector reform. *BMC Public Health* 2, no., Epub January 29.

Secretary's Advisory Committee on Genetic Testing. 2000. Enhancing the oversight of genetic tests: recommendations of the SACGT. Bethesda, MD: National Institutes of Health, available at http://www4.od.nih.gov/oba/sacgt/reports/oversight_report.pdf (accessed December 31, 2007).

Seilor, Naomi, Holly Taylor, and Ruth Faden. 2004. Legal and ethical considerations in government compensation plans: A case study of smallpox immunization. *Indiana Health Law Review* 1: 1–27.

Selgelid, Michael J. 2005. Ethics and infectious disease. *Bioethics* 19, no. 3: 272–289.

Selgelid, Michael J. 2007. Dual use discoveries: Censorship policy making. Lecture, Uehiro Center, Oxford University, Oxford, England, July 4.

Selgelid, Michael J. 2007. Ethics and drug resistance. *Bioethics* 21, no. 4 (May): 218–229, citing U.S. Congress, Office of Technology Assessment. 1995. *Impacts of antibiotic-resistant bacteria*, OTA-H-629. Washington, DC: Government Printing Office.

Selgelid, Michael J. 2007. Personal communication to Francis and Battin.

Selgelid, Michael J., and Margaret P. Battin, eds. 2005. Ethics and infectious disease. *Bioethics Special Issue* 19, no. 4 (August).

Selgelid, Michael J., Margaret P. Battin, and Charles B. Smith, eds. 2006. *Ethics and infectious disease.* Oxford: Blackwell.

Sen, Amartya. 1999. *Development as Freedom.* New York: Alfred A. Knopf.

Seppa, Nathan. 2007. Patch guards against Montezuma's revenge. *Science News* 172, no. 22 (December 1): 350.

Shal, D.J., ed. 1996. *Cystic fibrosis.* London: BMJ Publishing Group.

Shilts, Randy. 1987. *And the band played on: politics, people, and the AIDS epidemic.* New York: St. Martin's Press.

Shindell, Sidney. 1980. Legal and ethical aspects of public health. In *Maxcy-Rosenau preventive medicine and public health*, ed. Jerald A. Last and Philip E. Sartwell, 1834–1845. 11th ed. New York: Appleton Century Crofts.

Sidel, V.W., R.M. Gould, and H.W. Cohen. 2002. Bioterrorism preparedness: Cooptation of public health. *Medicine and Global Survival* 7, no. 2: 82–89.

Singer, Peter A. et al. 2007. Grand challenges in global health: The ethical, social and cultural program. *PLoS Medicine* 4, no. 9 (September 11), e265.

Sipress, Alan. 2004. Bird flu upends industry, livelihoods in Thailand. *Washington Post*, sec. A, January 25, 1.

Skocpol, Theda. 1992. *Protecting soldiers and mothers: The political origins of social policy in the United States.* Cambridge: Harvard University Press.

Small, P.M., and P.I. Fujiwara. 2001. Management of tuberculosis in the United States. *New England Journal of Medicine* 345, no. 3 (July 19): 189–200.

Smith, J. David, and Alison L. Mitchell. 2001. Sacrifices for the miracle: The polio vaccine research and children with mental retardation. *Mental Retardation* 39, no. 5: 405–409.

Smith, Patricia. 1998. *Liberalism and affirmative obligation*. New York: Oxford University Press.

Socialist Republic of Vietnam. 2006. *Vietnam integrated national operational program for avian and human influenza 2006–2010*. May. Available at http://microbiology.mtsinai.on.ca/avian/plans/Vietnam.pdf (accessed July 5, 2008).

Specter, Michael. 2007. Annals of science: "Darwin" surprise. *New Yorker*, December 3, 64–73.

Starace, F. 1993. Suicidal behavior in people infected with human immunodeficiency virus: A literature review. *International Journal of Social Psychiatry* 39: 64–70.

State of Alaska, Division of Public Health. 2008. *Pandemic influenza response plan*. February. Available at http://www.pandemicflu.alaska.gov/panfluplan.pdf (accessed July 5, 2008).

State of Illinois. 2006. *Illinois pandemic influenza preparedness and response plan*. Version 2.05, October 10. Available at http://www.idph.state.il.us/pandemic_flu/Illinois%20Pandemic%20Flu%20Plan%20101006%20Final.pdf (accessed July 1, 2008).

Statue of Liberty—Ellis Island Foundation, Inc. Ellis Island—History. Available at http://www.ellisisland.org/genealogy/ellis_island_history.asp (accessed January 22, 2008).

Stern, Howard, and Alexandra Minna Stern. 2002. The foreignness of germs: The persistent association of immigrants and disease in American society. *Millbank Quarterly* 80, no. 4: 757–788.

Stein, Rob. 2005. Cervical cancer vaccine gets injected with a social issue. Some fear a shot for teens would encourage sex. *Washington Post*, sec. A, October 31, 3.

Steinbrook, Robert. 2007. One Step Forward, Two Steps Back—Will There Even Be an AIDS Vaccine? *New England Journal of Medicine* 257, no. 26 (December 27): 2653–2655.

Stenseth, Nils, et al. 2008. Plague: Past, present, and future. *PLoS Medicine* 5, no. 1: 9–13.

Stolberg, Sherly Gay. 2008. Bush, Facing Troubles, Focuses on War and Taxes. *New York Times*, sec. A, January 28, 1.

Stolberg, Sheryl Gay. 2008. In global battle on AIDS, Bush creates legacy. *New York Times*, sec. A January 5, 1.

Stoto, Michael A., Donna A. Almario, and Marie C. McCormick. 1999. *Reducing the odds: Preventing perinatal transmission of HIV in the United States*. Washington, DC: National Academy Press.

Studdert, David M., and Troyen A. Brennan. 2001. Toward a workable model of "no-fault" compensation for medical injury in the United States. *American Journal of Law & Medicine* 27: 225–252.

Sumartojo, E. 1993. When tuberculosis treatment fails: A social behavioral account of patient adherence. *American Review of Respiratory Disease* 147, no. 5 (May): 1311–1320.

Summers, Lawrence H. 1989. Some simple economics of mandated benefits. *American Economic Review* 79, no. 2: 177–183.

Svoboda, Tomislav et al. 2004. Public health measures to control the spread of the severe acute respiratory syndrome during the outbreak in Toronto. *New England Journal of Medicine* 350, no. 23 (June 3): 2352–2361.

Swift, Mike. 2007. MediaNews. Travelers sought in TB case. *Palo Alto (CA) Daily News*, December 29, available at http://www.paloaltodailynews.com/article /2007-12-29-pa-tb (accessed January 22, 2008).

Swoyer, Chris. Relativism and the constructive aspects of perception. In *The Stanford Encyclopedia of Philosophy (Spring 2003 Edition)*, ed. Edward N. Zalta, available at http://plato.stanford.edu/entries/relativism/supplement1.html (accessed December 29, 2007).

Tabery, James, Charles W. Mackett III, and the UPMC Pandemic Influenza Task Force's Triage Review Board. 2008. "The Ethics of Triage in the Event of an Influenza Pandemic." *Disaster Medicine and Public Health Preparedness* 2(2): 114–118 (June).

Taglibue, John. 2001. Mad cow disease (and anxiety). *New York Times*, sec. C, February 1, 1.

Taha, T.E., N.I. Kumwenda, D.R. Hoover, S.A. Fiscus, G. Kafulafula, C. Nkhoma, S. Nour, et al. 2004. Nevirapine and Zidovudine at birth to reduce perinatal transmission of HIV in an African setting: A randomized controlled trial. *Journal of the American Medical Association* 292, no. 2 (July 14): 202–209.

Taiwo, B. O., A.D. Thrasher, C.L. Ford, K.A. Nearing, E. da Silveira, G.D. Sanders, A.M. Bayoumi, et al. 2005. Cost-effectiveness of screening for HIV. *New England Journal of Medicine* 352, no. 20 (May 19): 2137–2139.

Taylor, James Stacey, ed. 2005. *Personal autonomy: New essays on personal autonomy and its role in contemporary moral philosophy*. Cambridge: Cambridge University Press.

Tayman, John. 2006. *The colony: The harrowing true story of the exiles of Molokai*. New York: Scribner.

Teixeira, P.R., M.A. Vitoria, and J. Barcarolo. 2004. Antiretroviral treatment in resource-poor settings: The Brazilian experience. *AIDS* 18, supplement 3: S5–S7.

Temmerman, M., J. Ndinya-Achola, J. Ambani, and P. Piot. 1995. The right not to know HIV-test results. *Lancet* 345, no. 8955 (April 15): 969–970.

Tennessee Department of Health. 2006. *Pandemic influenza response plan*. July, available at http://health.state.tn.us/CEDS/PDFs/2006_PanFlu_Plan.pdf (accessed July 5, 2008).

Terry, Nicolas P., and Leslie P. Francis. 2007. Ensuring the privacy and confidentiality of electronic health records. *Illinois Law Review* 2007: 681–735.

Texas Department of State Health Services. 2005. *Pandemic influenza preparedness plan*. October. Available at http://www.dshs.state.tx.us/idcu/disease/influenza/pandemic/Draft_PIPP_10_24_web.pdf (accessed July 5, 2008).

Thomas, James C. 2007. *Ethical concerns in pandemic influenza preparation and responses*. Southeast Regional Center of Excellence for Emerging Infections and Biodefense, Policy, Ethics and Law Core, available at http://www.serceb .org/wysiwyg/downloads/pandemic_flu_white_paper.May_25.FORMATTED .pdf (accessed Sept. 2007).

Thomas, James C., Nabarun Dasgupta, and Amanda Martinot. 2007. Ethics in a pandemic: A survey of the state pandemic influenza plans. *American Journal of Public Health* 97 (April): S26–S31.

Thomas, M., P. Gilbert, et al. 2007. The Emergence of HIV/AIDS in the Americas and Beyond. *Proceedings of the National Academy of Sciences* 104, no. 47 (November 20): 18566–18570.

Titball, R. 2004. *Plague vaccines and assessment of immune responses.* Paper presented at the Public Workshop on Animal Models and Correlates of Protection for Plague Vaccines, Gaithersburg, Maryland. October 13.

Toronto Public Health. 2006. *Toronto public health plan for an influenza pandemic.* November 2005, updated March, available at http://www.toronto.ca/health /pandemicflu/pandemicflu_plan.htm (accessed February 2007).

Tramont, E.C. 2004. The impact of syphilis on humankind. *Infectious Disease Clinics of North America* 18: 101–110.

Tramont, E.C. 2005. Treponenion pallidum (Syphilis). In *Principle and practice of infectious diseases,* ed. G.L. Mandell, J.E. Bennett, and R. Dolin, 2 vols. 6th ed. Philadelphia: Elsevier.

Treanor, John D. 2007. Influenza—the goal of control. *New England Journal of Medicine* 357, no. 14: 1440.

Trujillo, Alfonso Cardinal Lopez. 2003. Family Values Verses Safe Sex. (December 1). Available at http://www.vatican.va/roman_curia/pontifical_councils/family/ documents/rc_pc_family_doc_20031201_family-values-safe-sex-trujillo_en. html (accessed February 16, 2008).

Tuberculosis Coalition for Technical Assistance. 2006. *International standards for tuberculosis care.* Available at http://www.who.int/tb/publications/2006/istc_ report.pdf (accessed December 29, 2007).

Tuckett, Anthony G. 2004. Truth telling in clinical practice and the arguments for and against: A review of the literature. *Nursing Ethics* 11, no. 5: 500–513.

Tuomala, R.E., and S. Yawetz. 2006. Protease inhibitor use during pregnancy: Is there an obstetrical risk? *Journal of Infectious Diseases* 193: 1191–1194.

U.K. Department of Health. 2007. *Pandemic flu: A national framework for responding to an influenza pandemic.* November. Available at http://www.dh.gov.uk /en/Publicationsandstatistics/Publications/PublicationsPolicyAndGuidance/DH_ 080734 (accessed February 7, 2008).

Ungchusak, K., P. Auewarakul, S.F. Dowell, et al. 2005. Probable person-to-person transmission of avian influenza A (H5N1). *New England Journal of Medicine* 352: 333–340.

United Nations Economic and Social Council, U.N. Sub-Commission on Prevention of Discrimination and Protection of Minorities. 1984. *Siracusa principles on the limitation and derogation of provisions in the international covenant on civil and political rights.* Annex, UN Doc E/CN.4/1984/4, available at http://hei.unige.ch/~clapham/hrdoc/docs/siracusa.html (accessed January 27, 2008).

United States Mexico Border Health Commission. *Early warning infectious disease surveillance project.* Available at http://www.borderhealth.org/ewids.php? curr=programs (accessed January 24, 2008).

United States of America. 2005. *Statement for the record by the Government of the United States of America concerning the World Health Organization's revised*

International Health Regulations. May 23, available at http://usinfo.state.gov/ usinfo/Archive/2005/May/23–321998.html (accessed February 7, 2008).

University of Pennsylvania, Center for Bioethics, Ethics of Vaccines Project. 2008. Vaccines: A Timeline. Available at http://www.bioethics.upenn.edu/vaccines/ ?pageId=3&sub page=196 (accessed May 9, 2008).

University of Toronto Joint Centre for Bioethics Pandemic Influenza Working Group. 2005. *Stand on guard for thee: Ethical considerations in preparedness planning for pandemic influenza.* Toronto: University of Toronto Joint Centre for Bioethics, available at http://www.utoronto.ca/jcb/home/documents/ pandemic.pdf (accessed January 27, 2008).

U.S. Department of Health and Human Services. Request for information: Guidance for prioritization of pre-pandemic and pandemic influenza vaccine, available at http://aspe.hhs.gov/PIV/RFI/ [URL no longer valid] (accessed February 2007).

U.S. Department of Health and Human Services. 2005. *HHS Pandemic Influenza Plan.* November, available at http://www.hhs.gov/pandemicflu/plan/pdf/ HHSPandemicInfluenzaPlan.pdf (accessed July 5, 2008).

U.S. Department of Health and Human Services. *About the commissioned corps: history.* Available at http://commcorps.shs.net/aboutus/history.aspx (accessed January 2007).

U.S. Department of Health and Human Services. *PandemicFlu.gov: State pandemic plans.* Available at http://www.pandemicflu.gov/plan/states/stateplans.html (accessed February 7, 2008).

U.S. Department of Health and Human Services, Health Resources and Services Administration. 2007. Women's health USA 2007: HIV in pregnancy. Rockville, MD: U.S. Department of Health and Human Services, available at www.mchb.hrsa.gov/whusa_07/healthstatus/maternal/0330hp.htm (accessed January 1, 2008).

U.S. Department of Health and Human Services. *HHS pandemic influenza implementation plan.* Available at http://www.hhs.gov/pandemicflu/implementationplan/intro.htm#bookmark_6 (accessed February 2007).

U.S. Department of Health and Human Services. *Medical privacy—national standards to protect the privacy of personal health information.* Available at http:// www.hhs.gov/ocr/hipaa/ (accessed January 2007).

U.S. Department of Health and Human Services, Health Resources and Services Administration, HIV/AIDS Bureau. The 2006 Ryan White CARE act progress report. Available at http://hab.hrsa.gov/publications/careactreport06/ careacttoday.htm (accessed January 3, 2008).

U.S. Department of Health and Human Services, Health Resources and Services Administration. National vaccine injury compensation program: Statistics reports. Available at http://www.hrsa.gov/vaccinecompensation/statistics_ report.htm (accessed January 4, 2008).

U.S. Department of Health and Human Services, National Institutes of Health, National Heart, Lung and Blood Institute. Diseases and conditions index: What is cystic fibrosis? Available at http://www.nhlbi.nih.gov/health/dci /Diseases/cf/cf_what.html (accessed December 31, 2007).

U.S. Federal Government. 2007. *Draft guidance on allocating and targeting pandemic influenza vaccine.* October 17, available at http://www.pandemicflu.gov/vaccine/prioritization.pdf (accessed February 6, 2008).

U.S. Food and Drug Administration. 2005. *FDA announces final decision about veterinary medicine.* News release (July 28), available at http://www.fda.gov/bbs/topics/news/2005/new01212.html (accessed January 3, 2008).

U.S. Food and Drug Administration. 2006. *FDA licenses new vaccine for prevention of cervical cancer and other diseases in females caused by human papillomavirus.* News release, June 8, available at http://www.fda.gov/bbs/topics/NEWS/2006/NEW01385.html (accessed January 5, 2008).

U.S. Food and Drug Administration. *Facts about antibiotic resistance.* Available at http://www.fda.gov/oc/opacom/hottopics/antiresist_facts.html (accessed January 3, 2008).

U.S. Food and Drug Administration. *OraQuick rapid HIV-1 antibody test: Frequently asked questions (FAQs).* Available at http://www.fda.gov/cber/faq/oraqckfaq.htm (accessed January 3, 2008).

U.S. General Accounting Office. 2003. *Newborn screening: Characteristics of state programs.* Report number GAO–03–449, March. Available at http://www.gao.gov/new.items/d03449.pdf (accessed December 31, 2007).

U.S. Government. 2008. *Federal Guidance to Assist States in Improving State-Level Pandemic Influenza Operating Plans,* March. Available at http://www.health.state.nm.us/flu/FEDERAL%20GUIDANCE%20TO%20ASSIST%20STATES.pdf (accessed July 1, 2008).

U.S. National Library of Medicine and National Institute of Health, Medline Plus, Medical Encyclopedia. Congenital syphilis. Available at www.nlm.nih.gov/medlineplus/ency/article/001344.htm (accessed December 31, 2007).

The Urban Institute. 1985. The Siracusa principles on the limitation and derogation provisions in the international covenant on civil and political rights. *Human Rights Quarterly* 7: 3–14.

Uscher-Pines, Lori et al. 2006. Priority setting for pandemic influenza: an analysis of national preparedness plans. *PLoS Medicine* 3, no. 10: e436.

Utah Department of Health. 2007. *Utah Pandemic Influenza Response Plan.* August 28. Available at http://pandemicflu.utah.gov/plan/CorePanFlu-10012007.pdf (accessed July 5, 2008).

van den Hoven, Mariette A., and Marcel F. Verweij. 2003 Should we promote influenza vaccination of health care workers in nursing homes? Some ethical arguments in favour of immunization. *Age and Ageing* 32: 487–489.

van der Steen, Jenny T. 2002. *Curative or palliative treatment of pneumonia in psychogeriatric nursing home patients: Development and evaluation of a guideline, decision-making, and disease course.* Wageningen, the Netherlands: Ponsen & Looijen.

van Kammen, Jessika, Don de Savigny, and Nelson Sewankambo. 2006. Using Knowledge Brokering to Promote Evidence-Based Policy-Making: The Need for Support Structures. *Bulletin of the World Health Organization* 84, no. 8 (October 3): 608–612.

Vazquez, M., P.S. LaRussa, A.A. Gershon, L.M. Niccolai, C.E. Muehlenbein, S.P. Steinberg, et al. 2004. Effectiveness over time of varicella vaccine. *Journal of the American Medical Association*, 291(7), 851–855.

Veatch, Robert M. 1977. *Case studies in medical ethics*. Cambridge: Harvard University Press.

Veatch, Robert M. 2005. *Disrupted dialogue: Medical ethics and the collapse of physician–humanist communication, 1770–1980*. Oxford: Oxford University Press.

Viani, R.M., M.R. Araneta, J. Ruiz-Calderon, P. Hubbard, G. Lopez, E. Chacón-Cruz, and S.A. Spector. 2006. Perinatal HIV counseling and rapid testing in Tijuana, Baja California, Mexico: Seroprevalence and correlates of HIV infection. *Journal of Acquired Immune Deficiency Syndromes* 41, no. 1 (January 1): 87–92.

Vinson, E. 2007. Managing bioterrorism mass casualties in an emergency department: lessons learned from a rural community hospital disaster drill. *Disaster Management Response* 5, no. 1: 18–21.

Virginia Department of Health. 2006. *Emergency operations plan attachment pandemic influenza*. March. Available at http://www.vdh.virginia.gov/PandemicFlu/pdf/DRAFT_Virginia_Pandemic_Influenza_Plan.pdf (accessed July 7, 2008).

von Radowitz, John. 2006. Animals spreading many more diseases to humans. *Press Association Newsfile*, February 20.

Wade, Nicholas. 2007. Genome of DNA discoverer is deciphered. *New York Times*, sec. A., June 1, 19.

Walensky, Rochelle P., Elena Losina, Laureen Malatesta, George E. Barton, Catherine A. O'Connor, Paul R. Skolnik, Jonathan M. Hall, Jean F. McGuire, and Kenneth A. Freedberg. 2005. Effective HIV case identification through routine HIV screening at urgent care centers in Massachusetts. *American Journal of Public Health* 95, no. 1 (January): 71–73.

Walker, D.G., and G.J.A. Walker. 2002. Forgotten but not gone: The continuing scourge of congenital syphilis. *Lancet Infectious Disease* 2: 432–436.

Wang, T.H., K.C. Wei, C.A. Hsiung, S.A. Maloney, R.B. Eidex, D.L. Posey, W.H. Chou, W.Y. Shih, and H.S. Kuo. 2007. Optimizing severe acute respiratory syndrome response strategies: Lessons learned from quarantine. *American Journal of Public Health* 97 Supplement 1 (April): S98–S100.

Washington, Harriet A. 2006. *Medical apartheid: The dark history of medical experimentation on black Americans from colonial times to the present* New York: Doubleday.

Wear, Stephen, James J. Bono, Gerald Logue, and Adrianne McEvoy. 2000. *Ethical issues in health care on the frontiers of the twenty-first century*. Dordrecht, the Netherlands: Kluwer Academic.

Webb, P.M., G.D. Zimet, R. Mays, and J.D. Fortenberry. 1999. HIV Immunization: Acceptability and anticipated effects on sexual behavior among adolescents. *Journal of Adolescent Health* 25: 320–322.

Webby, Richard J. and Robert G. Webster. 2003. Are we ready for pandemic influenza? *Science* 302, no. 5650: 1519 – 1522.

Webster, Robert G., and Elena A. Govorkova. 2006. Focus on research: H5N1 influenza—Continuing evolution and spread. *New England Journal of Medicine* 355, no. 21 (November 23): 2174–2177.

Weiler, P.C., H. H. Hiatt, J. P. Newhouse, W. G. Johnson, T. A. Brennan, and L. L. Leape. 1993. *A measure of malpractice*. Cambridge: Harvard University Press.

Weintraub, Arlene. 2007. Making her mark at Merck. *Business Week*, January 8, available at http://www.businessweek.com/magazine/content/07_02/b4016074.htm?chan=top±news_top±news±index_technology (accessed January 5, 2008).

Wendo, Charles. 2001. Caring for the survivors of Uganda's Ebola epidemic one year on. *Lancet* 358: 1350.

Wertz, DC, S.R. Janes, J.M. Rosenfield, and R.W. Erbe. 1992. Attitudes toward the prenatal diagnosis of cystic fibrosis: Factors in decision making among affected families. *American Journal of Human Genetics* 50, no. 5: 1077–1085.

Wesolowski, L.G., D.A. MacKellar, S.N. Facente, et al. 2006. Post-marketing surveillance of OraQuick whole blood and oral fluid rapid HIV testing. *AIDS* 20(12)(August 1):1661-1666.

White, Stuart, 2004. Social Minimum. In *Stanford Encyclopedia of Philosophy*. Available at http://plato.stanford.edu/entries/social–minimum/(accessed December 1, 2007).

Whitehouse, Peter J. 2003. The rebirth of bioethics: Extending the original formulations of Van Rensselaer Potter. *American Journal of Bioethics* 3, no. 4: W21–W26.

Whitley, R.J., and A.S. Monto. 2006. Seasonal and pandemic influenza preparedness: A global threat. *Journal of Infectious Diseases* 194, supplement 2: S65–S69.

Whitman, Jim, ed. 2000. *The politics of emerging and resurgent infectious diseases*. New York: St. Martin's Press.

Wikler, Daniel, and Dan W. Brock. 2004. Ethical Issues in Population Health: Mapping a New Agenda, paper delivered at the 7th World Congress of Bioethics, International Association of Bioethics, University of New South Wales, Sydney, Australia (November).

Wilfert, C.M. 1994. Mandatory screening of pregnant women for the human immunodeficiency virus. *Clinical Infectious Diseases* 19: 664–666.

Wilfond, B.S., and E.J. Thomson. 2000. Models of public health genetic policy development. In *Genetics and public health in the 21st century*, eds. M.J. Khoury, W. Burke, and E.J. Thomson. New York: Oxford University Press.

Williams, Vickie J. 2007. Fluconomics: preserving our hospital infrastructure during and after a pandemic. *Yale Journal of Health Policy, Law & Ethics* 7: 99–152.

Williamson, Ian G. et al. 2007. Antibiotics and Topical Nasal Steroid for Treatment of Acute Maxillary Sinusitis, *Journal of the American Medical Association* 298, no. 21 (December 5): 2487–2496.

Wilson, Jane. 2005. To know or not to know: Genetic ignorance, autonomy and paternalism. *Bioethics* 19, nos. 5–6: 492–504.

Wilson, Kumanan, Christopher MacDougall, and Ross Upshur. 2006. The new international health regulations and the federalism dilemma. *PLoS Medicine* 3, no. 1 (January): e1.

Winslow, Charles E.A. 1920. The untilled fields of public health. *Science* 51: 23–33.

Winston, Pamela, Olivia Golden, Kenneth Finegold, Kim Rueben, Margery Austin Turner, and Stephen Zuckerman. 2007. Federalism after hurricane Katrina: How can social programs respond to a major disaster? *Tulane Law Review* 81: 1219–1261.

Wisconsin Bureau of Communicable Diseases. 2004. *Wisconsin pandemic influenza preparedness*. Wisconsin Division of Public Health, Department of Health and Family Services. Available at http://dhfs.wisconsin.gov/prepared ness/pdf_files/WIPandemicInfluenzaPlan.pdf (accessed July 5, 2008).

Wise, Jacqui. 2006. Southern Africa is moving swiftly to combat the threat of XDR-TB. *Bulletin of the World Health Organization* 84, no. 12 (December): 924–925, available at http://www.who.int/bulletin/volumes/84/12/news.pdf (accessed February 9, 2008).

Wittgenstein, Ludwig. 2003 [2001]. *Philosophical Investigations*. Trans. G.E.M. 3rd ed. Cornwall, UK: Blackwell.

Wolinsky, Howard. 2006. The battle of Helsinki: Two troublesome paragraphs in the Declaration of Helsinki are causing a furore over medical research ethics. *EMBO Reports* 7, no. 7: 670–672.

Working Group on HIV Testing of Pregnant Women and Newborns. 1991. HIV infection, pregnant women, and newborns: A policy proposal for information and testing. In *AIDS, women and the next generation*, ed. R.R. Faden, G. Geller, and M. Powers. New York: Oxford University Press.

World Care Council. *Patients' Charter for Tuberculosis Care*. Available at http:// www.worldcarecouncil.org/pdf/PatientsCharterEN2006.pdf (accessed December 29, 2007).

World Health Organization. 1980. Global eradication of smallpox. *Bulletin of the World Health Organization* 58: 161–163.

World Health Organization. 2001. *The world health report*. Geneva: World Health Organization.

World Health Organization. 2002. Antimicrobial resistance. Fact Sheet No. 194 (January), available at http://www.who.int/mediacentre/factsheets/fs194/en /(accessed January 3, 2008).

World Health Organization. 2002. *Use of antimicrobials outside human medicine and resultant antimicrobial resistance in humans. Fact Sheet No. 268*. January, available at http://www.who.int/mediacentre/factsheets/fs268/en/ (accessed January 3, 2008).

World Health Organization. 2004. *HIV assays: Operational characteristics report* 14 */simple/rapid tests*. Geneva: World Health Organization, available at http:// www.who.int/diagnostics_laboratory/publications/hiv_assays_rep_14.pdf (accessed January 3, 2008).

World Health Organization. 2005. *International health regulations*. Available at http:// www.who.int/csr/ihr/IHRWHA58_3-en.pdf (accessed January 28, 2008).

World Health Organization. 2005. *WHO global influenza preparedness plan*. Geneva: World Health Organization, available at http://www.who.int/csr/re sources/ publications/influenza/GIP_2005_5Eweb.pdf (accessed February 7, 2008).

World Health Organization Writing Group. 2006. Nonpharmaceutical interventions for pandemic influenza, national and community measures. *Emerging Infectious Diseases* 12, no. 1 (January): 88–94.

World Health Organization. 2006. *Tough choices: investing in health for development.* Geneva: World Health Organization, available at http://www.who.int/macrohealth/documents/report_and_cover.pdf (accessed December 29, 2007).

World Health Organization. 2007. *Ethical considerations in developing a public health response to pandemic influenza.* Geneva: WHO Press, available at http://www.who.int/csr/resources/publications/WHO_CDS_EPR_GIP_2007_2c.pdf (accessed January 21, 2008).

World Health Organization. 2007. The global MDR-TB and XDR-TB response plan 2007–2008. Available at http://whqlibdoc.who.int/hq/2007/WHO_HTM_TB_2007.387_eng.pdf (accessed December 29, 2007).

World Health Organization. 2007. *New plan to contain drug-resistant TB.* http://www.who.int/mediacentre/news/releases/2007/pr32/en/index.html (accessed June 2007).

World Health Organization. 2007. *Outbreak of ebola haemorrhagic fever in DRC.* October 10, available at http://www.who.int/features/2007/ebola_cod/en/index.html (accessed December 29, 2007).

World Health Organization. 2007. *Towards universal access: Scaling up priority HIV/AIDS interventions in the health sector: Progress report, April 2007.* Geneva: World Health Organization, available at http://www.who.int/hiv/mediacentre/uni versal_access_progress_report_en.pdf (accessed January 1, 2008).

World Health Organization. 2007. *What are the key health dangers for children?* (October), available at http://www.who.int/features/qa/13/en/index.html (accessed January 26, 2008).

World Health Organization. 2007. *The world health report 2007—A safer future: Global public health security in the 21st century.* Available at http://www.who.int/whr/2007/overview/en/index1.html (accessed January 22, 2008).

World Health Organization. 2008. *Cumulative number of confirmed human cases of avian influenza A/(H5N1) reported to WHO.* February 5, available at http://www.who.int/csr/disease/avian_influenza/country/cases_table_2008_02_05/en/in dex.html (accessed February 6, 2008).

World Health Organization. 2008. *H5N1 Influenza: Timeline of Major Events.* January 14, available at http://www.who.int/csr/disease/avian_influenza/Timeline_08%2001%2014.pdf (accessed February 7, 2008).

World Health Organization. *Drug resistance.* Available at http://www.who.int/topics/drug_resistance/en/ (accessed January 3, 2008).

World Health Organization. *Fact sheet: Smallpox.* Available at http://www.who.int/mediacentre/factsheets/smallpox/en/ (accessed January 5, 2008).

World Health Organization. *National influenza pandemic plans.* Available at http://www.who.int/csr/disease/influenza/nationalpandemic/en/index.html (accessed July 1, 2008).

World Health Organization, "New Rapid Tests for Drug-Resistant TB for Developing Countries," http://www.who.int/mediacentre/news/releases/2008/pr21/en/index.html (accessed July 1, 2008).

World Health Organization. *World Health Organization report on infectious diseases 2000: Overcoming antimicrobial resistance.* Available at http://www.who.int/infectious-disease-report/2000/index.html (accessed January 3, 2008).

World Medical Organization Declaration of Helsinki. *Ethical principles for medical research involving human subjects.* Available at http://www.wma.net/e/policy/b3.htm (accessed November 2007).

Wright, A.A., and I.T. Katz. 2006. Home testing for HIV. *New England Journal of Medicine* 354, no. 5 (February 2): 437–440.

Writing Committee of the World Health Organization Consultation on Human Influenza A/5. 2005. Avian influenza A (H5N1) infections in humans. *New England Journal of Medicine* 353, no. 13, (September 29): 1374–1385.

Writing Committee of the Second World Health Organization Consultation on Clinical Aspects of Human Infection with Avian Influenza A (H5N1) Virus. 2008. Update on avian influenza A (H5N1) virus infection in humans. *New England Journal of Medicine* 358, no. 3 (January 17): 261–273.

Wynia, M.K. 2004. Civic obligations in medicine: Does "professional" civil disobedience tear, or repair, the basic fabric of society? *Virtual Mentor.* Vol. 6, no. 1, (January), available at http://virtualmentor.ama-assn.org/2004/01/pfor1-0401.html.

Yarney, Gavin. 2004. Roll back malaria: A failing global health campaign. *British Medical Journal* 328, no. 7448 (May 8): 1086–1087.

York, Geoffrey. 2005. Human bird flu in China; After initially dismissing their illnesses, Beijing admits H5N1 has infected people. *Globe & Mail (Canada),* sec. A1, November 17.

Zilinskas, Ray. 2007. Assessing the bioterrorism threat: Problems and possibilities. Lecture, Uehiro Center, Oxford University, Oxford, England, July 4.

Zimet, G.D., N. Liddon, S.L. Rosenthal, E. Lazcano-Ponce, and B. Allen. 2006. Chapter 24: Psychosocial aspects of vaccine acceptability. *Vaccine* 24, supplement 3 (August 21): S201–S209.

Zimmerman, M. 2006. Ethical analysis of HPV vaccine policy options. *Vaccine* 24: 4812–4820.

Zuger, Abigail. 2003. What did we learn from AIDS? *New York Times,* sec. F, November 11, 8.

Zuk, Marlene. 2007. *Riddled with life: Friendly worms, ladybug sex, and the parasites that make us who we are.* Orlando, FL: Harcourt.

ACKNOWLEDGMENTS

An earlier version of Chapter 3 appeared as:

Charles B. Smith, Margaret P. Battin, Jay A. Jacobson, Leslie P. Francis, Jeffrey R. Botkin, Emily P. Asplund, Gretchen J. Domek, and Beverly Hawkins, "Are There Characteristics of Infectious Diseases that Raise Special Ethical Issues?" *Developing World Bioethics*, no. 1 (May 2004): 1–16.

An earlier version of Chapter 4 appeared as:

Leslie P. Francis, Margaret P. Battin, Jay A. Jacobson, Charles B. Smith, and Jeffrey Botkin, "How Infectious Disease Got Left Out—and What this Omission Might Have Meant for Bioethics," *Bioethics*, special issue on ethics and infectious disease, ed. Michael J. Selgelid and Margaret P. Battin, also in Michael J. Selgelid, Margaret P. Battin, and Charles B. Smith, eds., *Ethics and Infectious Disease*. Oxford: Blackwell, 2006.

An earlier version of Chapter 5 appeared as:

Leslie P. Francis, Margaret P. Battin, Jay A. Jacobson, Charles B. Smith, "Closing the Book on Infectious Disease: The Mischievous Consequences for Bioethics and for Public Health," in Angus Dawson, ed., *The Philosophy of Public Health*. Aldershot: Ashgate, 2008.

An earlier version of Chapter 10 appeared as:

Leslie P. Francis, Margaret P. Battin, Jeffrey R. Botkin, Jay A. Jacobson, and Charles B. Smith, "Infectious Disease and the Ethics of Research: The Moral Significance of Communicability," in Matti Häyry, Tuija Takala and Peter Herissone-Kelly, eds., *Ethics in Biomedical Research: International Perspectives*. Amsterdam and New York: Rodopi, 2007, pp. 135–150.

An earlier version of Chapter 11 appeared as:

Jay A. Jacobson, Margaret P. Battin, Jeffrey Botkin, Leslie P. Francis, James O. Mason, Charles B. Smith, "Vertical Transmission of Infectious Disease and Genetic Disorders," in Angus Dawson and Marcel Verweij, eds., *Ethics, Prevention, and Public Health*. Oxford: Clarendon Press, 2007, pp. 145–159.

An earlier version of Chapter 12 appeared as:

Charles B. Smith, Margaret P. Battin, Leslie P. Francis, Jay A. Jacobson, "Should Rapid Tests for HIV Infection Now Be Mandatory During

Pregnancy? Global Differences in Scarcity and a Dilemma of Technological Advance," *Developing World Bioethics*, special issue, Reproductive Health Ethics: Latin American Perspectives, ed. Debora Diniz, Florencia Luna, and Juan Guillermo Figueroa, 7, no. 2 (August 2007): 86–103.

An earlier version of Chapter 15 is to appear as:

Margaret P. Battin, Charles B. Smith, Larry Reimer, Jay A. Jacobson, Leslie P. Francis, "Rapid Tests for Infectious Disease: A Thought Experiment about Universal Use and Public Surveillance," in *Cutting Though the Surface: Philosophical Approaches to Bioethics (Festschrift for Matti Häyry)*, ed. Tuija Takala, Peter Herissone-Kelly, and Søren Holm, Rodopi, forthcoming 2008.

An earlier version of material from several chapters appeared as:

Margaret P. Battin, Leslie P. Francis, Jay A. Jacobson, and Charles B. Smith, "The Patient as Victim and Vector: The Challenge of Infectious Disease for Bioethics," in R. Rhodes, A. Silvers, L. Francis, *Blackwell Guide to Medical Ethics*. New York: Blackwell, 2007, pp. 269–288.

An earlier version of material from several chapters appeared as:

Leslie Pickering Francis, Margaret P. Battin, Jay A. Jacobson, and Charles B. Smith, "The Patient as Victim and Vector: The Significance of Contagious, Infectious Disease for Bioethics," *ASBH Exchange*, newsletter of the American Society for Bioethics and Humanities, vol. 9, no. 1, Winter 2006, pp. 1, 4–5.

An earlier version of material from several chapters appeared as:

Margaret P. Battin, Linda S. Carr-Lee, Leslie P. Francis, Jay A. Jacobson, Charles B. Smith, "The Patient as Victim and Vector: Bioethics and the Challenge of Infectious Disease," in *Principles of Health Care Ethics* (second edition), edited by Richard Ashcroft, Angus Dawson, Heather Draper, and John McMillan. Chichester, UK: Wiley, April 2007.

Material from chapters 16–19 appeared as:

Leslie P. Francis, Jay A. Jacobson, Charles B. Smith, Margaret P. Battin, "Privacy, Confidentiality, or Both?" *ASBH Exchange*, 11, no. 2 (Spring 2008): 1, 8–9, 2008.

Material from chapter 19 will appear as:

Leslie P. Francis, Margaret P. Battin, Jay A. Jacobson, Charles B. Smith, "Pandemic Planning and Distributive Justice in Health Care," in *Law and Bioethics*, Michael Freeman, ed. Aldershot: Ashgate, forthcoming 2008.

Chapter 20 is a modified and extended version of Margaret P. Battin, Charles B. Smith, Leslie P. Francis, and Jay A. Jacobson, "Toward the Control of Infectious Disease: Ethical Challenges for a Global Effort," in *International Public Health Policy and Ethics*, ed. Michael Boylan. Dordrecht, Netherlands: Springer, 2008, pp. 191–214. By kind permission of Springer Science and Business Media.

INDEX

vaccine prioritization, 385–89
See also Avian flu pandemic planning;
 Pandemic planning, ethical issues;
 Violations of justice

King, Martin Luther, Jr., 406
Know–do gap in infectious disease, 437
Kotalik, Jaro, 314
Kuru, 445

Last, John, 65
Lazarini, Zita, 71
Leischmaniasis (sandfly fever), 421
Leprosy (Hansen's Disease)
 bioethical issues, 32, 472–74
 eliminability, 424
 fear and panic related to disease, 32
 Hawaiian leper colony at Molokai, 318,
  323–24, 350, 473–74, 481
 in scriptures of religious traditions, 442
 "leper," meaning of, 472
 shunning and belling of lepers, 61, 442,
  460, 472–73
 vaccine, 419
Lerner, Barron, 146
Levinson, A-J Rock, 53
Liao, Matthew, 122 n. 17, 416 n. 15
Liberal theory
 harm principle, 68, 85–89, 306, 468–69
 implications of PVV view, 468–69
 Mill, John Stuart, 463
 paradigm of autonomous individual, 7,
  77–78, 305, 468–69
 See also Autonomy; Bioethics, early issues
Liberty, 24, 71–72, 83–87, 122, 124–125, 248,
  276 n.111, 283, 285, 288–289, 291–
  296, 299, 302–303, 309–318, 373
  n.15, 469, 471, 476, 481
Lice or crabs, 17
Linezolid, 236–37
Lo, Bernard, 265–66
London, Alex John, 178
Love, and infectious disease, 467–468

Macklin, Ruth, 6 n. 11, 43, 507
Macroeconomics and Health Report, 39
Mad cow disease. *See* Variant
  Creutzfeldt-Jakob Disease
  (vCJD, "mad cow disease")
Maine, pandemic plan, 357
Malaria
 deaths in children, 382, 458
 deaths worldwide, 458
 incidence, 420, 458

mosquitoes as vectors, 18, 20, 423–24
plasmodia, 18
prevention, 405, 418
Roll Back Malaria campaign, 412
Mallon, Mary (Typhoid Mary), 21, 447,
  475, 476
Mandatory
 immunization, ch. 14, *passim*
 testing or screening, definition, ch. 11
  passim, 202
 see also chs. 12, 15, *passim*
Mann, Jonathan, 66, 67, 72
Mann, Thomas (*The Magic Mountain*),
  145–46
Marburg, 421
Mariner, Wendy, 63, 127, 417, 448
Maryland, pandemic plan, 338
Massachusetts
 addressing needs of uninsured, 383
 compulsory smallpox vaccination law, 253
 Jacobson v. Massachusetts, 253–54, 270, 273
 pandemic planning, 352, 357, 375, 376, 394
*Maxcy-Rosenau Preventive Medicine and
  Public Health*, 64–65
May, Thomas, 59, 78, 386
Mbeki, Thabo, 447
McGuire, James G., 310
McKenna, J. J., 200 n. 1, 203 n. 12, 204, 215,
  220, 227
MDR-TB. *See* Tuberculosis, Multiple
  drug-resistant tuberculosis
Measles
 contagiousness, 24
 deaths worldwide, 405 n. 59
 German, *see* Rubella
 immunization, 254–55, 262, 405 n. 59, 419
 outbreaks in unvaccinated populations,
  270–71, 448–49
 transmission to Native America
  populations, 471–72
Medicare, Medicaid, 41, 54, 227, 262, 379–80
Médicins sans Frontieres, 346
Meningitis (meningococcal)
 acuity, 30–31
 difficulties in diagnosing, 137
 fear and panic related to disease, 22, 30–31
 high incidence in central Africa, 37
 informed consent and the refusal of a
  spinal tap, 117–21
 transmission mechanisms, 22
 vaccine, 419
Merck, 259, 261–62, 264–65, 265 n. 76, 267,
  270; *see also* Gardasil, Human
  Papillomavirus Vaccine

See also Cystic fibrosis; Prenatal HIV
testing
Veterans Administration medical system, 395
"Victim and Vector" view, *see* PVV view.
Violations of bodily integrity and physical
security, 291–92, 306–8
Violations of justice, 296–301, 312–13
See also Justice of health-care distribution
Violations of liberty and consent, 292–94,
306–8
Violations of privacy and confidentiality,
291, 311–12
Vioxx, 261
Virginia, pandemic plan, 338, 361
Viruses, overview, 19–20

Walter Reed Army Research Institute, 426
Watchful waiting, 138, 242, 246
"Way-station self," xi, 6, 9,77, 85, 89, 101,
244–45, 306–7, 384, 434, 461
antimicrobial resistance, 244–45
colonization by microorganisms, 80–81
theoretical uncertainty perspective about
infectious disease, 93, 101–7, 384
vulnerability, 77
"Web of disease," ix, 6, 7, 82, 83, 91, 102,
133, 158–159, 279, 302, 430, 434, 440,
443, 457, 461, 468, 471
West Nile, 90, 104, 403
Whipworm, 420, 431
White, Ryan, 33; Ryan White Fund, 227
Whooping cough, *see* Pertussis
Wikler, Daniel, 5, 64, 66, 532
Wilfert, C. M., 204
Willowbrook experiment, 4, 45–46, 48, 172
See also Research ethics in infectious
disease
Winslow, Charles, 61

Wittgenstein, Ludwig (duck-rabbit figure),
94–97, 109
World Bank, 426
World Health Organization (WHO), 28, 34,
39, 100, 143, 162, 176, 207, 220, 229
n. 13, 230, 231, 232, 244, 245 n. 39,
286 n. 4, 314, 336, 382, 416, 426, 428,
432–33, 458, 484
International Health Regulations,
345, 346
pandemic planning, 336–37, 339, 342,
346–47
"3 by 5 initiative," 100, 410, 412
World Medical Association *Declaration of
Helsinki,* 167–68
World Organization for Animal Health, 426

XDR-TB. *See* Tuberculosis, Extensively
drug-resistant tuberculosis
Xenotransplantation, 177, 179–80
Xhosa, 442

Yager, Paul, 301–2
Yeasts, 18
Yellow fever
epidemic in U.S. South in 1878, 318–19
mosquitoes as vectors, 424
public health focus, 56, 72
reemergence, 421
vaccine, 419
Walter Reed's vaccine trials, 164

Zimmerman, M., 265–66
Zoonoses, 9, 53 n. 52, 182, 422, 425, 454 n.
93, 461
see also Animals and animal diseases;
specific diseases, transmission
Zuger, Abigail, 5, 171